Laryngology

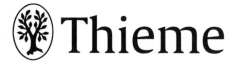

Laryngology

Series Editors

Professor Emeritus Milind V. Kirtane, M.S. (ENT)
Seth G. S. Medical College & KEM Hospital
P. D. Hinduja National Hospital & Research Centre
Breach Candy Hospital
Prince Aly Khan Hospital
Saifee Hospital
Mumbai, India

Chris E. de Souza, M.S., D.O.R.L., D.N.B., F.A.C.S.
ENT Consultant
Lilavati Hospital
Holy Family Hospital
Holy Spirit Hospital
Tata Memorial Hospital
Mumbai, India

Visiting Assistant Professor
Department of Otoloaryngology
SUNY Brooklyn, New York, USA
Department of Otolaryngology
LSUHSC, Shreveport, Louisiana, USA

Volume Editor

Abir K. Bhattacharyya, M.S., D.N.B., F.A.C.S., F.R.C.S., F.R.C.S.(O.R.L.)
Consultant Otolaryngologist & Head and Neck Surgeon
Associate Director Medical Education (Surgery) &
Royal College Surgical Tutor, Whipps Cross University
Hospital, Barts Health
Consultant ENT Surgeon at Spire Roding Hospital,
Holly House Hospital & Wellington Hospital
Consultant Surgeon to the High Commission of India
London, United Kingdom

Associate Editor

Nupur Kapoor Nerurkar M.S., D.O.R.L.
Laryngologist and Voice Surgeon
Bombay Hospital and Medical Research Center
Mumbai, India

Thieme Medical and Scientific Publishers Private Limited
A-12, Second Floor, Sector - 2
Noida, Uttar Pradesh - 201 301, India
Email: customerservice@thieme.in
www.thieme.com

Thieme
Delhi • Stuttgart • New York • Rio

Thieme Medical and Scientific Publishers Private Limited
A-12, Second Floor, Sector- 2
Noida, Uttar Pradesh - 201 301, India

Editorial Services Director: Sangeeta PC
Assistant Manager - Editorial Production: Kumar Kunal
Sales and Marketing Director: Harish Singh Bora
Chief Executive Officer: Ajit Kohli

Laryngology / [edited by] Abir K. Bhattacharyya, Nupur Kapoor Nerurkar.

Includes bibliographical references and index.

ISBN 978-93-82076-02-5

Bhattacharyya, Abir K. II. Nerurkar, Nupur Kapoor.

5 4 3 2 1

ISBN: 978-93-82076-02-5
eISBN: 978-93-82076-08-7

Laryngology
Published by Thieme Medical and Scientific Publishers Private Limited
A-12, Second Floor, Sector- 2, Noida, Uttar Pradesh - 201 301, India
Email: customerservice@thieme.in
www.thieme.com
Printer: Gopsons Papers Limited, Noida

Dedication

I wish to dedicate this volume to my parents for instilling the virtues of honesty, integrity, and hard work.

I thank my teachers for their motivation and "If I have seen further it is by standing on the shoulders of giants."

I acknowledge the help from my residents and students (past and present) for the inspiration they provide.

And finally my gratitude and appreciation to my family - my wife Rinku for her encouragement and understanding, and our children Anudeep and Amrita for the little joys with which they fill our lives.

Abir K. Bhattacharyya

The loving memory of my father, Kewal Kapoor, who taught me to "hold the bull by the horns",

My mother, Dr. Indira Kapoor, elegance personified,

My darling daughters, Kanika and Anaaya, who are the center of my universe and

their father and my husband, Dr. Rajeev Nerurkar, without whom I would not dare to dream!

Nupur Kapoor Nerurkar

Laryngology

Table of Contents

Foreword

The boundaries of otorhinolaryngology continue to widen, and Laryngology in all its aspects has been dealt within this volume in the six-volume series of otorhinolaryngology books. The eight sections of the book present a complete and thorough review of the most up-to-date aspects of Laryngology. The editors have called on a tremendous panel of world authorities who are among the most outstanding, experienced, and knowledgeable doctors in their respective fields. The addition of sections on clinical insights, pearls and pitfalls, and evidence-based medicine are highly recommended and provide stimulation for the full range of laryngologists from those just beginning in the discipline to those at the senior end of the spectrum.

The world of otorhinolaryngology books has become a highly competitive one but the quality of the editors and contributors to this particular book series leaves me in no doubt that they have made a significant contribution to our specialty and will be a very popular source of reference. This has to be the simple but defining requirement for any book.

Professor David Howard
Founding Member & President
British Laryngological Association

Preface

I do not know what I may appear to the world, but to myself I seem to have been only like a boy playing on the sea-shore, and diverting myself in now and then finding a smoother pebble or a prettier shell than ordinary, whilst the great ocean of truth lay all undiscovered before me.

This Newtonian quote remains as relevant today in the 21st century as it was over 400 years ago. Our quest for knowledge remains unabated; we are still picking pebbles and the vast ocean lies ahead.

The one feature that distinguishes humans or mankind is their ability to communicate with speech (and song) for other species can also see, hear, or smell; and it is the human larynx that gives us this unique edge. Laryngology has encompassed the fascinating science behind breathing, swallowing, and most importantly phonation which sets us apart.

Laryngology is one of the traditional medical specialties studied since the time of Hippocrates. A genuine spurt in interest was understandable when the vocal cords were first visualized in the 1850s. The recent surge in interest and reemergence as a subspecialty in this century has more to do with scientific and technological advances far beyond the field of Laryngology, such as development of tissue engineering and real-time imaging. It is befitting that Thieme decided to commission a separate volume on "Laryngology" in its six-volume series as Laryngology with its distinct following has now matured from its teenage years to adulthood with a dedicated volume!

There are quite a few excellent reference textbooks in this ever-expanding field of Laryngology—our idea was to have a single volume which could "stand on its own feet." In between the first section on "Historical Developments" and the concluding section on "New Frontiers" we have attempted to cover the fundamental principles and core concepts that govern present-day thinking on modern Laryngology. We hope we have a comprehensive, state-of-the-art book on the subject spread across eight sections. The building blocks of anatomy and physiology in the "Basic Sciences" section underpins the multidisciplinary approach and evaluation described in detail in the "Clinical Assessment and Diagnostic Procedures" section. A section on "Therapeutic Principles" outlines the broad concepts and helps in better understanding of the management principles in "Disorders of the Larynx." There is a separate section on "Professional Voice" with inputs from laryngologists across three different continents, each providing a unique perspective. The chapters have been interspersed with "Clinical Insights," where relevant, to communicate with the reader more effectively.

We wanted to design a book that informs, enthuses, and serves as a reference to laryngologists all over the world, whether beginners or established "connoisseurs" in the field. We hope and believe that the authors, all respected and established leaders in their field, have delivered on this premise. We would welcome your comments, reviews (critical or otherwise), and any questions on this first edition.

We would like to extend our gratitude to the Series Editors, Dr. Kirtane and Dr. de Souza, for their help and encouragement at all stages in the production of this book. Finally we would like to thank the team at Thieme Publishers, especially Sangeeta PC and Kumar Kunal for their dedication and professionalism in bringing together such a large, six-volume reference series to fruition.

Abir K. Bhattacharyya
Nupur Kapoor Nerurkar

A Note from Series Editors

This book is written by the world's best practitioners in the field of Laryngology. Each chapter has been chosen carefully. The editors and authors have striven to be lucid and comprehensive. Laryngology, like most disciplines, has seen considerable development. Disorders of the voice are emerging as a major subspecialty. The wish of the Series Editors, the editors, and the authors is to provide the readers with a good reliable roadmap in this discipline, especially where the landmarks keep on changing so quickly.

Milind V. Kirtane, M.S. (ENT)
Chris E. de Souza, M.S., D.O.R.L., D.N.B., F.A.C.S.

Contributor List

Jahangir Ahmed, M.R.C.S.
Department of Ear, Nose and Throat Surgery
St. Bartholomew's Hospital
Barts Health National Health Service Trust
London, England, United Kingdom

Shalini Arulanandam, M.B.B.S., M.M.E.D.
Department of Otorhinolaryngology
Tan Tock Seng Hospital
Singapore

Yogesh Bajaj, M.D., F.R.C.S.
Department of Otorhinolaryngology – Head and Neck Surgery
St. Barts and Royal London Hospitals
Barts Children's Hospital
London, England, United Kingdom

Anca M. Barbu, M.D.
Division of Laryngeal Surgery
Massachusetts General Hospital
Harvard Medical School
Boston, Massachusetts, USA

Abir K. Bhattacharyya, M.S., D.N.B., F.R.C.S., F.R.C.S. (ORL), F.A.C.S.
Department of ENT and Head & Neck Surgery
Royal College Surgical Tutor
Whipps Cross University Hospital
Barts Health & Barts and The London School of Medicine
London, England, United Kingdom

Martin A. Birchall, M.D., F.Med.Sci.
UCL Ear Institute
Royal National Throat, Nose and Ear Hospital
University College London
London, England, United Kingdom

James A. Burns, M.D.
Department of Surgery
Center for Laryngeal Surgery
Massachusetts General Hospital
Boston, Massachusetts, USA

Natasha Choudhury, B.Sc., D.O.H.N.S., M.D., F.R.S.C. (ORL-HNS)
Department of Ear, Nose and Throat, and Head & Neck Surgery
Barts Health National Health Service Trust
London, England, United Kingdom

Matthew S. Clary, M.D.
Department of Otolaryngology
University of Colorado School of Medicine
Aurora, Colorado, USA

Declan Costello, M.A., M.B.B.S., F.R.C.S.
Department of Otorhinolaryngology – Head and Neck Surgery
Queen Elizabeth Hospital
Birmingham, England, United Kingdom

Mark S. Courey, M.D.
Department of Otolaryngology – Head and Neck Surgery
University of California, San Francisco
Division of Laryngology
University of California, San Francisco
San Francisco, California, USA

Cathal Coyle, Ph.D.
Department of Clinical Biochemistry and Metabolic Medicine
University of Liverpool
London, England, United Kingdom

Taryn Davids, M.D., F.R.C.S.C.
Division/ Department of
University of Toronto
Toronto, Ontario, Canada

Mriganka De, F.R.C.S.
Department of Head and Neck Surgery
Derby Royal Hospitals NHS Foundation Trust
Derby, England, United Kingdom

Venu Divi, M.D., F.A.C.S.
Department of Otolaryngology
Torrance Memorial Medical Center
Torrance, California, USA

Chee-Yean Eng, F.R.C.S.
Department of Otorhinolaryngology – Head and Neck Surgery
Royal Hallamshire Hospital
Sheffield Teaching Hospitals NHS Foundation Trust
South Yorkshire, England, United Kingdom

Ruth Epstein, Ph.D., M.R.C.S.L.T.
Department of Speech and Language Pathology
Royal National Throat, Nose and Ear Hospital
University College London NHS Foundation Trust
London, England, United Kingdom
Voice Pathology Unit
Ear Institute
University College London
London, England, United Kingdom

D. Gregory Farwell, M.D., F.A.C.S.
Department of Otolaryngology – Head and Neck Oncology Surgery, and Microvascular Surgery
University of California, Davis
Sacramento, California, USA

Sachin Gandhi, M.S.
Department of Laryngology
Deenanath Mangeshkar Hospital and Research Centre
University of Pune
Pune, Maharashtra, India

C. Gaelyn Garrett, M.D.
Department of Otolaryngology
Vanderbilt Voice Center
Vanderbilt University
Nashville, Tennessee, USA

Khalid Ghufoor, F.R.C.S., B.Sc., M.B.B.S.
Department of Otorhinolaryngology – Head and Neck Surgery
St. Bartholomew's and The Royal London Hospital
Smithfield, London, United Kingdom
The Royal National Throat, Nose and Ear Hospital
London, England, United Kingdom

Nicholas Gibbins, F.R.C.S. (ORL-HNS), M.D.
Department of Otolaryngology – Voice Disorders Unit and Laryngological Surgery
University Hospital Lewisham
Lewisham, London, United Kingdom

Meredydd Harries, F.R.C.S., M.Sc.
Department of Ear, Nose and Throat, and Laryngology
Royal Sussex County Hospital
Brighton National Health Service Trust
Brighton, England, United Kingdom

Ben Hartley, F.R.C.S., M.B.B.S., B.Sc.
Department of Ear, Nose and Throat, and Pediatric Otolaryngology
Great Ormond Street Hospital
London, England, United Kingdom

Sonna Njideka Ifeacho, M.B.Ch.B.
Department of Ear, Nose and Throat Surgery
Whipps Cross University Hospital
Barts Health National Health Service Trust
London, England, United Kingdom

Michael M. Johns, M.D.
Department of Otolaryngology – Head and Neck Surgery
Emory Voice Center
Emory University Hospital Midtown
Atlanta, Georgia, USA

Jeevendra Kanagalingam, M.A., F.R.C.S. (ORL-HNS), F.A.M.S.
Lee Kong Chian School of Medicine
Singapore

Gauri Kapre, M.S.
Department of Ear, Nose and Throat
Bombay Hospital Institute of Medical Sciences
Mumbai, Maharashtra, India

Neil Mackenzie Kernohan, M.D., Ph.D., F.R.C.Path.
Department of Pathology
Ninewells Hospital
University of Dundee
Dundee, Scotland, United Kingdom

Milind V. Kirtane, M.S. (ENT)
Professor Emeritus
Department of Otolaryngology
Seth Gordhandas Sunderdas Medical College and King Edward Memorial Hospital
Consultant - P. D. Hinduja National Hospital and Medical Research Centre
Breach Candy Hospital
Prince Aly Khan Hospital
Saifee Hospital
Mumbai, Maharashtra, India

Samit Majumdar, B.M. B.S., B.D.S. (Hon), B.Med. Sci. (Hon), F.R.C.S. Ed., F.D.S. R.C.P.S., F.R.C.S. (ORL-HNS)
Academic Department of Otolaryngology – Head and Neck Surgery
Ninewells Hospital
University of Dundee Medical School
Dundee, Scotland, United Kingdom

Julian A. McGlashan, F.R.C.S.
Department of Otorhinolaryngology – Head and Neck Surgery
Queen's Medical Centre Campus
Nottingham University Hospitals
Nottingham, England, United Kingdom

Jayakumar R. Menon, M.S., D.N.B., F.R.C.S., D.L.O.
Department of Laryngology
Kerala Institute of Medical Sciences
Thiruvananthapuram, Kerala, India

Sharat Mohan, F.R.C.S.I., D.L.O.R.C.S.
Department of Head and Neck Surgery
Voice Clinic
Royal Derby Hospital and Medical School
Derby, United Kingdom

Nupur Kapoor Nerurkar, M.S., D.O.R.L.
Division of Laryngology
Department of Ear, Nose and Throat Surgery
Bombay Hospital and Medical Research Center
Mumbai, Maharashtra, India

S. A. Reza Nouraei, M.A.(Cantab), M.B.B.Chir., Ph.D., M.R.C.S.
Department of Ear, Nose and Throat Surgery
The National Centre for Airway Reconstruction
Charing Cross Hospital
Anglia Ruskin University
London, England, United Kingdom

Curtis Offiah, B.Sc., M.B., Ch.B., F.R.C.S., F.R.C.R.
Department of Neuroradiology
St. Bartholomew's and The Royal London Hospitals
Barts Health NHS Trust
London, England, United Kingdom

Muhammad Shahed Quraishi, F.R.C.S., F.R.C.S. (ORL-HNS)
Department of Otolaryngology – Head and Neck Surgery
Doncaster Royal Infirmary
University of Sheffield
South Yorkshire, England, United Kingdom

Marc Remacle, M.D., Ph.D.
Department of Otorhinolaryngology – Head and Neck Surgery
Louvain University Hospital of Mont-Godinne
Mont-Godinne, Yvoir, Belgium

John Rubin, M.D., F.R.C.S., F.A.C.S.
Department of Ear, Nose and Throat Surgery
Royal National Throat, Nose and Ear Hospital
Neurological Voice and Swallow Clinic
National Hospital for Neurology and Neurosurgery
University College London Hospitals National Health Service Trust
London, England, United Kingdom

Guri S. Sandhu, M.D., F.R.C.S., F.R.C.S. (ORL-HNS)
Department of Otorhinolaryngology – Head and Neck Surgery
Charing Cross Hospital
Imperial College
London, England, United Kingdom

Sarah L. Schneider, M.S., C.C.C.-S.L.P.
Department of Speech-Language Pathology
Voice and Swallowing Center
Department of Otolaryngology – Head and Neck Surgery
University of California, San Francisco
San Francisco, California, USA

Purushotam Sen, F.R.C.S.
Department of Ear, Nose and Throat Surgery
Whipps Cross University Hospital
London, England, United Kingdom

Kevin Shields, M.B., B.Ch., B.A.O., B.A., Ph.D., M.R.C.P.I.
Department of Neurology and Clinical Neurophysiology
The National Hospital for Neurology and Neurosurgery
The Whittington Hospital
University College London Hospitals National Health Services Foundation Trust
London, England, United Kingdom

Anita Sonsale, F.R.C.S. (ORL-HNS), M.Sc. (Voice Pathology)
Department of Ear, Nose and Throat
Derby Royal Hospitals National Health Service Foundation Trust
Derby, England, United Kingdom

Paul Stimpson, M.B.Ch.B., M.Sc., F.R.C.S.
Department of Otorhinolaryngology – Head and Neck Surgery
Whipps Cross University Hospital
London, England, United Kingdom

Rishi Talwar, B.Sc. (Hons), M.B.B.S. (Lond), M.R.C.S. (Eng), D.O.H.N.S. (RCS Eng), F.R.C.S. (ORL-HNS)
Department of Otorhinolaryngology
St. Bartholomew's and the Royal London Hospitals
London, England, United Kingdom

Taranjit Singh Tatla, B.Sc., M.B.B.S., D.L.O., F.R.C.S. (Eng)
Department of Otorhinolaryngology – Head and Neck Surgery
Northwick Park Hospital
North West London Hospitals National Health Service Trust
London, England, United Kingdom

James Thomas, M.D.
Department of Laryngology
Portland, Oregon, USA

Kimberly N. Vinson, M.D.
Department of Otolaryngology
Vanderbilt Voice Center
Vanderbilt University
Nashville, Tennessee, USA

Brittany C. Weber, M.D.
Department of Otolaryngology – Head and Neck Surgery
Eastern Virginia Medical School
Norfolk, Virginia, USA

Neil Weir, M.D., M.A., F.R.C.S.
British Society for the History of ENT
London, England, United Kingdom

Peak Woo, M.D., F.A.C.S.
Department of Otolaryngology
Mount Sinai School of Medicine
New York, New York, USA

Katherine Young, B.Sc. (Hons)
Department of Speech and Language Therapy, and Voice/Head & Neck Surgery
Voice and Dysphagia Clinic
Royal Derby Hospital and Medical School
Derby, United Kingdom

Steven M. Zeitels, M.D., F.A.C.S.
Eugene B. Casey Professor of Laryngeal Surgery
Harvard Medical School
Center for Laryngeal Surgery and Voice Rehabilitation
Massachusetts General Hospital
Boston, Massachusetts, USA

Section A

Laryngology –
Historical Developments

1 Laryngology—A Historical Perspective

Neil Weir

It is tempting to think that the specialty of laryngology was born with the invention of indirect laryngoscopy in the mid-1850s. This view, though, would not do justice to the understanding of the anatomy, physiology, and pathology of the larynx which had been accrued since the time of Hippocrates. By the mid-19th century, the management of throat diseases relied on intuition, extreme manual dexterity, and good fortune, as none of the practitioners were yet able to visualize lesions of the larynx despite many valiant attempts to do so.

The stimulus given, however, to laryngology with the introduction of indirect laryngoscopy by Manuel Garcia in 1854 and its clinical application by Ludwig Türck in 1857 and Johann Czermak in 1858 was evidenced by the mass of literature on intralaryngeal lesions which abounded from the early 1860s. The application of the anesthetic and analgesic properties of cocaine to the mucous membrane of the pharynx and larynx demonstrated in 1884 by Edmund Jelinek and the replacement of the oxyhydrogen incandescent light by electric light invented in 1879 by Thomas Edison enabled mirror-guided surgical manipulation of the larynx to become commonplace.

Laryngoscopy enabled visually controlled surgical intervention for airway obstruction secondary to infectious membranous laryngeal diseases, which were rife in the 19th and early 20th centuries, and transoral biopsy of laryngeal tumors.

The unhappy case of the management of Crown Prince Frederick's laryngeal cancer in the late 19th century, which in the earlier stages had necessitated repeated inconclusive biopsies, dissuaded many laryngologists and surgeons from performing biopsies of the larynx for fear of inducing infection, malignant transformation, or metastasis. Felix Semon in 1888–1889 demonstrated, in a large, elegant, and comparative series, that there was no significant difference in the development of cancer between a biopsied and a nonbiopsied group. Despite this work and the strong support for laryngeal biopsy from other leading laryngologists, these misconceptions continued well into the early 20th century.

By this time, the technique of direct laryngoscopy promoted by Kirstein (1895), Killian (1898), Jackson (1907), and Brünings (1910) had become well established. Initially local anesthesia was used, but with the pioneering work on intubation by Ivan Magill (1921),[1] there was a move toward the use of general endotracheal anesthesia with paralyzing agents.

A greater understanding of the function of the larynx and voice production coupled with the use of the binocular operating microscope fitted with a 400-mm objective lens (Albrecht 1954, Kleinsasser 1962) opened the way to microlaryngoscopy, which enhanced the new discipline of phonosurgery, defined as any surgery designed primarily for the improvement or restoration of the voice. Although the term phonosurgery was first suggested by von Leden and Arnold in 1963, several functional procedures such as surgery for vocal fold paralysis had been described over 50 years before.

Further improvements in lighting, produced by fiberoptic systems (Hopkins 1954, Hirschowitz 1958);[2] magnification; stroboscopy (first invented by Oertel in 1878); and the introduction of lasers (light amplification by stimulated emission of radiation; Strong and Jako, 1972), together with new functional techniques aimed at altering the pitch, intensity, and quality of the voice, have advanced phonosurgery.

Laryngeal malignant tumors have been traditionally treated by a combination of radical or conservative surgery, radiotherapy, and/or chemotherapy. The total removal of the larynx (laryngectomy), first performed for cancer by Theodor Billroth (1873), gave rise to a host of different voice reconstruction techniques from that of Gussenbauer (1874) to those of Singer and Blom (1980). The replacement of the whole larynx by transplantation was first performed by Paul Kluyskens in 1969, but the need for immune suppression presently precludes its use for laryngeal cancer patients postlaryngectomy. Techniques that use stem cell regeneration and are not reliant on immune suppression are showing early promise.

Ancient History

In 1936, two slabs were discovered dating from the beginning of the first dynasty, one in Abydos relating to King Aha and the other, taken from the tomb of Hemaka at Saqqara, relating to King Dyer. Each slab depicts a seated person, presumably a physician, with a knife poised in an upheld arm in front of a patient whose head is extended backward. The signs above both operators and the heads of the patients indicate that life is being given from one to the other. Many scholars think this could be an illustration of an impending tracheotomy rather than a human sacrifice[3] (**Fig. 1.1**). In the oldest known surgical treatise, the Edwin Smith Papyrus written ca. 1550 BC there is, in Case 28, a description of a crush injury to the neck which resulted in a pharyngeal fistula and loss of speech.[4]

Within the *Corpus Hippocraticum or Hippocratic Collection*, the writings of followers of Hippocrates (ca. 460–?377–359 BC), there is, apart from the epiglottis, no account of laryngeal anatomy, but the human voice is described as clear, hoarse, or shrill. Hippocrates speculated that the lungs

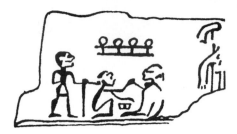

Figure 1.1   King Dyer slab dating from the first dynasty depicting tracheotomy.
Source: Pahor AL. Ear, nose and throat in Ancient Egypt. J Laryngol Otol 1992;106(9):773–779. Printed with permission.

and trachea played a role in voice production and that the lips and tongue were articulators.[5] Aristotle (384–322 BC), recognizing that the cartilage tube in front of the neck was used for the passage of air, reasoned that the voice was produced within the trachea or windpipe by the impact of air against it—inspired by the soul that lay between the heart and the lungs (*De Anima, II, viii*). This observation has given rise to the expression that "the voice is the mirror of the soul."[6]

In India, various remedies for disorders of the voice were included in the medical knowledge compiled in the *Sushruta Samhita* (ca. 300 BC) and the *Charaka* (ca. 100 BC).[7,8]

From Greece, the seat of learning eventually passed to Alexandria where Herophilus (ca. 335–280 BC) and Erasistratus (ca. 350–250 BC) practiced as physicians and anatomists. Erasistratus by dissecting the human body studied the larynx and "trachea arteria" (to differentiate it from the adjacent "carotid arteria") through which he believed air entered the lungs and then the heart, where it was changed into the "Vital Spirit" and then carried through the body by the arteries (the word "trachea" alone was not introduced until the 16th century). With the sacking of Alexandria, Greek medicine began to infiltrate Rome.

The Roman Period

The Roman period reached its climax with the appearance of a man whose teaching was to dominate medicine for the next 1200 years. Claudius Galen (ca. AD 129–200) regarded the body as the mere vehicle of the soul, a view which was warmly received by those of both Christian and Moslem faiths. Galen, in practice, followed the Hippocratic method and accepted the doctrine of the "humors." His strength lay in his anatomical and physiological studies. The former had largely to be based on pigs and apes as the dissection of the human body had become illegal. It is said that his appointment as surgeon to the school of gladiators in Pergamon had given him an insight into the human anatomy. Thus by transferring his experimental discoveries to the human anatomy, he inevitably perpetuated many errors. Galen distinguished six pairs of intralaryngeal muscles and defined which ones opened and closed the

larynx. Although he described three laryngeal cartilages (the thyroid, the cricoid, and the arytenoid), he assumed the arytenoid to be a single mass. Galen claimed to be the first to point out the ventricles of the larynx and reported the vocal folds as being of a membranous substance constituted so as to resist the impact of air and lubricated by mucus to prevent injury from vibrations of a dry surface. He taught that "the trachea-arteria prepares and prearranges the voice for the larynx … [The cartilages] increase it, and it is still further augmented by the vault of the throat, which acts like a sounding board" (*De usu partium* VII, 5).[9] He demonstrated in pigs that section of the recurrent laryngeal nerve led to the loss of voice. Galen's work was voluminous but many of his manuscripts, including those on the voice, were destroyed by fire. Galen did, however, cross-refer to these in other volumes.

No one dared to dispute Galen, such was his authority, until the early 16th century, when Paracelsus (1493–1541) used to preface his lectures by burning Galen's works and Andreas Vesalius (1514–1564), by dissecting the human body, disposed of many anatomical myths.

The Renaissance

Anatomy of the Larynx

With the awakening and renewal of culture implied in the Renaissance (late 14th century to 16th century) came an appreciation of the beauty of the human body. Those inspired artists, such as Michelangelo, Raphael, Dürer, and above all Leonardo da Vinci, turned to dissection of the human body. Despite correcting many of Galen's anatomical errors, Vesalius in *De Humanis Corporis Fabrica* hesitated to confirm that the arytenoids were actually two cartilages and that there were two paired (internal and external) cricothyroid muscles.[10] There was no doubt in the mind of Gabriel Fallopius (1523–1562) who confirmed that there were two arytenoid cartilages and only two complete cricothyroid muscles.[11] Fabricius ab Acquapendente (1537–1619) in 1600 described branches of the recurrent laryngeal nerve and for the first time the thyrohyoid ligament.[12]

The knowledge of the anatomical structure of the larynx was completed by Giovanni Battista Morgagni (1682–1771) who, in *Epistolae Anatomicae* (1740), noticed the oblique fibers of the thyroarytenoid muscle, described the ventricular folds (bands), and elaborated on the structure and function of the laryngeal ventricles which he observed acted as a reservoir of mucus for lubrication of the vocal folds.[13] Morgagni demonstrated that the organ (in this case the larynx) is the site of disease, and with careful examination of the postmortem larynx he reported on a wide range of laryngeal pathologies including trauma from hanging, infections such as syphilis and small pox, and cancerous growths.

In his anatomical descriptions, Morgagni made only one error—he classified the cuneiform cartilages as "laryngeal glands." This was later corrected in 1780 by Heinrich August Wrisberg (1739–1808) of Göttingen, whose name they now bear. Giovanni Domenico Santorini (1681–1737), professor of anatomy in Venice, discovered the "capitula" or corniculate cartilage, a cartilage that rests on the apex of the arytenoids, and the oblique fibers of the interarytenoid muscle.

Physiology of the Larynx

The anatomist/physiologist Antoine Ferrein (1693–1769) of Paris was the first to make acoustic experiments on the natural larynx.[14] He established that vibration of the vocal folds by a blast of air was the essential factor in the production of voice and that the intensity of the voice depended on the force of the blast of air. He proved that traction applied to the vocal folds produced variations in pitch and demonstrated the tensor function of the cricothyroid muscle. By likening the sound produced by the vibrating edge of the vocal folds to the effect of a bow on the strings of a violin (for which he originated the term vocal cords), he failed to appreciate the acoustic nature of the larynx as a reed instrument which was described later in 1806 by René Joachim Henri Dutrochet (1776–1847) who repeated Ferrein's experiments. Coincidentally he and Jean Baptiste Biot (1774–1862), professor of physics at the Collège de France, determined that sound arose from a series of puffs of air caused by the reed (vocal folds) alternately opening and closing as a steam of air passed through them. François Magendie (1783–1855), professor of medicine at Paris, reinforced the previously held view that the concavities of the mouth and nose acted as resonators. By experimenting on dogs, he observed the protective sphincter mechanism of the larynx in swallowing. He believed that the muscles closing the glottis were supplied by the superior laryngeal nerves and the dilators by the recurrent laryngeal nerves.[15] John Reid, professor of medicine at St Andrews, in 1838 showed conclusively that the internal branch of the superior laryngeal nerve supplies the larynx and the external branch supplies the cricothyroid muscle. All the remaining laryngeal muscles noted were activated by the recurrent (inferior) laryngeal nerve.[16]

Pathology of the Larynx

During the late 18th and the early 19th centuries, the various kinds of ulceration of the larynx were differentiated. Hitherto the word "phthisis" was applied to almost any wasting condition and not specifically to tuberculosis of the lung or larynx. Because of the indecisive origin of "laryngeal phthisis," the Academy of Medicine in Paris in 1836 offered a prize for the best essay on "The history of laryngeal phthisis." It was won jointly by Armand Trousseau (1801–1867) and Hippolyte Belloc (1779–1853) with their essay "Traité Practique de la Phtisie Laryngée, de la Laryngite Chronique, et des Maladies de la Voix" (1837), in which they classified laryngeal phthisis into four types: (1) "simple" (severe or hypertrophic chronic laryngitis), (2) "syphilitic," (3) "cancerous," and (4) "tuberculous."[17]

It was Karl Freiherr von Rokitansky (1804–1878), professor of pathology at Vienna, who in his *Handbuch der Pathologschen Anatomie* (1842) confirmed that laryngeal tuberculosis almost always follows lung tuberculosis.[18]

Dr. Francis Home (1719–1813) of Edinburgh, in *An Enquiry into the Nature, Causes and Cure of the Croup* (1765), was almost certainly describing diphtheria,[19] but the term itself was not defined until 1826 when Pierre Fidèle Bretonneau (1778–1862) published *Des Inflammations Spéciales du Tissu Muqueux et en Particulier de la Dipthérite, ou Inflammation Pelliculaire.*[20] The bacillus of diphtheria was discovered in 1883 by Edwin Klebs (1834–1913) of Zurich and was cultivated in the following year by Friedrich Loeffler (1852–1915).

Horace Green (1802–1866) of New York is credited with the first attempt to remove a laryngeal growth (a pedunculated polyp) *per viam naturales*. He described a further eight cases in his book *On the Surgical Treatment of Polypi of the Larynx and Oedema of the Glottis* published in 1852.[21] His innovative work on the direct treatment of laryngeal lesions in the prelaryngoscopic era was met with frank incredulity and savage attack. Eventually it was accepted that he was able to introduce instruments into the laryngeal inlet, but his more controversial treatment of lung disorders via the larynx was not accepted.

The History of Tracheotomy

Tracheotomy, or "laryngotomy" or "pharyngotomy" or "bronchotomy," was a subject of much speculation from the time of Asclepiades of Bithynia (120–40 BC), who was the first to recommend incision of the windpipe (which he called laryngotomy)[22] in cases of "angina," to the great anatomist/surgeons of the late Renaissance. Antyllus (AD 3rd–4th century) recommended incision through the third and fourth rings of the trachea (which he called "pharyngotomy") for relief of airway obstruction above the level of the larynx.[23] Fabricius ab Acquapendente (1537–1619) extolled the advantages of the operation but criticized the transverse incision because of the potential danger of cutting the great blood vessels of the neck and because of the restricted view of the trachea. His pupil and successor Julius Casserius (1561–1616) published his *De Vocis Auditusque Organis Historia Anatomicae* (1600),[24] which, apart from containing a wealth of comparative anatomy of the larynx, also illustrated the operation of tracheotomy with intubation with a curved silver tube (**Figs. 1.2** and **1.3**). Nicholas Habicot (1550–1624) performed four cases of "bronchotomy," but the illustration in his short volume, with the long title *Question Chirurgicale par Laquelle il est Démontré que le Chirurgien Doit Assurément Practiquer l'Opération de le Bronchotomie, vulgairement dicte Laryngotomie ou Perforation de la Fluste ou Tuyan du Poulmon*, clearly showed a horizontal incision.

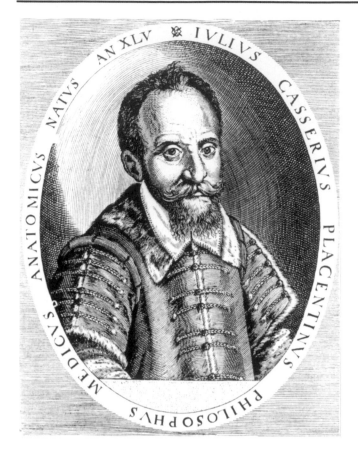

Figure 1.2   Julius Casserius (1561–1616).

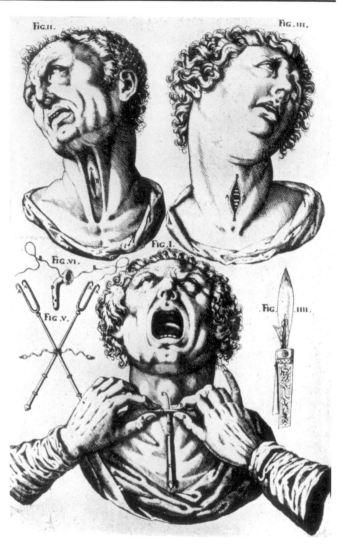

Figure 1.3   The operation of tracheotomy, figures I–VI.
Adapted from Casserius J. *De Vocis Auditusque Organis Historia Anatomicae.* Ferrara, Italy: Baldinus; 1600.

The word "tracheotomy" had first appeared in *Libri Chirurgiae XII*, which was written in 1649 by Thomas Fienus (1567–1631), professor of medicine at Louvain, but its use was lost for nearly a century. It was reintroduced in later editions of *Chirurgie* (1743) by Lorenz Heister (1683–1758), professor of physic and surgery at the University of Helmstadt and fellow of the Royal Society, who unsuccessfully recommended abandoning other terms.[25] Both Pierre Fidèle Bretonneau and Armand Trousseau used the term in relation to their work on diphtheria. Pierre Joseph Desault (1738–1795) clearly distinguished between "laryngotomy" and "bronchotomy." He defined the former as cutting transversely through the cricothyroid membrane or vertically through the cricoid cartilage and the latter as cutting transversely between the rings of the trachea or vertically through them.[26] For Desault it would seem that the terms bronchotomy and tracheotomy were still synonymous.

In his important article "The story of tracheotomy," published in the *British Journal of Children's Diseases* in 1934, Goodall was able to find only 28 successful cases of tracheotomy recorded up to the time of Pierre Fidèle Bretonneau. The chief indications were acute inflammations of the pharynx and larynx and removal of foreign bodies.[27] The earliest tracheotomy on a child was performed by Jean Charles Félix Caron (1745–1824) of Paris, who in 1776 removed an inhaled bean from a 7-year-old boy. Tracheotomy

for children suffering from diphtheria did not become accepted until the mid-19th century, but interestingly a century earlier Dr. Francis Home had recommended the use of tracheotomy in cases of croup.

The later part of the 19th century saw a huge increase in the numbers of tracheotomies performed. In 1884, Alois Monti (1839–1909) of Vienna perused the world literature and collected 12,736 cases of tracheotomy for diphtheria alone. By the end of the century, these figures had reduced significantly principally because of the discovery, in 1894, of diphtheria toxin by Emil von Behring (1854–1917).

With the introduction of direct laryngoscopy and bronchoscopy, the need for tracheotomy in cases of foreign body inhalation diminished. But in the 1930s, a new indication for the operation was found in the treatment of removal of bronchial secretions in cases of bulbar poliomyelitis, myasthenia gravis, and tetanus. Tracheotomy, combined with positive pressure respiration in the management of poliomyelitis during the epidemics of the early 1950s, helped reduce the mortality from 80 to 40%.[28] Prolonged use of polyvinyl chloride tubes with stiff cuffs tended to result in tracheal stenosis, but later soft cuffs solved this problem. Tracheotomy is still a life-saving operation, but in the emergency situation intubation or cricothyrotomy, if possible, is a preferable procedure.

The Laryngoscope

Prelaryngoscopic Era

Many strides had been taken in the understanding of the anatomy and physiology of the larynx and the management of laryngeal diseases before the arrival of successful laryngoscopy in 1854. All the earlier workers shared a desire to see the glottis and many efforts were made. Philipp Bozzini (1773–1809), working in Frankfurt in 1807, invented his *lichtleiter*, which was a double cannula with two mirrors placed at 45 degrees at the end.[29] Light from a wax candle was transmitted through one compartment and reflected onto the part to be examined. The image was received on the other mirror and reflected back to the eye through the second compartment. This instrument was used to inspect a variety of canals including the larynx. While it is doubtful whether Bozzini ever viewed the glottis, his concept of visualizing an interior organ using an external light source laid down

the principle for all endoscopies. Benjamin Babington (1794–1866), a physician at Guy's Hospital, London, presented his "glottiscope" (**Fig. 1.4**) to the Hunterian Society in 1829.[30] It was a combined tongue depressor and oblong piece of mirror that was placed against the soft palate. Bright sunlight was required and the mirror needed to be dipped in water to prevent clouding by the patient's breath. The epiglottis and the upper part of the larynx were visualized. A colleague at Guy's, Thomas Hodgkin, coined the phrase "speculum laryngis or the laryngoscope."

John Avery (1807–1855), a surgeon at Charing Cross Hospital, London, came nearer than most to viewing the vocal folds. He used a head mirror illuminated by candlelight and a laryngeal mirror housed within a cumbersome speculum (**Fig. 1.5**). Avery never reported his work but after Garcia described his successful autolaryngoscopy in 1854 (reported on May 24, 1855, to the Royal Society on his behalf by the secretary and physiologist William Sharpey[31]), claims were made that Avery had anticipated his discovery in 1846.[32]

Manuel Patricio Rodriguez Garcia (1805–1906) of Spanish origin and a professor of singing at the Conservatoire de Paris and later at the Royal Academy of Music in London nursed one desire which was to see a "healthy glottis exposed in the very act of singing." The inspiration for autolaryngoscopy came to him in 1854 while he was strolling in the gardens of the Palais Royal in Paris. He observed sunlight being reflected off window panes set in a quadrangle. He sought

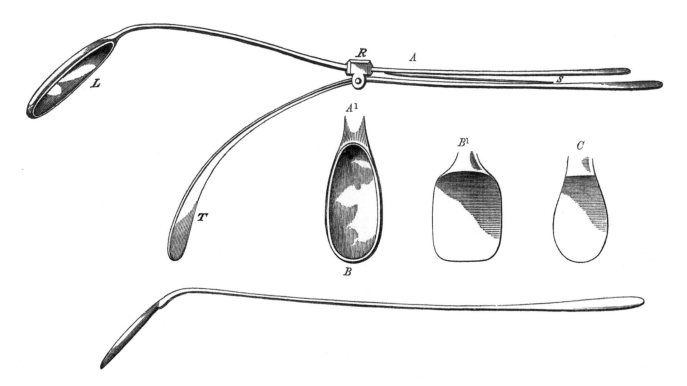

Figure 1.4 Dr. Babington's laryngeal mirrors.
Adapted from Mackenzie M. *The Use of the Laryngoscope in Diseases of the Throat.* 3rd ed. London: Longmans, Green & Co.; 1871:14.

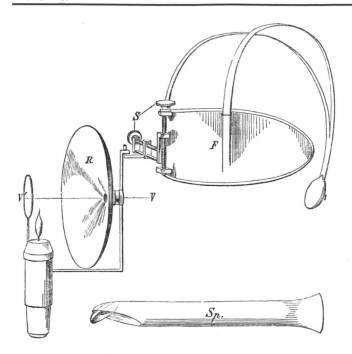

Figure 1.5   Avery's laryngoscope.
Adapted from Mackenzie M. *The Use of the Laryngoscope in Diseases of the Throat*. 3rd ed. London: Longmans, Green & Co.; 1871:24.

a hand mirror and a dental mirror. Having warmed the dental mirror and placed it against his uvula, he flashed a ray of sunlight onto this and to his excitement viewed his own glottis. His success was due to his own well-controlled capacious pharynx and his choice of a small simple mirror to introduce into his throat.

Postlaryngoscopic Era

The first clinical application of indirect laryngoscopy was made by Ludwig Türck (1810–1868), a neurologist in Vienna. Initially unaware of Garcia's discovery, he used small long-handled mirrors and sunlight to examine patients at the Allgemeine Krankenhaus in the summer of 1857. In the winter he put aside his mirrors and loaned them to Johann Czermak (1828–1873), a physician in Budapest. In a communication in April 1858, Türck stated that he was: "very far from having any exaggerated hopes about employment of the laryngeal mirror in practical medicine."[33]

Johann Czermak modified Türck's mirrors and developed his own technique of indirect laryngoscopy using a fenestrated head mirror and artificial light.[34] He demonstrated this technique on himself (**Fig. 1.6**) and his patients throughout Europe and incurred the displeasure of Türck who claimed that he was the first to use the mirror for diagnostic purposes. The "Turckish War", as the disagreement was called, successfully helped publicize laryngoscopy. In summary, it can be said that Manuel Garcia was the first to perform a successful mirror laryngoscopy, Johann Czermak developed and popularized the technique, and Ludwig Türck founded the specialty of laryngology.

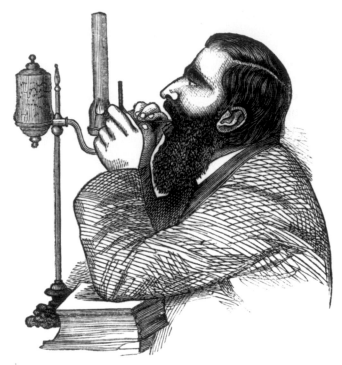

Figure 1.6   Autolaryngoscopy. The right hand holds the laryngeal mirror and the left hand holds the flat mirror, represented here in profile.
Adapted from Czermak JN. *On the Laryngoscope and Its Employment in Physiology and Medicine*. Translated from French by Gibb GD. London: New Sydenham Society; 1861:18.

Early Laryngeal Surgery after the Introduction of the Laryngoscope

Intralaryngeal Surgery

The stimulus given to laryngology by the introduction of laryngoscopy is readily seen in the mass of literature on intralaryngeal lesions that abounded from the early 1860s. Georg Richard Lewin (1820–1896) in 1861 reported on 50 to 60 cases of laryngeal neoplasms, which represented only 5 or 6% of all cases of laryngeal disorders.[35] He operated on his first case in July 1860 and used either cutting devices or caustics. Thomas J. Walker of Peterborough, England, reported a case to the *Lancet* in 1861 in which he described the removal of a polypoidal growth from the larynx of a 14-year-old boy using a twisted loop wire snare under laryngoscopic guidance.[36] He had visited Vienna and had observed the technique of indirect laryngoscopy. He published *The Laryngoscope and its Clinical Application* in 1864.[37]

Carl Stoerk (1832–1899) became the first full-time lecturer in laryngology and rhinology in Vienna in 1864. He developed many laryngeal instruments and possessed a skillful technique, which enabled him to successfully operate on the larynx in the era before the discovery in 1884 of the application of cocaine as a local anesthetic by Edmund Jelinek (1852–1928) who worked in the Clinic of

Laryngoscopy, founded in 1870 as the first of its kind in the world, at the Allgemeine Krankenhaus with Leopold Schrötter von Kristelli (1837–1908) as its head. Edmund Jelinek remarked on the high cost of cocaine at the end of his article entitled "Cocaine as an anesthesia and analgesia for the mucous membrane of the pharynx."[38]

In the United States, Louis Elsberg (1837–1885) of New York had been influenced by Johann Czermak who had sent him his book *On the Laryngoscope and Its Employment in Physiology and in Medicine* published in German in 1859 and in English in 1861.[39] Louis Elsberg published his essay "Laryngoscopal surgery, illustrated in the treatment of morbid growths within the larynx" in 1866 for which he was awarded the gold medal of the American Medical Association.[40] Jacob da Silva Solis-Cohen (1838–1927) of Philadelphia reported on the intralaryngeal removal of polyps in 1867. Four years later, the number of published cases of laryngeal polyps had reached 189 to which Morell Mackenzie (1837–1892) of London added a further 100 cases of his own.[41] In Paris, Charles Henri Fauvel (1830–1885) reported a personal series of 100 cases in his book *Traité Pratique des Maladies du Larynx* (1876).[42]

Among these cases were ones of early vocal fold cancer. The principles for their removal were laid down by Bernhard Fraenkel (1836–1911) of Berlin, who in 1886 noted that early vocal fold cancer is likely to arise on the superior surface of the vocal fold, to be of small volume, to present with hoarseness, and to be amenable to transoral resection.[43] In those cases where the tumor had extended anteriorly or posteriorly along the vocal fold or below the glottis, consideration was given to the much more risky operations of thyrotomy or laryngofissure.

Thyrotomy or Laryngofissure

Quoted in Albers,[44] the credit for the first thyrotomy or laryngofissure is normally given to Brauers of Louvain who performed the operation in 1833 without a preliminary tracheotomy to cauterize a papillomatous growth of the larynx.[44] Laryngofissure was first performed in the United States in 1851 by Gordon Buck (1807–1876), who, 2 days before the operation, performed a tracheotomy,[45] and in England in 1865 by Sir George Duncan Gibb (1821–1876) who used chloroform anesthesia.[46] The operation was not a bounding success. Morell Mackenzie on the strength of 28 published cases concluded that: "Thyrotomy does not even affect such complete evulsion as laryngoscopic treatment."[47] Perhaps these remarks were tainted by the fact that, as a physician, he did not perform the external operation but entrusted it to a surgeon. From his observations, the space in which to operate was limited by the need for and the restrictions of retraction of the two halves of the larynx. In his view this made surgical removal of lesions of the larynx more difficult than via the transoral route for which he was an acknowledged master. Even the eminent surgeon Sir Henry Trentham Butlin (1843–1912) in 1883 was disenchanted: "The disease is evidently far too deeply seated to admit of removal by so slight an operation".[48] He worked closely with Felix Semon (1849–1921) who agreed that: "Thyrotomy yields very bad results in cases of malignant growths and should not be attempted".[49] Their view started to change at the end of the 19th century as their results improved with better patient selection.[50] By 1930, Sir St Clair Thomson (1859–1943) was able to report only two operative deaths and a 76% 3-year survival rate in a series of 74 patients.[51]

First Laryngectomy

The operation of total laryngectomy for cancer was one which was held in awe. The general surgeon Professor Theodor Billroth (1829–1894), head of the Second Surgical University Clinic at the Allgemeine Krankenhaus, Vienna, was presented with a 36-year-old theology teacher who had been found by the laryngologist Carl Stoerk to have a histologically proven left-sided subglottic epithelioma. Theodor Billroth (**Fig. 1.7**) elected to remove the tumor by laryngofissure after a preliminary tracheotomy. The tumor was excised with preservation of the right vocal fold. A month later, as the patient became increasingly breathless, the tracheotomy track was reopened and a cannula was inserted. At a further laryngofissure, it was found that the tumor had spread into the perichondrium of the thyroid cartilage. The anesthetic was lightened and the patient was woken to be told that a total laryngectomy was the only option open to him. He consented and Theodor Billroth removed the larynx above the third tracheal ring and below

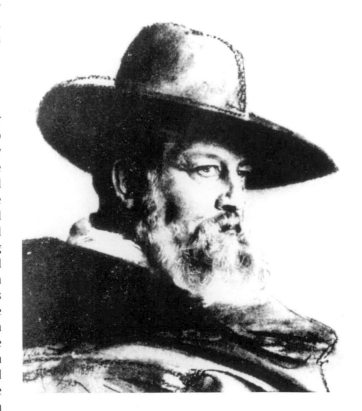

Figure 1.7   Theodore Billroth (1829–1894). From a hologravure of a drawing by Lenbach (1884).

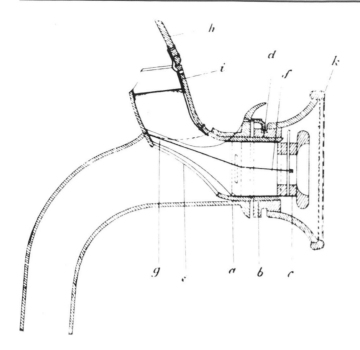

Figure 1.8 Carl Gussenbauer's "artificial larynx."
Adapted from Gussenbauer C. Über die erste durch Theodor Billroth am Menschen ausgeführte Kehlkopt-Extirpation und die Anwendung eines künstlichen Kehlkopfes. Langenbecks Arch Klin Chir 1874;17:343–356.

the epiglottis. He sutured the edges of the hypopharynx and the trachea to the skin. The open pharynx initially leaked liquid and food but gradually diminished in size such that more and more food went down the esophagus, and by 18 days he was able to swallow solid food. Theodor Billroth's assistant Carl Gussenbauer (1842–1903), who reported the case, designed an "artificial larynx", which was a T-shaped tube with one limb being placed in the trachea and the other passing through the fistula into the pharynx (**Fig. 1.8**). Both limbs had one-way valves such that the expiratory stream was forced into the pharynx but food did not enter the trachea.[52]

The patient was free of tumor for 4 months before a recurrence developed in the residual epiglottis. He died 7 months after the operation. In December 1887 a review of the first 103 total laryngectomies for cancer was published in the *Journal of Laryngology and Rhinology*. Of these, 40 (39%) died within 8 weeks of the operation and recurrence was noted in 21 (20%).[53] Total laryngectomy was only regarded as a success if a patient's life had been extended by at least 12 months as it was believed that this length of survival could be achieved by palliative tracheotomy alone. Only nine (8.5%) cases fulfilled these criteria and the surgeon in one third of the successful cases was Carl Gussenbauer.

Case of Crown Prince Frederick of Prussia

Morell Mackenzie in 1859 visited Johann Czermak in Budapest and from him learned the art of laryngoscopy. He

rapidly became the foremost British laryngologist. In 1863 he had founded the Metropolitan Free Dispensary for Diseases of the Throat and Loss of Voice, which 2 years later had moved to 32 Golden Square, London, and had been renamed the Hospital for Diseases of the Throat, the first of its kind in the world. With the publication and translation in French and German of his books—*The Use of the Laryngoscope in Diseases of the Throat* (1864), *Growths in the Larynx* (1871), and the two-volume *Diseases of the Throat and Nose* (1880, 1884)—Morell Mackenzie's skills had become widely known.

It was therefore not surprising that the German physicians and surgeons attending to the Crown Prince Frederick (**Fig. 1.9**), who was married to Queen Victoria's eldest daughter, Princess Victoria, had called in Morell Mackenzie as a consulting laryngologist (**Fig. 1.10**). The Crown Prince had been suspected of suffering from laryngeal cancer. Morell Mackenzie had rightly insisted on biopsy of the lesion on the left vocal fold but unfortunately the pieces removed on three separate occasions had been reported by the renowned surgical pathologist Rudolf Virchow (1821–1902) to be histologically inconclusive. Morell Mackenzie had counseled that the lesion should be removed by him by a transoral route

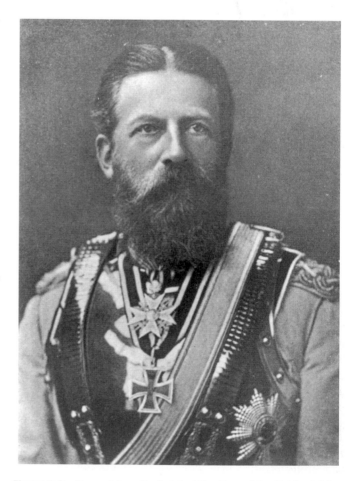

Figure 1.9 Crown Prince Frederick at the time of the Golden Jubilee of Queen Victoria, 1887.
Adapted from Stevenson RS. *Morell Mackenzie: The Story of a Victorian Tragedy*. London: William Heinemann Medical Books Ltd.; 1946.

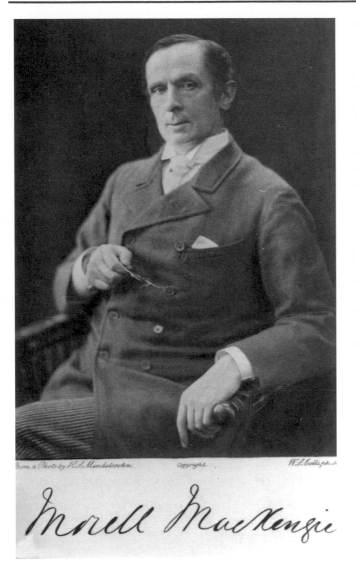

Figure 1.10 Morell Mackenzie (1837–1892).
Adapted from a photograph by HS Mendelsohn—frontispiece of Haweis HR. *Sir Morell Mackenzie, Physician and Operator—A Memoir.* London: WH Allen and Co Ltd., 1893.

must never be forgotten that Morell Mackenzie was the father of British laryngology.[54,55]

What were the lessons learned from the case of Crown Prince Frederick? First, Rudolf Virchow believed that cancer arose from connective tissue and invaded the epithelial layer to cause a raised lesion.[56] In contrast, Heinrich Wilhelm Waldeyer (1836–1921) held the view that a carcinoma arose from the epithelial layer and invaded deeper tissues.[57] When Rudolf Virchow's original reports were reviewed in this light, it became apparent that his descriptions were compatible with a diagnosis of laryngeal cancer. Second, an unfortunate theory was put about that Morell Mackenzie's biopsies had activated the cancer. The consequence of this belief was that the young specialty of laryngology had become threatened. In an attempt to combat this threat, Felix Semon (**Fig. 1.11**) published in 1888 and 1889 a large series of over 10,000 cases of laryngeal lesions (documented by mirror examination) that he divided into two groups.[58,59] He showed that there was no significant difference in the development of cancer between the group of 8000 who underwent biopsy, of whom 40% developed cancer, and the group of 2500 who were only observed, of whom 47% developed cancer. Despite this work and the strong support for

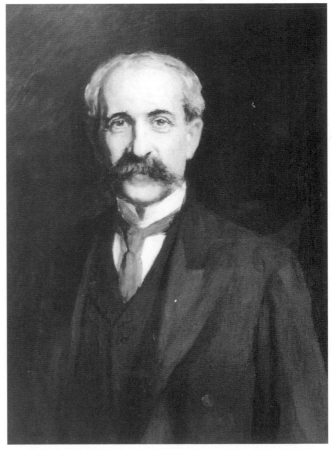

Figure 1.11 Sir Felix Semon (1849–1921). Artist: Sir Hubert von Herkomer.
Adapted from Sakula A. *The Portraits, Paintings and Sculpture of the Royal Society of Medicine.* London: Royal Society of Medicine Services Ltd., 1988:111.

and only if this method failed should an external operation such as thyrotomy or laryngofissure be considered. Sadly, within a few months, it became certain that the royal patient had cancer and a palliative tracheotomy was performed by Dr. Bramann. Two months later, the aged Emperor Wilhelm I died and the Crown Prince succeeded as Emperor (Kaiser) Frederick III. He reigned for 99 days and died on June 15, 1888. His death had been blamed by the Germans on Morell Mackenzie, but the patient himself had held his English doctor in great esteem and Queen Victoria had honored him with a knighthood in 1887. Sir Morell Mackenzie had served his patient well and had protected his interests both medically and socially to the extent that he himself had suffered both physically and mentally from the long ordeal. Morell Mackenzie, who was an asthmatic, died prematurely of influenza pneumonia at the age of 54. Despite the unhappy saga of Frederick the Noble, it laryngeal biopsy given by other leading laryngologists, these misconceptions continued into the early 20th century.

Direct Surgical Laryngoscopy

Enormous strides in the field of endoscopy were made in the last 20 years of the 19th century and the first decade of the 20th century. The major factors that enabled this development were the use of cocaine as a local anesthetic; the application of chloroform, ether, and nitrous oxide as general anesthetics; and the invention of the electric light. Alfred Kirstein (1863–1922) of Berlin, using a flat spatula and an electroscope designed by Caspar, with the patient's head extended and by depressing the tongue and the epiglottis, on April 23, 1895, for the first time saw the interior of the larynx by direct examination (**Fig. 1.12**). He called this examination "autoskopie."[60] He later substituted his own design of headlamp as the light source. The concept of intubation of the larynx followed the pioneering work of Joseph O'Dwyer (1841–1898), an obstetrician of New York, who 10 years before had published his method of intubation in an article in the *New York Medical Journal* entitled "Two cases of croup treated by tubage of the glottis" (1885).[61]

Gustav Killian (1860–1921) of Freiberg and later Berlin, stimulated by the work of Kirstein, devoted much of his time to endoscopy. His main contribution in the field of direct laryngoscopy was in 1911 to introduce the dorsal (as

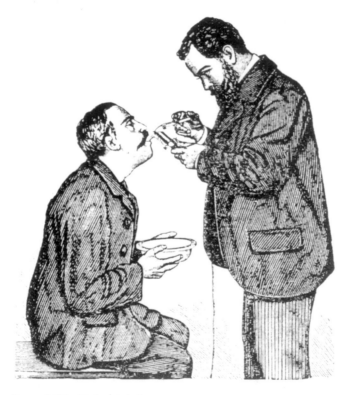

Figure 1.12 "Autoskopie."
Adapted from Kirstein A. Autoskopie des Larynx und der Trachea (Laryngoscopia directa, Euthyskopie, Besichtigung ohne Spiegel). Arch Laryngol Rhinol 1895;3:156–164.

opposed to the previous sitting) position for the patient and suspension laryngoscopy that enabled the operator to free both his hands.[62]

Wilhelm Brünings (1876–1958) of Jena, who had been Gustav Killian's assistant, reported the idea of mechanically placing external pressure on the larynx to give a better view of the anterior vocal folds and the anterior commissure.[63]

Frank Haslinger (1891–1966) described two measures aimed at enlarging the view of the larynx. These were to move the proximal lighting from the axis of the tube to the side and the creation of a bivalved speculum.[64] Richard Clyde Lynch (1880–?) refined suspension laryngoscopy and developed intralaryngeal techniques for the treatment of early cancer of the larynx.[65] He exhibited his pioneering laryngeal photography in 1920.

Perhaps the greatest and most lasting contribution to the field of direct surgical laryngoscopy came from Chevalier Jackson (1865–1958). Originally inspired by Gustav Killian, Chevalier Jackson went on to design his own endoscopy instruments that were fitted with distal lighting in an auxiliary tube.[66,67] Elected professor of laryngology in Pittsburgh in 1909, he moved to the chair of laryngology at Jefferson Medical College, Philadelphia, in 1916 and, such was his ability as a teacher, held three other chairs at the Graduate School of Medicine (1919), the University of Pennsylvania (1924), and the Women's Medical College of Pennsylvania. He possessed great dexterity, inventiveness, and communication skills.

Shortly after the First World War, Victor Ewings Negus (1887–1974) trained with Chevalier Jackson and on his return to London adopted Chevalier Jackson's techniques but devised his own set of endoscopes. He subsequently was appointed laryngologist at King's College Hospital, London.[68]

With the basic requirements for direct surgical laryngoscopy determined, the only modalities open to variation and improvement were laryngoscopes designed to give the largest safe access to the vocal folds, brighter lighting and magnification, and more refined instrumentation including the use of lasers. By the early 1960s, these advances led to a new era of microlaryngoscopy, which in turn made possible the refined goals of phonosurgery. The term phonosurgery had been first suggested by Hans von Leden and Arnold in 1963 to describe any surgery designed primarily for the improvement or restoration of the voice.[69,70]

Microstructure and Examination of the Vocal Fold

Voice production involves a complex and precise control by the central nervous system of a series of events in the peripheral phonatory organs. The phonosurgeon requires a thorough understanding of the process of voice production which especially includes the microanatomy of the vocal fold. John Bishop, without ever visualizing the larynx, aptly wrote in *The London Edinburgh Philosophical Magazine and Journal of Science* in 1836: "The true vibrating surface of

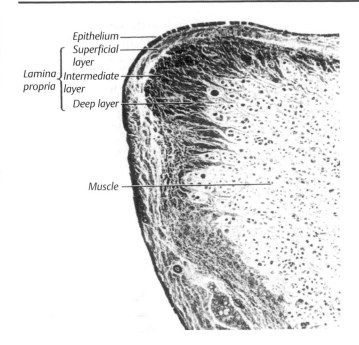

Epithelium
Superficial layer
Lamina propria { Intermediate layer
Deep layer
Muscle

Figure 1.13 A frontal (coronal) section of a human vocal fold through the middle of the membranous part.
Adapted from Hirano M. Clinical Examination of the Voice. Monograph 5 of Disorders of Communication (Arnold GE, Winckel F, Wyke BD, eds.) Wien, New York : Springer-Verlag, 1981;5.

the glottis is the mucous membrane. The vocal cords confer on it the tension, resistance, position and probably other conditions necessary for vibration."[71]

Much later in the last quarter of the 20th century, Minoru Hirano, professor of otolaryngology at Kurume University, Japan, by microanatomical and physiological studies, described the layers of the vocal folds.[72] He found that each fold consisted of a "cover" (epithelial layer and underlying superficial lamina propria of a soft gelatinous material), a "transition zone" (the intermediate lamina propria consisting of elastic tissue and the deep lamina propria consisting of collagen), and a "body" (the vocalis muscle). This knowledge explained why deep biopsies of the vocal fold could lead to scar tissue formation as the biopsy could penetrate the medial and deep lamina propria, both of which layers are abundant in fibroblasts (**Fig. 1.13**).

The assessment of the movement of vocal folds by stroboscopy is an integral part of the investigation of vocal disorders. Stroboscopy that optically slows down the movement of the vocal folds was first introduced in 1878 by Max Joseph Oertel (1835–1897). His apparatus (**Fig. 1.14**) consisted of a simple perforated disk, interspersed between a light source and the examiner's head mirror. The light to the mirror was pulsed by rotating the disk at variable speeds.[73] With the technological advances of the 1960s, more sophisticated stroboscopes have been developed, which give the clinician the opportunity to assess the biomechanical activity of the vocal folds' intrinsic layers and also to compare their movement preoperatively and postoperatively.

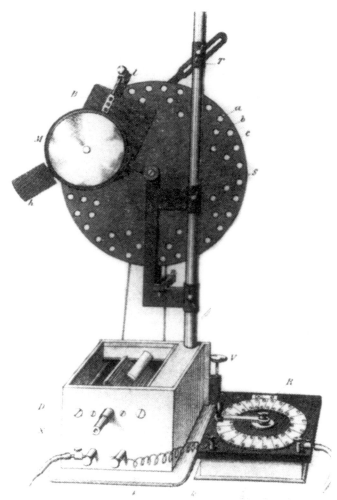

Figure 1.14 Oertel's stroboscope.
Adapted from Oertel M. Das Laryngo-Stroboskop und die Laryngo-Stroboskopische Untersuching. Arch Laryngol Rhinol (Berlin) 1895;3:1–16.

Microlaryngoscopy and Phonosurgery

Professor Rosemarie Albrecht of the Medical Academy in Erfurt (then in East Germany) was in 1954 the first to microscopically visualize the larynx using a colposcope borrowed from her gynecologic colleagues.[74] Scalco et al of Tulane University, New Orleans, described microscopic suspension laryngoscopy in 1960.[75] The major clinical applications of this technique, however, were developed and popularized in 1963 by the extensive work of Oskar Kleinsasser (1929–2001) initially at the University of Cologne and later as professor of otolaryngology at the University of Marburg in Germany. He encouraged Zeiss, the optical manufacturers, to make a 400-mm focal length lens and designed a completely new set of micro instruments for laryngeal surgery.[76]

Following the practice of Chevalier Jackson, most American laryngologists used local anesthesia. Any movement of the patient was not compatible with microsurgery; thus, new general anesthetic techniques were developed employing either jet delivery or the use of narrow endotracheal tubes.

The seminal article by Harold Hopkins (1918–1994) and Narinder Singh Kapany (b.1926) of Imperial College, London, published in 1954 and entitled "A flexible fiberscope, using static screening", heralded a new era of lighting by means of solid or flexible bundles of light fibers, connected to a proximal "cold light" source. This technique was later adapted for use in diagnostic laryngoscopy or laryngeal microsurgery.[77]

The principle of the laser (light amplification by stimulated emission of radiation) was discovered by Théodore Harold Maiman in 1960.[78] The carbon dioxide laser beam was found experimentally to behave as a scalpel and as a coagulator. Géza J. Jakó, working in the department of M. Stuart Strong in Boston, introduced the carbon dioxide laser into microlaryngeal surgery in 1972.[79] The laser was coupled to the surgical microscope. The main drawback of the carbon dioxide laser was the heat-induced trauma to the underlying vocal fold tissues. As a consequence, in the early 1990s there was a return to "cold steel" instrumentation.[80,81]

Phonosurgery also includes laryngeal framework procedures, laryngeal injection techniques, and the management of neural disorders of the larynx. Erwin Payr is credited with the first description, in 1915, of surgical medialization of the vocal fold,[82] but in his definitive article, Nobuhiko Isshiki et al, in 1974, described four stages of thyroplasty aimed at altering the shape of the laryngeal skeleton and thus the resulting voice.[83] Type I thyroplasty is a medialization technique used principally in cases of vocal fold paralysis. To achieve a similar goal, Wilhelm Brünings first described injection medialization with paraffin in 1911.[84] In 1961, Godfrey Arnold advocated the use of diced autologous nasal cartilage and others have Teflon paste (Du Pont Co., West Virginia, United States),[85] Gelfoam (Pfizer, New York City, United States), or autologous fat.

The management of laryngeal dystonias such as spasmodic dysphonia was revolutionized by the use of botulinum toxin (Botox , Allergan Inc., Irvine, CA, United States) by Andrew Blitzer et al in the mid-1980s.[86] The more complex procedure of selective adductor denervation–reinnervation treatment for adductor spasmodic dysphonia was described in 1999 by Berke et al.[87]

Treatment of Laryngeal Cancer

By the late 1920s, the results of laryngofissure (or thyrotomy) had improved significantly with the selection of patients with tumors on the free edge of a mobile vocal fold. More conservative approaches had been devised by Jacob Solis-Cohen who in 1907 described subperichondrial dissection,[88] and by Harry Lambert Lack (1871–1943) of London[89] who in 1916 removed part of the thyroid ala to excise a laryngeal tumor without performing a laryngofissure.

In the 1950s, Jean Leroux-Robert of Paris reported on a 100 cases of laryngeal cancer treated by partial vertical laryngectomy, of which 50% survived 5 years,[90] and Max Som

of New York reintroduced hemilaryngectomy,[91] which had first been performed in 1878 by Theodor Billroth and standardized by Themistokles Gluck (1853–1942) with Johannes Soerensen (1862–1939). Justo M. Alonso of Montevideo performed a two-stage supraglottic laryngectomy in 1939[92] and Joseph Ogura of St Louis refined the operation to one stage in 1958.[93]

Gluck and Soerensen improved the technique of total laryngectomy by severing the trachea and suturing it to the skin. The larynx was then removed from above. Their results greatly improved and by 1920 they were able to report on a series of 100 laryngectomies, of which 98 patients survived their operation.[94]

Surgery of Rehabilitation of the Voice Postlaryngectomy

Partial vertical and horizontal laryngectomy operations retain part of the glottis, and although the voice in the former case will never be normal, with the latter operation there is often little impairment. The initial deprivation of voice in patients who have undergone total laryngectomy presents a challenge in vocal rehabilitation to the laryngologist, to the speech therapist, and above all to the patient.

Methods of vocal rehabilitation include the development of "esophageal" or "pharyngeal" speech, the use of mechanical or electronic vibrators, and a variety of surgical voice restoration procedures.

Earlier mention has been made of the "artificial larynx" created in 1874 by Carl Gussenbauer for the first patient to undergo a total laryngectomy.[52] The patient was said to have developed a loud, clear but monotonous voice. Most of the early artificial larynxes suffered from problems of aspiration of saliva and food. Only Julius Wolff (1836–1902) of Berlin in 1893 was able to create different sounds in his artificial larynx as a result of a rubber tongue that could be elongated or shortened at the turn of a screw.[95]

Nicolas Taptas (1871–1955) of Constantinople, in 1900, rehabilitated a patient using an external laryngeal prosthesis connected between the tracheotomy tube and a deliberately created pharyngeal fistula. The patient, by occluding the tracheotomy cannula, diverted air through a flexible tube to the y-shaped pharyngeal part of the prosthesis. A valve, placed before the junction of the Y, prevented food and liquid from being aspirated. The patient was able to produce a sufficiently strong whispering voice.[96]

Many modifications of this principle were made during the first 50 years of the 20th century, culminating in the simple tracheoesophageal puncture and valved prosthesis introduced by Mark I. Singer and Eric D. Blom in 1980[97] and William R. Panje in 1981.[98]

Laryngeal Transplantation

The desire to perform human laryngeal transplantation started with dog experimental models in the 1960s.[99] In 1969, Kluyskens and Ringoir attempted to reconstruct the aerodigestive tract in a patient who had undergone a total laryngectomy for cancer.[100] They used a cadaveric transplant which was subtotal and preserved the recipient's perichondrium to revascularize the donor organ without the use of vascular or neural anastomoses. Unfortunately, the tumor recurred within a short period of time.

After 10 years of preliminary studies using a rat model, Robert R. Lorenz and Marshall Strome of Cleveland, Ohio, and New York, on January 4, 1998, performed a total laryngeal transplant in a man whose larynx had been severely traumatized in a road traffic accident.[101] The donor larynx was perfused by the recipient's blood while the damaged larynx was being removed. First, both the donor and recipient superior thyroid arteries were anastomosed and the donor's middle thyroid veins were joined to the recipient's internal jugular veins. Both superior laryngeal nerves were located and re-anastomosed, but only the recipient's right recurrent laryngeal nerve could be located. The patient made remarkable progress such that by 36 months after transplantation, all the subjective and objective measurements of phonation were within the normal range.

Twelve years passed before the next laryngeal transplant took place in October 2010 at the UC Davis Medical Center, Sacramento.[102] The female patient had lost the use of her larynx during surgery in 1999. She had a tracheotomy and, as she was unable to swallow, had been fed through a percutaneous gastrostomy. Her surgery entailed the replacement of her damaged larynx and pharynx by a donor larynx with the thyroid glands, blood vessels and nerves, and pharyngeal tissue attached. She had experienced a satisfactory restoration of her voice and swallow at 18 months posttransplantation.

Also in 2010, a 10-year-old British boy, suffering from congenital tracheal narrowing, became the first child in the world to receive a transplanted trachea which had been rebuilt inside his body using his own stem cells. The collagen scaffold donor trachea, stripped of its own cells, was injected 4 hours before implantation with the patient's own stem cells programmed with growth factors. The boy's body acted as a living bioreactor. By using his own stem cells, rejection was eliminated and immunosuppressant drugs were not needed. This pioneering technique had been devised by a European team led by Professor Paulo Macchiarini from Florence and Sweden and Professor Martin Birchall from the University College, London.[103]

Radiotherapy

Radium was discovered in 1898 by Pierre Curie (1859–1906) and his wife Marie Sklodowska Curie (1867–1934) and X-rays by Wilhelm Conrad Röntgen (1845–1923) in 1895. The effects of radiation on living tissues were initially applied to a variety of inflammatory and neoplastic conditions for which no other effective medical treatment was available at the time. The first radiotherapists were surgeons and dermatologists. Whereas the early developments of

laryngeal surgery for malignancy are associated with the names of Felix Semon and Henry Butlin, the pioneering efforts in radiotherapy are linked with the names Henri Coutard, Neville Finzi, and William Harmer.

Sir St Clair Thomson (1859–1943), writing with Lionel Colledge (1883–1948) in 1930, reported that: "the early history of radium in laryngeal cancer was a record of disappointment and disaster, of burns, necrosis or cartilage, toxemia, and increase in the rate of growth" [of the tumor].[104] Previous radium therapy increased the risks of delayed healing and secondary hemorrhage following subsequent surgery. In 1928, the physical measurement of ionizing radiation became practicable, and a unit of radiation exposure, the Roentgen (R), was defined.

William Douglas Harmer (1873–1962) working at St Bartholomew's Hospital, London, was aware that the supporting tissues surrounding a cancerous growth were more affected by radium than the growth itself. In his "Radium treatment of carcinoma of the larynx and tongue" (1932), he considered it necessary to screen the radium and ensure that the dose was evenly distributed throughout the tumor.[105] Louis Ledoux (1876–1947) of Brussels had already accomplished this, in 1923, by cutting a window in the thyroid cartilage and applying radium-filled needles into the growth.[106] This method, however, carried a potential for spreading the growth. William Harmer with his colleague Neville Samuel Finzi (1881–1968), in 1928, modified the technique of interstitial irradiation by placing the needles adjacent to but not penetrating the growth (**Fig. 1.15**).[107] Henri Coutard (1876–1950), working in the Curie Foundation, in 1932, published the results of external irradiation for squamous cell carcinomas of the tonsil, larynx, and hypopharynx treated between 1920 and 1926. He found that local recurrences were rare after 15 months, but that distant metastases could occur later. His few female patients did better than male patients.[108]

François Baclesse (1896–1967) of Paris, in 1949, and Manuel Lederman (1912–1984) of the Royal Marsden Hospital, London,

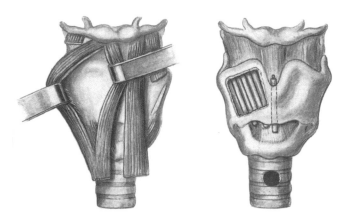

Figure 1.15 Harmer-Finzi radium needle technique for cancer of the larynx.
Adapted from Thomson St C, Colledge L. *Cancer of the Larynx*. London: Kegan Paul, Trench, Trubner & Co. Ltd.; 1930:223.

in 1952, divided laryngeal tumors into supraglottic, glottic, and subglottic. Hypopharyngeal tumors were classified separately. This concept together with the tumor-node-metastasis (TNM) classification, first proposed by Pierre Denoix in France in 1943, was accepted, with a few modifications, by the International Union Against Cancer (UICC) and the International Congress of Radiology in 1953 and later by the American Joint Committee on Cancer Staging and End Result Reporting (AJCC) in 1977. In 1988, the AJCC reached an agreement with the UICC for a common TNM and stage classification system. Both systems are now identical.[109,110]

Manuel Lederman in 1975 described the range of different techniques and increasing sophistication of radiotherapeutic technology in his article entitled "History of radiotherapy in the treatment of cancer of the larynx 1893–1939."[111] With cobalt units, 2 MV generators, and later linear accelerators, radiotherapy, particularly for tumors involving the vocal fold alone, became a serious alternative treatment to surgery. There were the potential drawbacks of mucositis, drying, and restriction of movement of the mucosal layer of the vocal folds with consequent vocal changes, but with ever-increasing refinement in delivery, radiotherapy in many countries is a treatment of choice for early laryngeal cancers where a cure can be expected.

For more advanced tumors with evidence of lymphatic spread, the choice of treatment rests between laryngeal surgery, including if necessary combined neck dissection, radiotherapy, chemotherapy, and combinations of each modality.

Summary

In the 21st century where communication is paramount, the inability to converse because of vocal impairment has a devastating effect on an individual's social interaction and work. Ever since laryngoscopy was born in 1854, physicians have been able to examine the larynx and determine the cause of hoarseness. For the last 30 years, the care of vocal disorders has been in the hands of multidisciplinary teams led by a laryngologist or a phoniatrician. Many causes of vocal impairment are treated by speech therapists (speech pathologists), vocal coaches, or singing teachers. Phonomicrosurgical techniques are employed for benign vocal fold pathology. In cases of laryngeal malignancy, the options of treatment range from vocal fold microsurgery or laser therapy to more extensive surgical procedures, radiotherapy, and/or chemotherapy depending on the classification of the tumor.

While total replacement of the larynx is still in the early experimental stage, three cases have so far been reported. There is significant hope that techniques will be developed which can, by using stem cell technology, dispense with the use of immunosuppressant drugs.

The maxim that "anyone who has suffered from a hoarse voice for more than a month must have a laryngoscopy" remains the gold standard for the management of all vocal disorders.

Bibliography

Karmody CS. The history of laryngology. In: Fried MP, Ferlito A, eds. The Larynx. Volume 1, 3rd ed. San Diego, CA: Plural Publishing Inc.; 2009:3–16

von Leden H. A cultural history of the larynx and voice and the history of phonosurgery. In: Sataloff RT, ed. Professional Voice: The Science and the Art of Clinical Care. 2nd ed. San Diego, CA: Singular Publishing Group Inc.; 1977:7–86, 561–580

Weir N, Mudry A. Otorhinolaryngology—An Illustrated History. 2nd ed. Ashford: Headley Bros. Ltd.; 2013

Zeitels SM. The history and development of phonomicrosurgery. In: Sataloff RT, ed. Professional Voice: The Science and the Art of Clinical Care. 2nd ed. San Diego, CA: Singular Publishing Group Inc.; 1977:581–602

References

1. Magill I. Endotracheal anaesthesia. Proc R Soc Med 1928;22(2): 83–88
2. Hirschowitz BI, Curtiss LE, Peters CW, Pollard HM. Demonstration of a new gastroscope, the fiberscope. Gastroenterology 1958;35(1):50, discussion 51–53
3. Pahor AL. Ear, nose and throat in Ancient Egypt. J Laryngol Otol 1992;106(9):773–779
4. Breasted JH. The Edwin Smith Surgical Papyrus. Chicago, IL: The University of Chicago Press; 1930
5. Potter P, Jones WHS, Withington ET, Smith WD. Hippocrates: with an English translation by W.H.S. Jones and E.T. Withington. In: Translation and Edition of Works of Hippocrates from Ancient Greek (to 1453) to English (1923). Volumes 1, 2, 3, 4; Medicine, Greek and Roman: Withington, London: Loeb Classical Library. Heinemann, London; Cambridge, MA: Harvard University Press; 1923–1931
6. Hamlyn DW. Aristotle De Anima. Books 11 and 111. Oxford: Clarendon Press; 1968
7. Muthu C. A short review of the history of ancient Hindu medicine. Proc R Soc Med 1913;6(Sect Hist Med):177–190
8. Bhishagratna KL. (Kaviraj), ed. An English translation of the Sushruta Samhita: Uttara-tantra. In: Medicine, Ayurvedic; Volume 3 of An English Translation of the Sushruta Samhita, Suśruta: Based on Original Sanskrit Text, with a Full and Comprehensive Introd., Additional Texts, Different Readings, Notes, Comparative Views, Index, Glossary and Plates. The University of Michigan: Chowkhamba Sanskrit Series Office; 1963;(2):535–538
9. May MT. Translation of Galen's De Usu Partium Corporis Humani. Ithaca, NY: Cornell University Press; 1968
10. Vesalius A. De Humanis Corporis Fabrica. Basel, Switzerland: J Oporini; 1543
11. Fallopius G. Observationes Anatomicae. Venetiis: Ulmus: 1561
12. Acquapendente F. De Visione, Voce, Auditu. Venetiis: Bolzetta: 1600
13. Morgagni GB. Valsalvae Opera, hoc est tractatus de aure humana [...] Epistolas addidit duodeviginti Johannes Baptista Morganus. 2 vols. Venetiis : Pitterei, 1740
14. Ferrein A. De la Formation de la Voix de l'Homme. In: Histoire de l'Académie Royale des Sciences (Paris): Imprimerie Royale; 1741, 409–430
15. Magendie F. Mémoire sur l'usage de l'épiglotte dans la déglutition. Paris:Méquignon-Marvis, 1813
16. Reid J. An experimental investigation into the glosso-pharyngeal, pneumo-gastric and spinal nerves. Edinburgh Med Surg J 1838;49: 109–176, ibid 1839;50:269–330

17. Trousseau A, Belloc JH. Traité pratique de la phtisie laryngée, de la laryngite chronique, et des maladies de la voix. Paris: Baillière; 1837: 26–27

18. Rokitansky K. Handbuch der Speciellen Pathologischen Anatomie. Vol. II. Wien: Braumüller & Seidel; 1842; 26–27

19. Home F. An Inquiry into the Nature, Cause, and Cure of the Croup. Edinburgh: Kincaid & Bell; 1765

20. Bretonneau PF. Des Inflammations Spéciales du Tissu Muqueux et en particulier de la Diphthérite, ou Inflammation Pelliculaire. Paris: Crevot; 1826

21. Green H. On the Surgical Treatment of Polypi of the Larynx and Oedema of the Glottis. New York, NY: Putnam; 1852

22. Guthrie D. Early records of tracheotomy. Bulletin of the History of Medicine 1944;15:59–64

23. Quoted by Paulus Aeginata. Adam F. The Seven Books of Paulus Aeginata. II. London: Sydenham Society; 1846:Lib. VI, Sect. XXXIII, 301–303

24. Casserius J. De Vocis Auditusque Organis Historia Anatomicae. Ferrara, Italy: Baldinus; 1600

25. Heister L. A General System of Surgery. English translation, London: Innys,Davis, Clark,Manby&Whiston,1743

26. Desault PJ. Oeuvres Chirurgicales de Desault (1798-1799). In: Bichat MFX, ed. Œuvres Chirurgicales Vol 1, Paris: Méquignon,1801: 180–196

27. Goodall EW. The story of tracheotomy. Brit J Child Dis 1934;31: 167–176, 253–272

28. Lassen HCA. A preliminary report on the 1952 epidemic of poliomyelitis in Copenhagen with special reference to the treatment of acute respiratory insufficiency. Lancet 1953;261(6749):37–41

29. Bozzoni P. Lichtleiter, eine Erfindung zur Anschaung innerer Theile und Krankheiten nebst der Abbildung. Practischen Arzneykunde und Wundarzneykunst (Berlin) 1806;24:107–124

30. Babington BG. Description of the Glottiscope. Lond Med Gaz 1829;3:555

31. Garcia M. Physiological observations on the human voice. Proc R Soc Lond 1855;7:399–410

32. Mackenzie M. The Use of the Laryngoscope in Diseases of the Throat. 3rd ed. London: Longmans, Green & Co.; 1871:25

33. Türck L. On the laryngeal mirror and its mode of employment, with engravings on wood. Zeitschrift der Gesellschaft der Ärzte zu Wien 1858;26:401–409

34. Czermak JN. Über den Kelhlkopfspiegel. Wien Med Wochenschr 1858;8:196–198

35. Lewin GR. Beiträge zur Laryngoscopie. Über Neubildungen, namentlich Polypen des Kehlkopfes. Dtsch Klinik 1862;14:114–116, 121-124, 171-175, 183-186, 191-194, 199-204, 223-227, 239-246, 257-260

36. Walker TJ. Report of a case of Polypoid Growth of the Larynx Diagnosed and Removed by aid of the Laryngoscope. Lancet 1861;ii:444–445

37. Walker TJ. On the Laryngoscope and its Clinical Application. London: Richards; 1864

38. Jelinek E. Das Cocain als Anästheticum und Analgeticum für den Pharynx und Larynx. Wien Med Wochenschr 1884;34:1334–1337, 1364–1367

39. Czermak JN. On the Laryngoscope and Its Employment in Physiology and Medicine. Translated from French by Gibb GD. London: New Sydenham Society; 1861

40. Elsberg L. Laryngoscopical Surgery Illustrated in Treatment of Morbid Growths within the Larynx. Philadelphia, PA: Collins; 1866

41. Mackenzie M. Essay on Growths in the Larynx. London: J&A Churchill; 1871

42. Fauvel C. Traité Pratique des Maladies du Larynx. Paris: Delahaye; 1876

43. Fraenkel B. First Healing of a Laryngeal Cancer taken out through Natural Passages. Archiv Klinische Chirurgie 1886;12:283–286

44. Albers JFH. Über die Geschwülste im Kehlkopf. J Chir Augenheilk 1834;21:517–536

45. Buck G. On the Surgical Treatment of Morbid Growths within the Larynx. Trans Am Med Assoc 1853;6:509–535

46. Gibb GD. The First Attempt in England to Remove a Growth from the Larynx through Division of the Pomum Adami. Brit Med J 1865;2: 327–331

47. Mackenzie M. A Manual of Diseases of the Throat and Nose. Volume 1. London: J&A Churchill; 1880:334

48. Butlin HT. On Malignant Disease, Sarcoma and Carcinoma of the Larynx. London: Churchill; 1883

49. Semon F. Larynx, growths in the. In: Heath C. Dictionary of Practical Surgery. Vol. 1. London: Smith Elder& Co.; 1886:892–898

50. Semon F. Some points in the diagnosis and treatment of laryngeal cancer: being an introduction to a discussion held in the Medical Society on January 28th, 1907. Brit Med J 1907;1:241–248

51. Thomson St C, Colledge L. Cancer of the Larynx. London: Kegan Paul, Trench, Trubner & Co. Ltd.; 1930:121

52. Gussenbauer C. Über die erste durch Theodor Billroth am Menschen ausgeführte Kehlkopt-Extirpation und die Anwendung eines künstlichen Kehlkopfes. Langenbecks Arch Klin Chir 1874;17: 343–356

53. Wolfenden NR. On Extirpation of the Larynx. J Laryngol Rhinol 1887;1:441–451

54. Stevenson RS. Morell Mackenzie: The Story of a Victorian Tragedy. London: William Heinemann Medical Books Ltd.; 1946

55. Mackenzie M. The Fatal Illness of Frederick the Noble. London: Sampson Low, Marston, Searle & Rivington; 1888

56. Lin JI. Virchow's pathological reports on Frederick III's cancer. N Engl J Med 1984;311(19):1261–1264

57. Waldeyer HM. Report of Dr Waldeyer. In: Case of Emperor Frederick III: Full Official Reports by the German Physicians and by Sir Morell Mackenzie. New York: Edgar S Werner; 1888:72–75

58. Semon F. Bezüglich des Überganges gutartiger Kehlkopf-Geschwülste in bosartiger nach intralaryngealen Operationen. Internationales Centralblatt für Laryngologie Rhinologie 1888;4:245–246

59. Semon F. Die Frage des Über ganges gutatiger Kehlkopf-Geschwüste in bosartiger, speciell nach intralaryngealen Operationen. Internationales Centralblatt für Laryngologie Rhinologie 1889;5:271–279

60. Kirstein A. Autoskopie des Larynx und Trachea (Laryngoscopia directa, Euthyskopie, Besichtigung ohne Spiegel). Arch Laryngol Rhinol 1895;3:156–164

61. O'Dwyer J. Two cases of croup treated by tubage of the glottis. N Y Med J 1885;46:146–151

62. Killian G. Die Schwebelaryngoscopie. Arch Laryngol Rhinol 1912;26:277–317

63. Brünings W. Direct Laryngoscopy, Bronchoscopy, and Esophagoscopy.(Translated by Howarth W.) London: Baillière, Tindall & Cox; 1912:110–115

64. Haslinger F. Die Diagnose und Therapie der Erkrankungen des Tracheo-bronchial baumes durch das Bronchoskop. Wien Klin Wochenschr 1931;44:1195

65. Lynch RC. Suspension laryngoscopy and its accomplishments. Ann Otolaryngol 1915;24:429–446

66. Jackson C. Instrumental aids to bronchoscopy and esophagoscopy. Laryngoscope 1907;17:492–494

67. Jackson C. Peroral Endoscopy and Laryngeal Surgery. St Louis: The Laryngoscope Co.; 1915:77–88

68. Weir N. Sir Victor Negus (1887–1974). In Oxford Dictionary of National Biography (Mathew HCG, Harrison B eds.). Oxford: Oxford University Press. 2004;40:341–343

69. von Leden H. The history of phonosurgery. In: Ford CN, Bless DM, eds. Phonosurgery: Assessment and Surgical Management of Voice Disorders. New York, NY: Raven Press Ltd.; 1991:3–24

70. von Leden H. Fono-cirugia. Acta ORL Iber-Americ 1971;22:291–299

71. Bishop J. Experimental Researches into the Physiology of the Human Voice. London and Edinburgh Philos Mag Third Series 1836;9(54):269–277

72. Hirano M. Structure of the vocal fold in normal and disease states: anatomical and physical studies. In: Ludlow CL, Hart MO, eds. Proceedings of the Conference on the Assessment of Vocal Pathology. Bethesda, MD: The American Speech-Language-Hearing Association; 1977: 11–30; Hirano M. Clinical Examination of the Voice. Monograph 5 of Disorders of Communication (Arnold GE, Winckel F, Wyke BD eds.) Wien, New York: Springer-Verlag, 1981

73. Oertel M. Das Laryngo-Stroboskop und die Laryngo-Stroboskopische Untersuching. Arch Laryngol Rhinol (Berlin) 1895;3:1–16

74. Albrecht R. Über den Wert Kolkoskopischer Untersuchungsmethoden bei Leukoplakien und Carcinomen des Mundes und Kehlkopfes. Arch Ohrenheilk 1954;164:459–463

75. Scalco AN, Shipman WF, Tabb HG. Microscopic suspension laryngoscopy. Ann Otol Rhinol Laryngol 1960;69:1134–1138

76. Kleinsasser O. Mikrolaryngoscopie und Endolaryngeale Mikrochirurgie. Stuttgart: Schattauer-Verlag, 1968

77. Hopkins HH, Kapany NS. A flexible fibrescope using static scanning. Nature 1954;173:39–41

78. Maiman TH. Stimulated optical radiation in ruby. Nature 1960;187:493–494

79. Jako GJ. Laser surgery of the vocal cords. An experimental study with carbon dioxide lasers on dogs. Laryngoscope 1972;82(12): 2204–2216

80. Zeitels SM. Laser versus cold instruments for microlaryngoscopic surgery. Laryngoscope 1996;106(5 Pt 1):545–552

81. Bouchayer M, Cornu G. Instrumental microscopy of benign lesions of the vocal folds. In: Ford CN, Bless DM, eds. Phonosurgery: Assessment and Surgical Management of Voice Disorders. New York, NY: Raven Press Ltd.; 1991:143–165

82. Payr E. Plastik am Schildknorpel zur Behebung der Folgen einseitiger Stimmbandlähmung. Dtsch Med Wochenschr 1915;43:1265–1270

83. Isshiki N, Morita H, Okamura H, Hiramoto M. Thyroplasty as a new phonosurgical technique. Acta Otolaryngol 1974;78(451-457):451–457

84. Brünings W. Über eine neue Behandlungsmethode der Rekurrenslähmung. 18. Verhandl Deutsch Laryngol 1911;93:151

85. Arnold GE. Vocal rehabilitation of paralytic dysphonia. VI. Further studies of intracordal injection materials. Arch Otolaryngol 1961;73:290–294

86. Blitzer A, Brin MF, Fahn S, Lange D, Lovelace RE. Botulinum toxin (BOTOX) for the treatment of "spastic dysphonia" as part of a trial of toxin injections for the treatment of other cranial dystonias. Laryngoscope 1986;96(11):1300–1301

87. Berke GS, Blackwell KE, Gerratt BR, Verneil A, Jackson KS, Sercarz JA. Selective laryngeal adductor denervation-reinnervation: a new surgical treatment for adductor spasmodic dysphonia. Ann Otol Rhinol Laryngol 1999;108(3):227–231

88. Solis-Cohen J. Modern procedures in excision of intrinsic malignant growths of the larynx. Laryngoscope 1907;17:365–369

89. Lack HL. Partial excision of the thyroid cartilage as an alternative to thyrotomy in malignant disease of the vocal cords. Proc R Soc Med 1916;9(Laryngol Sect):62–66

90. Leroux-Robert J. La chirurgie conservative par laryngofissure ou laryngectomie partielle dans le cancer du larynx. Ann Otol Laryngol (Paris) 1957;74:40–47

91. Som ML. Hemilaryngectomie—a modified technique for cordal carcinoma with extension posteriorly. AMA Arch Otolaryngol 1951;54(5):524–533

92. Alonso JM. Conservation of function in surgery of cancer of the larynx: bases, techniques, and results. I. Uruguayan technics. Trans Am Acad Ophthalmol Otolaryngol 1952;56:722–730

93. Ogura JH. Supraglottic subtotal laryngectomy and radical neck dissection for carcinoma of the epiglottis. Laryngoscope 1958;68(6):983–1003

94. Gluck T, Soerensen J. Die Resektion und Extirpation des Larynx, Pharynx und Ösophagus. In: Katz L, Preysing H, Blumenfeld F, eds. Handbuch der Speziellen Chirurgie des Ohres und der oberen Luftwege. Volume 1V. Würzburg: Verlag Curt Kabitzsch; 1922:1–70

95. Wolff J. Über den Künstlichen Kehlkopf und die Pseudo-stimme. Berl K Wochenschr 1893;30:1009–1013

96. Taptas N. Un Cas de Laryngectomie Totale pour Sarcome. Larynx Artificiel Externe. Ann Oreille. Larynx 1900;26:38–45

97. Singer MI, Blom ED. An endoscopic technique for restoration of voice after laryngectomy. Ann Otol Rhinol Laryngol 1980;89(6 Pt 1): 529–533

98. Panje WR. Prosthetic vocal rehabilitation following laryngectomy. The voice button. Ann Otol Rhinol Laryngol 1981;90(2 Pt 1):116–120

99. Work WP, Boles R. Larynx: replantation in the dog. Arch Otolaryngol 1965;82(4):401–402

100. Kluyskens P, Ringoir S. Follow-up of a human larynx transplantation. Laryngoscope 1970;80(8):1244–1250

101. Strome M, Stein J, Esclamado R, et al. Laryngeal transplantation: a case report with a three year follow up. N Engl J Med 2001;344:1676–1679

102. Farwell DG, Birchall MA, Macchiarini P, et al. Laryngotracheal Transplantation: Technical Modifications and Functional Outcomes. Laryngoscope 2013 doi: 10.1002/lary.24053

103. Elliott MJ, De Coppi P, Speggiorin S, et al. Stem-cell-based, tissue engineered tracheal replacement in a child: a 2-year follow-up study. Lancet 2012;380(9846):994–1000

104. Thomson St C, Colledge L. Cancer of the Larynx. London: Kegan Paul, Trench, Trubner & Co. Ltd.; 1930:219

105. Harmer D. The relative value of radiotherapy in the treatment of cancers of the upper air-passages. London: Murray, 1932

106. Ledoux L. Traitement Curie-chirurgical du Cancer Laryngé. Cancer (Brux) 1924;1:100–106

107. Finzi NS, Harmer D. Radium treatment of intrinsic carcinoma of the larynx. BMJ 1928;2(3541):886–889

108. Coutard H. Roentgenthérapie des épithéliomas de la région amygdalienne, de l'hypopharynx et du larynx au cours des années 1920 à 1926. Radiophysiol Radiothér 1930–1932;2:541–575

109. American Joint Committee on Cancer. AJCC Cancer Staging Manual. New York, NY: Springer-Verlag; 2002

110. UICC International Union Against Cancer. TNM Classification of Malignant Tumours. Committee on TNM Classification. Geneva; 1968

111. Lederman M. Panel discussion: the historical development of laryngectomy. VI. History of radiotherapy in the treatment of cancer of the larynx, 1896-1939. Laryngoscope 1975;85(2):333–353

Section B

Basic Sciences

2 Anatomy of the Larynx
Neil Weir

By the end of the 17th century, knowledge of the gross anatomy of the larynx was complete. The remaining detail of the nerve supply and structure of the epithelial lining emerged during the 18th and early 19th centuries well before the discovery of the laryngoscope by Manuel Garcia in 1854.[1]

Development of the Larynx, Trachea, Bronchi, and Lungs

During the 4th week of embryonic development, the rudiment of the respiratory tree appears as a median laryngotracheal groove in the ventral wall of the pharynx (**Fig. 2.1A, B**). The groove subsequently deepens, and its edges fuse to form a septum, thus converting the groove into a splanchnopleuric laryngotracheal tube. This process of fusion commences caudally and extends cranially but does not involve the cranial end where the edges remain separate, bounding a slit-like aperture through which the tube opens into the pharynx.

The tube is lined with endoderm from which the epithelial lining of the respiratory tract is developed. The cranial end of the tube forms the larynx and the trachea, and the caudal end produces two lateral outgrowths from which

the bronchi and right and left lung buds develop. These grow into the pleural coelomas and are thus covered with splanchnic mesenchyme from which the connective tissue, cartilage and nonstriated muscles, and the vasculature of the bronchi and lungs are developed.

Larynx and Trachea

The primitive larynx is the cranial end of the laryngotracheal groove, bounded vertically by the caudal part of the hypobranchial eminence and laterally by the ventral folds of the sixth branchial arches. The arytenoid swellings appear on both sides of the groove, and as they enlarge they become approximated to each other and to the caudal part of the hypobranchial eminence from which the epiglottis develops. The opening into the laryngeal cavity is at first a vertical slit or cleft, which becomes т-shaped with the appearance of the arytenoids. However, the epithelial walls of the cleft soon adhere to each other, and the aperture of the larynx is thus occluded until the 3rd month when its lumen is restored. The arytenoid swellings grow upward and deepen to produce the primitive aryepiglottic folds. This, in turn, produces a further aperture above the level of the primitive aperture that itself becomes the glottis. During the 2nd month of fetal life, the arytenoid swellings differentiate into the arytenoid and

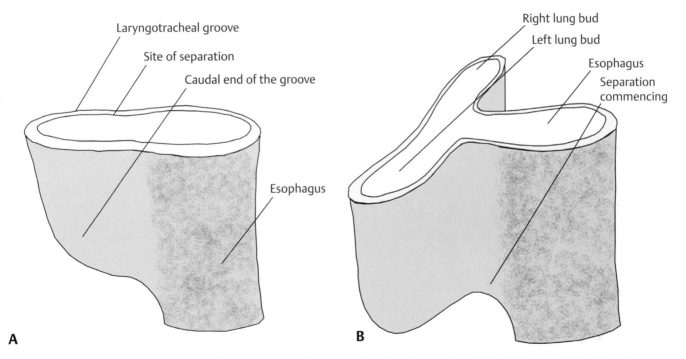

A　　　　　　　　　　　　　　　　**B**

Figure 2.1　(A) The closure of the laryngotracheal groove and (B) its separation from the esophagus in the latter part of the 4th week.

corniculate cartilages (derivatives of the sixth arch), and the folds joining them to the epiglottis become the aryepiglottic folds in which the cuneiform cartilages are developed as derivatives of the epiglottis. The thyroid cartilage develops from the ventral ends of the cartilages of the fourth branchial arch, appearing as two lateral plates, each with two chondrification centers. The cricoid cartilage and cartilages of the trachea develop from the sixth branchial arch during the 6th week. The trachea increases rapidly in length from the 5th week onward.

The branchial nerves of the fourth and sixth arches, namely the superior laryngeal and recurrent laryngeal nerves, supply the larynx (**Fig. 2.2**).

Each visceral arch is traversed by an artery (aortic arch). Each aortic arch connects the ventral and dorsal aortae of its own visceral arch. The primitive recurrent laryngeal nerve enters the sixth visceral arch, on each side, caudal to the sixth aortic arch. On the left side, the arch retains its position as the ductus arteriosus and the nerve is found caudal to the ligamentum arteriosum after birth. On the right side, the dorsal part of the sixth aortic arch and the whole of the fifth arch disappear. The nerve is, therefore, found on the caudal aspect of the fourth aortic arch, which becomes the subclavian artery. Piersol[2] described the "complete persistence of the distal portion of the right aortic arch associated with the disappearance of its proximal part." Here, the right subclavian artery originates from the descending aorta and passes right behind the esophagus.

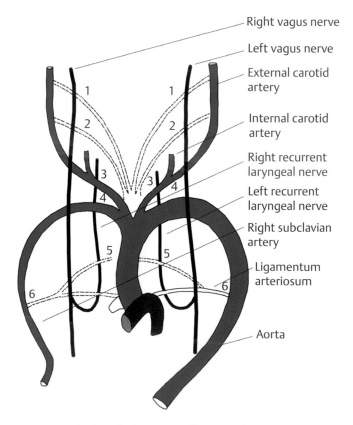

1
2
3
4
5
6

1
2
3
4
5
6

Right vagus nerve

Left vagus nerve

External carotid artery

Internal carotid artery

Right recurrent laryngeal nerve

Left recurrent laryngeal nerve

Right subclavian artery

Ligamentum arteriosum

Aorta

Figure 2.2   The branchial arteries and recurrent laryngeal nerves.

In the absence of the proximal portion of the right fourth aortic arch, no structure remains in contact with the right recurrent nerve. Instead of being pulled down into its usual position, the nerve passes directly from the main vagal trunk to enter the larynx.[3] In this context, the nerve is called the *nonrecurrent laryngeal nerve*. The incidence is variously reported to be between 0.3 and 1.0%. For a left nonrecurrent nerve to exist, there would have to be either a loss of the ductus arteriosus in fetal life or a right-sided aorta. A case of the latter situation was reported by Berlin.[4]

For further reading on the development of the trachea and lungs, consult O'Rahilly and Boyden[5] and Reid.[6]

Larynx

Comparative Anatomy and Modification of Olfaction and Deglutition

The prime reason for the existence of the larynx is not to make phonation possible, but to provide a protective sphincter at the inlet of the air passages. This can be seen in a lung fish, where the larynx takes the form of a simple muscular sphincter surrounding the opening of the air passage in the floor of the pharynx. In birds, the rima glottidis in the floor of the mouth shuts to close the air inlet, but it makes no sound; phonation is produced from a dilatation, the syrinx, at the lower end of the trachea just above its bifurcation.

The first breathers of air, the amphibia, do, however, phonate. They achieve this by "swallowing air" that, as there is no separate nasal cavity, is drawn in through valvular "nostrils" that open anteriorly into the roof of the mouth. In mammals, a nasal cavity develops with the appearance of a palate. The separation of a respiratory and olfactory chamber from the mouth has considerable advantages: predatory mammals can still breathe while the mouth is obstructed by prey, and herbivorous prey can still sense warning odors while feeding. In aquatic vertebrates, such as crocodiles, dolphins, and whales, an intranarial larynx has been developed where the inlet of the larynx is suspended within the nasopharynx and clasped by the sphincter of the nasopharyngeal inlet (the palatopharyngeus). Thus, respiration and olfaction can continue at the water surface even with the mouth submerged, open, and ready for prey.

The larynx of humans is still an essential sphincter, preventing the entry of swallowed food and other foreign bodies and providing a blockade to build up pressure for coughing or for aiding extreme muscular efforts. However, humans differ from other mammals in the ability to produce speech by the highest integrations of the nervous and locomotive systems.

Descriptive Anatomy

The larynx is situated at the upper end of the trachea; it lies opposite the third to sixth cervical vertebrae in men, while being somewhat higher in women and children. The average

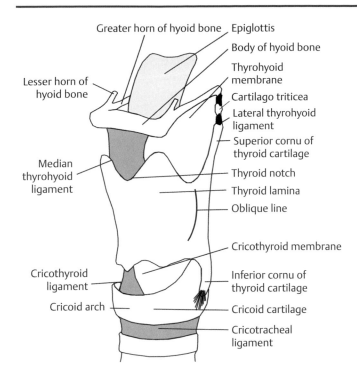

Figure 2.3   The cartilages and ligaments of the larynx.

length, transverse diameter, and anteroposterior diameter are 44, 43, and 36 mm, respectively, in men and 36, 41, and 26 mm, respectively, in women.

There is little difference in the size of the larynx in boys and girls until after puberty when the anteroposterior diameter in men almost doubles. The skeletal framework of the larynx (**Figs. 2.3** and **2.4**) is formed of cartilages, which are connected by ligaments and membranes and are moved in relation to one another by both intrinsic and extrinsic muscles. It is lined with mucous membrane that is

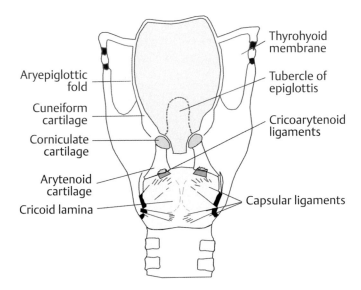

Figure 2.4   Ligaments, membranes, and cartilages of the larynx seen from behind.

continuous above and behind with that of the pharynx and below with that of the trachea.

The infantile larynx is both absolutely and relatively smaller than the larynx of the adult. The lumen is therefore disproportionately narrower. It is more funnel-shaped and its narrowest part is at the junction of the subglottic larynx with the trachea. A very slight swelling of the lax mucosa in this area may thus produce a very serious obstruction to breathing. The laryngeal cartilages are much softer in the infant and therefore collapse more easily in forced inspiratory efforts. The infantile larynx starts high up under the tongue and with development assumes an increasingly lower position.

Laryngeal Cartilages

Thyroid Cartilage

The shield-like cartilage (see **Figs. 2.3** and **2.4**) is the longest of the laryngeal cartilages and consists of two laminae that meet in the midline inferiorly, leaving an easily palpable notch, the thyroid notch, between them above. The angle of fusion of the laminae is approximately 90 degrees in men and 120 degrees in women. In men, the fused anterior borders form a projection, again easily palpable, which is the laryngeal prominence or Adam's apple. A small narrow strip of cartilage, the intrathyroid cartilage, separates the two laminae anteriorly in childhood. Posteriorly, the laminae diverge and the posterior border of each is prolonged as two slender processes, the superior and the inferior cornua. The superior cornu is long and narrow and curves upward, backward, and medially, ending in a conical extremity to which the lateral thyroid ligament is attached. The inferior cornu is shorter and thicker and curves downward and medially. On the medial surface of its lower end, there is a small oval facet for articulation with the cricoid cartilage.

On the external surface of each lamina, an oblique line curves downward and forward from the superior thyroid tubercle, situated just in front of the root of the superior horn, to the inferior thyroid tubercle on the lower border of the lamina. This line marks the attachments of the thyrohyoid, sternothyroid, and inferior constrictor muscles. The inner aspects of the laminae are smooth and are mainly covered by loosely attached mucous membrane. The thyroepiglottic ligament is attached to the inner aspect of the thyroid notch, and below this, and on each side of the midline, the vestibular and vocal ligaments and the thyroarytenoid, thyroepiglottic, and vocalis muscles are attached. The fusion of the anterior ends of the two vocal ligaments produces the anterior commissure tendon, which is of importance in the spread of carcinoma.

The superior border of each lamina gives attachment to the corresponding half of the thyrohyoid ligament. The inferior border of each half is divided into two by the inferior tubercle. The cricothyroid membrane is attached to the inner aspect of the medial portion of the inferior border of the thyroid cartilage.

Cricoid Cartilage

The cricoid cartilage (see **Figs. 2.3** and **2.4**) is the only complete cartilaginous ring present in the air passages. It forms the inferior part of the anterior and lateral walls and most of the posterior wall of the larynx. Likened to the signet ring, it comprises a deep broad quadrilateral lamina posteriorly and a narrow arch anteriorly. Near the junction of the arch and lamina, an articular facet is present for the inferior cornu of the thyroid cartilage. The lamina has sloping shoulders, which carry articular facets for the arytenoids. These joints are synovial with capsular ligaments. Rotation of the cricoid cartilage on the thyroid cartilage can take place about an axis passing transversely through the joints. A vertical ridge in the midline of the lamina gives attachment to the longitudinal muscle of the esophagus and produces a shallow concavity on each side for the origin of the posterior cricoarytenoid muscle. The entire surface of the cricoid cartilage is lined with mucous membrane.

Arytenoid Cartilages

The two arytenoid cartilages (see **Fig. 2.4**) are placed close together on the upper and lateral borders of the cricoid lamina. Each is an irregular three-sided pyramid with a forward projection, the vocal process, attached to the vocal folds and also a lateral projection, the muscular process, to which the posterior cricoarytenoid and lateral cricoarytenoid muscles are attached. Between these two processes is the anterolateral surface that is irregular and divided into two fossae by a crest running from the apex. The upper triangular fossa gives attachment to the vestibular ligament and the lower to the vocalis and lateral cricoarytenoid muscles. The apex is curved backward and medially and is flattened for articulation with the corniculate cartilage to which the aryepiglottic folds are attached. The medial surfaces are covered with mucous membrane and form the lateral boundary of the intercartilaginous part of the rima glottidis. The posterior surface is covered entirely by the transverse arytenoid muscle.

The base is concave and presents a smooth surface for articulation, with the sloping shoulder on the upper border of the cricoid lamina. The capsular ligament of this synovial joint is lax, allowing both rotatory and medial and lateral gliding movements. In humans, the cylindrical articulating surfaces permit a greater range of gliding movement than of rotatory movement, and the shape of the open human glottis resembles a "V." A firm posterior cricoarytenoid ligament prevents forward movement of the arytenoid cartilage.

Corniculate and Cuneiform Cartilages

The corniculate cartilages (see **Fig. 2.4**) are two small conical nodules of elastic fibrocartilage that articulate as a synovial joint, or which are sometimes fused, with the apices of the arytenoid cartilages. They are situated in the posterior parts of the aryepiglottic folds of the mucous membrane.

The cuneiform cartilages are small, paired, elongated flakes of elastic fibrocartilages placed in each margin of the aryepiglottic fold.

Cartilage of the Epiglottis

The epiglottis is a thin, leaf-like sheet of elastic cartilage that projects upward behind the tongue and the body of the hyoid bone (see **Figs. 2.3** and **2.4**). The narrow stalk is attached by the thyroepiglottic ligament to the angle between the thyroid laminae, below the thyroid notch. The upper broad part is directed upward and backward, and its superior margin is free.

The sides of the epiglottis are attached to the arytenoid cartilages by the aryepiglottic folds of the mucous membrane that, together with the free edge of the epiglottis, form the anterior boundary to the inlet of the larynx. The posterior surface of the epiglottis is concave and smooth but a small central projection, the tubercle, is present in the lower part. The bare cartilage is indented by a number of small pits into which mucous glands project. The anterior surface of the epiglottis is free and is covered with mucous membrane that is reflected on to the pharyngeal part of the tongue and the lateral wall of the pharynx, forming a median glossoepiglottic fold and two lateral glossoepiglottic folds. The depression formed on each side of the median glossoepiglottic fold is the vallecula. An elastic ligament, the hypoepiglottic ligament, connects the lower part of the epiglottis to the hyoid bone in front. The space between the epiglottis and the thyrohyoid membrane is filled with fatty tissue and is named the preepiglottic space. The epiglottis is not functionally developed in humans in that respiration, deglutition, and phonation can take place almost normally even if it has been destroyed. In neonates and infants, however, the epiglottis is omega-shaped. This long, deeply grooved, "floppy" epiglottis more closely resembles that of aquatic mammals and is more suited to its function of protecting the nasotracheal air passage during suckling.

Calcification of Laryngeal Cartilages

The corniculate and cuneiform cartilages, the epiglottis, and the apices of the arytenoids consist of elastic fibrocartilage, which shows little tendency to calcify. The thyroid, cricoid, and greater part of the arytenoids consist of hyaline cartilage, which begins to calcify in a person's late teens or early twenties. Calcification of the thyroid cartilage starts in the region of the inferior cornu and proceeds anteriorly and superiorly until the entire rim is involved. A central translucent window persists into old age.

Calcification of the posterior part of the lamina of the cricoid and of the posterior part of the arytenoid may be confused at radiology with a foreign body (see also section "Applied Anatomy of the Larynx" later in the chapter). Calcification of the body and muscular process of the arytenoid takes place later in the 4th decade, but the vocal process tends not to ossify.

Ligaments

Extrinsic Ligaments

The extrinsic ligaments (**Fig. 2.5**; see also **Figs. 2.3** and **2.4**) connect the cartilage to the hyoid bone and trachea.

The thyrohyoid membrane stretches between the upper border of the thyroid and the upper border of the posterior surfaces of the body and greater cornu of the hyoid bone. The membrane is composed of fibroelastic tissue and is strengthened anteriorly by condensed fibrous tissue called the median thyrohyoid ligament. The posterior margin is also stretched to form the lateral thyrohyoid ligament that connects the tips of the superior cornu of the thyroid cartilage to the posterior ends of the greater cornu of the hyoid bone. The ligaments often contain a small nodule, the cartilago triticea. The membrane is pierced by the internal branch of the superior laryngeal nerve and by the superior laryngeal vessels. The cricotracheal ligament unites the lower border of the cricoid cartilage with the first tracheal ring. The hypoepiglottic ligament connects the epiglottis to the back of the body of the hyoid bone.

Intrinsic Ligaments

The intrinsic ligaments (see **Fig. 2.5**) connect the cartilages themselves, and together they strengthen the capsule of the intercartilaginous joints and form the broad sheet of fibroelastic tissue, the fibroelastic membrane, which lies beneath the mucous membrane of the larynx and creates an internal framework.

The fibroelastic membrane is divided into an upper and lower part by the laryngeal ventricle. The upper quadrilateral membrane extends between the border of the epiglottis and the arytenoid cartilage. The upper margin forms the frame of the aryepiglottic inlet; the lower margin

is thickened to form the vestibular ligament that underlies the vestibular fold or false cord. The lower part is altogether a thicker membrane, containing many elastic fibers. It is commonly called the cricovocal ligament, cricothyroid ligament, or, by a more loose term, the conus elasticus. It is attached below to the upper border of the cricoid cartilage and above is stretched between the midpoint of the laryngeal prominence of the thyroid cartilage anteriorly and the vocal process of the arytenoid behind. The free upper border of the membrane constitutes the vocal ligament and the framework of the vocal fold or true cord. Anteriorly, there is a thickening of the membrane, the cricothyroid ligament, which links the cricoid and the thyroid cartilage in the midline. (For cricothyrotomy, see section "Applied Anatomy of the Larynx" later in the chapter.)

Interior of the Larynx

The cavity of the larynx extends from the pharynx at the laryngeal inlet to the beginning of the lumen of the trachea at the lower border of the cricoid cartilage and is divided by the vestibular and vocal folds into three compartments. The superior vestibule is above the vestibular folds, the ventricle or sinus of the larynx lies between the vestibular and vocal folds, and the subglottic space extends from the vocal folds to the lower border of the cricoid cartilage (see **Fig. 2.5**). The fissure between the vestibular folds is called the rima vestibuli and that between the vocal folds is the rima glottidis or glottis. The paraglottic and preepiglottic spaces, which are of importance in the spread of tumors, lie within the larynx.

The laryngeal inlet is bound superiorly by the free edge of the epiglottis and on each side by the aryepiglottic folds. Posteriorly, the inlet is completed by the mucous membrane between the two arytenoid cartilages. This region of the larynx was formerly termed the posterior commissure but is now correctly called the posterior glottis.[7] There is a plentiful supply of mucous glands in the margins of the aryepiglottic folds.

The superior vestibule lies between the inlet of the larynx and the level of the vestibular folds. It narrows as it extends downward, and the anterior wall, which is the posterior surface of the epiglottis, is much deeper than the posterior wall, which is formed by mucous membrane covering the anterior surface of the arytenoid cartilages. The lateral walls are formed by the inner aspect of the aryepiglottic folds.

The pre-epiglottic space is a wedge-shaped space lying in front of the epiglottis and is bound anteriorly by the thyrohyoid ligament and the hyoid bone. Above a deep layer of fascia, the hypoepiglottic ligament connects the epiglottis to the hyoid bone. It is continuous laterally with the paraglottic space that is bound by the thyroid cartilage laterally, the conus elasticus and quadrangular membrane medially, and the anterior reflection of the pyriform fossa mucosa posteriorly. It embraces the ventricles and saccules.

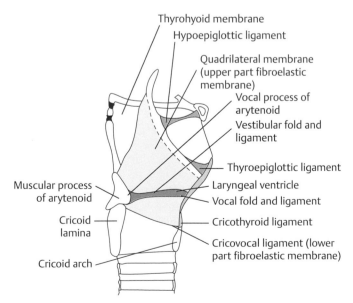

Thyrohyoid membrane
Hypoepiglottic ligament
Quadrilateral membrane (upper part fibroelastic membrane)
Vocal process of arytenoid
Vestibular fold and ligament
Thyroepiglottic ligament
Laryngeal ventricle
Vocal fold and ligament
Cricothyroid ligament
Cricovocal ligament (lower part fibroelastic membrane)
Muscular process of arytenoid
Cricoid lamina
Cricoid arch

Figure 2.5   Ligaments and membranes of the larynx seen laterally.

Laryngeal Ventricle and the Vestibular Folds

The middle part of the cavity (and ventricle) lies between the vestibular and vocal folds that cover the ligaments of the same name. On each side, it opens, through a narrow horizontal slit, into an elongated recess, the laryngeal ventricle or sinus. From the anterior part of the ventricle, a pouch, the saccule of the larynx, ascends between the vestibular folds and the inner surface of the thyroid cartilage.

It may extend as far as the upper border of the cartilage; indeed, in some monkeys and apes, it extends even further into the neck, as far as the axilla. In humans, the saccule occasionally protrudes through the thyrohyoid membrane. The mucous membrane lining the saccule contains numerous mucous glands, lodged in submucous alveolar tissue. Fibrous tissue surrounds the saccule and a limited number of muscle fibers pass from the apex of the arytenoid cartilage across the medial aspect of the saccule to the aryepiglottic fold. The muscle is presumed to compress the saccule and to express the secretion of its mucous glands over the surface of the vocal folds.

The vestibular folds are two thick, pink folds of mucous membrane, each enclosing a narrow band of fibrous tissue, the vestibular ligament, which is fixed in front to the angle of the thyroid cartilage, just below the attachment of the epiglottic cartilage, and behind to the anterolateral surface of the arytenoid cartilage, just above the vocal process.

Vocal Folds

The vocal folds are defined as two fold-like structures that extend from the middle of the angle of the thyroid cartilage to the vocal processes of the arytenoid cartilages. Each fold is a layered structure. The vocal fold consists of mucosa and muscle. The mucosa is subdivided into the epithelium, which is of the stratified squamous type, and the lamina propria, which consists of superficial, intermediate, and deep layers (**Fig. 2.6A**). The superficial layer of the lamina propria, referred to as Reinke space, is made of loose fibrous substance that can be likened to a mass of soft gelatin. It is this layer that vibrates most significantly during phonation. If it becomes stiff due to some pathological state, such as inflammation, tumor, or scar tissue, its vibrations are disturbed and voice problems result. The intermediate layer, consisting mainly of elastic fibers, and the deep layer, consisting of collagenous fibers rich in fibroblasts, together form the vocal ligament, deep to which is the vocalis muscle that constitutes the main body of the vocal fold.

Around the edge of the vocal fold, the elastic and collagenous fibers in the lamina propria and the muscle fibers of the vocalis muscle run parallel to the edge. The layered structure is not uniform along the length of the vocal fold (refer to **Figs. 2.6B** and **2.7**). At the anterior end, there is a mass of collagenous fibers that appear to be connected to the inner perichondrium of the thyroid cartilage anteriorly and to the deep layer of the lamina propria posteriorly. Posterior to this mass of collagenous fibers, there is another mass of elastic fibers, continuous with the intermediate layer of lamina propria, called the anterior

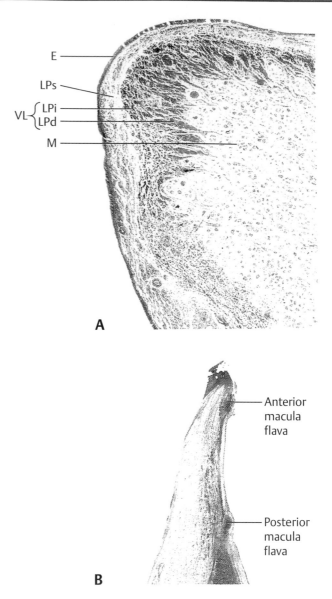

Figure 2.6 (A) Coronal section of the vocal fold at the mid-membranous part. (B) Horizontal section of the anterior and posterior ends of the membranous part of the vocal fold. E, epithelium; LP, lamina propria; LPd, deep; LPi, intermediate; LPs, superficial layers; VL, vocal ligament; M, vocal muscle.

macula flava. A similar picture is seen at the posterior end of the membranous part of the vocal fold. These structures at both ends of the membranous vocal folds appear to serve as cushions to protect the ends from mechanical damage caused by vocal fold vibration.

The vocal fold is a multilayered vibrator that, from a mechanical point of view, can be reclassified into three layers: the *cover*, consisting of the epithelium and the superficial layer of the lamina propria; the *transition*, consisting of the intermediate and deep layers of the lamina propria; and the *body*, consisting of the vocalis muscle. The blood vessels in the mucosa at the edge of the vocal fold run parallel to the edge. All the vessels are very small and therefore do not impede vibration.

Histological Variation in the Structure of the Vocal Fold in Children and the Elderly

The structure of the edge of the vocal fold in the newborn differs markedly from its adult form. The main difference is in the lamina propria that is very thick relative to the length of the vocal fold and is uniform in structure. There is no evidence of a vocal ligament, as almost the entire lamina propria is loose and liable. Some fibrous tissue, immature macula flava, is present near the anterior and posterior ends of the membranous vocal fold.

An immature vocal ligament emerges between the ages of 1 and 4 years. Differentiation between the two layers of the vocal ligament starts between 6 and 12 years of age and the ligament becomes thicker. Near the end of adolescence, the three-layered structure of the lamina propria is clearly evident.

There is great individual variation in changes in the structure of the vocal fold with increasing age. There is a little change in the epithelium, but the superficial layer of the lamina propria tends to become edematous and thicker with age. Elastic fibers in the intermediate layer become loose and atrophied and the layer thus becomes thinner. The collagenous fibers of the deep layer become thicker and denser and the vocalis muscle tends to atrophy with age.

Glottis

The rima glottidis or glottis is an elongated fissure between the vocal folds anteriorly and the vocal processes and bases of the arytenoid cartilages posteriorly. It is limited behind by the mucous membrane between the arytenoid cartilages with the top portion of the cricoid lamina as its base. The region between the vocal folds accounts for three-fifths of the length of the aperture and is termed the "intermembranous part." The remainder lies between the vocal processes and is called the intercartilaginous part. The average length of the glottis varies between 23 mm in men and 16 to 17 mm in women. In the resting state, the vocal processes are usually 8 mm apart. The glottis alters the shape with phonation and respiration.

Subglottis

The lower part of the laryngeal cavity or subglottic space extends from the level of the vocal folds to the lower border of the cricoid cartilage. Its upper part is elliptical in form, but its lower part widens and becomes circular in shape and continuous with the cavity of the trachea. It is lined with mucous membrane, and its walls consist of the cricothyroid ligament above and the inner surface of the cricoid cartilage below.

Muscles

The muscles of the larynx may be divided into extrinsic, which attach the larynx to neighboring structures and maintain the position of the larynx in the neck and intrinsic, which move the various cartilages of the larynx and regulate the mechanical properties of the vocal folds.

Extrinsic Muscles

The extrinsic muscles may be divided into those below the hyoid bone (infrahyoid muscles) and those above the hyoid bone (suprahyoid muscles). The infrahyoid muscles include the thyrohyoid, sternothyroid, sternohyoid, and omohyoid.

The thyrohyoid muscle arises from the oblique line of the thyroid lamina and is inserted into the inferior border of the greater cornu of the hyoid bone. It is supplied by C1 fibers by way of the hypoglossal nerve and elevates the larynx if the hyoid is fixed or depresses the hyoid if the larynx is fixed.

The sternothyroid muscle arises from the posterior surface of the manubrium sterni and from the edge of the first, and occasionally the second, costal cartilage and is inserted into the oblique line on the anterolateral surface of the thyroid lamina. It is supplied by the ansa cervicalis (C2 and C3) and depresses the larynx.

The sternohyoid muscle originates from the clavicle and the posterior surface of the manubrium sterni and is inserted into the lower edge of the body of the hyoid bone. It is supplied by a branch of ansa cervicalis (C1, C2, and C3) and depresses the larynx by lowering the hyoid bone.

It is likely that a more significant role of the infrahyoid muscles is to oppose the elevators of the larynx (the suprahyoid muscles) by "paying out rope" during contraction of the elevators; descent of the larynx after elevation is due to elastic recoil of the trachea.

The suprahyoid muscle originates from the mylohyoid line on the inner aspect of the mandible and is inserted into a midline raphe with fibers from the opposite side. The midline raphe and the posterior fibers are attached to the body of the hyoid bone. Its nerve supply is derived from the motor root of the trigeminal nerve by way of the mylohyoid branch of the inferior alveolar nerve and its action is to raise the hyoid bone and pull it anteriorly.

The geniohyoid muscle extends from each inferior genial tubercle to the upper border of the body of the hyoid bone. It is supplied by C1 fibers by way of the hypoglossal nerve and raises and pulls forward the hyoid bone.

The stylohyoid muscle arises from the back of the styloid process. It bifurcates around the intermediate tendon of the digastric muscle and is inserted by two slips into the base of the greater cornu of the hyoid bone. It is supplied by the facial nerve and acts as a retractor and elevator of the hyoid bone, used in swallowing.

The digastric muscle originates from the digastric notch on the medial surface of the mastoid process. Its posterior belly tapers to an intermediate tendon, held beneath a fibrous sling attached near the lesser cornu of the hyoid bone. The anterior belly connects the intermediate tendon to the digastric fossa on the lower border of the mandible. The posterior belly is supplied by the facial nerve and the anterior by the mylohyoid nerve (trigeminal). The anterior belly pulls the hyoid bone anteriorly and raises it, whereas the posterior belly pulls the hyoid bone posteriorly and also raises it.

The stylopharyngeus muscle arises from the deep aspect of the styloid process and sloping down crosses the lower border of the superior constrictor and passes down inside the middle constrictor. Here, it lies behind the palatopharyngeus and is inserted into the posterior border of the lamina of the thyroid cartilage and the side wall of the pharynx. The muscle is supplied by the glossopharyngeal nerve and helps elevate the larynx.

The palatopharyngeus is inserted into the posterior border of the thyroid ala and cornua. Some of the posterior fibers merge with the surrounding fibers of the inferior constrictor. It is supplied by the accessory nerve through the pharyngeal plexus. Although its main action is to raise and shorten the wall of the pharynx, it probably also helps in tilting the larynx forward, thus enabling food to pass straight into the esophagus during the act of swallowing.

The salpingopharyngeus muscle arises from the tubal elevation and passes vertically down inside the pharynx to be inserted into the posterior border of the thyroid cartilage and the side wall of the pharynx. It is supplied by the pharyngeal plexus and elevates the larynx and the pharynx in the second (involuntary) stage of swallowing.

Intrinsic Muscles

The intrinsic laryngeal muscles (**Figs. 2.7** and **2.8**) are of great importance in regulating the mechanical properties of the vocal folds as they control not only the position and shape of the vocal folds but also the elasticity and viscosity of each layer of the vocal fold. They may be divided into: (1) those that open and close the glottis, namely the posterior cricoarytenoids, the lateral cricoarytenoids, and the transverse and oblique arytenoids; (2) those that control the tension of the vocal folds, namely the thyroarytenoids (vocalis) and cricothyroids; and (3) those that alter the shape of the inlet of the larynx, namely the aryepiglotticus and the thyroepiglotticus. With the exception of the transverse arytenoid, all these muscles are paired.

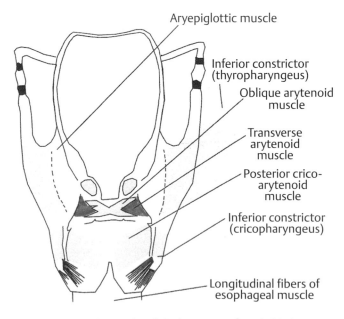

Figure 2.7   Intrinsic muscles of the larynx seen from behind.

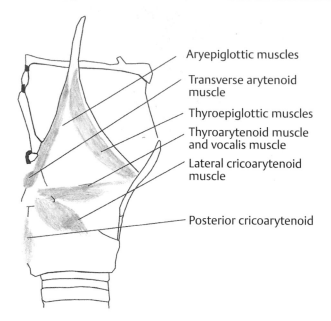

Figure 2.8   Intrinsic muscles of the larynx seen laterally.

The lateral cricoarytenoid arises from the superior border of the lateral part of the arch of the cricoid cartilage and inserts into the front of the muscular process of the arytenoid. It adducts and lowers the tip of the vocal process of the arytenoid by rotating the arytenoid medially. The entire vocal fold is thus adducted, lowered, elongated, and thinned. The edge of the vocal fold becomes sharp, and all layers are passively stiffened.

The posterior cricoarytenoid, which is the only muscle to open the glottis, arises from the lower and medial surface of the back of the cricoid lamina and fans out to be inserted into the back of the muscular process of the arytenoid cartilage. Its upper fibers are almost horizontal, while its lateral fibers are almost vertical. The horizontal action rotates the arytenoids and moves the muscular process toward each other, thus separating the vocal processes and abducting the vocal folds. The vertical action (lateral fibers) draws the arytenoids down the sloping shoulders of the cricoid cartilage, thus separating the arytenoids from each other. These actions take place simultaneously, although in humans there is greater proportion of vertical movement, thus opening the glottis in a V shape. The posterior cricoarytenoid abducts and elevates the tip of the vocal process of the arytenoid cartilage and therefore the entire vocal fold becomes markedly elongated and thin. The edge of the vocal fold is rounded and all layers are passively stiffened.

The weight of the abductor muscles of the larynx is not more than 25% of that of the adductors,[8] which may explain the greater vulnerability of the abductors in the event of partial injury to the recurrent laryngeal nerve. In a study of the intrinsic muscles of 54 normal postmortem larynges, it was observed that while no significant alterations had developed in the cricothyroid, interarytenoid, lateral cricoarytenoid, or thyroarytenoid muscles, all the larynges from patients 13 years or older revealed microscopic changes in the posterior cricoarytenoid muscles, and in many patients older

46 years, there had also been some necrosis and associated reactive changes.[9] Because the posterior cricoarytenoid muscle is the sole abductor of the vocal folds, the changes may be a manifestation of the continuous activity of this muscle. The change starts with the deposition of coarse lipofuscin granules near the sarcolemma. Similar granules are found in the tongue muscle and in myocardial fibers from an early age. Only in the posterior cricoarytenoid muscles, however, do concomitant muscle and other sarcoplasmic changes take place.

The interarytenoid muscles comprise the unpaired transverse arytenoid muscle and the paired oblique arytenoid muscles. The transverse arytenoid muscle arises from the posterior surface of the muscular process and the outer edge of one arytenoid and passes to similar attachments on the other cartilage. The oblique arytenoid muscles lie superficial to the transverse arytenoid and pass from the posterior aspect of the muscular process of one arytenoid cartilage to the apex of the other, thus crossing each other. Some of the fibers pass around the apex of the arytenoid cartilage and are prolonged into the aryepiglottic fold as the aryepiglottic muscle that acts as a rather weak sphincter of the laryngeal inlet. The interarytenoid muscle adducts the vocal fold chiefly at the cartilaginous portion. It controls the position of the vocal fold, but does not significantly affect its mechanical property.

The thyroarytenoid (vocalis) muscle extends from the back of the thyroid prominence and from the cricothyroid ligament to the vocal process of the arytenoid and to the anterolateral surface of the body of the cartilage. Each muscle is in the form of a broad sheet that lies lateral to and above the free edge of the cricovocal ligament (see section "Intrinsic Ligaments"). The lower part of the muscle is thicker and forms a distinct bundle called the vocalis muscle, contraction of which adducts the vocal folds, especially at the membranous portion. It lowers, shortens, and thickens the vocal fold, causing the edge of the vocal fold to be rounded. The body (muscular layer) of the vocal fold is actively stiffened but the cover and transition layers are passively slackened. Considerable numbers of fibers of the thyroarytenoid are prolonged into the aryepiglottic fold, some continuing to the margin of the epiglottis as the thyroepiglottic muscle that tends to widen the inlet of the larynx by pulling the aryepiglottic folds slightly apart. Occasionally, a very fine muscle is present, the superior thyroarytenoid, which lies on the lateral surface of the main mass of the thyroarytenoid and extends obliquely from the angle of the thyroid cartilage to the muscular process of the arytenoid cartilage.

The cricothyroid muscle (**Fig. 2.9**) is the only intrinsic laryngeal muscle that lies outside the cartilaginous framework. It is fan-shaped and arises from the lateral surface of the anterior arch of the cricoid cartilage. Its fibers then diverge and pass backward in two groups. The lower, oblique fibers pass backward and lateral to the anterior border of the inferior cornu of the thyroid cartilage, and the anterior, straight fibers ascend to the posterior part of the lower border of the thyroid lamina. The cricothyroid muscle rotates the cricoid cartilage about the horizontal axis passing through the cricothyroid joint (**Fig. 2.10**).

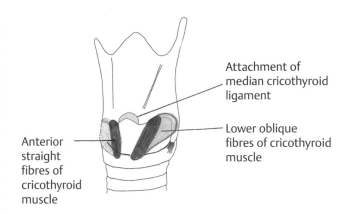

Anterior straight fibres of cricothyroid muscle

Attachment of median cricothyroid ligament

Lower oblique fibres of cricothyroid muscle

Figure 2.9 The cricothyroid muscle.

The question whether the thyroid cartilage moves on a fixed cricoid cartilage, as in phonation when the cricoid cartilage is held immovably against the vertebral column by the action of cricopharyngeus, or whether the cricoid cartilage moves on the thyroid cartilage, as in swallowing, is immaterial because the action of the cricothyroid muscle in each case is to lengthen the vocal folds by increasing the distance between the angle of the thyroid cartilage and arytenoids. When the cricoarytenoid muscle contracts; the vocal folds are brought into a line between the anterior commissure and the posterior cricoarytenoid ligament, namely the paramedian position. The level of the vocal folds is lowered and the entire fold is stretched, elongated, and thinned. The edge of the vocal fold becomes sharp and all the layers are thereby passively stiffened.

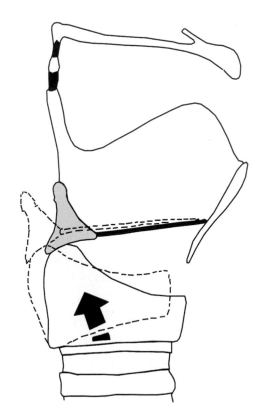

Figure 2.10 Movements of the cricothyroid muscle.

Movements of the Vocal Folds and the Anatomy of Speech

The vocal folds usually vibrate at 100 to 300 Hz during normal conversation, and even at 1000 Hz or more during singing. The observation and interpretation of such vibrations was enhanced by the high-speed film made by Bell Telephone Laboratories, (New Jersey, New York, United States) in 1937. The classic film, shot at 4000 frames per second, has been analyzed by many observers.[10,11] Other methods of observing vocal fold movements during phonation include frontal tomography[12,13] and stroboscopy.[14–16] A schematic presentation of vocal fold vibration is shown in **Fig. 2.11** and of the function of the laryngeal muscles in **Fig. 2.12**.[17] Movement of the vocal folds, whether in quiet respiration or in phonation, is controlled by the combined activity of all the muscles described above.

In quiet respiration, the intermembranous part of the glottis is triangular, and the intercartilaginous part is rectangular as the medial surfaces of the arytenoids are parallel (**Fig. 2.13A**).

In forced respiration (**Fig. 2.13B**), the vocal folds undergo extreme abduction; the arytenoid cartilages are rotated laterally and their vocal processes move widely apart.

Abduction of the vocal folds (**Fig. 2.13C**) is effected by the pull of the posterior cricoarytenoid muscles. The arytenoids are laterally rotated and thus the glottis becomes triangular.

Preparatory to phonation, the intermembranous and intercartilaginous part of the glottis is reduced to a linear chink by the adduction of the vocal folds and adduction and medial rotation of the arytenoid cartilages. The crude adduction is effected by the cricothyroid and lateral cricoarytenoid muscles (**Fig. 2.13D**) and the fine tension of the vocal fold is produced by the tonic contraction of the vocalis muscle. The interarytenoid muscles, by pulling the arytenoid cartilages together, complete adduction by closing the posterior glottic chink (**Fig. 2.13E**).

The vocal folds are lengthened by the cricothyroid muscles. Because of the nature of the felted membrane of fibroelastic tissue within the vocal folds, squares of this network are converted into diamonds by increasing the length of the vocal folds without a corresponding increase in tension. The tension of the vocal fold is a function of the tonic contraction of the vocalis muscle that is well designed to produce a wide range of tension in many small steps.[18]

Changes in length and tension control the pitch of the voice and are produced normally only when the vocal folds are in contact for phonation.

Three forces act to bring the vocal folds in contact with each other. They are as follows: (1) the tension in the fold; (2) the decrease in subglottic air pressure, which happens with each vibratory opening of the glottis; and (3) the sucking-in effect of escaping air (the Bernoulli effect). The result of this rapidly repeating cycle of opening and closing at the glottis is the release of small puffs from the subglottic air column, which forms sound waves.

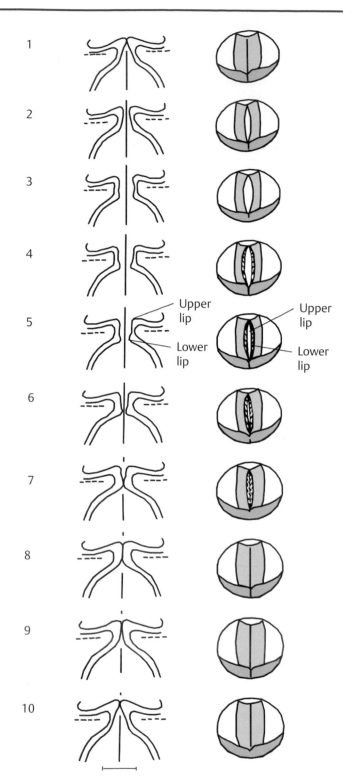

Figure 2.11 Schematic presentation of vocal fold vibration. Left column: frontal section; right column: view from above.

Printed with permission from Hirano M. *Clinical Examination of Voice.* New York, NY: Springer-Verlag; 1981:44.

Frontal tomography shows that the area of vocal fold surface in contact with its partners varies according to the pitch; at low pitches, the cross-sectional area of the

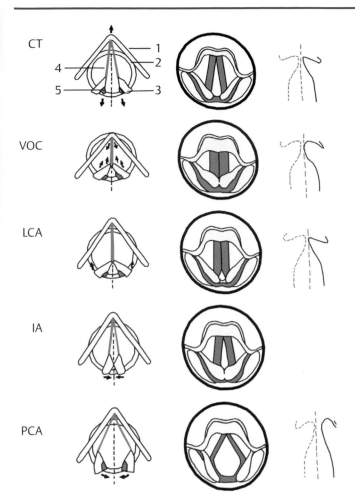

Figure 2.12 A schematic presentation of the function of the laryngeal muscles. The left column shows the location of the cartilages and the edge of the vocal folds when the laryngeal muscles are activated individually. The arrow indicates the direction of the force exerted. The middle column shows the views from above. The right column presents contours of frontal sections at the middle of the membranous portion of the vocal fold. The dotted line shows a control wherein the muscle is activated. 1, the thyroid cartilage; 2, the cricoid cartilage; 3, the arytenoid cartilage; 4, the vocal ligament; 5, the posterior cricoarytenoid ligament; CT, cricothyroid LCA, lateral cricoarytenoid; IA, interarytenoid; VOC, Vocalis; PCA, posterior cricoarytenoid.

Printed with permission from Hirano M. *Clinical Examination of Voice.* New York, NY: Springer-Verlag; 1981:8.

vocal folds is large, but as the pitch rises, the folds become thinner.[13]

Stroboscopy allows observation and description of fundamental frequency, symmetry of bilateral movements, regularity (periodicity), glottal closure, amplitude, mucosal wave, and nonvibrating portions. In the normal vocal fold, the mucosal wave travels on the mucosa from its inferior to the superior surface. This is observed during vibration except for falsetto and is a function of the soft and pliant superficial layer of the lamina propria.

The function of the vocal folds is to produce sound varying only in intensity and pitch. This is then modified by various resonating chambers above and below the larynx and is ultimately converted into phonemes by the articulating action of the pharynx, tongue, palate, teeth, and lips.

Techniques of spectral analysis of the voice show that the vocal tract (larynx, pharynx, mouth, and nasal cavities) acts as an intricately selective filter and resonator that propagates a remarkably similar pattern irrespective of the fundamental frequency. This is essential to speech as it ensures that, in spite of a continuously varying tone of voice, a constant quality or timbre is maintained.

Consonants of speech are associated with particular anatomical sites, from which they usually take their designations in the terminology of phonetics; for example, "p" and "b" are labials, "t" and "d" are dentals, and "m" and "n" are nasals. These sites have two factors in common. They cause partial obstruction or constriction at some level in the vocal tract, and they produce an aperiodic vibration or noise that is superimposed on or interrupts the flow of laryngeal tones. For example, dental consonants result from apposition of the top of the tongue to the back of the teeth. This momentarily constricts the passage of escaping air, modifies the resonant parameters of the "vocal tract," and also generates a local noise.

The extreme complexity of speech is reflected in the multiplicity of laryngeal, pharyngeal, hyoid, palatal, lingual, and circumoral muscular movements, which are combined in rapidly changing combinations to produce phonation and articulation.

Mucous Membranes of the Larynx

The mucous membrane lining the larynx is continuous above with that of the pharynx and below with that of the trachea. It is closely attached over the posterior surface of the epiglottis, over the corniculate and cuneiform cartilages, and over the vocal ligaments. Elsewhere, it is loosely attached and therefore liable to become swollen.

The epithelium of the larynx is squamous, ciliated columnar, or transitional. The upper half of the posterior surface of the epiglottis, the upper part of the aryepiglottic folds, and the posterior commissure are covered with squamous epithelium. The vocal folds are also covered with squamous epithelium. The height of the vocal fold diminishes toward the anterior commissure mainly because the inferior edge of the vocal fold slopes upward. The lower edges of the anterior end of the folds form the apex of the triangular fixed part of the subglottis. Thus, a tumor reaching or spreading across the anterior commissure has been found to involve the subglottic space in 50% of postmortem larynges taken from nonsmokers.[19] Stell et al,[19] in the same study, reported that although the remainder of the epithelium of the laryngeal mucous membrane is ciliated columnar, islands of squamous metaplasia have been found in the subglottic space. Mucous glands are

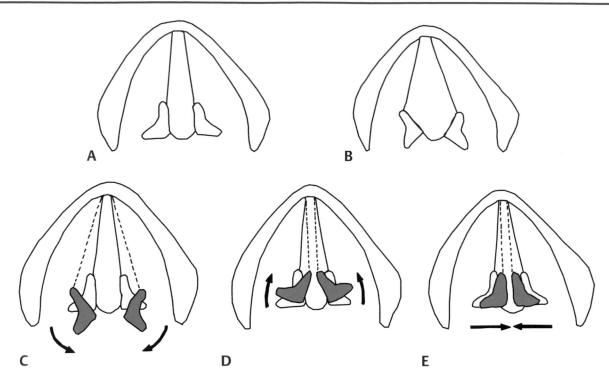

Figure 2.13 Diagrams to show the different positions of the vocal folds and arytenoid cartilages. (A) Position at rest in quiet respiration; (B) forced inspiration; (C) abduction of the vocal folds; (D) adduction of the vocal folds; and (E) closure of the posterior glottic chink.

freely distributed throughout the mucous membrane and are particularly numerous on the posterior surface of the epiglottis, where they form indentations into the cartilage, in the margins of the lower part of the aryepiglottic folds, and in the saccules. The vocal folds do not possess any glands, and the mucous membrane is lubricated by the glands within the saccules. The squamous epithelium covering the vocal folds is, therefore, vulnerable to desiccation. Scanning electron microscopy has demonstrated the existence not only of microvilli but also of microridges (microplicae) on the surface cells of the epithelium of the folds and elsewhere in the larynx.[20] Such features have been observed in other epithelia subjected to drying out (e.g., the corneal epithelium), and microplicae are regarded as being conducive to the retention of surface secretions.

Some taste buds, similar to those in the tongue, are scattered over the posterior surface of the epiglottis and in the aryepiglottic folds.

Blood Supply

The blood supply is derived from the laryngeal branches of the superior and inferior thyroid arteries and the cricothyroid branch of the superior thyroid artery. The superior thyroid artery arises from the external carotid artery, and the inferior thyroid artery arises from the thyrocervical trunk of the first part of the subclavian artery. On the left side, the thoracic duct is an important relation to the thyrocervical trunk, crossing from the medial to the lateral side.

The superior laryngeal artery arises from the superior thyroid artery. It passes deep to the thyrohyoid muscle and, together with the internal branch of the superior laryngeal nerve, pierces the thyrohyoid membrane to supply the muscles and mucous membrane of the larynx and to anastomose with branches of its opposite side and with those of the inferior laryngeal artery. The latter arises from the inferior thyroid artery at the level of the lower border of the thyroid gland and ascends on the trachea, together with the recurrent laryngeal nerve. It enters the larynx beneath the lower border of the inferior constrictor muscle and supplies the muscles and mucous membrane. The cricothyroid artery passes from the superior thyroid artery, across the upper part of the cricothyroid ligament, and anastomoses with the branch of the opposite side.

The veins leaving the larynx accompany the arteries; the superior vessels enter the internal jugular vein by way of the superior thyroid or facial vein, and the inferior vessels drain by way of the inferior thyroid vein into the brachiocephalic veins. Some venous drainage from the larynx is by way of the middle thyroid vein into the internal jugular vein.

Lymphatic Drainage

The lymphatics of the larynx are separated by the vocal folds into an upper and lower group. The part of the larynx above the vocal folds is drained by vessels that accompany the superior laryngeal vein, pierce the thyrohyoid membrane, and empty into the upper deep cervical lymph nodes, whereas the zone below the vocal folds drains, together with the inferior vein, into the lower part of the deep cervical chain often through the prelaryngeal and pretracheal nodes.

The vocal folds are firmly bound down to the underlying vocal ligaments and this results in an absence of lymph vessels, a fact that accounts for the clearly defined watershed between the upper and lower zones.

Nerve Supply

The nerve supply of the larynx is from the vagus by way of its superior and recurrent laryngeal branches.

The *superior laryngeal nerve* arises from the inferior ganglion of the vagus and receives a branch from the superior cervical sympathetic ganglion. It descends lateral to the pharynx, behind the internal carotid, and, at the level of the greater horn of the hyoid bone, divides into a small external branch and a larger internal branch. The external branch provides motor supply to the cricothyroid muscle while the internal branch pierces the thyrohyoid membrane above the entrance of the superior laryngeal artery and divides into two main sensory and secretomotor branches. The upper branch supplies the mucous membrane of the lower part of the pharynx, epiglottis, vallecula, and vestibule of the larynx. The lower branch descends in the medial wall of the pyriform fossa beneath the mucous membrane and supplies the aryepiglottic fold and the mucous membrane down to the level of the vocal folds.

The internal branch of the superior laryngeal nerve also carries fibers from the neuromuscular spindles and other stretch receptors in the larynx. There, the nerve ends by piercing the inferior constrictor muscle of the pharynx and unites with an ascending branch of the recurrent laryngeal nerve. This branch is called Galen's anastomosis or loop and is purely sensory.

The *recurrent laryngeal nerve* on the right side leaves the vagus as the latter crosses the right subclavian artery and then loops under the artery and ascends to the larynx in the groove between the esophagus and the trachea. On the left side, the nerve originates from the vagus as it crosses the aortic arch. It then passes under the arch and the ligamentum arteriosum to reach the groove between the esophagus and the trachea. In the neck, both nerves follow the same course and pass upward accompanied by the laryngeal branch of the inferior thyroid artery, deep to the lower border of the inferior constrictor, and enter the larynx behind the cricothyroid joint. The nerve then divides into motor and sensory branches.

The motor branch has fibers derived from the cranial root of the accessory nerve with cell bodies lying in the nucleus ambiguous; these supply all the intrinsic muscles of the larynx with the exception of the cricothyroid. The sensory branch supplies the laryngeal mucous membrane below the level of the vocal folds and also carries afferent fibers from stretch receptors in the larynx.

As the recurrent laryngeal nerve curves around the subclavian artery or the arch of the aorta, it gives off several cardiac filaments to the deep part of the cardiac plexus.

As it ascends in the neck, it gives branches, which are more numerous on the right than the left, to the mucous membrane and the muscular coat of the esophagus and trachea and some filaments to the inferior constrictor.

Applied Anatomy of the Larynx

Surface Anatomy and Cricothyrotomy (Laryngotomy)

In the midline, from above to downward, it is possible to palpate the hyoid bone, the thyroid cartilage with the laryngeal prominence (Adam's apple), the cricoid cartilage, and the trachea. The level of the vocal folds is approximately at the midpoint of the anterior surface of the thyroid cartilage. By rolling the finger upward over the cricoid cartilage, it is possible to feel a soft depression between the cricoid and thyroid cartilages. This is the cricothyroid ligament (**Fig. 2.14**) and is the site at which a cricothyrotomy (laryngotomy) is performed to relieve upper airway obstruction. This is preferable, as an emergency procedure, to a tracheostomy because of the increased depth of soft tissue associated with an approach to the trachea and the greater likelihood of bleeding from the thyroid isthmus.

Laryngoscopic Examination

The larynx and surrounding structures can be examined by either indirect or direct laryngoscopy. With a cooperative patient, indirect laryngoscopy (**Fig. 2.15**), using the laryngeal mirror, will give a good view of the back of the tongue, the valleculae, the epiglottis (which is seen foreshortened),

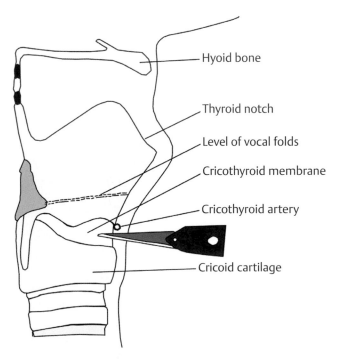

— Hyoid bone

— Thyroid notch

— Level of vocal folds

— Cricothyroid membrane

— Cricothyroid artery

— Cricoid cartilage

Figure 2.14 The site for cricothyrotomy.

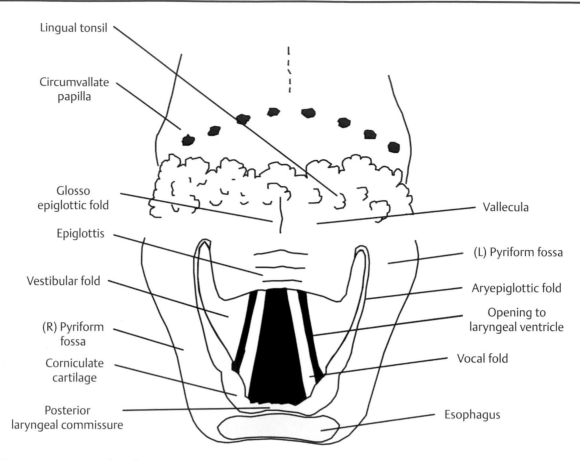

Lingual tonsil

Circumvallate papilla

Glosso epiglottic fold

Epiglottis

Vestibular fold

(R) Pyriform fossa

Corniculate cartilage

Posterior laryngeal commissure

Vallecula

(L) Pyriform fossa

Aryepiglottic fold

Opening to laryngeal ventricle

Vocal fold

Esophagus

Figure 2.15   Larynx seen on indirect laryngoscopy.

the pyriform fossae, and the structures of the larynx. If the patient will not tolerate the laryngeal mirror, there are two options open to the examiner. First, the flexible fiberoptic nasopharyngoscope can be passed along the floor of a previously locally anesthetized nasal cavity and then suspended above the larynx to give a direct view. This technique affords an excellent view of the nose and nasopharynx as well as the larynx and adjacent structures. The laryngeal position is natural in that the patient's tongue is not being pulled out, and the examination is well tolerated by the patient. Second, if a pathological lesion is seen or suspected and a biopsy or removal of tissue is required, then direct laryngoscopy with or without microscopy under general anesthesia is recommended. This technique will afford a better view of the laryngeal ventricles and of the subglottis.

Injuries to the Laryngeal Nerves

There is an intimate and important relationship between the nerves that supply the larynx and the vessels that supply the thyroid gland. In a postoperative study of voice function in 325 patients who had undergone thyroidectomy, Kark et al[21] found that permanent changes had been sustained by 35 (25%) patients after a subtotal thyroidectomy and

by 19 (11%) patients after lobectomy. The commonest cause of voice change appeared to be injury to the external branch of the superior laryngeal nerve on one or both sides. Damage to the recurrent laryngeal nerve, which was routinely identified and protected, was rare as a cause. They found that when the external branch of the superior laryngeal nerve, which descends over the inferior constrictor muscle immediately deep to the superior thyroid artery and vein as these pass to the superior pole of the gland, was identified and preserved, permanent voice changes were recorded in only 5% of the cases (**Fig. 2.16**). This was similar to an incidence of 3% in control patients after endotracheal intubation alone. The functional effect of damage to the external laryngeal nerve is a lower pitched, husky voice that is easily fatigued and has a reduced range. The laryngoscopic changes are much less obvious than those that are seen after palsy of the recurrent laryngeal nerve, and their identification may be helped by the use of a stroboscopic light. The edge of the affected vocal fold may be irregular or wavy and usually lies at the lower level, producing an oblique glottic aperture. Recovery after palsy of the external nerve is poor and prognosis is not good.[22]

The recurrent laryngeal nerve comes into close relationship with the inferior thyroid artery as the latter

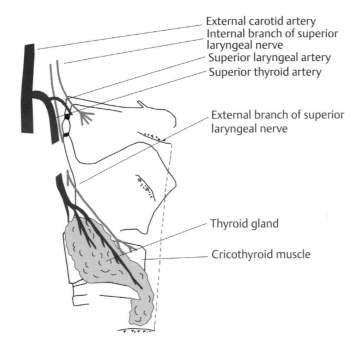

Figure 2.16 Anatomy of the external branch of the superior laryngeal nerve.

passes medially, behind the common carotid artery, to the gland. The artery may cross posteriorly or anteriorly to the nerve, or the nerve may pass between the terminal branches of the artery (**Fig. 2.17**). On the right side, there is an equal chance of locating the nerve in each of these three situations; on the left side, the nerve is more likely to lie posterior to the artery.[23] Injury to the recurrent nerve is enhanced due to its displacement from the normal anatomical location by the diseased thyroid gland.

Apart from injury complicating thyroidectomy, the nerve can also be affected by benign or malignant enlargement of the thyroid gland, by enlarged lymph nodes, or by cervical trauma. Paralysis of the left nerve, by virtue of its intrathoracic course, is twice as likely to happen as that of the right nerve. It may be involved by malignant tumors of the lung or esophagus, by malignant or inflamed nodes, by an aneurysm of the aortic arch, or by left atrial hypertrophy associated with mitral stenosis.

The anomalous position of a nonrecurrent laryngeal nerve predisposes to injury during thyroidectomy and to compression by a thyroid mass. Symptoms range from hoarseness associated with a vocal fold paralysis to a vague pressure sensation over the larynx, a need to clear the throat or a chronic cough. Recognition of this uncommon anomaly, which is usually right-sided, is necessary and no structure passing medial from the carotid sheath, except the middle thyroid vein, should be ligated until the recurrent laryngeal nerve is identified.[24]

The functional effect of damage to one recurrent laryngeal nerve is hoarseness, which later resolves itself almost completely in 50% of patients, either by a return of function on the affected side or by compensatory overadduction of the opposite normal vocal fold. Bilateral paralysis, however, results in complete loss of vocal power and a marked inspiratory stridor often necessitating tracheostomy. Respiratory obstruction following a thyroidectomy can also result from collapse of the tracheal cartilages (tracheomalacia) associated with a large goiter or with carcinoma of the thyroid or from external pressure on the trachea from postoperative hemorrhage.

It is generally accepted that the concept embodied in Semon law, namely that the abductor nerves or muscle

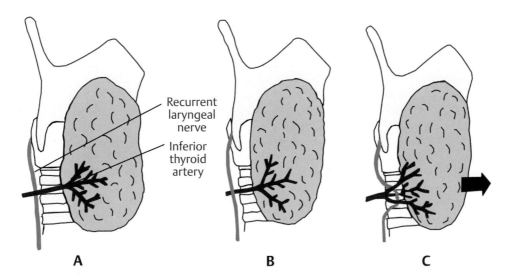

Figure 2.17 Variations in the relationship of the recurrent laryngeal nerve and the inferior thyroid artery.[23] The nerve may cross (A) posterior to the artery or (B) anterior to the artery or (C) through the branches of the artery. The lateral lobe of the thyroid has been pulled forward as it would be during thyroidectomy.

fibers are generally more susceptible to injury, is no longer valid. The "law," after several amendments, stated that:

> [i]n the course of a gradually advancing organic lesion of the recurrent nerve or its fibers in the peripheral trunk, three stages can be observed. In the first stage, only abductor fibers are damaged and the vocal folds approximate in the midline and adduction is still possible. In the second stage, additional contracture of the adductors occurs so that the vocal folds are immobilized in the median position. In the third stage, the adductor becomes paralysed and the vocal fold assumes the cadaveric position.

Descriptions of multiple positions assumed by paralyzed vocal folds still cause confusion.

The hypothesis, attributed to Wagner[25] and Grossman,[26] is the one preferred by more recent laryngologists[27] states:

> [...] first, that total paralysis of the recurrent laryngeal nerve immobilizes the vocal fold in the paramedian position because of the adduction action of the intact cricothyroid muscles, and second, that a 'combined' recurrent laryngeal nerve and superior laryngeal nerve paralysis causes the fold to be immobilized in the intermediate (open or cadaveric) position

This hypothesis is supported by electromyographic and photographic studies of both the human and canine larynx, which confirm that the adduction and lengthening effect of an intact cricothyroid muscle is the primary force that holds a paralyzed vocal fold in the paramedian position. A vocal fold in the paramedian position is, therefore, paralyzed only by a defective recurrent laryngeal nerve, while a vocal fold immobilized in the intermediate position is usually paralyzed by a lesion affecting both the recurrent and superior laryngeal nerves (**Fig. 2.18**). The apparent small variations of positions can be attributed to compensation provided by the normal vocal fold crossing the midline or to atrophy and scarring of the paralyzed vocal fold.

Kirchner[28] stated that if the ipsilateral vagus nerve, as well as the recurrent laryngeal nerve, was injured, the vocal fold might assume the intermediate position because of the loss of adductor function of the cricothyroid muscle brought about by the interruption of vagal afferent fibers originating in pulmonary stretch receptors. These receptors exert a monitoring effect on the respiratory center, which, in turn, allows reflex adjustments of laryngeal resistance in breathing. These adjustments involve moment-to-moment changes in the area of the glottis aperture that require normally innervated laryngeal muscles. Interruption of the motor innervation to the laryngeal muscles, even if unilateral, disturbs one arm of this finely adjusted reflex system and provides an explanation of the intermediate position of the paralyzed vocal fold under such conditions.

Acknowledgments

The author and the editor kindly acknowledge the permission from the copyright holders Hodder Education to use reference material from Weir N. Anatomy of the larynx and tracheobronchial tree. In: Kerr AG, ed. *Scott Brown's Otolaryngology*. Vol. 1. 6th ed. London: Butterworth-Heinemann; 1997: Chap12.

They also acknowledge the technical skills of Ms. Andrea Pisesky in coloring the line drawings originally created by Mr. Stephen Metcalfe FRCS.

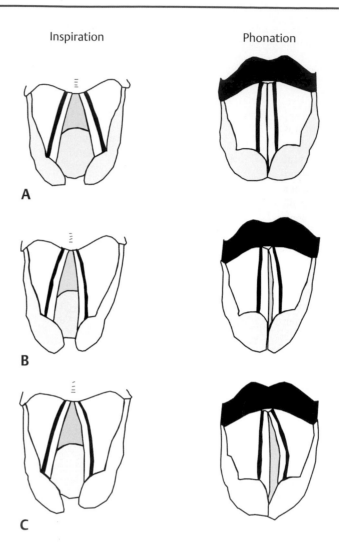

Inspiration   Phonation

Figure 2.18 Vocal fold positions in inspiration and phonation. (A) Normal. (B) Paramedian. (C) Intermediate.

References

1. Weir N, Mudry A. Otorhinolaryngology- An Illustrated History. 2nd ed. Ashford: Headley Brothers; 2013:130–132
2. Piersol GA. Human Anatomy. 9th ed. Philadelphia, PA: JB Lippincott; 1930:724
3. Work WP. Unusual position of the right recurrent laryngeal nerve. Ann Otol Rhinol Laryngol 1941;50:769–775
4. Berlin DD. The recurrent laryngeal nerves in total ablation of the normal thyroid gland: an anatomical and surgical study. Surg Gynecol Obstet 1935;60:19–26
5. O'Rahilly R, Boyden EA. The timing and sequence of events in the development of the human respiratory system during the embryonic period proper. Z Anat Entwicklungsgesch 1973;141(3): 237–250

6. Reid L. Visceral cartilage. J Anat 1976;122(Pt 2):349–355

7. McIlwain JC. The posterior glottis. J Otolaryngol 1991;20(Suppl 2): 1–24

8. Bowden REM, Scheuer JL. Weights of abductor and adductor muscles of the human larynx. J Laryngol Otol 1960;74(12):971–980

9. Guindi GM, Michaels L, Bannister R, Gibson W. Pathology of the intrinsic muscles of the larynx. Clin Otolaryngol Allied Sci 1981;6(2):101–109

10. Farnsworth DW. High-speed motion pictures of the vocal cords. Bell Lab Rec 1940;18:203–208

11. Pressman JJ. Physiology of the vocal cords in phonation and respiration. Arch Otolaryngol 1942;35(3):355–398

12. Fink BR, Kirschner F. Observations on the acoustical and mechanical properties of the vocal folds. Folia Phoniatr (Basel) 1959;11:167–172

13. Hollien H, Curtis JF. A laminagraphic study of vocal pitch. J Speech Hear Res 1960;3:361–371

14. Smith S. Remarks on the physiology of the vibrations of the vocal cords. Folia Phoniatr (Basel) 1954;6(3):166–178

15. Beck J, Schönhärl E. [A new microphone-controlled light-flash stroboscope]. [in German] HNO 1953-1954-1954;4(7):212–214

16. Schönhärl E. Die Stroboskopie in der praktischen laryngologie. Stuttgart: Thieme; 1960

17. Hirano M. Clinical Examination of Voice. Wien and New York: Springer-Verlag; 1981

18. Zenker W. Vocal muscle fibres and their motor endplates. In: Brewer DW, ed. Research Potentials in Voice Physiology. New York, NY: New York State University Press; 1964:256–271

19. Stell PM, Gregory I, Watt J. Morphology of the human larynx. II. The subglottis. Clin Otolaryngol Allied Sci 1980;5(6): 389–395

20. Andrews PM, Hackenbrock CR. Microplicae: characteristic ridge-like folds of the plasmalemma. J Cell Biol 1976;68(3): 420–429

21. Kark AE, Kissin MW, Auerbach R, Meikle M. Voice changes after thyroidectomy: role of the external laryngeal nerve. Br Med J (Clin Res Ed) 1984;289(6456):1412–1415

22. Arnold GE. Vocal rehabilitation of paralytic dysphonia. VII. Paralysis of the superior laryngeal nerve. Arch Otolaryngol 1962;75: 549–570

23. Bowden REM. The surgical anatomy of the recurrent laryngeal nerve. Br J Surg 1955;43(178):153–163

24. Friedman M, Toriumi DM, Grybauskas V, Katz A. Nonrecurrent laryngeal nerves and their clinical significance. Laryngoscope 1986;96(1):87–90

25. Wagner R. Die medianstellung der stimmbander bei der Rekurrenslahmung. Arch Pathol Anat Physiol 1890;120:437–459

26. Grossman M. Experirnentelle Beitrage zur Lehre von der 'Posticuslähmung'. Arch Laryngol Rhinol 1897;6:282–360

27. Dedo DD, Dedo HH. Vocal cord paralysis. In: Paparella MM, Shumrick DA, eds. Otolaryngology. Vol. 111. Philadelphia, PA: WB Saunders; 1980:2489–2503

28. Kirchner JA. Semon's law a century later. J Laryngol Otol 1982;96(7):645–657

3 Microanatomy and Cellular Physiology

Kimberly N. Vinson and C. Gaelyn Garrett

The human vocal folds are unique structures. The microanatomy of these structures dictates the fluidity of the vibration and the quality of sound they produce. An understanding of vocal fold histology and cellular physiology is necessary to understand, diagnose, and treat pathology of the vocal folds.

Vocal Fold Histology

Hirano elegantly described the unique multilayered structure of the vocal folds in 1974 (**Fig. 3.1**).[1] This layered structure has relevance not only in the maintenance of the mechanical properties of the vocal folds but also in the development of benign vocal lesions. These layers include the epithelium, the lamina propria, and the vocalis muscle. The lamina propria is further subdivided into superficial, intermediate, and deep layers. Each layer has distinct structural and mechanical properties that contribute to the characteristic vibration seen on laryngeal videostroboscopy or high-speed videography. An understanding of the structure and the varying mechanical properties of each layer is necessary to fully understand vocal fold vibration.

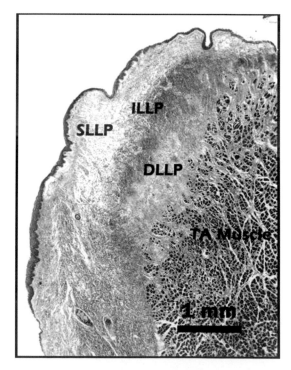

Figure 3.1 Coronal section of the human vocal fold. Movat stain highlights layers of the lamina propria. DLLP, deep layer of the lamina propria; ILLP, intermediate layer of the lamina propria; SLLP, superficial layer of the lamina propria; TA, thyroarytenoid.

Epithelium

The epithelium of the vocal folds is composed of stratified squamous cells that maintain the shape of the vocal folds. The remainder of the glottis, however, has ciliated pseudocolumnar epithelium. Unlike most squamous cells, such as normal skin, the vocal fold epithelium remains metabolically active throughout its life cycle. The surface cells slough off into the laryngeal lumen as new cells migrate superiorly and medially to replace them. The luminal cells exhibit a "microridge" pattern, thus increasing the surface area to better maintain the mucus blanket that covers the vocal fold surface. This bilayer mucus blanket is vital to ensure adequate moisture and lubrication of the vocal folds. The luminal layer of the blanket is mucinous. This layer, which is primarily composed of mucin molecules, is the thicker of the two layers and acts to prevent dehydration of the surface epithelium. The inner, serous layer is thinner due to its higher water content. This layer is in direct contact with the squamous cells of the vocal fold epithelium and the cilia of the pseudocolumnar cells of the glottis and facilitates the mucociliary transport of secretions up from the trachea and through the glottis for expectoration. Inhibition of mucociliary clearance can lead to impaired function of the upper respiratory tract.

The epithelium is secured to the lamina propria by the basement membrane zone (BMZ). This zone is a collection of protein and nonprotein structures and is composed of two layers, the lamina lucida and the lamina densa. The lamina lucida is the low-density, clear zone medial to the basal epithelial cells, while the lamina densa is a zone of increased type IV collagen fibers adjacent to the lamina propria. These two layers provide structural support, connecting the epithelium to the underlying lamina propria through anchoring fibers.[2] The BMZ is also essential for repair and maintenance of the epithelium. Chronic disruption of this layer may lead to the formation of a vocal fold nodule.[3]

Clinical Insight

The BMZ is an area of clinical importance to differentiate between carcinoma in situ (CIS) and invasive carcinoma of the vocal folds. CIS of the vocal fold is defined as the presence of atypical cells within the epithelial layer of the vocal fold without evidence of invasion through the BMZ. Once cancerous cells infiltrate the BMZ, the process becomes invasive and the risk of regional and distant metastases increases. Therefore, great care must be taken to dissect below the BMZ when performing a biopsy of a suspicious vocal lesion to ensure that the correct diagnosis is made.

Superficial Layer of the Lamina Propria

The superficial layer of the lamina propria (SLLP), or Reinke space, is a potential space composed of loose, fibrous tissue in an extracellular matrix (ECM). It is extremely pliable and often compared to soft gelatin. Owing to its structure, the SLLP offers little resistance to vibration. The ECM is the key component of the SLLP that allows this motion. The ECM is a mixture of fibrous and interstitial proteins that serve as a scaffold for the SLLP. It provides strength and resilience in allowing the vocal fold to vibrate freely, while allowing the SLLP to maintain its structure. The fibrous proteins, namely collagen type I and elastin, provide the tensile strength needed to maintain the SLLP, while the interstitial proteins, such as hyaluronic acid, decorin, and versican, provide the viscoelastic characteristics of the vocal fold for vibration.[2] These interstitial proteins also give the vocal fold the ability to absorb the shock of repeated impact from phonation. Understanding the microanatomy and the mechanical properties of this layer is extremely important as the majority of benign vocal fold lesions occur in this layer. Vocal fold polyps, nodules, cysts, and polypoid corditis, or Reinke edema, all form in the SLLP.[4]

Hyaluronic acid, or hyaluronan, is perhaps the most important of the ECM proteins. It is a glycosaminoglycan polymer of disaccharides composed of repeating units of glucuronic acid and acetylglucosamine.[5] Owing to its high charge at physiologic pH, hyaluronic acid readily binds water to form a gel-like substance that affects the viscoelasticity of the lamina propria, determining tissue viscosity, osmosis, and flow resistance.[6] This most likely determines the biomechanics of vocal fold vibration.

Clinical Insight

Polypoid corditis, or Reinke edema, most often occurs in the setting of heavy cigarette smoking and, less often, in severe hypothyroidism. Patients typically complain of lowered vocal pitch. Physical examination with indirect laryngoscopy reveals varying degrees of edema of the vocal folds due to the abnormal accumulation of fluid in the SLLP (**Fig. 3.2**). The marked edema likely occurs as a response to the chronic irritation of the cigarette smoke or as a manifestation of myxedema in the setting of hypothyroidism. This edema typically involves the entire membranous vocal fold from the vocal process to the anterior commissure, causing it to become floppy. Increased mucosal wave is observed on laryngovideostroboscopy. The fundamental frequency during phonation is decreased due to the increased mass of the affected vocal fold, according to the equation $\omega = \sqrt{(k/m)}$, where ω is frequency, k is constant, and m is mass. The initial treatment for polypoid corditis is to remove the chronic irritant, in the case of smoking, or to correct the hormone deficiency, as in hypothyroidism. If a patient continues to have significant dysphonia despite these measures, surgical treatment may be considered. Typically, microflap excision is performed to remove the excess SLLP and redundant mucosal cover. More recently, angiolytic lasers have been used to treat polypoid corditis in-office. Occasionally, extensive bilateral disease may cause airway compromise. Surgical treatment should occur in this setting despite the patient's smoking status.

Intermediate and Deep Layers of the Lamina Propria

The intermediate layer of lamina propria (ILLP) and the deep layer of lamina propria (DLLP) together comprise the vocal ligament, or the transition layer between the overlying epithelium and the SLLP and the underlying vocalis muscle. The ILLP comprises roughly one-half of the lamina propria and contains a high concentration of reticular type III collagen fibers. It is less densely organized than the DLLP, which is composed of type I and type III collagen fibers that penetrate the superficial bundles of the vocalis muscle.[7] The vocal ligament is the free, superior margin of the conus elasticus, which is an elastic membrane that connects the cricoid cartilage to the thyroid and arytenoid cartilages. The ILLP is thickened at the anterior and posterior ends of the membranous vocal fold. These areas are known as the anterior and posterior macula flava. The anterior macula flava serves as a transition zone between the stiff thyroid cartilage and the pliable membranous vocal fold, while the posterior macula flava serves as a transition between the membranous vocal fold and the stiff vocal process of the arytenoid cartilage.[8] This structure allows for the support of increased tensile stress that occurs in vocal tasks that require high-pitched sounds. The vocal ligament is a key landmark for the depth of dissection of a benign laryngeal lesion in laryngeal microflap surgery. Once the epithelium has been incised and the SLLP bluntly elevated, the vocal ligament appears laterally as a shiny, yellow-white strip of elastic tissue.

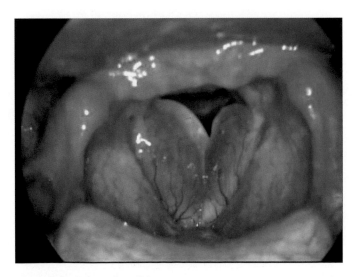

Figure 3.2 Polypoid corditis.

It is hypothesized that hyaluronic acid may play a role in the maintenance of the ECM. The hyaluronic cell receptor CD44 is most concentrated in the vocal fold epithelium and the lamina propria, that is, the areas of greatest vibration. Studies have shown that 95% of the cells of the macula flava stain positively for CD44 in phonated larynges, while only 10% of the cells stain for CD44 in nonphonated larynges. These data suggest that hyaluronic acid is a cellular signal for the maintenance of the lamina propria in response to stress.[9]

Vocalis Muscle

The vocalis muscle is composed of the most medial fibers of the thyroarytenoid muscle. Its medial insertion is the vocal ligament. The vocalis is stiff compared with the other layers of the vocal fold and has contractile properties that allow for the modification of the effective overall tension of the vocal folds.

Cover-Body Theory of Vocal Fold Motion

The five histological layers of the vocal fold work in three increasingly stiffer mechanical layers during vibration. The "cover" is composed of the epithelium and the SLLP. The intermediate and deep layers of the lamina propria comprise the "transition" layer, and the vocalis muscle act as the "body."

The cover-body theory was proposed by Hirano in 1974 and describes the mucosal wave of the vocal fold. As air passes between the vocal folds, the loose "cover" moves in a wave-like motion over the stiffer "body." The cover is pliable and elastic, while the body uses its contractile properties to allow for the adjustment of the stiffness of the vocal fold. The overall tension of the vocal fold is dependent on the coupling of cover to the adjustable, muscular body.[1]

Vocal Fold Wound Healing

When considering the cellular physiology of the vocal fold, wound healing is perhaps the most important phenomenon to discuss. However, before examining the unique characteristics of vocal fold wound healing, a brief review of the general principles of wound healing should be done. Basic knowledge of this process is crucial for the voice clinician, as most of the treatment that is offered is aimed at improving injured tissue.

The wound-healing process is a complex cascade that involves inflammation, proliferation, epithelialization, and remodeling. During the inflammation stage, several processes must take place. Hemostasis must be achieved at the wound site. Tissue deficits resulting from the injury must be filled and a matrix to facilitate migration of cells into the wound bed must be formed. All of these processes are achieved with the formation of a fibrin clot. Macrophages and neutrophils then invade the area to clear the wound of contaminants. Cell

signaling calls for fibroblasts to migrate into the wound bed to lay down collagen, elastin, and hyaluronic acid to establish a new ECM. Epithelial cells create a watertight seal over the wound bed. Finally, tissue remodeling occurs and persists up to 12 months after injury. Early scar formation occurs in the first 3 months following injury. During early scar formation in the first 3 months, the scar is thick and stiff. As it matures, it becomes more pliable as reorganization of collagen and elastin fibers occurs.[10]

Pearls and Pitfalls

Iatrogenic vocal fold scarring can be a devastating complication of vocal fold surgery, causing permanent dysphonia. It may result from over-resection of the SLLP along with surface epithelium during the excision of a benign vocal fold lesion. This most often occurs with a technique called vocal fold stripping. In this technique, the vocal fold epithelium and the SLLP are literally stripped away from the underlying vocal ligament to remove the benign lesion. As this vocal fold wound heals, remucosalization occurs over the area devoid of the SLLP. The result is scarring of the epithelium to the underlying vocal ligament (**Fig. 3.3**). With the loss of the loose vocal fold cover that typically vibrates over the vocal fold body and the resultant scar to the vocal ligament, the mucosal wave is disrupted. As there is then no way to adequately reconstruct the SLLP, the resulting dysphonia is often permanent.

To avoid iatrogenic scar when excising benign vocal fold lesions, it is imperative to preserve as much as possible all normal epithelium and superficial lamina propria and to avoid trauma to the vocal ligament. With microflap excision of a benign lesion, the epithelium overlying the lesion and the normal surrounding SLLP are preserved as the lesion is excised. This reduces the scarring observed with remucosalization after vocal fold stripping.

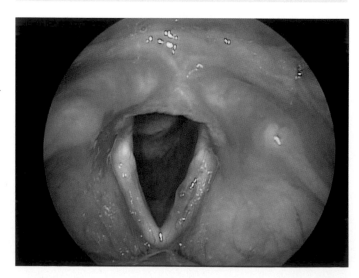

Figure 3.3   Sulcus vocalis. The image demonstrates sulcus vocalis of the right vocal fold in a patient who also has a left vocal fold polyp.

Human vocal folds are unique because they are subjected to nearly continuous mechanical trauma resulting from the phonation that takes place on a daily basis. It is thought that vocal fold tissues have developed specialized functions to withstand the constant stress of phonation. Recently, a great deal of research has been performed to characterize these functions. As it is difficult to study these processes in vivo in humans, animal models have been developed to study the effects of phonotrauma on cellular physiology of the vocal folds.

Changes to the ECM of the lamina propria have great impact on the voice. The lamina propria is maintained by the constant degradation and synthesis of ECM components. Gene expression of a variety of lamina propria proteins, including matrix metalloproteinases (MMPs) and cytokines, is being explored.

MMPs are enzymes that play an important role in wound healing by acting against certain ECM components. The two important MMPs are MMP-1 and MMP-9. MMP-1 is an interstitial collagenase that catalyzes the first step in the degradation of fibrillar collagen types I and III. MMP-9 is both a collagenase and a gelatinase that breaks down basement membrane collagens and gelatins. MMPs are essential for maintaining ECM homeostasis.[11]

Cytokines are cell-signaling proteins that attract inflammatory cells to an area of injury to initiate the inflammatory phase of the wound-healing cascade. Proinflammatory cytokines interleukin-1 (IL-1) and tumor necrosis factor α (TNF-α) and the pro-cytokine cyclooxygenase-2 (COX-2) play a role in the initiation of the inflammatory response in the vocal fold. IL-1 is activated by macrophages, neutrophils, and fibroblasts and induces the synthesis of procollagen types I and III. TNF-α is produced primarily by macrophages and stimulates the phagocytosis of contaminants in the wound bed. COX-2 is an enzyme that is undetectable in most normal tissues, but becomes abundant in activated macrophages during the inflammatory process to stimulate the conversion of arachidonic acid to prostaglandins.[12,13]

When considering wound healing in the vocal fold, the differences between acute and chronic phonotrauma should be considered. Acute phonotrauma typically manifests as vocal fold edema or laryngitis. With this type of injury, the vascular network, basement membrane, and ECM are all likely impacted. In 2008, Rousseau et al[11] demonstrated an increase in the gene expression of MMP-1 in rabbits receiving acute experimental phonation compared with controls that did not. His group did not find a significant increase in the expression of MMP-9 of IL-1β. In 2010, Rousseau's laboratory demonstrated an increase in the expression of IL-1β, tumor growth factor β1 (TGF-β1), and COX-2 in the setting of acute raised-intensity phonation as compared with modal phonation and sham control in the rabbit model.[14] Another group found IL-1 and prostaglandin E_2 (PGE$_2$) to be associated with acute wound healing in the rabbit model. Both markers were found to be significantly elevated in the injured vocal fold compared with normal vocal fold.[15] Significant changes in TNF-α and MMP-8 have also been observed.[16] As discussed previously, data also suggest that hyaluronic acid is a key cellular signal for the maintenance of the lamina propria in response to stress.

Chronic phonotrauma occurs in the setting of repeated episodes of acute phonotrauma that result in long-standing vocal fold damage. This damage could present in the form of vocal fold scarring as seen in benign vocal fold lesions, such as nodules, polyps, and cysts. Vocal fold nodules occur with repeated injury of the basement membrane. Kotby et al[3] report intercellular junction gaps, disruption and duplications of the basement membrane, and focal collagen deposition in nodules. Fibronectin, an adhesion molecule primarily located in the basement membrane, is also thought to be increased in nodules. It is also believed that the disruption of the basement membrane places the nodule at an increased risk for repeated injury, leading to propagation of scar over time. Polyps, however, occur in the setting of repeated acute vascular trauma instead of disruption of the basement membrane and have less deposition of fibronectin. While nodules appear to be the end result of wound healing with the deposition of fibronectin as early scar, polyps may be an arrest of the wound-healing process following the inflammatory phase.

Controversy exists when considering vocal fold cysts as the result of the wound-healing process from chronic phonotrauma. Generally, two types of cysts are thought to exist, epithelial-filled cysts and mucus retention cysts. The epithelial-filled cysts that are found at the impact zone of the membranous vocal fold are likely due to repeated phonotrauma at that site.[10]

Biochemical markers involved in wound healing in the setting of chronic phonotrauma have been studied. In contrast to acute trauma, IL-1 is not upregulated. This supports the hypothesis that the products of chronic phonotrauma demonstrate the entire process of the wound-healing cascade. In the case of polyps, it demonstrates at least progression of the cascade beyond the acute inflammatory phase before arresting. PGE$_2$, however, remains increased even in the setting of chronic phonotrauma, as it is an inflammatory mediator that is ubiquitous in wound healing.[17]

References

1. Hirano M. Morphological structure of the vocal cord as a vibrator and its variations. Folia Phoniatr (Basel) 1974;26(2):89–94
2. Gray SD. Cellular physiology of the vocal folds. Otolaryngol Clin North Am 2000;33(4):679–698
3. Kotby MN, Nassar AM, Seif EI, Helal EH, Saleh MM. Ultrastructural features of vocal fold nodules and polyps. Acta Otolaryngol 1988;105(5–6):477–482
4. Gray SD, Hammond E, Hanson DF. Benign pathologic responses of the larynx. Ann Otol Rhinol Laryngol 1995;104(1):13–18
5. Ruoslahti E. Structure and biology of proteoglycans. Annu Rev Cell Biol 1988;4:229–255

6. Gray SD, Titze IR, Chan R, Hammond TH. Vocal fold proteoglycans and their influence on biomechanics. Laryngoscope 1999;109(6): 845–854

7. Prades JM, Dumollard JM, Duband S, et al. Lamina propria of the human vocal fold: histomorphometric study of collagen fibers. Surg Radiol Anat 2010;32(4):377–382

8. Hirano M, Sato K, Nakashima T. Fibroblasts in human vocal fold mucosa. Acta Otolaryngol 1999;119(2):271–276

9. Sato K, Umeno H, Nakashima T, Nonaka S, Harabuchi Y. Expression and distribution of hyaluronic acid and CD44 in unphonated human vocal fold mucosa. Ann Otol Rhinol Laryngol 2009;118(11):773–780

10. Branski RC, Verdolini K, Sandulache V, Rosen CA, Hebda PA. Vocal fold wound healing: a review for clinicians. J Voice 2006;20(3): 432–442

11. Rousseau B, Ge PJ, French LC, Zealear DL, Thibeault SL, Ossoff RH. Experimentally induced phonation increases matrix metalloproteinase-1 gene expression in normal rabbit vocal fold. Otolaryngol Head Neck Surg 2008;138(1):62–68

12. Dinarello CA. Proinflammatory cytokines. Chest 2000;118(2): 503–508

13. Dinarello CA. Interleukin-1. Cytokine Growth Factor Rev 1997;8(4):253–265

14. Swanson ER, Ohno T, Abdollahian D, Garrett CG, Rousseau B. Effects of raised-intensity phonation on inflammatory mediator gene expression in normal rabbit vocal fold. Otolaryngol Head Neck Surg 2010;143(4):567–572

15. Branski RC, Rosen CA, Verdolini K, Hebda PA. Biochemical markers associated with acute vocal fold wound healing: a rabbit model. J Voice 2005;19(2):283–289

16. Verdolini K, Rosen CA, Branski RC, Hebda PA. Shifts in biochemical markers associated with wound healing in laryngeal secretions following phonotrauma: a preliminary study. Ann Otol Rhinol Laryngol 2003;112(12):1021–1025

17. Branski RC, Rosen CA, Verdolini K, Hebda PA. Markers of wound healing in vocal fold secretions from patients with laryngeal pathology. Ann Otol Rhinol Laryngol 2004;113(1):23–29

4 Physiology of Phonation

Venu Divi and Brittany C. Weber

The capacity to produce complex phonatory behavior appears to be a recent evolutionary phenomenon limited to human beings.[1] Phonation, or the production of voice, involves a power source, oscillator, and resonance chamber, each with different anatomical parts and specialized roles. Together, these three subsystems produce sound perceived as voice.

Power Source

Air is the power source of voice. Coordinated functions of the diaphragm, abdominal and chest muscles, lungs, and chest cavity work in concert to inspire air, filling the pulmonary reserve. This is followed by the movement of air superiorly toward the vocal folds. In expiration, as air flows past adducted vocal folds, the folds are set into motion leading to their vibration.[2]

Oscillator

Although almost all body systems can affect the voice, the larynx is the most sensitive and expressive component of the vocal mechanism.[3] The four main parts of the larynx involved in phonation are the skeleton, mucosa, intrinsic muscles, and extrinsic muscles.

Laryngeal Anatomy and Structure

Skeleton

The main cartilages of the larynx that have importance in phonation are the cricoid, thyroid, and arytenoid cartilages.

Musculature of the Vocal Fold

The intrinsic laryngeal muscles are paramount in the functioning of the vocal folds as they control the position and shape of the folds along with the elasticity and viscosity of each layer.[4]

The fibers of the thyroarytenoid muscle run parallel to the vocal ligament. The part of the muscle that borders the vocal ligament is called the vocalis muscle. Contraction of the thyroarytenoid muscle lowers, shortens, adducts, and thickens the vocal fold, bringing the arytenoid and thyroid cartilages closer. The body of the vocal fold is actively stiffened, and the cover and transition are passively slackened, resulting in rounding of the vocal fold edge.[3,4] When the thyroarytenoid muscle is activated, the length and tension of the vocal ligament are decreased, lowering the pitch of the voice. The vocalis muscle can provide fine control of the tension in the vocal ligaments enabling rapid variation in the pitch. Depending on tension in the rest of the thyroarytenoid, contraction of the vocalis may result in either raising or lowering of the vocal pitch.

The posterior cricoarytenoid muscle abducts, elevates, elongates, and thins the vocal fold by rocking the arytenoid cartilage posterolaterally.[3] The vocal fold elongates and thins. The size of the rima glottidis, the opening between the vocal folds, is increased. The lateral cricoarytenoid muscle adducts, lowers, elongates, and thins the vocal fold, making the edge of the vocal fold sharp while passively stiffening all layers.[4]

The interarytenoid muscle serves to adduct the cartilaginous portion of the vocal folds altering the position of the vocal folds, but has little influence on the stiffness of the membranous section.

The extrinsic muscles of the larynx, mainly the strap muscles, serve an important function of preserving the position of the larynx in the neck. The extrinsic muscles are responsible for maintaining a stable laryngeal skeleton to ensure the intrinsic musculature can work effectively.[3]

Innervation of the Larynx

The vagus nerve (cranial nerve [CN] X) provides sensory and motor innervation to the larynx. The two main nerves supplying sensory and motor innervation to the larynx are the superior laryngeal nerve (SLN) and the recurrent laryngeal nerve (RLN). The SLN is divided into the internal and external branches. The internal branch carries sensory fibers (pain, touch, and temperature) from the mucosa superior to the glottis and provides secretomotor fibers to the same area. The external branch provides motor innervation to the cricothyroid muscle.

The RLN contains motor fibers that innervate all of the intrinsic muscles of the larynx except for the cricothyroid muscle as well as sensory innervations to the infraglottis, subglottis, and trachea.

Structure of the Vocal Fold Edge

The vocal folds are two infoldings of mucous membrane stretched horizontally across the larynx. The most important aspect of voice production is vibration of the vocal folds that converts aerodynamic energy into acoustic energy. The nature of the sound produced is primarily dictated by the condition of the vocal folds, or the vibrators.[4]

The unique properties of sound from the larynx are determined by the inherent properties and manipulation

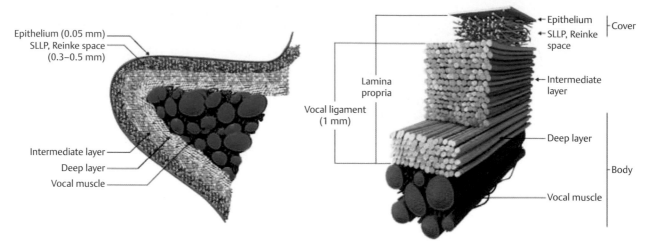

Figure 4.1   Cross-section of a true vocal fold.
Reprinted with permission from Elsevier. Finck C, Lejeune L. Structure and oscillatory functions of the vocal fold. In: Stefan M. Brudzynski, ed. *The Handbook of Mammalian Vocalization: An Integrative Neuroscience Approach*. Chapter 10.2. Figure 2. Copyright Elsevier (2009).

of the vocal folds. The cross-section of the vocal fold reveals a five-layered structure, with each layer having a different mechanical property (**Fig. 4.1**). The outer four layers are controlled passively and the innermost layer is controlled both actively and passively.[3,4] Functionally, the vocal fold acts as three separate layers consisting of the cover (epithelium and Reinke space), the transition (intermediate and deep layers of the lamina propria), and the body (vocalis muscle). The vibratory margin of the vocal fold consists of a stratified squamous epithelium with the purpose of maintaining the shape of the vocal fold and withstanding the trauma of vocal fold contact.[3] The superficial layer of the lamina propria, or Reinke space, consists of loose fibrous components and a matrix of elastic fibers. The rheological properties of this layer allow for dynamic spectrum of sound production. The intermediate and deep layers of the lamina propria constitute the vocal ligament, with the intermediate layer composed mainly of elastic fibers and the deep layer made up primarily of collagenous fibers.[4] The thyroarytenoid or vocalis muscle constitutes the body of the vocal fold.[3]

Clinical Insight

In most instances of vocal fold injury, such as that seen with nodules or polyps, the area of insult is limited to the epithelium and superficial layers of the lamina propria. The healing process in these two areas results in a minimal effect on vocal fold function because the fibers of the lamina propria are generally restored in an orientation parallel to the epithelium. If the injury or surgery involves both the epithelium and the deep layer of the lamina propria, then the scar can develop perpendicular to the epithelium, resulting in stiffness of the vocal fold leading to reduction of the vocal wave.[5,6] This can result in striking and possibly permanent changes in voice.[7]

Pearls and Pitfalls

No other animal has a deep layer of the lamina propria. This could contribute to the distinctions between phonation of humans and other species. The deep layer of the lamina propria, or the vocalis ligament, is not present at birth and starts to thicken around age 8, fully developing around the age of 11 or 12.[8,9] The larynges of children are more resistant to developing dysphonia (abnormal voice), but they are less able to perform fine vocal articulations compared with adults.[9] The changes in voice that occur with age are due to a reduction in the thickness of the lamina propria and the density of epithelial cells.[8]

Physiology of Vocal Fold Vibration

Three important steps must happen before the production of voice. The first two steps are development of tension in the vocal folds and adduction to the midline (also known as the phonatory attack phase). This is accomplished by the lateral cricoarytenoid and interarytenoid muscles. The final step is the production of airflow from the lungs.

While there are several models describing vocal vibration in various amounts of detail, the myoelastic-aerodynamic theory of phonation provides an appropriate description of the basic forces involved in voice production.[10] As air emerges from the lungs, the pressure in the subglottis increases. Once the subglottic pressure exceeds the myoelastic tension between the vocal folds, the lower lips of the vocal folds separate followed by the upper lips. The myoelastic tension is determined by both the volitional contraction of the laryngeal musculature and the intrinsic elastic properties of the vocal folds. Once the vocal folds are completely separated, air escapes superiorly and the subglottic pressure subsequently

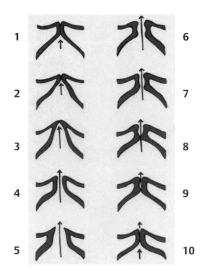

Figure 4.2 (1) Air pressure generated by the power source moves superiorly toward the adducted vocal folds. (2 and 3) Once subglottic pressure exceeds the myoelastic tension between the vocal folds, maintaining them in adduction, the bottom lips of the vibrating vocal folds begin to separate. (4 and 5) The column of air pressure continues to move superiorly opening the top lips of the vocal folds. (6 to 10) The increased velocity of air flow causes a drop in air pressure creating a Bernoulli effect. The inferior lips of the vocal folds adduct in the lower pressure system followed by the superior lips. This completes one glottic cycle.

drops. When the myoelastic tension exceeds the subglottic pressure, the vocal folds will again approximate. This is assisted by aerodynamic forces known as Bernoulli principle. As air passes through a narrowed opening, such as the glottis, an increase in speed of airflow results in a decrease in pressure, which draws the vocal folds together. Once the vocal folds close, the subglottic pressure begins to increase pushing the vocal folds apart again. This completes one glottic cycle.[2,7] This entire sequence is illustrated in **Fig. 4.2**. The number of cycles that occur per second determines the frequency in hertz (Hz) or pitch of the sound produced.

There are several important factors that contribute to the pitch including the mass of the vocal fold, the tension of the vocal folds, and the level of subglottic pressure. A heavier vocal fold will vibrate slower than a lighter vocal fold, accounting for the lower pitched voice of a smoker with edematous vocal folds or a patient with masses on their vocal folds. Decreased mass, increased vocal fold tension, and increased subglottic pressure will all increase the pitch, while increased vocal fold mass, decreased tension, and decreased subglottic pressure will all serve to decrease the pitch.[11]

Resonance Chamber

In isolation, the larynx produces an uninteresting sound similar to a reed played apart from its woodwind instrument. Sound produced from vocal fold vibration is modified or amplified by the resonating cavities of the pharynx, oral cavity, nose, sinuses, and chest.[7] The fundamental frequency

(f_o) is defined as the number of glottal vibratory cycles per second. Along with f_o, laryngeal vibration results in the production of multiple frequencies at regular intervals from f_o. The f_o is the lowest frequency produced, and the other frequencies are known as overtones. Partials (fundamental plus overtones) are accentuated and diminished by the vocal tract. The vocal tract includes the entire upper aerodigestive tract from the ventricular folds (false vocal folds) to the lips, acting as a resonator. A resonator acts to amplify certain frequencies known as resonances or resonant frequencies, thereby increasing their volume. In the vocal tract, these resonances are known as formants. This means that as sound emerges from the larynx and resonates the upper aerodigestive tract, certain overtones will be amplified and others will be diminished. This is accomplished by altering the shape and length of the vocal tract, which results in a change in the timbre, or color of the voice giving the voice a unique, recognizable sound.[12]

The "false vocal folds," located above the true vocal folds, do not make contact during normal speaking or singing. In certain conditions, they may contact in the midline and produce voice in a phenomenon called "dysphonia plica ventricularis." They are considered to be used for forceful laryngeal closure and cannot be removed without affecting phonation as they are a component of the resonance chamber.[3]

Functional Neuroanatomy of Phonation

Phonation requires complex and precise communication between the central nervous system and the peripheral phonatory organs.[4] The production of speech requires the integration of diverse information sources (auditory, somatosensory, and motor) to generate the intricate patterning of muscle activations required for fluency.[4,13] Even the simplest task such as producing a single syllable requires recruitment of a large portion of the cerebral cortex.[14]

The sequence of sound production starts with the activation of Broca area of the brain. The motor commands from the Broca area are transmitted to the motor cortex in the precentral gyrus, which then sends a series of commands to the motor nuclei in the brainstem and spinal cord. These nuclei project neurons that synapse with respiratory, laryngeal, and articulatory musculature to produce movement of the phonatory organs creating a series of sounds known as voice.[4,13] The voice is heard by the speaker and is immediately compared against the intended sound providing a feedback mechanism enabling voice modification. Sensory receptors also provide information about the movements of the phonatory organs, playing an important role in tuning the speech motor control system.[4] Additional refinement of motor activity is achieved by the extrapyramidal (cerebral cortex, cerebellum, and basal ganglion) and autonomic nervous system. The movement of the phonatory organs represents the composite signaling within the central nervous system that plans, executes, and modifies muscular activity to produce voice.[3]

Physiology of Deglutition

Deglutition, more commonly known as swallowing, is a complex and highly coordinated activity involving muscles of the oral cavity, oropharynx, pharynx, and esophagus. Swallowing includes volitional and reflexive activities involving more than 30 nerves and muscles. Generally, swallowing is divided into four stages: oral preparation, oral propulsive, pharyngeal, and esophageal.[15]

Oral Preparation Stage

The oral preparation stage is responsible for taking food and pulverizing it into a bolus that can be easily swallowed. The oral stage is under voluntary motor control. Mastication requires several coordinated muscular movements, with the tongue playing a paramount role. The most important aspect of the oral phase is the lateral excursion of the tongue, which continuously moves food from the middle of the oral cavity to a more lateral position between the teeth for further breakdown.[16] Rotary and lateral jaw movements are necessary to chew the food, modifying its consistency. The soft palate also moves forward, which simultaneously prevents the food from spilling posteriorly and increases the amount of air available to enter through the nasal cavity. While patients with restricted jaw motion, poor dentition, and reduced buccal and oral tension are still able to chew the food, those patients who lack lateral tongue rolling motion are unable to effectively chew owing to the inability to keep food between the teeth for pulverization. The tongue then gathers the food within the oral cavity into a cohesive bolus and holds it against the soft palate or floor of the mouth. The bolus is then ready to be moved into the oropharynx.[15]

Oral Propulsive Stage

In the oral propulsive stage of swallowing, the bolus of food moves posteriorly into the oropharynx and initiates the pharyngeal phase of swallowing. The tongue is again the most critical part of the oral propulsive stage of swallowing. Given the unique arrangement of its muscle fibers, the tongue is able to perform a variety of movements and functions. In the oral stage, the tongue pushes laterally against the alveolus as the midline of the tongue moves the bolus posteriorly along the hard palate. Once the bolus has reached the base of the tongue, the pharyngeal phase is triggered. The oral phase lasts from 1 to 1.5 seconds, partly depending on the consistency of the bolus.[15]

Pharyngeal Stage

The pharyngeal phase is perhaps the most important stage of swallowing. While the importance of the first two stages can be reduced by the administration of different consistencies, the pharyngeal phase cannot be bypassed as it is critical in the function of airway protection. Pharyngeal swallow is a brisk sequential activity, occurring within 1 second. It has two main events that include food passage, or propelling the food bolus through the pharynx and upper esophageal sphincter (UES) to the esophagus, and protecting the airway by insulating the larynx and trachea from the pharynx during food passage to prevent the food from entering the airway. There are five highly coordinated motions that occur during this phase of swallowing. Initially, the soft palate raises, which results in velopharyngeal closure preventing food from entering the nasal cavity. This is followed by propulsion of the bolus posteriorly by the base of the tongue and sequential contraction of the pharyngeal musculature to move the bolus inferiorly toward the esophagus. There are multiple protective layers that prevent food from entering the airway. The vocal folds close to seal the glottis (space between the vocal folds), and the arytenoids tilt forward to contact the epiglottic base before opening of the UES.[17,18] The hyoid bone and larynx are pulled upward and forward by contraction of the suprahyoid muscles and the thyrohyoid muscle. This displacement tucks the larynx under the base of the tongue. The epiglottis tilts backward to seal the laryngeal vestibule. Airway protection is primarily provided by the closure of the false vocal folds and the anterior tilt of the arytenoid cartilages. The closure of the vocal folds provides only a brief cessation in respiration, which resumes as soon as the bolus enters the esophagus.[16]

Respiration ceases briefly during swallowing not only because of the physical closure of the airway by elevation of the soft palate and tilting of the epiglottis but also because of neural suppression of respiration in the brainstem.[19] The respiratory pause continues for 0.5 to 1.5 seconds during swallowing, and respiration usually resumes with expiration.[20–22]

The pharyngeal stage ends with the relaxation of the UES. This muscle, also known as the cricopharyngeus, is the lowest aspect of the inferior constrictor. There are three main factors that contribute to the opening of the UES. Relaxation of the cricopharyngeus muscle precedes opening of the UES or arrival of the bolus. The contraction of the suprahyoid muscles and thyrohyoid muscles pulls the hyolaryngeal complex forward, opening the sphincter. The pressure of the descending bolus distends the UES, physically assisting its opening.[23] At rest, the UES is in tonic contraction to prevent entry of air into the esophagus during respiration and simultaneously to avoid gastric contents from entering the pharynx. As the constrictor muscles propel the bolus inferiorly and the larynx elevates, the UES relaxes to admit the bolus into the esophagus and immediately contracts again to avoid retrograde movement of the food. The pharyngeal phase typically lasts 1 second in the normal individual and does not have significant variation despite the consistency of the food.

Esophageal Stage

The esophageal stage begins after the bolus passes through the UES into the esophagus.[15] The cervical esophagus (upper one-third) is composed of striated muscle, but the thoracic esophagus (lower two-thirds) is made up of smooth muscle. Bolus transport in the thoracic esophagus is different from that in the pharynx because true peristalsis occurs there, regulated by the autonomic nervous system. Initially, a wave of relaxation accommodates the bolus, followed by a wave of contraction propelling the bolus inferiorly.[16]

Neurophysiology of Swallowing

There are many highly coordinated neural actions that take place for feeding and swallowing. Smell and taste, via CNs I, VII, and IX, all provide essential feedback for the feeding process. Sensory input is relayed via CNs V, IX, and X.[24] The three primary functions of sensory input to the swallowing tract are to assist in initiating swallowing, to modify the threshold for a pharyngeal swallow, and to alter the level of muscle recruitment during swallowing. The most important sensory contribution for swallow arises from the SLN, the first branch of CN X (**Table 4.1**).[25]

Neural control of swallowing recruits from all levels of the neurological system in a hierarchical manner.[24] The first level of control arises from the brainstem swallowing center with the central pattern generator.[26] The central pattern generator organizes the sequential excitation of motor neurons controlling the swallowing muscles. Subcortical structures such as the hypothalamus, amygdala, basal ganglia, and tegmental areas of the midbrain represent the second level of swallowing control. The third level of control is provided by the suprabulbar cortical swallowing centers.[27] Appropriate preparation of food relies on the continuous feedback of sensory information from receptors in the tongue, soft palate, floor of the mouth, and tooth pulp, which detect the size and texture of the bolus. These sensory

inputs help determine the chewing action required from the muscles of mastication.[28,29] Anesthetizing these mucosal regions locally has been shown to increase the time to evoke repeated swallows and may disrupt swallowing modulation, but does not eliminate swallowing completely.[30–32]

Clinical Insight

Swallowing function can be reduced in those patients affected by stroke, neurological disorders, and myopathies. Those patients suffering from dysphagia due to stroke are at increased risk for stroke mortality, increased hospital length of stay, dehydration, and malnutrition. Stroke patients with dysphagia have a threefold increased likelihood of developing aspiration.[33] Both central and peripheral neurological disorders can result in dysphagia. Some common causes include Parkinson disease, multiple sclerosis, amyotrophic lateral sclerosis, Alzheimer disease, and muscular dystrophies. All such patients should be evaluated with a clinical bedside swallowing evaluation (CSE).

CSEs involve several levels of evaluation. A thorough head and neck examination is performed with specific inspection of the dentition and oral mucosa, looking for pooling of secretions or retained food substance indicating dysphagia. A CN examination allows the assessment of specific sensory or motor deficits, which may lead to dysphagia or aspiration. Evaluation of motor and sensory integrity of the face, lips, tongue, and palate will allow the examiner to link clinical observations of the CN impairment with suspected oropharyngeal

Table 4.1   Sensory and Motor Functions of the Various Nerves Involved in Mastication and Deglutition

Cranial Nerve	Motor	Sensory	Special sensory	Secretomotor
CN V	Muscles of mastication	Anterior two-thirds of tongue, face, and mouth	–	–
CN VII	Muscles of face including orbicularis oris		Taste from anterior two-thirds of tongue	Minor salivary gland secretion
CN IX	Stylopharyngeus	Posterior one-third of tongue, oropharynx	Taste from posterior one-third of tongue	Parotid salivary secretion via lesser superficial petrosal nerve
CN X	Glossopalatine, levator veli palatini, pharyngeal constrictors, intrinsic laryngeal muscles, cricopharyngeal relaxation, esophageal muscles, and muscles of respiration	Velu, posterior and inferior pharynx, and larynx via superior and recurrent laryngeal nerves	–	–
CN XII	Intrinsic and extrinsic tongue muscles except palatoglossus	–	–	–

Adapted from reference 25.
CN, cranial nerve.

pathophysiology and thereby increase sensitivity for detecting dysphagia on the CSE.[34] The swallowing portion of the CSE includes administration of various consistencies and volumes over multiple trials. It is important to optimize the patient for the examination by ensuring appropriate positioning and mental alertness and rehydrating oral mucosa with ice chips or cotton swabs. The primary function of the CSE is to determine which patients are at risk for aspiration and therefore require instrumental examination.[33] Six clinical features (dysphonia, dysarthria, abnormal volitional cough, abnormal gag reflex, cough on trial swallow, and voice change on trial swallow) were associated with the risk of aspiration as identified using videofluoroscopy.[35] The presence of any two of these six clinical features could correctly identify the risk of aspiration with 92% accuracy.[36]

References

1. Tucker H. Gross and microscopic anatomy of the larynx. In: Benninger MS, Jacobson BH, Johnson AF, eds. Vocal Arts Medicine: The Care and Prevention of Professional Voice Disorders. New York, NY: Thieme Medical Publishers; 1994:11–29

2. Jiang J. Physiology of voice production: how does the voice work? In: Benninger MS, Murry T, eds. The Performer's Voice. San Diego, CA: Plural Publishing; 2006:22–32

3. Sataloff RT. Clinical anatomy and physiology of the voice. In: Sataloff RT, ed. Professional Voice: The Science and Art of Clinical Care. 2nd ed. San Diego, CA: Singular Publishing Group, Inc.; 1997:111–130

4. Hirano M. Clinical Examination of Voice. New York, NY: Springer-Verlag/Wien; 1981

5. Benninger MS. Microdissection or microspot CO_2 laser for limited vocal fold benign lesions: a prospective randomized trial. Laryngoscope 2000;110(2 Pt 2, Suppl 92):1–17

6. Benninger MS, Jacobson B. Vocal nodules, microwebs, and surgery. J Voice 1995;9(3):326–331

7. Benninger MS. The human voice: evolution and performance. Music Med 2010;2(2):104–108

8. Hartnick CJ, Rehbar R, Prasad V. Development and maturation of the pediatric human vocal fold lamina propria. Laryngoscope 2005;115(1):4–15

9. Prades JM, Dumollard JM, Duband S, et al. Lamina propria of the human vocal fold: histomorphometric study of collagen fibers. Surg Radiol Anat 2010;32(4):377–382

10. Van de Berg J. Myoelastic-aerodynamic theory of voice production. J Speech Hear Res 1958;1:222–244

11. Coulton RH. Physiology of phonation. In: Benninger MS, Jacobson BH, Johnson AF, eds. Vocal Arts Medicine: The Care and Prevention of Professional Voice Disorders. New York, NY: Thieme Medical Publishers; 1994:30–59

12. Sunberg J. Vocal tract resonance. In: Sataloff RT, ed. Professional Voice: The Science and Art of Clinical Care. San Diego, CA: Singular Publishing Group, Inc.; 1997:167–184

13. Guenther FH. Cortical interactions underlying the production of speech sounds. J Commun Disord 2006;39(5):350–365

14. Fiez JA, Petersen SE. Neuroimaging studies of word reading. Proc Natl Acad Sci USA 1998;95(3):914–921

15. Logemann J. Mechanisms of normal and abnormal swallowing. In: Cummings CW, Harker LA, Krause CH, et al., eds. Otolaryngology–Head and Neck Surgery. 3rd ed. St. Louis, MO: Mosby; 1998:1844–1853.

16. Matsuo K, Palmer JB. Anatomy and physiology of feeding and swallowing: normal and abnormal. Phys Med Rehabil Clin N Am 2008;19(4):691–707, vii

17. Shaker R, Dodds WJ, Dantas RO, et al. Coordination of deglutitive glottis closure with oro-pharyngeal swallowing. Gastroenterology 1998;98:1478–1484

18. Ohmae Y, Logemann JA, Kaiser P, Hanson DG, Kahrilas PJ. Timing of glottic closure during normal swallow. Head Neck 1995;17(5):394–402

19. Nishino T, Hiraga K. Coordination of swallowing and respiration in unconscious subjects. J Appl Physiol 1991;70(3):988–993

20. Selley WG, Flack FC, Ellis RE, Brooks WA. Respiratory patterns associated with swallowing: part 1. The normal adult pattern and changes with age. Age Ageing 1989;18(3):168–172

21. Klahn MS, Perlman AL. Temporal and durational patterns associating respiration and swallowing. Dysphagia 1999;14(3):131–138

22. Martin-Harris B, Brodsky MB, Michel Y, Ford CL, Walters B, Heffner J. Breathing and swallowing dynamics across the adult lifespan. Arch Otolaryngol Head Neck Surg 2005;131(9):762–770

23. Shaw DW, Cook IJ, Gabb M, et al. Influence of normal aging on oral-pharyngeal and upper esophageal sphincter function during swallowing. Am J Physiol 1995;268(3 Pt 1):G389–G396

24. Mistry S, Hamdy S. Neural control of feeding and swallowing. Phys Med Rehabil Clin N Am 2008;19(4):709–728, vii–viii

25. Miller AJ, Vargervik K, Phillips D. Neuromuscular adaptation of craniofacial muscles to altered oral sensation. Am J Orthod 1985;87(4):303–310

26. Martin RE, Sessle BJ. The role of the cerebral cortex in swallowing. Dysphagia 1993;8(3):195–202

27. Jean A. Brainstem control of swallowing: localization and organization of the central pattern generator for swallowing. In: Taylor A, ed. Neurophysiology of the Jaws and Teeth. London: MacMillan Press; 1990:294–321

28. Anderson DJ, Hannam AG, Mathews B. Sensory mechanisms in mammalian teeth and their supporting structures. Physiol Rev 1970;50(2):171–195

29. Luschei ES, Goodwin GM. Patterns of mandibular movement and jaw muscle activity during mastication in the monkey. J Neurophysiol 1974;37(5):954–966

30. Ertekin C, Aydogdu I. Neurophysiology of swallowing. Clin Neurophysiol 2003;114(12):2226–2244

31. Jean A. Brain stem control of swallowing: neuronal network and cellular mechanisms. Physiol Rev 2001;81(2):929–969

32. Månsson I, Sandberg N. Effects of surface anesthesia on deglutition in man. Laryngoscope 1974;84(3):427–437

33. González-Fernández M, Daniels SK. Dysphagia in stroke and neurologic disease. Phys Med Rehabil Clin N Am 2008;19(4):867–888, x

34. Daniels SK, Huckabee ML. Dysphagia Following Stroke. San Diego, CA: Plural; 2008

35. Daniels SK, Brailey K, Priestly DH, Herrington LR, Weisberg LA, Foundas AL. Aspiration in patients with acute stroke. Arch Phys Med Rehabil 1998;79(1):14–19

36. Daniels SK, McAdam CP, Brailey K, et al. Clinical assessment of swallowing and prediction of dysphagia severity. Am J Speech Lang Pathol 1997;6:17–24

5 Current Perspectives on the Molecular Biology of the Larynx

Samit Majumdar and Neil Mackenzie Kernohan

Although the larynx may be the site of origin for many different types of cancer, squamous carcinomas account for 95% of cases.[1] While the incidence of laryngeal carcinoma is increasing in some areas of the world, there are still notable geographic variations and epidemiological trends in the incidence. Laryngeal cancer is most commonly diagnosed in individuals over the age of 60, with diagnoses below the age of 40 being uncommon. In the United Kingdom, laryngeal cancer is the 18th most common type of cancer affecting men, with a male:female ratio of approximately 5:1 based on figures from 2008. The incidence of this form of cancer has remained approximately 1 in 100,000 for women. There has been some variation in the incidence of laryngeal carcinoma in men, but over the past 30 years the incidence in the United Kingdom has been between 5 and 7 per 100,000 and recently has remained around 5.3 per 100,000.[2]

Laryngeal Cancer

- Squamous carcinomas account for 95% of cases of laryngeal malignancies.
- Laryngeal cancer is most commonly diagnosed in individuals over the age of 60, with diagnoses below the age of 40 being uncommon.
- Incidence in the United Kingdom has been between 5 and 7 per 100,000.
- Male:female ratio is approximately 5:1.

The development of laryngeal squamous cell carcinoma (SCC) may be viewed in the same manner as the paradigm for stepwise carcinogenesis defined by significant pathological and molecular rate-limiting steps in cellular proliferation, described originally for colorectal carcinoma.[3] As with sporadic colorectal carcinoma, the epidemiological data are compatible with cumulative exposure to carcinogenic agents that result in neoplastic transformation of cell(s) within the laryngeal epithelium. It is proposed that laryngeal SCC emerges after a prolonged period of time during which there is an accumulation of genetic abnormalities within a transformed cell and its progeny consequent upon the action of carcinogenic agents. As a result, the affected cells acquire morphologically identifiable changes. An initial hyperplastic phase is followed by a period during which the affected epithelial cells exhibit cytological changes associated with architectural disarray of variable severity within the epithelium that the pathologist recognizes as dysplasia. Such dysplastic lesions are represented by a spectrum of lesions that can be collectively termed squamous intraepithelial lesions. These changes could progress further as within the abnormal cell population the increasing mutational load may lead to the emergence of a clone of cells with invasive properties, thus heralding the onset of SCC.

Stepwise Carcinogenesis

- The development of laryngeal SCC may be viewed in the same manner as the paradigm for stepwise carcinogenesis defined by significant pathological and molecular rate-limiting steps in cellular proliferation, described originally for colorectal carcinoma.[3]
- The epidemiological data are compatible with cumulative exposure to carcinogenic agents that result in neoplastic transformation of cell(s) within the laryngeal epithelium.
- Dysplastic lesions are represented by a spectrum of lesions that can be collectively termed squamous intraepithelial lesions.
- Increasing mutational load may lead to the emergence of a clone of cells with invasive properties, thus heralding the onset of SCC.

These models of cancer development are likely to represent a rather simplistic view for what is an incredibly complex process. Indeed the paradigm of colorectal carcinoma now reflects this notion as it is now evident that the original model does not seem to apply in all cases. In this particular system, it is now accepted that there are distinct routes by which various molecular alterations can be acquired within cells, leading ultimately to the onset of malignancy.[3–5]

It seems likely that a similar argument could be advanced for laryngeal SCC, especially as now several important and distinct etiological factors have been recognized. Furthermore, with regard to the larynx, although the model systems proposed might suggest that lesions will necessarily progress to SCC, it is evident that this need not be the case, particularly for lesions showing relatively minor histological abnormalities. Nevertheless, it is equally well recognized that in some cases lesions with low-grade histological change can progress rapidly to invasive disease.[6] However, an important challenge for clinicians at this time is to appreciate which lesions are likely to progress to malignancy and over what time frame might this occur. Having an awareness of environmental factors that might perpetuate these events may offer further scope for intervention that will moderate or attenuate progression of the disease.

In an attempt to understand the basis for the etiology, pathogenesis, and behavior of laryngeal squamous carcinoma and its precursor lesions, the molecular pathogenesis of laryngeal SCC has been an area of keen interest in the recent years. The epidemiological data would suggest a strong influence of environmental factors in the pathogenesis of this form of cancer. As important environmental risk factors become more widely appreciated, this has served to reinforce the perception that this disease is potentially preventable.

Etiological Factors for Laryngeal Squamous Cell Carcinoma

Established Etiological Factors

Many environmental factors have been linked to the development of laryngeal squamous carcinomas. Foremost among these and the most widely recognized are smoking and alcohol usage, and in virtually all populations, most cases of SCC occur in patients with a history of tobacco use and consumption of alcohol. These two risk factors have a synergistic influence on the risk of developing laryngeal SCC. Smoking carries a greater risk of developing carcinomas arising from the glottis compared with other regions of the larynx. Conversely, alcohol consumption has stronger associations with carcinomas arising in the supraglottis and hypopharynx.[1,7] The body of evidence that now links smoking to laryngeal SCC is overwhelming, and many studies have shown that the risk of developing laryngeal SCC in smokers is proportional to the number of years over which an individual smokes, the degree to which the patient inhales their smoke, and the type of tobacco used. Smoking traditionally is associated with an increased risk of mutational events affecting genes (**Fig. 5.1**), such as *p53* that would predispose the cell to further errors of

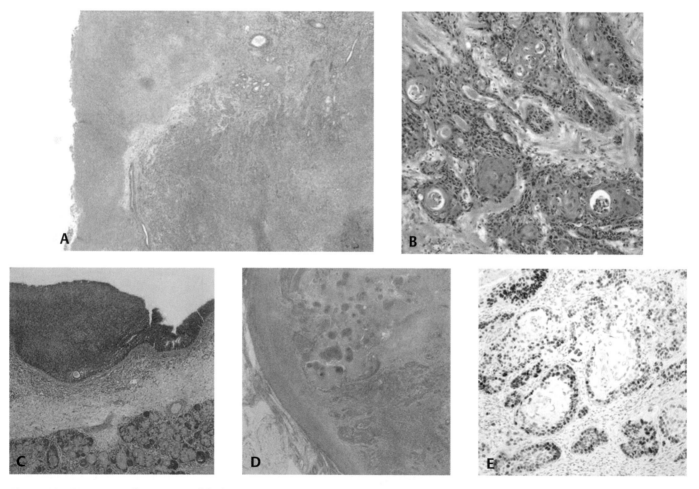

Figure 5.1   Squamous cell carcinoma of the larynx arises as a result of an accumulation of genetic damage within laryngeal squamous epithelial cells. Such tumors may present as locally advanced disease with ulcerated lesions of the vocal cord with underlying infiltration of the structures of the laryngeal wall by squamous carcinoma (A and B). However, it is well established that hyperplastic and dysplastic lesions precede the onset of overt malignancy (C). With invasive growth and progression of disease, lymph node metastasis may occur (D). In many laryngeal squamous carcinomas, mutation of the *p53* gene can be interred by the strong nuclear staining of the malignant cells for p53 protein using immunohistochemical staining (E). Such staining techniques can be used to investigate molecular events that may have led to malignant transformation of epithelial cells or provide clues to the etiology of some cancer types, for example, nuclear staining for p16 may indicate underlying infection with human papillomavirus (not shown).

proliferation culminating in the development of cancer.[8] The role of alcohol is less clearly understood, but it has been proposed that it acts as a promoter, driving the proliferation of abnormal cells and thus also accelerating the acquisition of further abnormalities.

However, several other environmental factors (dietary and occupational exposure to dusts and chemicals) have been linked with the risk of developing laryngeal SCC. Overall, it is likely that these will either be much less commonly identified in patients with SCC and/or a causal association with individual cases of SCC will be difficult to prove. Nevertheless, an extremely unusual condition associated with laryngeal SCC is worthy of note. Patients with Bloom syndrome appear to have an increased risk of developing laryngeal SCC.[9] This condition is a rare autosomal recessive genetic disorder caused by mutations in *BLM*, a member of the RecQ deoxyribonucleic acid (DNA) helicase family.[10] A characteristic feature of this condition is the accumulation of chromosomal abnormalities associated with chromosomal breaks and high rates of sister chromatid exchange. Although a rare association with laryngeal SCC in young patients, this condition provides a clear link between chromosome breakage, genetic damage, and the onset of malignancy at this site. This consolidates the popular models of carcinogenesis that propose that environmental carcinogens cause cancer in exposed cell populations by generating or facilitating an accumulation of genetic damage, that is, aberrations, of the tumor suppressor genes and oncogenes within cells, which is associated with an increased mutational load with consequent ability to drive the cells along the cell cycle (**Fig. 5.2**) and preventing their entry into the resting phase (G_0). These acquired mutations are responsible for the genetic infidelity that allows the cancer cells to bypass the natural control through apoptosis.

New Concepts in Laryngeal Carcinogenesis

Two other factors that have recently gained wide interest are infection with high-risk serotypes of the human papillomavirus (HPV) and laryngopharyngeal reflux (LPR)

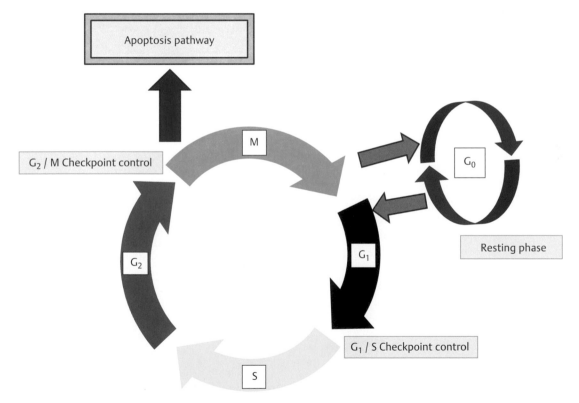

Figure 5.2 Simplified sketch of the cell cycle and its various phases. Progression through the cell cycle is dependent upon the sequential activation and degradation of cyclin/cyclin-dependent kinase complexes. Cyclin D/cdk4/6 activity early in G_1 gives way to cyclin E/cdk2 toward the G_1/S transition. Progression through the S and G_2 phases is associated with cyclin A/cdk2 activity, with cyclin B/cdk1 operating through mitosis. In addition, the cell cycle checkpoints must be permissive for progression to the next phase of the cell cycle. Restrictions are present in both the S phase and mitosis, but key tumor suppressor pathways operate at G_1/S and G_2/M. At the former, activation of p53 increases expression of p21 leading to arrest of the cells in G_1. In addition, sequestration of E2 promoter binding factor transcription factors by the retinoblastoma protein will prevent entry to S phase. The tumor suppressor p53 also operates at the G_2/M transition, its effects here being mediated by 14–3-3σ. G_1+S+G_2 = Interphase; M = Mitosis; S phase = DNA synthesis phase.

Note: (1) DNA damage can activate apoptosis pathways as well as pathways that act at key checkpoints to mediate cell cycle arrest. (2) Cancer cells do not enter the G_0 phase.

disease. These factors are of particular interest as they may account for most cases of laryngeal SCC in the subgroup of patients without any history of smoking or alcohol intake; therefore, it may point toward different and important molecular events and pathways that might be implicated in the etiology of laryngeal SCC.

Human Papillomavirus Infection

High-risk serotypes of HPV, particularly HPV 16, have been linked to carcinomas arising at various sites within the head and neck region, with the highest viral load being consistently identified within tonsillar tissue. This is consistent with studies that show that the strongest and clinically the most significant associations of HPV infection are with tonsillar carcinoma as well as those arising in the oral cavity.[11] In clinical terms, identification of HPV-associated cases of oropharyngeal squamous carcinoma is relevant; tumors associated with HPV have characteristic histological appearances, are often associated with strong expression of surrogate marker p16, are particularly responsive to chemotherapy/radiotherapy, and, paradoxically, have a relatively favorable prognosis.[12]

However, HPV does not carry the same degree of risk at all sites within the regions of the oral and upper aerodigestive tract, although it has been suggested that HPV may also be an important etiological factor for laryngeal carcinoma. There is considerable debate within the published literature regarding the frequency with which cases of laryngeal SCC are associated with HPV infection. Depending on the individual study, the frequency with which HPV is claimed to be associated with laryngeal SCC ranges from 3 to 85%. It might be argued that different techniques or reagents used in different studies could account for this striking variability in the results obtained, and the criteria by which cases are defined as HPV positive or negative may vary. Furthermore, it has been shown that in normal appearing larynges, both clinically and histologically, molecular evidence of HPV infection has been found in up to 25% of cases, which is a very intriguing finding indeed.

Despite all of these caveats, a meta-analysis of cases reported in the literature suggests that about one quarter of cases of laryngeal SCC may be HPV related.[11] Therefore, the prevailing opinion that HPV plays a relatively minor role in laryngeal SCC seems validated, but equally the role of HPV cannot be discounted, and consideration of the molecular events involved in HPV-related carcinogenesis will have some relevance to laryngeal SCC. However, laryngeal papillomatosis (recurrent respiratory papillomatosis) is an uncommon but well-recognized condition associated with HPV infection and yet malignant transformation in this setting is uncommon and most often associated with other recognized predisposing factors, such as smoking or following irradiation.[13] This suggests that HPV infection may be a cofactor in the progression to malignancy but in and of itself may not be sufficient to cause laryngeal SCC, although certain viral serotypes (types 11, 16, and 18) appear to be associated with more aggressive disease and an increased risk of progression to malignancy.

Laryngopharyngeal Reflux

The role of LPR in the pathogenesis of laryngeal carcinoma has also now gained wider recognition. Since early reports linking reflux diseases to the onset of laryngeal neoplasia and the increased risk of laryngeal carcinoma for patients after gastric surgery, it is interesting to note that in those cases of laryngeal carcinoma occurring in patients without exposure to the major risk factors of smoking and alcohol, evidence of reflux disease is now often identified.[14] Furthermore, reflux disease is associated with alcohol intake, raising the possibility that these factors may act synergistically as cofactors in laryngeal carcinogenesis.

Human Papillomavirus

- High-risk serotypes of HPV, particularly HPV 16, have been linked to carcinomas arising at various sites within the head and neck region, with the highest viral load being consistently identified within tonsillar tissue.
- Clinically the most significant associations of HPV infection are with tonsillar carcinoma as well as those arising in the oral cavity.[11]
- Tumors associated with HPV have characteristic histological appearances, are often associated with strong expression of surrogate marker p16, are particularly responsive to chemotherapy/radiotherapy, and, paradoxically, have a relatively favorable prognosis.[12]

Laryngopharyngeal Reflux

- The role of LPR in the pathogenesis of laryngeal carcinoma has also now gained wider recognition.
- Reflux disease is associated with alcohol intake, raising the possibility that these factors may act synergistically as cofactors in laryngeal carcinogenesis.
- In combination with acid, pepsin is believed to be a prime cause of injury to the laryngeal epithelium.
- Scientific studies have recognized that the composition of the refluxate is complex (**Fig. 5.3**) and have sought to define which component(s) of the refluxate have a pivotal role driving the onset and progression of esophageal neoplasia.
- Bile acids and their salts have gained wider recognition as agents implicated in the pathogenesis of a variety of cancers of the gastrointestinal (GI) tract.[29,32,45]

Reflux diseases are now very commonly diagnosed and represent a major issue in the development of disease of the upper GI tract and airways. An important association has been established between reflux gastroesophageal reflux disease

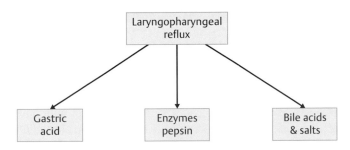

Figure 5.3 Principal components of refluxate implicated in laryngopharyngeal disease. Traditionally, the roles of acid and enzymes such as pepsin have been the focus of research into mechanisms of epithelial injury. Recent studies have highlighted the potential for bile acids to cause epithelial injury and to mediate intracellular events that might predispose exposed cells to neoplastic transformation and lead to the development of squamous epithelial malignancy.

(GERD) and Barrett esophagus and its attendant risk of esophageal adenocarcinoma. The epidemiology of esophageal malignancy has changed dramatically in the recent decades, thus supporting the impact of reflux disease, adenocarcinoma now being the most common type of esophageal malignancy. Scientific studies have recognized that the composition of the refluxate is complex (**Fig. 5.3**) and have sought to define which component(s) of the refluxate have a pivotal role driving the onset and progression of esophageal neoplasia. Further work has focused on the molecular mechanisms by which these substances might enhance or possibly moderate the risk of developing malignancy. These issues are now at the forefront of research into laryngeal neoplasia, and it is time to review the present evidence that links reflux disease to laryngeal neoplasia.

Laryngopharyngeal Reflux as a Risk Factor for Laryngeal Squamous Cell Carcinoma

Cases of laryngeal carcinoma occurring in patients without exposure to the major risk factors of smoking and alcohol are often associated with evidence of reflux disease.[14,15] As reflux disease can be associated with alcohol intake, there is a possibility that in some cases alcohol and reflux may act cooperatively in laryngeal carcinogenesis. As the association between LPR and laryngeal disease, including neoplasia, has gained wider acceptance, investigations have sought to provide a molecular explanation for the pathogenesis of laryngeal disease caused by LPR. This has been particularly challenging regarding the role of LPR in the molecular pathogenesis of neoplastic transformation of the laryngeal epithelium.

Laryngopharyngeal Reflux Disease

In terms of reflux diseases, it is now accepted that LPR and GERD are distinct pathophysiologically. Patients with LPR do not typically present with symptoms classically recognized as being those of GERD. Rather they manifest signs and symptoms related to the upper aerodigestive tract.[16] With respect to laryngeal disease, it has been shown that upper esophageal pH measurements demonstrate evidence of reflux in patients with these symptoms and signs. However, the mechanism(s) by which LPR might lead to laryngeal SCC have been debated. This debate recapitulates that related to the association between GERD and esophageal carcinoma, particularly adenocarcinoma arising on a background of Barrett esophagus.

LPR is now a major focus of research interest, with gathering evidence linking LPR to the onset of neoplastic disease of the larynx. The presence of refluxate within the upper esophagus can be strongly inferred by pH measurements. When combined with the demonstration of pepsin molecules within sputum by Western blotting and within laryngeal epithelial cells by immunohistochemistry, there is strong evidence that episodes of reflux genuinely occur and that the refluxate can wash over the laryngeal epithelium.[17–21] Furthermore, as fundoplication results in symptomatic improvement in patients with LPR,[22] and with antireflux surgery objective measures of the presence of refluxate within sputum decline,[21] the causal association between LPR and clinically significant laryngeal disease has acquired a sound footing for a greater debate.

Biochemical Effects of Refluxate on Laryngeal Epithelium—Acid and Pepsin

The chemical composition of refluxate is complex. For the most part, it will include acid, pepsins, and bile acids. The refluxate, by the nature of its component parts, introduces a harsh and toxic chemical environment to the larynx that is not adapted to protect itself from such attacks and as a result the epithelial cells are damaged. Morphologically, early evidence of reflux disease is manifested by disruption of intercellular junctions.[18]

Several components of the refluxate might be responsible for such an effect, either individually or in combination. However, in combination with acid, pepsin is believed to be a prime cause of injury to the laryngeal epithelium.

Early studies on esophageal epithelium have examined the response of squamous epithelial cells to acid stress both in vitro (cell lines) and in clinical samples. In the presence of reflux, squamous epithelial cells engage stress response pathways and in conditions of low pH downregulate expression of hsp70 but increase expression of two novel stress proteins,[23] sep53 and sep70. It is interesting to note that these responses are not strictly recapitulated in laryngeal epithelium as at this site although low pH does induce expression of sep53 and sep70, there is also strong expression of hsp70.[24] The present data suggest that in terms of sep53 and sep70, this response is characteristic of a low pH environment, but further studies of laryngeal epithelium have shown that in the presence of pepsin, although the level of expression of hsp70 is maintained, there is loss of expression of sep53 and sep70. High levels of hsp70 are characteristic of many types of cancer cells and confer some survival advantage indeed; a specific inhibitor of hsp70, 2-phenylethynesulphonamide, increases protein aggregation within cells, reduces autophagy and lysosomal function, and leads to increased cell death.[25,26] Pepsin is also associated with loss of expression of carbonic anhydrase III, an enzyme that can provide cytoprotection against acid injury, and depletion of E-cadherin with loss of localization to the cell surface membrane.[18,27]

Evidence from in vitro and in vivo studies therefore suggests that pepsin can significantly modify the level of expression of several proteins within laryngeal epithelial cells. To achieve these effects, pepsin must be in its active form and in that state appears able to mediate cell damage. The refluxate is not always highly acidic and therefore may not be assumed to support the catalytic activity of pepsin. However, there are several forms of pepsin whose activity is not restricted to the low pH present within the stomach, and this may permit some forms of pepsin to remain active within the larynx. It has also been shown that pepsin can be reactivated following receptor-mediated endocytosis by laryngeal squamous epithelial cells. When in its active form within the cell, there is evidence of cellular damage manifested by mitochondrial injury and expression of stress response proteins.[20,27]

Biochemical Effects of Refluxate on Laryngeal Epithelium—Bile Acids

Acid and pepsin may therefore account for epithelial damage and the onset of inflammatory changes within the larynx. However, other than through chronic inflammation and altered levels of expression of stress response proteins, an overt link to neoplastic transformation is not apparent. However, the refluxate can include bile acids and their salts[28]; otherwise known as nonacid reflux. Clinically, patients in this group do not respond adequately to conventional treatment with twice-daily proton pump inhibitor and alginate-based liquid medication.

Bile acids are acidic steroid molecules derived from cholesterol and are potentially profoundly damaging to epithelial cells of various types but can also affect exposed cells in many ways that are potentially deleterious and render them susceptible to neoplastic transformation.[29,30] Different bile acids have distinct properties, although collectively they have been associated with cytotoxicity, mitogenic activity, and mutagenicity linked to DNA damage. The presence of bile acids and their salts within refluxate is intriguing and suggests possible mechanisms for induction of inflammatory lesions within the larynx as well as for laryngeal carcinogenesis.

Bile Acids, Epithelial Damage, and Inflammation

The presence of bile acids has been associated with inflammatory conditions of the upper GI tract, namely, gastritis, esophagitis, and Barrett esophagus.[31-33] Bile acids as part of the refluxate have also been implicated in laryngeal disease.[34] Damage to cell membranes mediated by the detergent action of these molecules offers one mechanism by which they may exert cytotoxic effects and contribute to mucosal damage that is also associated with the presence of acid and pepsin. It has been shown that bicarbonate secretion by biliary epithelial cells protects cells against bile acid-mediated injury,[35] but depletion of carbonic anhydrase 3 by pepsin present in the refluxate might deprive epithelial cells of this cytoprotective mechanism. Early experimental models have clearly demonstrated that bile acids can mediate epithelial damage that leads to increased mucosal permeability associated with disruption of intercellular adhesion, damage to cell membranes, and induction of apoptosis.[36,37] In both animal models and human esophageal tissue, these effects are enhanced in the presence of acid.[38,39] Chen et al[40] have recently shown that the ability of bile acids to disrupt the integrity of an epithelial barrier as determined by transepithelial electrical resistance is associated with reduced levels of expression of claudin 1 and 4, adhesion molecules found in the vicinity of tight junctions. The importance of tight junctions in maintaining barrier integrity has been highlighted in animal models in which mice lacking claudin 1 dehydrate as a consequence of reduced barrier function.[41-43]

Cytotoxicity and cell death associated with bile acid-mediated membrane damage is associated with laryngeal disease, particularly inflammatory conditions. However, membrane damage associated with exposure to certain bile acids is not restricted to the cell surface—internal membranes may be damaged, either directly or as a result of the increased production of reactive oxygen species (ROS) associated with oxidative stress, as discussed below. Damage to mitochondrial membrane integrity by bile acids may be associated with increased cytosolic calcium levels. The stress response protein sep53 is believed to provide an important mechanism to protect against bile acid-induced injury associated with increased cytosolic calcium levels, a cellular defense mechanism that in the presence of acid and pepsin may be attenuated.[44] However, such damage would also permit the release of ROS from the mitochondria, a feature of cell damage that is potentially of more profound significance with regard to neoplastic transformation of laryngeal epithelium.

Bile Acids and Carcinogenesis

Bile acids and their salts have gained wider recognition as agents implicated in the pathogenesis of a variety of cancers of the GI tract.[29,32,45] Bile acids may also play a role in the pathogenesis of laryngeal carcinoma. The relationship between gastric surgery and laryngeal neoplasia also provides some circumstantial evidence linking biliary secretions with laryngeal neoplasia.[15] The association between gastric surgery and laryngeal neoplasia is reduced in patients with Roux-en-Y gastrectomy, a procedure that will carry the bile flow more distally to the jejunum and not allow direct access to the stomach where it may then form a more prominent component of refluxate that might gain entry to the larynx.

It is now recognized that bile acids have more widespread biochemical effects on cell function.[33,46] The induction of oxidative stress within cells associated with the production of ROS and reactive nitrogen species provides a key link between bile acid reflux and carcinogenesis. ROS can induce DNA damage and increase the burden of mutations within the genome.[29,45] Damage to internal membranes may lead to the release of ROS from the mitochondria that may therefore lead to DNA damage and acquisition of mutations and an increased risk of neoplastic transformation.[44] In experimental models, exposure of cell lines to deoxycholic acid (DCA) enhances nicotinamide adenine dinucleotide phosphate (NADPH) oxidase activity and increases production of ROS.[47,48] These consequences of exposure to (DCA) were abrogated by pretreatment of cells with either scavengers of ROS (N-acetyl cysteine) or chemical inhibitors (such as diphenyleneiodonium, apocynin, and neopterin) of NADPH oxidases, providing strong evidence that oxidative stress induced by exposure to DCA may be mediated by ROS generated through the activity of NADPH oxidases. The phenolic phytochemical rottlerin also inhibits these effects of DCA on epithelial cell lines, but although often quoted as being an inhibitor of protein kinase C, systematic analyses of its chemical properties have shown that it lacks specificity and does not therefore provide strong evidence for the involvement of this specific kinase pathway in the mediation of bile acid-induced oxidative stress.[47–50]

Bile acids are recognized as promoters of cancers of the GI tract, particularly colorectal carcinoma. This property of bile acids does not appear to depend upon activation of their natural receptor molecule, the orphan nuclear receptor farnesoid X receptor.[51] Increased production of ROS is associated with yes-dependent activating phosphorylation of epidermal growth factor receptor, a key transmembrane tyrosine kinase signaling molecule implicated in the regulation of proliferative responses in laryngeal squamous epithelial cells.[48] Other studies, however, have shown that exposure of normal colonic epithelial cells and colonic cancer cells to low doses of DCA increases expression of cyclin E, an effect that might contribute to increased proliferative activity within these cells and therefore suggest a mechanism that could contribute to bile acid-mediated promotion of tumor development.[52] It seems likely that this effect of bile acids will be observed in most cell types exposed as the ability of bile acids to stimulate cell proliferation has been demonstrated in other cell types; taurodeoxycholic acid can stimulate a proliferative response in an esophageal adenocarcinoma cell line, and in this system the proliferative response is associated with activation of phosphatidylinositol-specific phospholipase C gamma 2, extracellular signal-regulated kinase (ERK) 2/mitogen-activated protein kinase signaling pathways.[53]

These effects of bile acids may therefore be of significance in the pathogenesis of laryngeal carcinoma in those patients with LPR. In keeping with studies outlined above, Hong et al also noted that the cells exposed to bile acids were subject to oxidative stress with increased production of ROS that could then be associated with the acquisition of an increased mutational load within the cell population. Collectively, these properties and effects of bile acids were felt to be important contributors to the molecular pathogenesis of Barrett adenocarcinoma, but in principle, delivery of a mitogenic stimulus to cells exposed to increased mutational risk provides a fertile soil within which any form of cancer may develop.[53]

There are mechanisms available to cells to resist such damaging effects of potentially carcinogenic agents. Tumor suppressor proteins and DNA repair pathways are crucial in this regard. Bile acids have been shown to inhibit the activity of the tumor suppressor protein p53, also known as the guardian of the genome.[54] This protein is a stress-inducible nuclear phosphoprotein that when stabilized and activated by various forms of cell stress binds to DNA in a sequence-specific manner and regulates the expression of an array of downstream target genes that mediate the effector functions of the p53 response within the cell. These functions are critical for the integrity of the tumor suppressor function of p53, the tumor suppressor activity of this protein being most closely linked to its ability to induce either cell cycle arrest or apoptosis. It is therefore significant that ursoDCA and its taurine conjugate have been associated with proteasomal degradation of p53 mediated by binding to the E3 ubiquitin ligase mdm2. Depletion of cellular p53 in this way was associated with reduced levels of p53 bound to DNA as well as reduced expression of the proapoptotic p53-dependent gene *bax*.[46,55–57]

These studies suggest one mechanism by which bile acids can attenuate the capacity of a cell to engage apoptotic pathways. As it has also been shown that DCA can inhibit apoptosis through activation of nuclear factor κB-dependent pathways, it is evident that the effect of bile acids on biochemical events within the cell is complex; indeed, some forms of bile acid stimulate apoptosis.[32,58]

Conclusion

In terms of their clinical presentation and behavior, cancers are a diverse group of disorders that can be considered together because they all share certain fundamental biological properties. This notion was most eloquently defined by Willis (1948)[59] in his classic description of a neoplasm. The basic tenets that this definition advances have been borne out in the molecular era. Indeed, the seminal descriptions of the molecular era by Hanahan and Weinberg[60,61] reiterate and extend these principles in the context of molecular and cell biological parameters that are now widely accepted. In consideration of potential mechanisms by which reflux disease might be associated with an increased risk of laryngeal neoplasia, there is now a substantial and growing body of evidence by which reflux disease can be linked to many of these defining principles. Bile acids in particular have the capacity to engender an intracellular environment in which DNA damage with increased mutational load can occur. The present evidence also suggests that bile acids may attenuate important cellular defense mechanisms such as the function of p53 tumor suppressor activity, in particular p53-dependent apoptosis. In this context, the mitogenic signals may also be delivered to the cell through enhanced signaling through receptor tyrosine kinases, ERK/MAP kinase pathways, and increased expression of cyclin E. Other constituents of the refluxate may facilitate bile acid-mediated cell damage, and collectively these properties of bile acids and other components of refluxate have the potential to act in concert to drive changes within laryngeal epithelial cells that provide a molecular basis for the association of reflux disease with laryngeal cancer. Thus, the molecular biology of laryngeal cancer is becoming more intriguing as newer players in its mechanism are being identified and explored.

References

1. Barnes L, Tse LLY, Hunt JL, et al. Tumours of the hypopharynx, larynx and trachea: introduction. In: WHO Classification of Tumours: Head and Neck Tumours. Oxford: Oxford University Press; 2005:107–162

2. http://info.cancerresearchuk.org/cancerstats/types/larynx/incidence/

3. Fearon ER, Vogelstein B. A genetic model for colorectal tumorigenesis. Cell 1990;61(5):759–767

4. Smith G, Carey FA, Beattie J, et al. Mutations in APC, Kirsten-ras, and p53—alternative genetic pathways to colorectal cancer. Proc Natl Acad Sci U S A 2002;99(14):9433–9438

5. Söreide K, Janssen EA, Söiland H, Körner H, Baak JP. Microsatellite instability in colorectal cancer. Br J Surg 2006;93(4):395–406

6. Gale N, Michaels L, Luzar B, et al. Current review on squamous intraepithelial lesions of the larynx. Histopathology 2009;54(6):639–656

7. Tuyns AJ, Estève J, Raymond L, et al. Cancer of the larynx/hypopharynx, tobacco and alcohol: IARC international case-control study in Turin and Varese (Italy), Zaragoza and Navarra (Spain), Geneva (Switzerland) and Calvados (France). Int J Cancer 1988;41(4):483–491

8. Brennan JA, Boyle JO, Koch WM, et al. Association between cigarette smoking and mutation of the p53 gene in squamous-cell carcinoma of the head and neck. N Engl J Med 1995;332(11):712–717

9. Berkower AS, Biller HF. Head and neck cancer associated with Bloom's syndrome. Laryngoscope 1988;98(7):746–748

10. Ellis NA, Groden J, Ye TZ, et al. The Bloom's syndrome gene product is homologous to RecQ helicases. Cell 1995;83(4):655–666

11. Syrjänen S. The role of human papillomavirus infection in head and neck cancers. Ann Oncol 2010;21(Suppl 7):vii243–vii245

12. Dayyani F, Etzel CJ, Liu M, Ho CH, Lippman SM, Tsao AS. Meta-analysis of the impact of human papillomavirus (HPV) on cancer risk and overall survival in head and neck squamous cell carcinomas (HNSCC). Head Neck Oncol 2010;2:15

13. Gale N. Papilloma/Papillomatosis in WHO Classification of Tumours: Head and Neck Tumours. Oxford: Oxford University Press; 2005

14. Cammarota G, Galli J, Cianci R, et al. Association of laryngeal cancer with previous gastric resection. Ann Surg 2004;240(5):817–824

15. Galli J, Cammarota G, Calò L, et al. The role of acid and alkaline reflux in laryngeal squamous cell carcinoma. Laryngoscope 2002;112(10):1861–1865

16. Blumin JH, Merati AL, Toohill RJ. Duodenogastroesophageal reflux and its effect on extraesophageal tissues: a review. Ear Nose Throat J 2008;87(4):234–237

17. De Corso E, Baroni S, Agostino S, et al. Bile acids and total bilirubin detection in saliva of patients submitted to gastric surgery and in particular to subtotal Billroth II resection. Ann Surg 2007;245(6):880–885

18. Gill GA, Johnston N, Buda A, et al. Laryngeal epithelial defenses against laryngopharyngeal reflux: investigations of E-cadherin, carbonic anhydrase isoenzyme III, and pepsin. Ann Otol Rhinol Laryngol 2005;114(12):913–921

19. Johnston N, Knight J, Dettmar PW, Lively MO, Koufman J. Pepsin and carbonic anhydrase isoenzyme III as diagnostic markers for laryngopharyngeal reflux disease. Laryngoscope 2004;114(12):2129–2134

20. Johnston N, Wells CW, Blumin JH, Toohill RJ, Merati AL. Receptor-mediated uptake of pepsin by laryngeal epithelial cells. Ann Otol Rhinol Laryngol 2007;116(12):934–938

21. Wassenaar E, Johnston N, Merati A, et al. Pepsin detection in patients with laryngopharyngeal reflux before and after fundoplication. Surg Endosc 2011;25(12):3870–3876

22. Westcott CJ, Hopkins MB, Bach K, Postma GN, Belafsky PC, Koufman JA. Fundoplication for laryngopharyngeal reflux disease. J Am Coll Surg 2004;199(1):23–30

23. Yagui-Beltran A, Craig AL, Lawrie L, et al. The human oesophageal squamous epithelium exhibits a novel type of heat shock protein response. Eur J Biochem 2001;268(20):5343–5355

24. Johnston N, Dettmar PW, Lively MO, et al. Effect of pepsin on laryngeal stress protein (Sep70, Sep53, and Hsp70) response: role in laryngopharyngeal reflux disease. Ann Otol Rhinol Laryngol 2006;115(1):47–58

25. Leu JI, Pimkina J, Frank A, Murphy ME, George DL. A small molecule inhibitor of inducible heat shock protein 70. Mol Cell 2009;36(1):15–27

26. Leu JI, Pimkina J, Pandey P, Murphy ME, George DL. HSP70 inhibition by the small-molecule 2-phenylethynesulfonamide impairs protein clearance pathways in tumor cells. Mol Cancer Res 2011;9(7):936–947

27. Johnston N, Wells CW, Samuels TL, Blumin JH. Rationale for targeting pepsin in the treatment of reflux disease. Ann Otol Rhinol Laryngol 2010;119(8):547–558

28. Galli J, Calò L, Agostino S, et al. Bile reflux as possible risk factor in laryngopharyngeal inflammatory and neoplastic lesions. Acta Otorhinolaryngol Ital 2003;23(5):377–382

29. Bernstein H, Bernstein C, Payne CM, Dvorak K. Bile acids as endogenous etiologic agents in gastrointestinal cancer. World J Gastroenterol 2009;15(27):3329–3340

30. Monte MJ, Marin JJ, Antelo A, Vazquez-Tato J. Bile acids: chemistry, physiology, and pathophysiology. World J Gastroenterol 2009;15(7):804–816

31. Sobala GM, O'Connor HJ, Dewar EP, King RF, Axon AT, Dixon MF. Bile reflux and intestinal metaplasia in gastric mucosa. J Clin Pathol 1993;46(3):235–240

32. Bernstein H, Bernstein C, Payne CM, Dvorakova K, Garewal H. Bile acids as carcinogens in human gastrointestinal cancers. Mutat Res 2005;589(1):47–65

33. McQuaid KR, Laine L, Fennerty MB, Souza R, Spechler SJ. Systematic review: the role of bile acids in the pathogenesis of

gastro-oesophageal reflux disease and related neoplasia. Aliment Pharmacol Ther 2011;34(2):146–165

34. Galli J, Cammarota G, De Corso E, et al. Biliary laryngopharyngeal reflux: a new pathological entity. Curr Opin Otolaryngol Head Neck Surg 2006;14(3):128–132

35. Hohenester S, Wenniger LM, Paulusma CC, et al. A biliary HCO3- umbrella constitutes a protective mechanism against bile acid-induced injury in human cholangiocytes. Hepatology 2012;55(1):173–183

36. Lillemoe KD, Johnson LF, Harmon JW. Alkaline esophagitis: a comparison of the ability of components of gastroduodenal contents to injure the rabbit esophagus. Gastroenterology 1983;85(3):621–628

37. Bateson MC, Hopwood D, Milne G, Bouchier IA. Oesophageal epithelial ultrastructure after incubation with gastrointestinal fluids and their components. J Pathol 1981;133(1):33–51

38. Lillemoe KD, Johnson LF, Harmon JW. Role of the components of the gastroduodenal contents in experimental acid esophagitis. Surgery 1982;92(2):276–284

39. Hopwood D, Bateson MC, Milne G, Bouchier IA. Effects of bile acids and hydrogen ion on the fine structure of oesophageal epithelium. Gut 1981;22(4):306–311

40. Chen X, Oshima T, Tomita T, et al. Acidic bile salts modulate the squamous epithelial barrier function by modulating tight junction proteins. Am J Physiol Gastrointest Liver Physiol 2011;301(2):G203–G209

41. Morita K, Miyachi Y, Furuse M. Tight junctions in epidermis: from barrier to keratinization. Eur J Dermatol 2011;21(1):12–17

42. Furuse M, Hata M, Furuse K, et al. Claudin-based tight junctions are crucial for the mammalian epidermal barrier: a lesson from claudin-1-deficient mice. J Cell Biol 2002;156(6):1099–1111

43. Turksen K, Troy TC. Junctions gone bad: claudins and loss of the barrier in cancer. Biochim Biophys Acta 2011;1816(1):73–79

44. Darragh J, Hunter M, Pohler E, et al. The calcium-binding domain of the stress protein SEP53 is required for survival in response to deoxycholic acid-mediated injury. FEBS J 2006;273(9):1930–1947

45. Cronin J, Williams L, McAdam E, et al. The role of secondary bile acids in neoplastic development in the oesophagus. Biochem Soc Trans 2010;38(2):337–342

46. Amaral JD, Castro RE, Solá S, Steer CJ, Rodrigues CM. p53 is a key molecular target of ursodeoxycholic acid in regulating apoptosis. J Biol Chem 2007;282(47):34250–34259

47. Reinehr R, Becker S, Keitel V, Eberle A, Grether-Beck S, Häussinger D. Bile salt-induced apoptosis involves NADPH oxidase isoform activation. Gastroenterology 2005;129(6):2009–2031

48. Sommerfeld A, Reinehr R, Häussinger D. Bile acid-induced epidermal growth factor receptor activation in quiescent rat hepatic stellate cells can trigger both proliferation and apoptosis. J Biol Chem 2009;284(33):22173–22183

49. Longpre JM, Loo G. Protection of human colon epithelial cells against deoxycholate by rottlerin. Apoptosis 2008;13(9):1162–1171

50. Davies SP, Reddy H, Caivano M, Cohen P. Specificity and mechanism of action of some commonly used protein kinase inhibitors. Biochem J 2000;351(Pt 1):95–105

51. Modica S, Murzilli S, Salvatore L, Schmidt DR, Moschetta A. Nuclear bile acid receptor FXR protects against intestinal tumorigenesis. Cancer Res 2008;68(23):9589–9594

52. Ha YH, Park DG. Effects of DCA on cell cycle proteins in colonocytes. J Korean Soc Coloproctol 2010;26(4):254–259

53. Hong J, Behar J, Wands J, et al. Bile acid reflux contributes to development of esophageal adenocarcinoma via activation of phosphatidylinositol-specific phospholipase Cgamma2 and NADPH oxidase NOX5-S. Cancer Res 2010;70(3):1247–1255

54. Lane DP. Cancer. p53, guardian of the genome. Nature 1992;358(6381):15–16

55. Amaral JD, Viana RJ, Ramalho RM, Steer CJ, Rodrigues CM. Bile acids: regulation of apoptosis by ursodeoxycholic acid. J Lipid Res 2009;50(9):1721–1734

56. Amaral JD, Xavier JM, Steer CJ, Rodrigues CM. Targeting the p53 pathway of apoptosis. Curr Pharm Des 2010a;16(22):2493–2503

57. Amaral JD, Castro RE, Solá S, Steer CJ, Rodrigues CM. Ursodeoxycholic acid modulates the ubiquitin-proteasome degradation pathway of p53. Biochem Biophys Res Commun 2010;400(4):649–654

58. Huo X, Juergens S, Zhang X, et al. Deoxycholic acid causes DNA damage while inducing apoptotic resistance through NF-κB activation in benign Barrett's epithelial cells. Am J Physiol Gastrointest Liver Physiol 2011;301(2):G278–G286

59. Willis RA. Definition of tumour. In: Pathology of Tumours. London: Butterworth & Co.; 1948:1–8

60. Hanahan D, Weinberg RA. The hallmarks of cancer. Cell 2000;100(1):57–70

61. Hanahan D, Weinberg RA. Hallmarks of cancer: the next generation. Cell 2011;144(5):646–674

Section C

Clinical Assessment and Diagnostic Procedures

6 Clinical Assessment of Voice Disorders

Julian A. McGlashan

Normal and Disordered Voice

The human voice gives us our identity and personality, and it changes throughout our lives from birth through to senescence. It is actually difficult to simply define a normal voice, but it is usually described as having the following characteristics:

- It is audible, clear, or stable in a wide range of acoustic settings.
- It is appropriate for the gender and age of the speaker.
- It is capable of fulfilling its linguistic and paralinguistic functions.
- It does not fatigue easily.
- It is not associated with discomfort or pain on phonation.

Voice quality is an extremely important element in how well a message is communicated with positive and negative effects. A "good" voice can captivate our attention or stir our emotions and is an essential attribute for a performance-level professional voice user such as an entertainer, an actor, a singer, or a broadcaster. However, a "bad" voice, which may sound strained, weak, rough, monotonous, or inappropriate in pitch, can cause the listener to become distracted and bored or lose concentration. Variations in voice quality can provide valuable cues about our current emotions, physical health, and psychological well-being.

There is also a continuum between normal and disordered or pathological voice. Individuals, with what an objective listener would consider a pathological voice, may be quite comfortable with their voice quality considering it "their voice"—as long as it fulfills their functional needs.

Indeed, abnormal speaking and singing voice qualities can sometimes help determine the personality and character of a professional voice.

Patients seek help with their voice problem because they are suffering some form of disability that can take three main forms: (1) *impairment*, which is a structural problem with the vocal apparatus, for example, a laryngeal tumor causing an alteration in function such as hoarseness; (2) *limitation in activity*, for example, reduced vocal range in singing or voice tiring with use; and (3) *participation restriction*, for example, not being able to work or sing in a choir as a result of the voice problem (http://www.who.int/topics/disabilities/en/).[1] The consequences of voice problems can be physical, functional, psychosocial, occupational, or financial.

Normal and Disordered Voice Production

To understand the link between impairment, activity limitations, and participation restrictions, it is important to briefly review the normal mechanism of voice production and how this mechanism can be affected by pathological processes.

Normal Voice Production

Normal voice production (phonation) is discussed in detail in Chapter 4. Simplistically, voice production requires three processes: (1) an energy source—provided by the lungs; (2) a vibrating structure—usually the two vocal folds in normal voice production; and (3) a resonator—the vocal tract (**Table 6.1**). The vocal folds are adducted and the free edges of the

Table 6.1 Systematic Checking Process for Identification of Pathology in Voice Disorders and Their Relevance

Which Essential Element of Voice Production Is Affected?	Which Pathological Processes Are Present?

1. Energy source: provided by the lungs and causing the vocal folds to vibrate
2. Vibrating structure: the vocal folds—the sound source of the voice
3. Resonator: the vocal tract—modulating the acoustic properties of the sound source (vowels) and adding additional sounds (consonants) to produce recognizable speech and singing voice tones
	1. Structural/neoplastic abnormality
	  • Malignant
	  • Benign
	2. Inflammation
	  • Infective
	  • Noninfective
	3. Neuromuscular dysfunction
	  • Hyperfunctional
	  • Hypofunctional
	  • Mixed hyper-/hypofunctional
	  • Control/coordination issues
	4. Muscle tension imbalance
	  • Primary
	  • Secondary

mucosal surfaces start to vibrate causing compression followed by rarefaction of air molecules, which is the fundamental property of the generation of a periodic sound wave.[2]

The frequency of vibration of the vocal folds (fundamental frequency) is determined by their elastic properties and tensioning.[2] The actual sound that a listener hears, however, is determined by the resonance properties of the vocal tract. The resonance properties and the consequent filtering effect can be modulated by the shaping and structure of the vocal tract. The sound emitted from the mouth therefore consists of the fundamental frequency and the nonfiltered multiples of the fundamental frequency (harmonics or overtones). This filtering effect results in concentrations of sound energy at specific frequency bands (formants) that we interpret as individual vowel sounds. Additional sound elements can be added by constricting parts of the vocal tract in production of consonants.[3]

Pathological Processes Causing Voice Problems

There are four main pathological processes that can contribute to the voice becoming disordered (**Table 6.1**). It is essential that the presence or absence of these four processes is checked for systematically, particularly as voice disorders tend to be multifactorial (**Fig. 6.1**). This also reduces the chances of overlooking pathologies, for example, a vocal fold paresis in cases of apparent *muscle tension imbalance*. Each pathological process can affect any part of the three essential elements of voice production, that is, breath control, vocal fold vibration, and resonance. This is determined by careful history and examination, occasional specialist assessments, and probe therapy or empirical treatment. However, by looking for evidence for each of the four etiologic factors individually, the clinician is able to target the treatment more precisely.

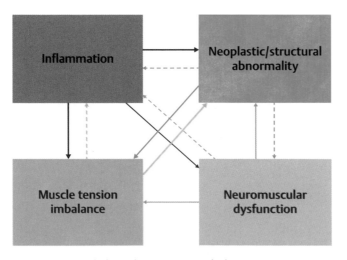

Figure 6.1 Pathological processes and their interactions. Voice disorders are often multifactorial in origin. More than one pathological process may be present or one can lead to another.

It is also important to try and ascertain which is the primary factor and which are secondary or compensatory factors affecting the voice quality. This is not always the same as the patient's complaint!

Clinical Example of Interaction

A patient with long-standing Reinke edema (*structural abnormality*) may develop laryngopharyngeal reflux (*inflammation*), which stiffens the tissues making them more difficult to vibrate. This in turn may require increased muscular effort (*muscle tension imbalance*) and a more strained voice quality. This increased muscular effort may be compounded by the patient's concern that he or she might have cancer from smoking. Treating the reflux and muscle tension elements may mean the Reinke edema does not require surgical treatment. In fact surgical treatment can be positively detrimental. In some cases, it can cause stiffened, scarred vocal folds (iatrogenic *impairment*), making voice production more difficult causing *activity limitations* and social *participation restrictions*.

Operating on the Reinke edema usually involves reducing the bulk of the vocal folds with the consequence of increasing the pitch of the voice. This can affect the patient's self-identity particularly in women, leading to further psychological issues. This is in contrast to the patient with Reinke edema who dislikes the sound of and the negative comments about the voice because it is too deep and who has given up smoking. Surgery, after appropriate counseling, can then have significant positive effects on the quality of life.

Inadequate Energy Input (Breath Support)

To vibrate, healthy vocal folds need an adequate flow of air from the lungs and generation of subglottic pressure to overcome the inertia and viscoelasticity of the apposed vocal folds to induce oscillation. This minimum pressure to initiate phonation is known as the phonation threshold pressure. Values of phonation threshold pressure are in the order of 3 to 5 cm H_2O but once oscillating the pressure can be reduced by 1 to 2 cm H_2O.[4] *Structural* or *inflammatory* changes in any part of the lower respiratory tract from alveoli to trachea or chest wall (polymyositis, poliomyelitis, severe chest wall, or diaphragmatic deficiencies) may potentially affect voice production secondary to hypoventilation. Similarly, weakness of the respiratory muscles may result from *neuromuscular disorders* such as Guillain-Barré syndrome, motor neuron disease, and myasthenia gravis.

Primary abnormal breathing patterns (*muscle tension imbalance* of respiratory muscles) are a common cause of voice disorders, resulting in inefficient speech-breathing patterns.[5,6] By relying on the accessory respiratory muscles (high clavicular breathing pattern) rather than the diaphragm, patients may feel they are running out of air when they talk.[7,8] In paradoxical vocal cord dysfunction, when there is adduction of the vocal cords during inspiration causing inspiratory stridor, there may be associated dysphonia.[9]

Disease processes may not be isolated to the respiratory muscles or the effects on the voice may be overshadowed by the respiratory symptoms. There is a huge amount of reserve in the system and also in the ability to compensate, so the effects of chest disease may not be apparent until they are quite severe. In the most extreme situation, the patient may be aphonic due to the effort required in breathing. When present, voice problems include running out of air while speaking, weakness or breathiness of the voice, an inability to control the pitch or loudness, a lack of volume, and/or an inability to project the voice.

Dysfunction of Vibratory Apparatus

To vibrate efficiently and effectively, the vocal cords need to come together and oscillate in a controlled regular manner. A gap between the vocal folds causes *breathiness*, whereas irregular vibration or involvement of supraglottic structures causes *roughness*. *Hoarseness* is the perception of voice abnormality, which can be due to breathiness, roughness, or a combination of the two.

To vibrate effectively, the vocal cords need an adequate driving (subglottic) pressure. This is determined by the airflow and resistance (gap) at the glottis (Pressure = Flow × Resistance). If the gap is too large (low resistance), the flow is too high to maintain the pressure necessary to vibrate the vocal folds. Air escapes giving a breathy voice and the poor vocal fold vibration does not lead to the generation of good-quality sound waves. The patient may not be able to produce a loud voice or be heard above background noise, the patient's voice may tire with use, or the patient may run out of air while talking and suffer throat dryness or paralaryngeal discomfort.

If the vocal folds are held too tightly together or there is an imbalance in tension or mass or if the layered structure of the vocal folds is abnormal, they will not be able to vibrate effectively, giving a hoarse, rough, or strained voice quality. They may also suffer with some of the above symptoms due to the increased effort in phonation and poor resonance.

In some cases of primary *muscle tension dysphonia*, there is excessive medial, anteroposterior, or concentric constriction at the glottic or supraglottic level (**Table 6.2**).[5] The vocal folds may be partially or sometimes completely obscured by the false folds during attempted phonation. Several patterns associated with distinct voice profiles have been identified.[10–14] The effect on the voice can vary in severity, be intermittent or constant, and be episodic. Muscle tension dysphonia (Type IIb) can also be secondary to a structural, neuromuscular, or inflammatory cause requiring increased laryngeal muscular effort to overcome the underlying defect (**Table 6.2**). Psychological issues can lead to either excessive vocal or false fold constriction (Type II) preventing air passing through the larynx or the vocal folds being excessively tensed and splinted apart but with little or no air flow (Type IV).

In *neuromuscular* cases, the degree of vocal fold contact during phonation can vary between being fully abducted, that is, in the "cadaveric" position (e.g. in brainstem injury) to reduced contact that may only be apparent with prolonged voice use (e.g. in myasthenia or a paresis). No contact or reduced contact affects the ability of the lungs to generate sufficient subglottal pressure to lead to sustained vocal fold vibration. The voice is whispery due to turbulent airflow through the glottis and from vocal tract constriction. In unilateral vocal fold palsies, the gap is variable and depends on many factors including the degree of compensation (**Table 6.3**). To achieve better closure, the larynx may become asymmetrical and the vocal folds may stretch, allowing better closure and loudness but at the expense of a rise in pitch. In unilateral superior laryngeal nerve palsy, the symptoms may be vague but there may be diplophonia and instability of the voice at higher pitches.[15] Findings can be subtle but include asymmetry of the posterior glottis and petiole of the epiglottis at higher pitches.[16]

Although the vocal folds can vibrate irregularly in neuromuscular disorders and muscle tension dysphonia due to tensioning abnormalities, the effects on the voice are often overshadowed by other perceptual features such as breathiness and abnormalities in pitch or loudness. Roughness is more common when there is evidence of *inflammation* or *structural abnormalities* of the vocal folds. Inflammation can cause surface exudate (thickened mucus and/or ulceration) or inflammatory changes in the vocal fold mucosa. Structural lesions have variable effects depending on which layer or layers of the lamina propria or vocal fold are affected, the resultant effect on the remaining normal structures, and the compensatory response. For example, an early cancer extending from the epithelium to the deeper underlying muscle on one vocal fold inhibits the mucosal wave so that it cannot vibrate and produce a sound wave. The main effect on the voice is actually the aperiodic vibration of the opposite normal vocal fold caused by the mass effect of the cancer, which is perceived as roughness. This can be seen on stroboscopy or high-speed recordings. An increase in the mass of the vocal folds will lower the pitch of the voice: other mass effects may lead to supraglottic structures vibrating, adding an additional deep rough quality to the sound. If the mass lesion prevents complete glottal closure, air will escape through the glottis causing added breathiness to the voice quality. Analyzing what structures can and cannot vibrate the size of the glottal gap and what can be realistically restored to normal underpins the surgical treatment principles of phonosurgery.

In summary, if air is allowed to escape through the vocal folds from incomplete closure (glottal gap), then a breathy quality will be added to the voice. Abnormalities of the mass, the layered structure, in tensioning, or the elasticity of the vocal folds will cause them to vibrate in a disordered and irregular (aperiodic) manner. This will cause roughness, strain, or pitch abnormalities. Supraglottic structures such as the false folds, aryepiglottic folds, and arytenoid mucosa may also be induced to vibrate. This may be in addition to, or more rarely replace vibration of the vocal folds causing deepening of the pitch and roughness of the voice.

Table 6.2 Different Patterns of MTD Based on Morrison Classification

	Glottis	Supraglottis	Paralaryngeal Structures	Profile	Voice
MTD Type I (laryngeal isometric pattern)	Anterior two-thirds of vibrating vocal folds pressed tightly together Large interarytenoid and posterior glottis chink May be associated with vocal nodules or edema	False cords retracted posteriorly Some medial constriction anterior half	Generalized increased tension, especially suprahyoid and pharyngeal muscles Closed cricothyroid visor due to excessive chronic cricothyroid muscle contraction	Professional voice users Poor vocal technique Excessive demands on voice Anxiety or other psychological factors Personality traits, extrovert	Breathy/harsh quality Constricted Low pitch Poor pitch control at upper part of range of voice Pitch and voice breaks
MTD Type IIa (lateral contraction glottal level)	Hyperadduction Prolonged closed phase Reduced vibratory amplitude of mucosal wave	Variable hyperaddution	In coordination with breathing Closed cricothyroid visor due to excessive chronic cricothyroid muscle contraction	Poor vocal habits, posture, or technique More likely psychogenic factors if false cord involvement	Harsh/strident quality Aggressive voice onsets Vocal fatigue Laryngeal discomfort Tender cricothyroid muscle, tight visor
MTD Type IIb (lateral contraction false cord level)	Tightly adducted *or* partially abducted *or* poor contact from bowed vocal folds	Variable hyperaddution: from midline contact to prominence above mid-membranous vocal folds	Variable paralaryngeal tenderness	Psychogenic dysphonia or *compensatory* for poor glottic closure, e.g., neurological weakness, sulcus vergeture, or presbyphonia	High-pitched squeaky, effortful voice or breathy, tense whisper
MTD Type III (anterosuperior supraglottal compression)	Vocal fold contact may be reduced Vocal folds appear shortened	Reduced space between epiglottis and arytenoids May be some false cord phonation	Backed tongue base May have habitually raised or lowered larynx Closed cricothyroid visor due to excessive chronic cricothyroid muscle contraction	Need to put on authoritative voice Nonpathological cases—often seen in vocal performers	Effortful voice, rapid fatigue Constricted, harsh phonation Low pitch Poor resonance due to pharyngeal constriction May be normal appearance in loud voice phonation
MDT Type IV (conversion aphonia/ dysphonia)	Vocal folds look normal but are splinted apart	Normal or stretched	May be tender in paralaryngeal muscles	May be anxious or depressed May have "*la belle indifference*" in conversion disorders Often underlying psychological issues	Aphonia or whispery May have normal cough and laugh

MTD, muscle tension dysphonia.

Table 6.3 Factors that Determine the Unpredictable Voice Outcome Following Damage to the Neural Supply to the Larynx

Factor	Comment
Patient factors: • Individual patient neuroanatomy	• There is considerable variability in the degree of anastomoses between right and left, superior and recurrent, laryngeal nerves. • This complex arrangement helps explain some of the variability in presentation, compensation, reinnervation, and recovery from patient to patient.

Injury factors:
• Level of injury
  ○ Recurrent laryngeal nerve (RLN)
  ○ Superior laryngeal nerve (SLN)
  ○ High vagal (RLN+SLN)
• Degree of neural damage
  ○ Complete transection or crush injury
  ○ Partial transection or infiltration
  ○ Segmental demyelination
  ○ Tumor infiltration/scarring
	• The degree and severity of the conduction block resulting from the injury also influence recovery.
	• The severity of the neural injury can vary from segmental demyelination (neuropraxia) to preservation of the neural conduits (axonotmesis) to complete severance (neurotmesis).
	• A full recovery is usual in neuropraxia as remyelination over the preserved axon restoring conduction and function. In neurotmesis, only a small proportion of fibers bridge the gap between proximal and distal ends being inversely proportional to the size of the gap.
	• To complicate matters further, the RLN carries mixed adductor and abductor fibers so reinnervation is a random process, which leads to synkinesis.
	• Other factors influencing recovery and the voice outcome include neurogenic muscle atrophy and vocal fold height disparity.

Ineffectiveness of the Vocal Tract Resonator

If air is blown through an excised human larynx with the vocal folds adducted, the sound produced has a buzzing quality unlike any recognizable voice quality. This is similar to blowing through an oboe reed that is not attached to the bore of the instrument. The shaping of the vocal tract allows standing waves to develop in the air column. The sound produced by resonance of the air column consists of the fundamental frequency (determined by the frequency of vibration of the vocal folds) and certain harmonics (multiples of the fundamental frequency). Some of these harmonics are effectively filtered out by reducing their intensity, which has the effect of enhancing the energy in certain bands of frequencies (formants). Our brain recognizes these patterns of sound energy concentrated in specific frequency bands as a specific sound character, that is, a vowel. By changing the length and the shape of the resonating chamber (vocal tract), the energy and intensity of sound in specific frequency bands (formants) change. Our brain recognizes the new pattern as a different vowel. It is important to recognize that the fundamental frequency and the harmonics generated by the vibration of the vocal folds may not have changed, rather it is only the effect of the filter of the harmonics that has changed. Consonant sounds in contrast are produced by passing air through constrictions in the vocal tract and can be associated either with vocal fold vibration (voiced) or without (voiceless). For a more in-depth discussion, see Kent et al (1996).[3]

Individual variations of the vocal tract (supraglottis, piriform fossae, oropharynx, palate, oral cavity, postnasal space, and nasal cavity) are largely responsible for giving us our unique voices. However, structural abnormalities, neuromuscular deficits, inappropriate excessive constriction (muscle tension imbalance), and inflammation of any part of the vocal tract will affect the resonance characteristics of the air column and hence the voice quality. In extreme cases of *structural abnormality* such as a cleft lip and palate, the resonance patterns and vocal tract constrictions are less precise, making both the vowel and consonant components of the speech sound more difficult to interpret.[17] *Neuromuscular* lesions such as a stroke have variable effects depending on the area and extent of the brain that is affected. The vocal tract can undergo structural changes (due to muscle atrophy or spasticity) and there can be a lack of control of the articulators causing dysarthria. The effect is imprecise consonants, distorted vowels, and hypernasality.[18,19]

Inflammation, for example, an upper aerodigestive tract infection, affects the resonance characteristics in two ways. The inflammatory process is likely to alter the elasticity of the mucous membranes and therefore the reflective properties of the lining of the vocal tract. Second, there may be changes due to certain resonance chambers, for example, the nasal passages and sinuses being narrowed or occluded. This may be in addition to any inflammatory effects on the vocal folds. The dominant effects on an individual's voice will vary depending on their anatomy and the nature and severity of the disease process. The voice tonal quality may change and become, for example, "hyponasal," with a reduction of higher frequency energy due to damping. This has been shown to affect speech intelligibility using automatic speech recognition software.[20] Attempts to overcome this effect may result in additional laryngeal effort (increased glottal contact), sometimes risking damage to the vocal fold mucosa.

For the standing waves to be generated efficiently, the lower end of the air column (glottis) needs to be closed. In other words, if there is a glottal gap, energy can escape back into the lungs, which reduces the energy in the transmitted sound from the lips. Muscular constriction of the pharynx, incorrect laryngeal height, too much tightness in the jaw, and tongue narrowing the oral cavity all reduce the effectiveness of the resonating chamber in voice projection, which is often found in cases of *muscle tension dysphonia*.

Clinical Assessment

A key responsibility as a health professional is to provide an accurate diagnosis to avoid injudicious surgery or prolonged voice therapy that can have detrimental effects on the voice or, at the very least, be a waste of time and resources. Other patient relevant factors that should be taken into consideration during a consultation are listed in **Table 6.4**.

Clinical Setting

Ideally, all voice disordered patients should be managed by an ENT surgeon and speech pathologist (SP) with a specialized interest in voice disorders. Different models of working exist such as independent working but an integrated team approach, a joint voice clinic (SP + ENT), parallel clinics (SP-led clinic with ENT input available), and SP alone (SP sees triaged referrals). The availability of these services is determined by the enthusiasm and collective experience of the team members, the types of referrals seen in the department, and pragmatism. Other members of a voice disorders service may include a singing teacher, clinical psychologist, osteopath, and physiotherapist. A key element

of a voice clinic is the availability of stroboscopy. This is a pragmatic tool for the detailed assessment of the vibrating vocal folds (see Chapter 7). Other imaging techniques such as high-speed digital video recording and videokymography are gaining in popularity and are useful in understanding complex vibratory behavior. Other common methods of assessment include acoustic analysis, electromyography, electrolaryngography, and aerodynamic measurements (see Chapter 7). These can be used to provide supporting evidence for the diagnosis, the objective evaluation of severity, and specific outcome measures.

History

In voice assessment, it is necessary to take a detailed history. It is important to determine the following:

- The nature and chronology of the voice problem.
- Exacerbating and relieving factors.
- Lifestyle, dietary, and hydration issues.
- Contributing medical conditions or the effects of their treatment.
- The patient's voice use and requirements.
- The impact on their quality of life and social and psychological well-being.
- Their expectations for outcome of the consultation and treatment.
- The patients' complaints which are most frequently related to changes in voice quality (hoarseness, roughness, and breathiness).

Table 6.4 Adapted General Medical Council Guidance on the Information Patients Have a Right to Know Following a Consultation About Their Voice

- The diagnosis

- Prognosis and the consequences if the condition is not treated

- Uncertainties in the diagnosis and possibilities for further investigation

- Options for treatment, including the option of not treating

- The purpose of proposed investigation or treatment, details of therapies, including subsidiary treatment such as pain relief, and details of what the patient can expect to experience

- Details of common side effects

- Explanations of the benefits of each option for treatment

- Details of serious or frequently occurring risks and lifestyle changes that may be necessary as a result of the treatment

- Advice as to whether the treatment is experimental (or evidence for treatment is poor)

- How the patient's condition and possible side effects may be monitored

- The name of the health professional in charge of the treatment and names of senior team members if appropriate

- Whether students or trainees may be involved

- The right to change their mind at any time

- The right to seek a second opinion

- Details of any costs or charges, if applicable

Adapted from http://www.gmc-uk.org/static/documents/content/Consent_0510.pdf.

- A pitch that is too high or too low, which is not appropriate for their age and sex.
- An inability to control the voice as required (pitch breaks, voice cutting out).
- An inability to raise the voice or make the voice heard in a noisy environment (reduced loudness).
- An increased effort and/or reduced stamina of the voice, or one that tires with use.
- Difficulties or restrictions in the use of the voice at different times of the day or related to specific daily, social or work-related tasks.
- A reduced ability to communicate effectively.
- Difficulty in singing.
- Throat-related symptoms (soreness, discomfort, aching, dryness, and mucus) particularly related to voice use.
- The consequent emotional and psychological effects caused by the above.

Patients generally use descriptive terms less precisely than clinicians, so a degree of interpretation is required. They will complain or have a voice problem that generally reflects impairment, limitations of activity, and occasionally lack of ability to participate in an activity (http://www.disabilitaincifre. it/documenti/ICF_18.pdf). Self-rating questionnaires such as the Voice Handicap Index,[21] Voice-Related Quality of Life,[22] and Voice Symptom Scale[23] have been developed on the basis of the complaints of patients attending with voice problems (see Chapter 10). The most common impairments relate to the quality of the voice, the pitch, the ability and effort required to produce a loud enough voice, and other throat symptoms. The following is a general guide to the interpretation of vocal complaints and their possible etiology.

Voice Quality

Patients may use the term hoarseness to describe any abnormality of voice quality including roughness, breathiness, weakness (asthenia), and strain. The clinician needs to decide which elements are present and which are most dominant by carefully listening to the voice. This can be quantified using the grade of hoarseness, roughness, breathiness, aesthenia, strain (GRBAS) perceptual rating scale (see Chapter 10).[24]

Hoarse, Croaky, Rough, Gruff, or "Rusty" Voice
This rough or harsh quality to the voice is usually due to irregular (aperiodic) vibration of the vocal folds. The sound may be coarser if supraglottic structures, for example, the false folds or aryepiglottic folds, are involved. It is one of the most common complaints in patients with structural or inflammatory lesions of the vocal folds and in some forms of muscle tension dysphonia.

Creaky Voice
A creaky voice is characterized by a low-pitched (7 to 78 Hz), "popping quality" voice. The vocal folds are normal but tend to close quickly and peel apart slowly resulting in prolonged vocal fold contact with a sudden short opening burst as part of a long vibratory cycle.[25] It is considered to be part of the normal range of voice qualities and appears to be becoming more used in everyday speech, particularly in young women at the end of utterances.[26,27] It can become a problem if it becomes habitual and the patient is required to project the voice or vary the pitch as the range is usually reduced. Raising the loudness of the voice is difficult in creaky voice, for example, while singing, without amplification.

Breathy Voice
Breathiness reflects an inability to bring the vocal folds together and there is a consequent leakage of air through the glottis. It most commonly results from neurological problems such as a vocal cord palsy or paresis,[28] structural problems such as sulcus vergeture,[29] and muscle tension dysphonia such as Morrison Type 4 pattern[13,14] and presbylaryngis.[30] Myasthenia gravis can rarely present with isolated phonatory and speech symptoms such as breathiness, reduced loudness, hypernasality, and dysarthria.[31]

Roughness with Breathiness
Breathiness can be associated with a degree of roughness if the vocal folds vibrate irregularly due to a lesion that physically prevents glottal closure such as a polyp or large ventricular cyst. Conversely, lesions such as vocal fold nodules may be secondary due to tensioning of vocal folds such that the shearing forces on the mucosa cause the localized tissue damage of the nodule. In some circumstances, inadequate glottal closure may also result in the false cords vibrating. If the vocal folds are flaccid due to atrophy, presbylaryngis, or a bilateral paresis, they may vibrate irregularly and with large amplitude, which can also add a rough quality to breathy voice.

Whispery Voice
A whispery voice is produced by turbulent airflow through adducted but nonvibrating vocal folds. If the vocal folds are severely inflamed and phonation is painful or difficult, whispering may be easier and more comfortable for the patient. Sometimes this pattern of speaking continues when the original illness has resolved. Splinting of the vocal folds apart can also be the result of a severe primary muscle tension imbalance (whispery dysphonia)[13,14] or secondary muscle tension imbalance due to poor coordination of breathing with phonation often due to psychogenic reasons.[32] If there is severe structural damage to the vibrating structures of the larynx from trauma and scarring, then there may be no alternative to using a whispery voice if supraglottic structures are not employed as a sound source.

"No Voice" or Aphonia
"No voice" or aphonia may rarely be an extreme form of a breathy voice due to a bilateral adductor vocal fold palsy secondary to a lesion in the brainstem or fixation of cricoarytenoid joints in an abducted position. More

commonly, this is due to a psychogenic muscle tension dysphonia.[32] The vocal folds can either be held together so tightly than no air can pass through or are splinted apart and the breath is held. In rare cases, there may be a dominant cerebral hemisphere lesion affecting Broca area causing an apraxia of phonation, while other widespread cortical lesions cause mutism.[33]

Voice Breaks

This can be in the form of pitch breaks where the voice cracks, squeaks, or becomes (usually) high pitched. Pitch breaks can be used with effect in singing when these are known as register transitions[34] or mode changes.[35] A patient, however, may have no control over what sound is going to come out. Alternatively, the voice may cut out all together. Voice breaks result when some parameter of the vibrating system is changed (e.g., lung pressure, vocal fold tension, or there is an asymmetry of tension or mass between the two vocal folds).[2] For example, failure to maintain an adequate subglottic pressure with adequate breath support is one cause. Voice breaks may also be present when the vocal folds are inflamed, there is a primary muscle tension imbalance such as puberphonia or secondary tensioning asymmetries such as a superior laryngeal nerve palsy. Structural abnormalities of the free edge of the vocal folds such as polyps and nodules can lead to vocal fold mass asymmetry or cause voice breaks from the lesion "catching" on the contralateral vocal fold.

Diplophonia

This is when two distinct pitches can be perceived simultaneously during phonation. It can result from tensioning imbalance in primary muscle tension dysphonia, secondary to a subtle neurological weakness such as a paresis,[36] or when there is a difference in mass between the two vocal folds due to a structural abnormality such as an intracordal cyst.[37] The cyst can act as a vibratory node causing one vocal fold to vibrate at a different phase anterior and posterior to the lesion or at different frequencies. There may also be associated voice breaks.

Tremor

Tremor is a regular wobble or shakiness of the voice (5 to 12 Hz). It is more common in the elderly in isolation or as one of several tremors affecting different parts of the body (essential tremor). It can be present together with other neurological conditions such as cerebellar ataxia (2 or 3 Hz), spasmodic dysphonia (irregular frequency),[38] and late-stage Parkinson disease (4 to 7 Hz).[39]

Fundamental Frequency and Pitch of the Voice

The fundamental frequency of the voice is the measurable vibratory frequency of the sound source, which is in most cases the vocal folds. Pitch is a psychoacoustic phenomenon defined as "that attribute of auditory sensation in terms of

which sounds may be ordered on a scale extending from low to high."[40] Pitch depends primarily on the frequency content of the sound stimulus, but it also depends on the sound pressure and the waveform stimulus.[41] In other words, although the pitch ascribed by our brains to a certain sound is most usually determined by the fundamental frequency, it is also influenced, and can be derived solely, from the higher harmonics and the loudness of the sound.[40] This leaves room for different perceptions of pitch level of the voice by different listeners, which can be at odds with measured fundamental frequency.

In addition to these psychoacoustic difficulties, there are many factors that determine what is perceived as a normal pitch for an individual's voice. These include anatomical, physiological, social, and cultural influences. As a rough guide, the mean fundamental frequency of adult men during speech ranges between 100 and 150 Hz, between 180 and 250 Hz for adult women, and between 205 and 290 Hz for children.[42]

Pragmatically, the inappropriateness of the pitch is defined as that judged by the patient and assessor to be outside the normal range based on the age and sex of the individual.

Too High

This is quite a common perceptual finding but is rarely a complaint in women except when the voice has changed or is associated with other vocal complaints. In women, the commonest cause is muscle tension imbalance (lateral compression or Morrison Type 2) resulting from habitual talking at the top of the range of the voice, a common tendency in primary school teachers.[13,14] This can result in chronic stretching of the vocal folds and pitch instability. In men, a high-pitched voice can cause negative comments about gender and lead to ridicule and psychological problems. It can result from muscle tension imbalance known as puberphonia or "mutational falsetto."[43] In these cases, the voice commonly never changed at puberty, although the laugh or cough may have a deep tone. Structural abnormalities and neurological problems need to be excluded. Structural problems include sulcus vergeture and an anterior glottis web. In sulcus vergeture, there is a longitudinal groove in the membranous portion of the vocal fold and is frequently bilateral. There is tethering of the epithelium to the underlying ligament or vocalis muscle.[44] The thin, stretched free lower edge of the vocal folds make contact, which allows more regular vibration than if the stiffened area is involved. The consequence is a high-pitched voice with reduced pitch range. The voice can also be breathy, lack power, and projection.[45] Anterior glottic webs can be congenital or acquired. Both can cause significant high-pitched voices and dysphonia.

In recurrent laryngeal nerves palsies, the compensatory unbalanced pull of the laryngeal muscles leads to asymmetry of the glottis and stretching of the vocal folds. This leads to a high-pitched voice with the breathiness from glottal gap. In advanced Parkinson disease, the mean speaking fundamental is raised compared with age-matched men but not in women and not for early-stage disease.[39]

Too Low

A low pitch to the voice is a much more common complaint in women who often get comments about sounding like a man, particularly on the phone. The most common cause is Reinke edema in which there is an increased amount of extracellular matrix produced in the superficial lamina propria.[46] This is strongly linked to smoking.[47] Large polyps, the use of the false folds during phonation, use of androgenic drugs, severe hypothyroidism, and some forms of muscle tension dysphonia will also result in a lower pitched voice.

Altered Pitch Range

The whole pitch range may have shifted, often becoming lowered. This can result from natural changes with age or from the structural effects of increasing the mass of the vocal folds, for example, from smoking. The pitch range may have become narrowed or monopitch, that is, lacks variation in speech. This can be due to personality issues, anxiety, and depression. It can also be a feature of neurological conditions such as Parkinson disease[39,48] and in recurrent laryngeal nerve palsy.[49] A patient may choose to limit the pitch variation if straying outside that range results in instability of the voice or is more effortful particularly in structural or neurological conditions.

Singers

Singers who are struggling with their pitch range may, for example, need to change key to sing a range of notes in a specific song. Loss of the top end of the range of the voice or difficulty with certain parts of their range may be because of inadequate technique in making transitions between registers or modes of the voice.[35]

Loudness of the Voice

Not Loud Enough

Reduced loudness of the voice may result from neuromuscular problems such as vocal fold palsies or paresis, Parkinson disease, or myasthenia gravis where there is a physical inability to oppose the vocal folds.[39,48] Muscle tension imbalance, structural abnormalities, and inflammation may have variable effects on the ability to produce a loud voice. Sometimes the loudness reduces with voice use. Alternatively, it may only be an issue in noisy environments or when there is a need to project the voice.

Too Loud

Most patients will not complain about this but it may be apparent to the listener. It is common in muscle tension dysphonia when it may be a manifestation of an extrovert personality, a need to be heard when there are other dominant siblings or when the voice cannot be regulated when there is an untreated hearing loss. Occasionally, it may be necessary to increase the subglottic pressure to overcome the inertia of the vocal folds from structural or inflammatory causes. The result can be uncontrolled regulation of loudness and may be associated with voice breaks.

Other Throat Symptoms

Throat symptoms may be present with any of the four etiologic conditions. These include paralaryngeal discomfort or soreness of the throat from the increased effort of phonation (**Table 6.5**). Dryness of the throat is a common complaint in many types of voice disorder. Specifically, it can be due to medications such as diuretics or antimuscarinics, not drinking enough fluids, too much consumption of sugary or caffeine-containing foods and drinks, a persistent glottic gap or excessive autonomic stimulation secondary to anxiety, throat clearing, and mucus in the throat.[50]

Endoscopic Laryngeal and Vocal Tract Examination

Based on the history, it should be possible to make a preliminary differential diagnosis. It is, however, virtually

Table 6.5 Summary of Some of Other Throat Symptoms Commonly Reported in Patients with Voice Disorders

Paralaryngeal discomfort or pain

Soreness, burning, or tickling in the throat

Feeling of a lump or something stuck in the throat (globus)

Tightness or feeling of being strangled

Throat dryness

Mucus or catarrh in throat

Needing to clear throat

Irritating cough

Choking episodes

Difficulty swallowing

impossible in most cases to make a confident diagnosis without examining the larynx. Both oral rigid (70 or 90 degrees) endoscopes and flexible or video nasendoscopes should be available and also a continuous (halogen or xenon) and stroboscopic light source and a digital imaging capture system for storage and replay.[51] Stroboscopic light used with a rigid endoscope gives the best quality image of the mucosal wave particularly when used with a high-definition camera. Nasendoscopes (diameter 3.2 to 4.8 mm) allow examination of the whole of the vocal tract, including the nasal cavity, and also examination of the patient during speech and nonphonatory tasks such as coughing and swallowing, for example, FEES (functional endoscopic evaluation of swallowing). Video nasendoscopes now allow much improved imaging with stroboscopy, which was previously limited with the fiberoptic nasendoscopes. High-speed digital imaging and videokymography can provide additional useful information when the vibratory patterns are complex, but are not in general use as yet.

The choice of examination technique depends on the quality and availability of the equipment and the specific aim of the assessment (**Table 6.6**). If a subtle abnormality of the mucosal wave is suspected, then good quality images using stroboscopy should be employed. If a neurological or muscle tension problem is likely, then nasendoscopy with continuous light source is more useful. Inflammation can be assessed with either method. Sometimes both methods need to be employed and patient preference needs to be considered. There are patients who hate anything in their nose and others who have too strong gag reflexes to tolerate a rigid endoscope. Rigid endoscopy can be used in many children from 5 years of age, although views are generally brief. Pediatric nasendoscopes (diameter 2.2 to 2.8 mm) allow neonates upward to be screened for pathology and laryngeal movement abnormalities such as vocal cord palsies and laryngomalacia.

As part of the assessment, it is essential to check each anatomical site and subsite for the presence or absence of the four etiologic factors together with a series of phonatory and nonphonatory tasks (**Table 6.7**). The phonatory tasks

include checking the degree of closure of the vocal folds and supraglottic structures on phonation and the change in the mucosal wave with change in pitch and loudness. Nonphonatory tasks include observing adduction and abduction of the vocal folds on coughing and repeated "i"/ sniffing looking for asymmetry and a lag in movement between the two sides.

Further Clinical Evaluation

Palpation of the neck is also another key part of the assessment. This is not only to detect enlarged lymph nodes or other structural abnormalities in the neck but also to detect evidence of muscle tension. In muscle tension dysphonia, the paralaryngeal and other anterior neck muscles are often chronically contracted and tender. The most consistently abnormal muscles are the cricothyroid, thyrohyoid, middle constrictor, and suprahyoid muscles.[52,53]

Further Evaluation

In spite of a detailed history and examination, it is sometimes still not possible to make an accurate diagnosis. In these cases, further investigations may be required including acoustic and electrolaryngographic analysis of the voice, laryngeal electromyography, a diagnostic microlaryngoscopy, and high-definition computed tomography scan of the larynx. Trials of medication and probe voice therapy are also useful and are covered in other chapters of the book.

Summary

Once the main types of etiologic factor have been identified by detailed history, careful voice assessment, neck palpation, and laryngostroboscopic examination, it is then possible to be more precise in the diagnosis. **Fig. 6.2** summarizes the steps in clinical assessment and **Table 6.8A–D** describes the more common conditions encountered in patients presenting with hoarseness.

Table 6.6 Relative Advantages and Disadvantages of Each Type of Endoscopic Examination Method of the Larynx

Advantages	Rigid (Oral) Scope (70 or 90 degrees)	Videonasendoscope	Flexible Nasendoscope
Best quality image with stroboscopy of mucosal wave	+++	++	+
Examination of whole of vocal tract	0	+++	++
Examination during speech and nonphonatory tasks	0	+++	++

Table 6.7   Key Endoscopic Features to Observe in the Diagnosis of the Four Main Etiologic Factors Responsible for Voice Disorders

Structural/Neoplastic	Inflammation	Neuromuscular	Muscle Tension Imbalance[a]

• Glottis
  ○ Mass lesion present?
  ○ Epithelial change?
  ○ Submucosal?
  ○ Vibratory appearance on stroboscopy
    – Aperiodicity?
    – Mucosal wave inhibition?
 	
• Posterior glottis
  ○ Lesion?
 	
• Supraglottis
  ○ False cord lesion?
  ○ Aryepiglottic fold lesion?
 	
• Hypopharynx
  ○ Piriform fossa lesion?
  ○ Posterior pharyngeal wall?
	• Vocal folds
	  ○ Localized?
	  ○ Prominent vessels?
	  ○ Erythema?
	  ○ Edema?
	  ○ Erythema + edema?
	  ○ Infraglottic edema?
	  ○ Thickened mucus?
	
	• Posterior glottis
	  ○ Interarytenoid region thickening/ pachydermia?
	  ○ Erythema?
	  ○ Thickened mucus?
	
	• Supraglottis
	  ○ Erythema?
	  ○ Edema?
	  ○ Ventricular obliteration?
	
	• Hypopharynx
	  ○ "Cobblestoning?"
		• On phonation to breathing and cough:
		  ○ Immobile vocal fold
		    – Unilateral?
		    – Bilateral?
		    – Reduced movement?
		  ○ Lag on repeated "i"/sniff?
		
		• Glottis
		  ○ Glottal gap?
		  ○ Reduced contact?
		  ○ Bowing of vocal fold?
		
		• Posterior glottis
		  ○ "Prolapsed" arytenoid
		  ○ Asymmetry between low and high pitch
		
		• Supraglottis
		  ○ Asymmetry
		    – False cords?
		    – Petiole of epiglottis?
		
		• Other abnormal movements
		  ○ Tremor
		    – At rest?
		    – On phonation?
		  ○ Dystonia?
		
		• Hypopharynx
		  ○ Asymmetry of movement of posterior pharyngeal wall?
		  ○ Pooling of saliva?
			• Vocal folds
			  ○ On breathing
			    – Normal appearance?
			  ○ On phonation variable patterns
			    – Anterior two-thirds of vocal folds pressed tightly together and posterior glottal chink?
			    – Stretched and thin?
			    – Splinted apart?
			    – No mucosal wave as no breath support?
			
			• Supraglottis (variable pattern)
			  ○ False cords
			    – Medial/lateral constriction?
			  ○ Arytenoids
			    – Tilted forward?
			    – Anteroposterior constriction?
			  ○ Concentric constriction? ˙
			  ○ Base of epiglottis obscures anterior vocal folds?
			
			• Laryngeal height in vocal tract
			  ○ Too high?
			  ○ Too low?
			
			• Pharynx
			  ○ Posterolateral wall constriction
			
			• Tongue
			  ○ Too high in oral cavity?
			  ○ Too backed?

Note: It must be remembered that more than one etiologic factor may be present. Once the factor has been identified, the precise condition, for example, the cause of the structural abnormality, inflammation, neuromuscular disorder, or reason for the muscle tension dysphonia, can be explored.

[a]Some of the findings in muscle tension imbalance overlap with findings in asymptomatic individuals and so must be interpreted in the context of the overall clinical picture.

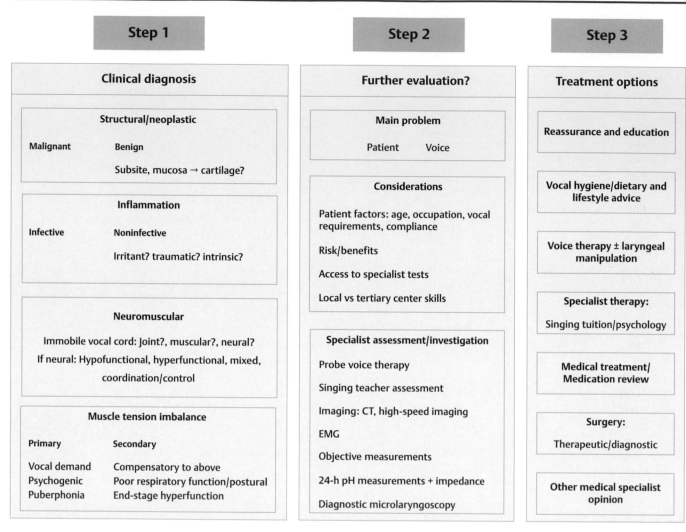

Figure 6.2 Summary of the steps in clinical assessment. Step 1 is identifying the four main etiological factors present and making the clinical diagnosis based on the history and examination. Step 2 is determining the factors that are relevant for the voice disorder and for the patient and whether further information through specialist assessment or investigation is required. Step 3 is then considering the treatment options and deciding with patients about options that would be most appropriate for their needs. CT, computed tomography; EMG, electromyography.

Table 6.8   Summary Tables of the Common Conditions Encountered in Patients Presenting with Hoarseness

(A) Structural/Neoplastic Abnormality

Benign
- Mucosal deposits/thickenings
  - Nodules
  - Pseudocyst
  - Polyp
  - Reinke edema/polypoid degeneration
- Deficits/tethering
  - Cysts
    - Mucus retention
    - Epidermoid
  - Sulcus vocalis
  - Sulcus vergeture
  - Mucosal bridge
- Scarring

Malignant/premalignant
- Epithelial
  - Hyperkeratosis
  - Dysplasia
  - Squamous cell carcinoma
- Salivary gland tumors
- Lymphoma
- Neuroendocrine tumors

Table 6.8   *(Continued)*

(A) Structural/Neoplastic Abnormality

- Microvascular lesions
  - Ectasia
- Endocrinological
  - Myxoedema
  - Androgenic changes
  - Inflammatory mass
    - Papillomatosis
    - Granuloma
    - Rheumatoid deposits
    - Amyloid
    - Sarcoid
- Framework trauma
- Benign neoplasms

(B) Inflammation

Infective	Noninfective
• Primary laryngeal	• Laryngopharyngeal reflux
○ Viral	• Allergy
– Acute	• Trauma
– (Chronic, e.g., human papilloma virus)	○ Irritant
○ Bacterial including tuberculosis	○ Fumes/chemical
○ Fungal	○ Smoke
– Candida	○ Laryngeal dehydration
• Secondary	○ Physical
○ Chest?	• Drugs
○ Rhinosinusitis?	• Autoimmune
	• Rheumatoid
	• Endocrinological
	• Nonspecific?

(C) Neuromuscular Abnormality

Hypofunctional	Mixed or variable hypo-/hyperfunctional
• Parkinson disease	• Vocal cord palsy/paresis
• Myasthenia gravis	• Motor neurone disease
• Bulbar palsy	• Multiple sclerosis

Hyperfunctional	Control/coordination
• Spasmodic dysphonia	• Tremor
• Pseudobulbar/spastic dysphonia	• Myoclonus
• Chorea	• Cerebellar lesions

(D) Muscle Tension Dysphonia

Primary	Secondary
• Vocal demands/strain	• Inflammation
○ Occupational	○ Including postinfection problems
○ Inadequate vocal skills	• Structural/neoplastic
• Psychogenic	○ Including end-stage hyperfunction
○ Anxiety/"stress"	• Neuromuscular
○ Conversion dysphonia/aphonia	• Breathing disorders
• Puberphonia/mutational voice disorder	• Postural abnormalities
• Presbylaryngis	• Congenital laryngeal anatomical abnormalities

References

1. International Classification of Functioning. Disability and Health (ICF). http://www.who.int/classifications/en/

2. Titze IR. Principles of Voice Production. Englewood Cliffs, NJ: Prentice Hall; 1994

3. Kent RD, Dembowski J, Lass NJ. The acoustic characteristics of American English. In: Lass NJ, ed. Principles of Experimental Phonetics. St. Louis, MO: Mosby-Year Book, Inc.; 1996:185–225

4. Baken RJ, Orlikoff RF. Airflow and volume. In: Clinical Measurements of Speech and Voice. 2nd ed. San Diego, CA: Singular Thomson Learning; 2000:337–391

5. Harris TM, Harris SC, Rubin JS, Howard DM. The Voice Clinic Handbook. London: Whurr Publishers Ltd.; 1998

6. Mathieson L. Hyperfunctional voice disorders. In: Mathieson L, ed. The Voice and Its Disorders. 6th ed. London: Whurr Publishers Ltd.; 2001:145–185

7. Gilbert C. Interaction of psychological and emotional effects with breathing dysfunction. In: Chaitow L, Bradley D, Gilbert C, eds. Multidisciplinary Approaches to Breathing Pattern Disorders. Edinburgh: Churchill Livingstone; 2002:111–129

8. Mathieson L. The lower respiratory tract. In: Mathieson L, ed. The Voice and Its Disorders. 6th ed. London: Whurr Publishers Ltd.; 2001:51–66

9. Kellman RM, Leopold DA. Paradoxical vocal cord motion: an important cause of stridor. Laryngoscope 1982;92(1):58–60

10. Koufman JA, Blalock PD. Classification and approach to patients with functional voice disorders. Ann Otol Rhinol Laryngol 1982;91(4 Pt 1):372–377

11. Belisle GM, Morrison MD. Anatomic correlation for muscle tension dysphonia. J Otolaryngol 1983;12(5):319–321

12. Koufman JA, Blalock PD. Functional voice disorders. Otolaryngol Clin North Am 1991;24(5):1059–1073

13. Morrison M, Rammage LA, Nichol H, Pullan B, Salkeld L, May P. Causes and classifications of voice disorders. In: Morrison M, Rammage LA, eds. The Management of Voice Disorders. 2nd ed. San Diego, CA: Singular; 2001:67–103

14. Harris S. Speech therapy for dysphonia. In: Harris T, Harris S, Rubin JS, Howard DM, eds. The Voice Clinic Handbook. London: Whurr Publishers Ltd.; 1998:139–206

15. Sulica L. The superior laryngeal nerve: function and dysfunction. [Review] Otolaryngol Clin North Am 2004;37(1): 183–201

16. Roy N, Smith ME, Houtz DR. Laryngeal features of external superior laryngeal nerve denervation: revisiting a century-old controversy. Ann Otol Rhinol Laryngol 2011;120(1):1–8

17. Schuster M, Maier A, Haderlein T, et al. Evaluation of speech intelligibility for children with cleft lip and palate by means of automatic speech recognition. Int J Pediatr Otorhinolaryngol 2006;70(10):1741–1747

18. Darley FL, Aronson AE, Brown JR. Clusters of deviant speech dimensions in the dysarthrias. J Speech Hear Res 1969;12(3): 462–496

19. Darley FL, Aronson AE, Brown JR. Differential diagnostic patterns of dysarthria. J Speech Hear Res 1969;12(2):246–269

20. Mayr S, Burkhardt K, Schuster M, Rogler K, Maier A, Iro H. The use of automatic speech recognition showing the influence of nasality on speech intelligibility. Eur Arch Otorhinolaryngol 2010;267(11):1719–1725

21. Jacobson BH, Johnson A, Grywalski C, Silbergleit A, Benninger MS. The Voice Handicap Index (VHI): development and validation. Am J Speech Lang Pathol 1997;6:66–70

22. Hogikyan ND, Sethuraman G. Validation of an instrument to measure voice-related quality of life (V-RQOL). J Voice 1999;13(4):557–569

23. Deary IJ, Wilson JA, Carding PN, MacKenzie K. VoiSS: a patient-derived Voice Symptom Scale. J Psychosom Res 2003;54(5): 483–489

24. Hirano M. Clinical Examination of Voice. Vienna: Springer-Verlag; 1981

25. Zemlin WR. Speech and Hearing Science: Anatomy and Physiology. 4th ed. Boston: Allyn and Bacon; 1997

26. Wolk L, Abdelli-Beruh NB, Slavin D. Habitual use of vocal fry in young adult female speakers. J Voice 2012;26(3):e111–e116

27. Yuasa IP. Creaky voice: a new feminine voice quality for young urban-oriented upwardly mobile American women? Am Speech 2010;85(3):315–337

28. Hajioff D, Rattenbury H, Carrie S, Carding P, Wilson J. The effect of Isshiki type 1 thyroplasty on quality of life and vocal performance. Clin Otolaryngol Allied Sci 2000;25(5):418–422

29. Giovanni A, Chanteret C, Lagier A. Sulcus vocalis: a review. Eur Arch Otorhinolaryngol 2007;264(4):337–344

30. Kendall K. Presbyphonia: a review. Curr Opin Otolaryngol Head Neck Surg 2007;15(3):137–140

31. Carpenter RJ III, McDonald TJ, Howard FM Jr. The otolaryngologic presentation of myasthenia gravis. Laryngoscope 1979;89(6 Pt 1):922–928

32. Butcher P, Elias A, Cavalli L. Understanding and Treating Psychogenic Voice Disorders—A CBT Framework. Chichester: John Wiley & Sons Ltd.; 2007

33. Aronson AE, Bless DM. Neurologic voice disorders. In: Aronson AE, Bless DM, eds. Clinical Voice Disorders. 4 ed. New York, NY: Thieme Medical Publishers Inc.; 2009:71–100

34. Miller DG, Schutte HK. "Mixing" the registers: glottal source or vocal tract? Folia Phoniatr Logop 2005;57(5–6):278–291

35. Sadolin C. Complete Vocal Technique. 2nd ed. Copenhagen: CVI Publications; 2012

36. Koufman JA, Postma GN, Cummins MM, Blalock PD. Vocal fold paresis. Otolaryngol Head Neck Surg 2000;122(4):537–541

37. Hong KH, Kim HK. Diplophonia in unilateral vocal fold paralysis and intracordal cyst. Otolaryngol Head Neck Surg 1999;121 (6):815–819

38. Ziegler W, Hoole P. Neurologic disease. In: Kent RD, Ball MJ, eds. Voice Quality Measurement. San Diego, CA: Singular Publishing Group; 2000:397–410

39. Holmes RJ, Oates JM, Phyland DJ, Hughes AJ. Voice characteristics in the progression of Parkinson's disease. Int J Lang Commun Disord 2000;35(3):407–418

40. Plack CJ. The Sense of Hearing. Mahwah, NJ: Lawrence Erlbaum Associates, Inc.; 2005

41. ANSI. American National Standard Acoustical Terminology. New York, NY: American National Standards Institute; 1994

42. Baken RJ, Orlikoff RF. Clinical Measurements of Speech and Voice. 2nd ed. San Diego, CA: Singular Thomson Learning; 2000

43. Dagli M, Sati I, Acar A, Stone RE Jr, Dursun G, Eryilmaz A. Mutational falsetto: intervention outcomes in 45 patients. J Laryngol Otol 2008;122(3):277–281

44. Lindestad PA, Hertegård S. Spindle-shaped glottal insufficiency with and without sulcus vocalis: a retrospective study. Ann Otol Rhinol Laryngol 1994;103(7):547–553

45. Hirano M, Yoshida T, Tanaka S, Hibi S. Sulcus vocalis: functional aspects. Ann Otol Rhinol Laryngol 1990;99(9 Pt 1):679–683

46. Volić SV, Klapan I, Seiwerth S, Ibrahimpašić T. Extracellular matrix of Reinke's space in some pathological conditions. Acta Otolaryngol 2004;124(4):505–508

47. Branski RC, Saltman B, Sulica L, et al. Cigarette smoke and reactive oxygen species metabolism: implications for the pathophysiology of Reinke's edema. Laryngoscope 2009;119(10):2014–2018

48. Gamboa J, Jiménez-Jiménez FJ, Nieto A, et al. Acoustic voice analysis in patients with Parkinson's disease treated with dopaminergic drugs. J Voice 1997;11(3):314–320

49. Murray T. Speaking fundamental frequency characteristics associated with voice pathologies. J Speech Hear Disord 1978; 43(3):374–379

50. Mathieson L. The Voice and Its Disorders. 6th ed. London: Whurr Publishers Ltd.; 2001

51. Woo P. Stroboscopy. San Diego, CA: Plural Publishing Inc.; 2007

52. Lieberman J. Principles and techniques of manual therapy: applications in the management of dysphonia. In: Harris T, Harris S, Rubin JS, Howard DA, eds. The Voice Clinic Handbook. London: Whurr Publishers Ltd.; 1998:91–138

53. Piron A. Techniques ostéopathiques appliquées à la phoniatrie: Biomécanique fonctionnelle et normalisation du larynx. Lyon: Symétrie; 2007

7 Objective Measures of Laryngeal Imaging and Laryngeal Electromyography

Peak Woo

The principle of using flashing lights for examination of rapidly moving but periodic oscillation using stroboscopy is well known for over a century. Today, videostroboscopy is one of the standard methods used to examine moving vocal folds. Laryngeal videostroboscopy is used extensively for the analysis of vocal folds and in the clinical practice for diagnosing voice disorders. Since the initial book on videostroboscopy by Schönharl,[1] the technique and interpretation of laryngeal videostroboscopy have been well formalized. Stroboscopic signs are associated with benign mucosal lesions and can also be systematically rated and characterized.[2] Laryngeal videostroboscopy is able to reveal several abnormalities, including abnormalities of laryngeal structure, absence of vibration, and vibratory asymmetry. The pliability of the vocal fold after surgical intervention can be assessed qualitatively by observation of vibratory characteristics using stroboscopy.[3] Objective measurement of the vocal fold vibration pattern dates back to the initial high-speed cinematography recordings of vocal fold vibration from the works of Timcke, von Leden, and Moore.[4–7]

Although the concept of objective measurements of vocal fold vibration is attractive, the actual clinical application of objective measurements has not been realized. This is because of multiple factors related to the complex vocal fold vibratory image.

With the availability of digital image processing, there are now possibilities for automated image extraction and quantification. High-speed imaging (HSI) of vocal fold vibration and clinical applications is now readily available within the time and cost constraints of a clinical practice.[8,9] Today, digital kymography from high-speed video images can be routinely captured and analyzed and compared. Such rapid capture and analysis of the vibratory capability of vocal fold vibration was a dream only a decade ago. Such tools today represent the ability for easy quantification of the vocal fold vibration image for the study of normal function and physiology of normal and pathologic laryngeal states and for the objective measure of surgical and therapeutic techniques.

The use of laryngeal electromyography (LEMG) has also become more popular for the investigation of mobile vocal fold and for central neurological disorders affecting voice. Much controversy continues to exist in the interpretation of the LEMG literature.[10] Much of this is due to the qualitative nature of the LEMG and interpretation. Because interpretation of the LEMG requires many years of practice, the experience necessary for good EMG interpretation is not easily acquired by the average laryngologist. The possibility of quantitative methods to reduce interpreter bias has been introduced in other EMG literature.[11] Quantitative and qualitative methods for LEMG interpretation and measurement have the potential of advancing electrodiagnosis of laryngeal movement disorders, improving prognostic indication for patients with vocal fold paralysis, and differentiation between myopathy and neuropathy.

The goal of this chapter is to summarize the objective measures that one can measure from stroboscopy and high-speed video. We will introduce the concept of the glottal area waveform (GAW). From digital kymographic tracing, we will introduce the concept of kymographic waveform analysis. We will also summarize the concept of quantitative LEMG.

Measurements from Stroboscopy Video

Videostroboscopy is a well-established technique in clinical applications for the evaluation of dysphonic patients. In the voice clinic, it is most useful for the identification of small lesions and mass lesions and for the verification of stiffness.[12] Laryngeal asymmetry during vocal fold oscillation is one of the most obvious abnormalities that one can identify during sustained phonation and points to asymmetric rheological changes in the vocal fold cover. Often, these asymmetrical changes are the indicators for recommendation for surgical intervention.[13] After surgical intervention, videostroboscopy examination often shows improvement in the vocal fold edge, configuration, phase closure, and return of amplitude and mucosal wave.[14] Objective measures of vibratory capability based on videostroboscopy examination are more challenging. The single-flash-timing laryngeal videostroboscopy is difficult to standardize from examination to examination. Control of the patient's phonatory volume, frequency, and the size of the laryngeal image must be standardized if one were to compare the vibratory pattern before and after treatment.[15] Some authors have recommended overlaying images from the prior examination over the current examination using a transparency tracing to standardize the distance of the endoscope from the vocal folds and to standardize the size of the laryngeal image.[16] Such an approach is practically reserved for the research laboratory where specific information is to be obtained.

Not all stroboscopy examinations can be useful for imaging analysis. This is because the stroboscopic image is a montage of many glottal cycles. By accepting the stroboscopy images as representative of the pattern of vocal fold oscillation, one is assuming that the multiple frames that are analyzed from the video captured is produced at the same fundamental frequency and the same loudness. Using the standard stroboscopic flash rate of 1.5 Hz above the fundamental frequency, a video frame rate of 30 frames per second will result in a complete glottal cycle in 20 video frames. If the patient can hold the steady phonation for 2 full seconds at this same fundamental frequency and loudness, then a montage of video frames can be acquired that is representative of the sustained phonation for that token. The stroboscopic images from the assembled three glottal cycles are a montage of the vibratory pattern for the vocal folds for those 2 seconds assembled from all the glottal cycles during the 2 seconds. For males, this would be approximately 250 glottal cycles, while for females, this would be approximately 500 glottal cycles. Provided the waveforms are quasiperiodic and repeatable from cycle to cycle on the visual inspection of the stroboscopy video, this sequence can be subject to analysis. **Fig. 7.1** is a montage of glottal cycles obtained by capturing every frame of the video cycle and limiting the frame of interest to the vibratory margin. This is assembled as a single image made up of many video frames with the area of interest. The vibratory pattern is regular and the completion of a glottal cycle shows the characteristic pattern of open and closed phase with the phase difference between the upper and lower lips of the vocal fold. If one compares this with other glottal cycles from the same stroboscopy token and it looks similar, then one

can assume that the stroboscopic montage is representative of the actual glottal cycle.

If the glottal cycle is not evenly illuminated, frame dropout will occur. This will result in a glottal cycle that is not suitable for automated image extraction. An inherent limitation of videostroboscopy is that not all patients can have the entire vocal fold margin visualized during video endoscopy. This is because some patients will have tilting of the epiglottis that obscures the anterior commissure. Some patients will have arytenoid hooding that prevents the posterior vocal fold from being visualized. In patients with mass lesions of the vocal folds, the vibratory pattern may not be delineated due to mass effect or due to ventricular hyperfunction. For patients with severe dysphonia who cannot sustain phonation for more than 2 seconds at a steady fundamental frequency, it is best not to attempt objective analysis using videostroboscopy methodology.

Although objective evaluation is difficult due to the montage nature of video recordings, some authors have tried to use the strobe image for quantification.[17] The mucosal wave propagation across the superior surface of the vocal fold can be identified for tracking and some information regarding mucosal pliability can be estimated.

In a comparison of 162 patients examined by videostroboscopy versus HSI, significant variation between subjective ratings was noted between both stroboscopy and HSI. This variation between subjective raters is one rational for need of objective imaging of vibratory movements.[18]

Developments in modern image processing techniques have led to the quantification of various aspects of vocal fold vibration. Stroboscopic images of the vocal fold were digitized and, subsequently, the glottal gap area, amplitude, and degree of bowing were analyzed quantitatively in relation to phonatory function. Measurement of the glottal gap probably represents the easiest and most reliable

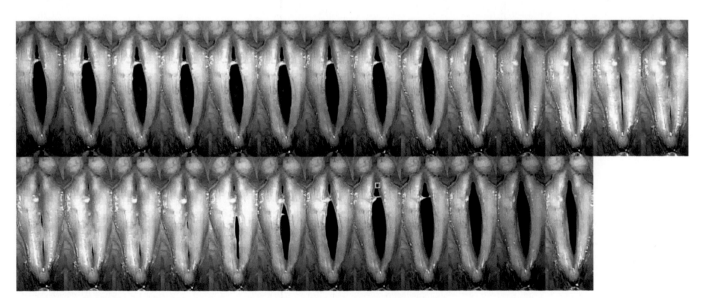

Figure 7.1 The glottal cycle can be assembled as a montage of video frames by clipping the area of interest and assembled as a series of glottal images. Typically, a minimum of 10 video frames is used to represent one glottal cycle. The montage image is ready for automated analysis.

quantitative measure. Because it is assumed that the vocal fold at its most closed phase should have no glottal gap during sustained phonation in modal voice, estimate of the glottal gap before and after surgical intervention has been obtained.[19] These studies do not require videostroboscopic analysis and are primarily based on digitized image of the vocal fold at its most closed phase. By measuring the glottal length and several pixels that are dark within the glottal gap, one can get a ratio of pixels to vocal fold length. This can then be compared with before and after surgical treatment. This normalized glottal gap estimate has been used in clinical studies to estimate the risk of aspiration in patients with vocal cord paralysis.[20]

One way to obtain an estimate of the vibratory function is the plot of GAW. The GAW is a measure of the glottal area function throughout the glottal cycle. The normal GAW has features that can be measured. These include the open and closed phase of vocal fold oscillation. The maximum glottal area and the minimum glottal area can also be measured. The rate of vocal fold opening and closing during all vocal fold oscillations can be calculated by measuring the slope of the GAW. The ability to rapidly change the configuration of the vocal fold or the opening and closing speed index is an indication of the vocal fold pliability and has been shown to change before and after phonosurgery.[14]

Quantification of the stroboscopic image comes from the initial manual measurements of the glottal cycle from high-speed cinematography.[21] With some regularity, one can trace the edge of the vocal fold visually to obtain the elliptical shape of the vocal fold margin. By dividing the area measured by the length of the vocal folds, one can get a normalized measure of the glottal area of function. When the glottal area of function is assembled over the glottal cycle, the GAW can be plotted versus time. The GAW can then be compared between subjects and between variations in amplitude and frequency. In a study of normal subjects, the GAW showed significant differences between the sexes in GAW, peak glottal area, closed period, closing slope, and size and incidence of the posterior glottal gap. Intensity and frequency changes significantly affected GAW. Intensity variations affected the steepness of the closing phase and the duration of the closed period. Frequency changes affected the open period and the relative duration of opening versus closing.[22] In the initial study of normal phonation, approximately 35% of the images were not suitable for objective quantification.

To reduce the subjective bias in tracing out the GAW from videostroboscopy images, several digital image analysis routines may be applied to the videostroboscopy image. The videostroboscopy image in modal phonation is complicated by having an upper and a lower lip that alternates in contact. Tracing of the vocal fold edge always alternates between tracing the upper lip and the lower lip. This can cause some confusion for the technician who is asked to trace out the vocal fold margin in a purely manual manner. Such difficulties may result in subjective bias and uneven results. One approach to reduce subjective selection

of the vocal fold margin is by routine use of digital image enhancement. Digital image analysis has become practical in biological sciences and has been used extensively. Some of the image analysis routines include contrast enhancement, edge detection, and image gradient analysis. Histogram equalization followed by maximum histogram gradient shift was found to be most effective in edge detection in a semiquantitative method for the detection of vocal fold vibratory pattern and reduces the subjective bias and identification of the GAW. Such an algorithm was used for the study referred to above.[22] Since that time, a variety of clinically available software have become available for the analysis of the videostroboscopy image. One of the common software packages is the KSIP software available with the digital stroboscopy unit (Kay-Pentax, Montvale, New Jersey, United States).

We will demonstrate the application of GAW extraction and analysis from a videostroboscopy image.

To verify that the stroboscopic image is suitable for image analysis, it is best to review the stroboscopy videotape to verify that the frequency recorded is stable and that the amplitude is sustained throughout the phonation of at least 2 seconds at steady frequency and amplitude. Once this is verified, this sequence of video image frames is suitable for image capture and analysis. Typically, modal phonation at comfortable pitch and loudness is used for analysis.

For males, the centering fundamental frequency is 110 to 120 Hz at 75 dB microphone output recorded at 6 inches from the mouth. For females, it is 200 to 250 Hz at 75 dB microphone output recorded at 6 inches from the mouth. The video frames are converted into Audio Video Interleave format for automated image extraction. Once the image is selected, the frame that represents the vocal fold in its most closed phase is used for defining the beginning of the glottal cycle sequence. The image cursor is used to define the area of interest for automated image extraction. By limiting the cursor to the area of vocal folds, the image analysis routine can be best utilized to analyze the changes in the GAW function. Typically, 10 frames of video image representing one glottal cycle are used for analysis. A minimum of two glottal cycles is used to verify the repeatability of glottal cycle measures. **Fig. 7.1** is an example of a glottal cycle that has been captured and assembled in a photomontage for image analysis.

Once the color image montage has been assembled, it is usually necessary to enhance the image before automated edge detection and area of detection. **Fig. 7.2** shows the image after it has been changed to a black and white image and subject to image brightening and contrast enhancement. Once the image has been treated, the image edge detection algorithm is applied to automatically trace the glottal edge based on maximum histogram gradient shift. **Fig. 7.3** shows the automated edge tracing that has been applied. During image analysis, the operator can visually check the area specified for image analysis and position the curser on the glottal area to be analyzed. This is shown in **Fig. 7.4**. The edge tracing of the glottal area is

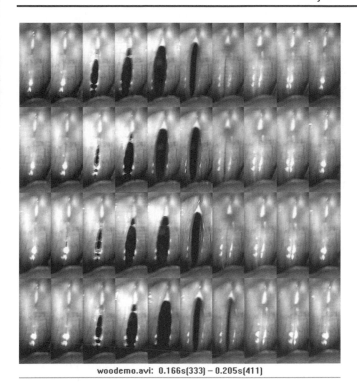

woodemo.avi: 0.166s[333] – 0.205s[411]

Figure 7.2 The image has been brightened and contrast enhanced and changed to a black and white image. Now the glottal area is quite sharp and ready for automated edge detection and area extraction.

then assembled as a GAW with the frame number in the *x*-axis. In addition to the GAW path, right versus left vocal fold movement relative to the defined midline can also be plotted. This is shown in **Fig. 7.5**.

From the GAW, one can obtain numeric values in peak glottal area, middle glottal area, opening and closing speed ratio, and the open and closed phase.

For abnormal vocal fold function, the relative displacement abnormality in patients with reduced amplitude can be demonstrated. Differences in amplitude can be displayed graphically and phase differences can be measured in degrees of phase shift. Measurement of this type can give the investigator data on the degree of phase shift between the two vocal folds as well as their relative amplitude difference between the two vocal folds. This has clinical implications as to relative stiffness of the vocal folds.

Despite the clinical availability of objective image analysis for clinical application, only limited literature support its routine use. One of the difficulties in using edge analysis alone is the lack of in-depth information about the vocal folds. Three-dimensional videostroboscopy can be obtained but its quantification would be difficult. Development of new automated image analysis routine is ongoing. Analysis of vertical contact should be taken into account when surgical intervention to improve hoarseness resulting from unilateral vocal fold immobility is performed. The future of standardized analysis of videostroboscopy and laryngeal image analysis are prerequisites to achieve objective measures of phonatory function before and after surgery.[23]

Stroboscopy will continue to be an easy clinical tool useful for the evaluation of the patient with dysphonia. As long as the clinician can recognize the deficiencies of stroboscopy, the use of a brief flashing light to freeze motion will see continued application in the clinic. With the new generation of high-definition videos and stroboscopy combined with special image filters such as narrowband imaging and florescence imaging, the role of imaging of the vocal fold is continuing to expand in the clinical diagnosis arena. As researchers come to some agreement as to which of the parameters from the stroboscopy image are most relevant

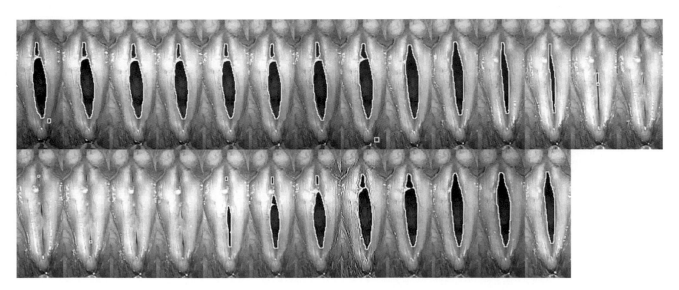

Figure 7.3 The glottal area has been traced out using the automated edge detection algorithm and the glottal area has been outlined for extraction. Note that the tracing is imperfect as mucous on the edge has been erroneously excluded from the vocal fold edge and will not be included in the area. These areas may need operator intervention to correct the deficiencies.

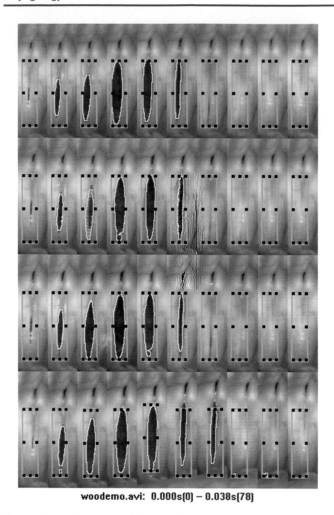

woodemo.avi: 0.000s(0) − 0.038s(78)

Figure 7.4 The image analysis software has selected the area of interest for analysis. Note that the operator can change the box placement and has excluded the small glottal gap posterior to the vocal process for image analysis.

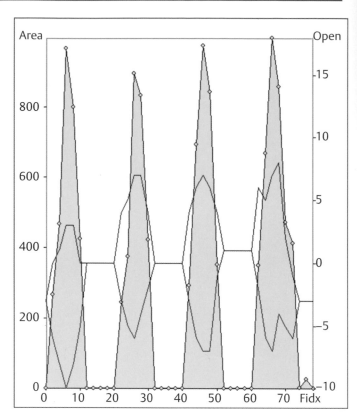

Figure 7.5 The extracted glottal area waveform (GAW) is the tracing in yellow and is depicted for four glottal cycles from a videostroboscopy. The frame number is plotted as the x-axis and the pixel/glottal length is represented in the y-axis. Note that the cycle-to-cycle repeatability is good with well-defined opening and closing speed, closed phase, and peak glottal area. These measures can be reliably obtained in normal patients. The other tracing is the plot of the right (upward) and the left (downward) excursion of the vocal fold edge at the mid-membranous portion of the defined glottal length.

in the evaluation of the vocal vibratory function, there is now a robust set of tools that could be applied. What will be needed for routine image measurements to be applicable to the clinician will be a set of automated software tools that can access the stroboscopy video, do preliminary analysis of the quality, and extract key parameters without extensive user input.

Digital Kymography and High-Speed Video

The deficiencies of using a videostroboscopy for imaging of vocal fold vibration are outlined in **Table 7.1**. Stroboscopy is based on the assumption that the vibration of the vocal folds is stable and regular. Irregular vibrations, which are common in voice pathology, cannot easily be studied and described in a reliable way. Because videostroboscopy depends on quasiperiodic vocal fold oscillation, many features of the phonatory gesture cannot be visualized (**Table 7.1**).

To correct the deficiencies of stroboscopy, HSI has been of importance since the 1970s.

Because high-speed cinematography is not practical for clinical purposes, the initial report using high-speed digital imaging was by Hirose.[24,25] This was limited to 100 × 100 pixels and had poor detail resolution. Nevertheless, many new observations are now available in terms of vibratory asymmetry as well as sources of vibration that could

Table 7.1 Features of Vocal Fold Behavior That Cannot Be Imaged with Stroboscopy

a. Voice breaks

b. Diplophonia

c. Vocal function during voice onset and voice offset

d. Vocal tremor and spasms

e. Extremely rough voice quality

f. Alternative laryngeal and pharyngeal sources of oscillation not be observed using standard videostroboscopy. Other authors have used high-resolution high-speed cameras to make observations regarding aperiodicity and asymmetry and have published the results.[26] With the continuing cost reduction of charge-coupled device (CCD) cameras, a commercially available high-speed video system became available in early 2000. This system initially had 256 × 256 pixel resolution in black and white. Today, such a system is available in 512 × 512 pixels in color (Kay-Pentax, Montvale, New Jersey, United States).

High-speed video overcomes some of the problems with stroboscopy. HSI allows thousands of pictures to be taken of the vibrating vocal folds per second. Rigid endoscopes are normally used for high-speed video. After clinical investigation of the patient, kymographic analysis from the video can be performed offline. In one clinical model, up to 8000 grayscale images of 256 × 256 pixels can be stored by the Wolf HS Endocam 5560 (Richard Wolf Medical Instruments Corporation, Vernon Hills, Illinois, United States). A maximum of 4000 images per second can be taken by the high-speed camera.[27] In contrast to stroboscopic investigations, aperiodic movements of the vocal folds can be visualized. The duration of a recording differs from 2 seconds to 4 seconds depending on the capture speed. The data transfer to the computer for archiving and analyzing the images takes a few minutes.

Using high-speed video, initial observations about laryngeal physiology were able to show that combining high-speed video with other measures such as electroglottography is very helpful in the visualization of voice onset and offset, singing gestures, and extremely high phonation. Furthermore, analysis of various singing styles could be realized.[28,29] Clinical report of high-speed video to identify diplophonia pattern consistent with vocal fold paresis was also reported as being important in the identification of a patient with previously undiagnosed vocal fold paresis.[30] Some of the foci in recent years have been to look for a way of automated analysis of the high-speed video. This is because at 4000 frames per second of acquisition, playback is usually at 20 frames per second. This means that a 2-second phonation acquisition will take 8000 frames. This will take 400 seconds or close to 7 minutes to review a 2-second video sample. Another deficiency of the high-speed system is the necessity to acquire the image sequence and then subject it to review. If the sample time is insufficient, a repeat examination must be done. The current system that is in use in our clinic permits an 8-second acquisition time with a pixel resolution of 256 × 125. Undoubtedly, system improvements and software for detection of the video frames for areas of interest will evolve, making review and analysis easier.

An alternative method for measurements of the vibratory capability of the vocal fold is by videokymography. The initial impetus for videokymography is the same realization of the deficiencies of videostroboscopy. Vocal fold vibration was observed with the aid of videokymography, during which images from a single transverse line can be recorded.

Successive line images were shown in real time on a monitor, with the time dimension displayed in the vertical direction. Videokymography, using a modified CCD video camera, works in two modes: standard and high speed. In standard mode, the vocal folds are displayed on a video monitor in the usual way, providing 50 images per second (or 60 in the National Television Standards Committee (NTSC) system). This is used for routine laryngoscopy and stroboscopic examination of the larynx. In high-speed mode (nearly 8000 images per second), only one line from the whole image is selected and displayed on the x-axis of the monitor; the y-axis represents the time dimension. This system enabled the assessment of left–right asymmetries, open quotient, and propagation of mucosal waves. Scanning camera using a single line can be placed on the area of interest of the laryngeal image and line scanning of that line is able to be achieved at high speed. This was initially reported by Svec and Schutte.[31] This was reported for routine laryngoscopy and stroboscopic examination of the larynx in clinical applications. They reported that all vocal fold vibrations, including those leading to pathological rough, breathy, hoarse, or diplophonic voice productions, can be observed.[32] Videokymography was able to detect small left–right asymmetries, open quotient differences along the glottis, lateral propagation of mucosal waves, and movements of the upper margin.

An example of a kymographic image is shown in **Fig. 7.6**. In this tracing, the voice onset during the beginning of vocal fold oscillation is captured. In this abnormal tracing, one can appreciate many glottal cycles that are aperiodic and asymmetric, with couplets and triplets of vocal fold vibration at the beginning of vocal fold vibration. After the established vocal fold vibration, the pattern becomes regular. This would not be appreciated using stroboscopy as tracking of the aperiodic vibrations would not be possible with stroboscopy.

Measurement of vocal fold movements can also be done either with HSI or with short-interval, color-filtered double strobe flash-stroboscopy. The strobe flashes are color filtered and are separated by a brief interval. By this means, a double exposure is created in each video frame. Real-time visualization of opening and closing velocities over the entire length of the vocal fold from anterior to posterior is possible. Quantification is possible offline after image calibration.[33] Another method for data reduction from high-speed motion is using multiline kymography. In this technique, the video is acquired at a high-speed mode. The line of interest across the mid-membranous vocal fold at several sites is selected for digital kymography extraction and a videokymography plot is generated. This technique is more practical than the line scanning camera because the line of interest can be defined after the high-speed images have been acquired.[34] Using multislice kymography, asymmetry and breaks can be compared and measured.[35]

The images obtained at high speed can be analyzed in the same way as the stroboscopy image. The major advantage

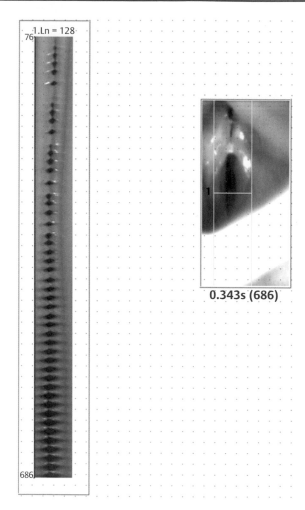

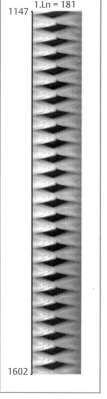

0.343s (686)

Figure 7.6 The digital kymography is shown on the left with the cursor line showing the line of interest of vocal fold on the right. This is from a high-speed video recording of the onset of vocal fold vibration in a pathological case of presbyphonia. The time axis is down. Note the chaotic irregular onset of vibration with many coupled triplophonic vibrations before steady oscillation is achieved. This will result in subharmonics with diplophonia and triplophonic sounds. This type of visualization is only possible with high-speed video or high-speed kymography.

is that the images are real-time images and not based on a montage. Because the images are acquired in such a brief period with steady light illumination, the images are very stable for image analysis. In the following, we will demonstrate some tools that can be used to measure the digital kymographic waveform.

Once the video image has been acquired, the curser is placed on the mid-membranous vocal fold. Multiple lines may be placed to obtain multiple digital kymography lines. **Fig. 7.7** is a photo of the videokymography for a short token of phonation. In this illustration, the cross line at the vocal fold is the image of the line displayed against time. Time axis is read from the top down with the vocal fold movement along the line shown on the video image on the right.

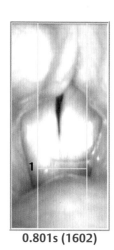

0.801s (1602)

Figure 7.7 Another way to analyze the digital kymography is to obtain the kymography image and convert it into a phonation vibrogram by edge detection and automated waveform extraction. This has the advantage of analyzing every oscillation of the vocal fold.

Once the videokymography display is done, the image can be converted into the digital kymographic waveform using edge detection software. **Fig. 7.8** is the line tracing of the digital kymographic waveform based on edge detection. **Fig. 7.9** is the glottogram waveform extracted from the edge detection in **Fig. 7.8**. One can appreciate two lines, with one line representing the right vocal fold and the other line representing the left vocal fold. The vibratory patterns can be transformed into a numerical waveform suitable for signal analysis. The typical way it can be analyzed is to subject the waveform to power spectrum analysis and fast Fourier transformation to derive the frequency versus power plot. This is shown in **Fig. 7.10**. Note that there are two lines, with one line representing the left and the other line representing the right. Other features are typical of the normal power spectral plot. These include the following: the energy is limited to the fundamental frequency and its harmonics, there is little subharmonic energy and interharmonic energy, and there is symmetry of the spectral plot between the two vocal folds.

Fig. 7.11 is a six power spectral plots of kymography waveform. The top three figures (**Fig. 7.11A** to **C**) are normal spectrograms. They are showing symmetry of vocal fold with energy in the fundamental frequency and

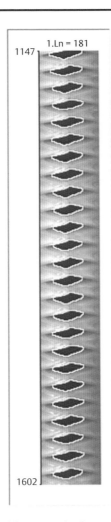

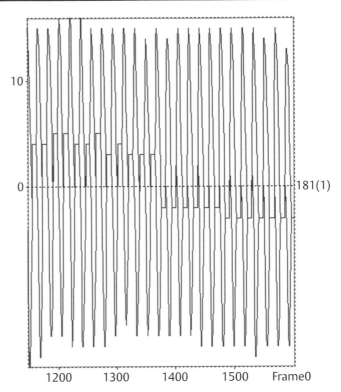

Figure 7.9 The right and the left vocal fold edges have been extracted and plotted as opposing waveform tracings. The time axis is the x-axis and the right vocal fold excursion is upward while the left vocal fold excursion is downward.

Figure 7.8 The digital kymography figure has been submitted for automated edge detection and the edge of the fold has been traced out.

its first three harmonics. There is also spectral energy in the second to fourth harmonic. There is little energy in the interharmonic area. The bottom three figures show three spectral plots from pathological vocal folds in vibration. The lower left figure (**Fig. 7.11D**) shows graph of a patient with a rough voice. This shows the energy peak to be limited to only the fundamental frequency. There is now energy in the low frequency area and large amount of interharmonic energy. The first and second harmonics above the fundamental frequency have very little power. The middle lower figure is a patient with unilateral stiffness (**Fig. 7.11E**). Now note that the side with normal vibration has a nice power spectral peak, whereas the opposite vocal fold has almost no energy in the fundamental. The lower right figure shows a patient with diplophonia (**Fig. 7.11F**). Each vocal fold has different fundamental frequency of vocal fold vibration. With sustained phonation, the vocal folds come in and out of phase, resulting in subharmonic energy. Using such analysis, diplophonia may be revealed as discreet vocal fold oscillations or subharmonics of the fundamental frequency.

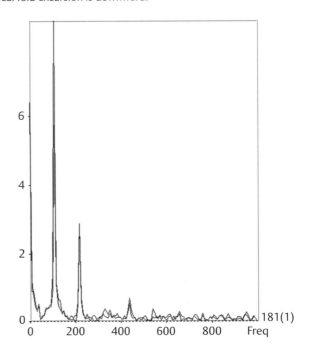

Figure 7.10 A spectrogram of normal vocal fold oscillation with the red line representing the right vocal fold and the black line representing the left vocal fold. Note that the spectral power plot shows the energy limited to the fundamental frequency of vocal fold oscillation and the first three harmonics. The spectral peaks are symmetric with the right versus left. There is little interharmonic energy and low-frequency energy.

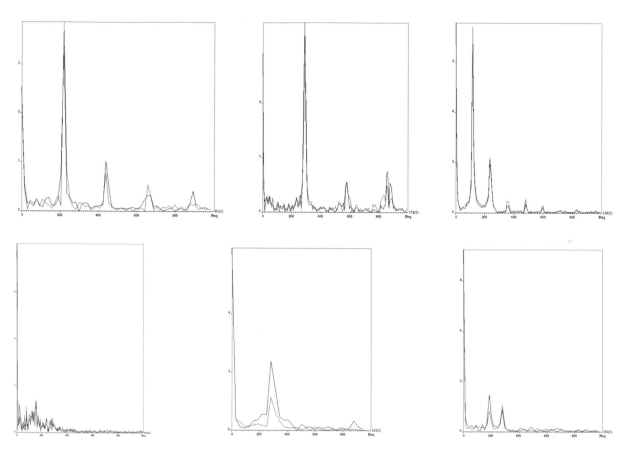

Figure 7.11 Spectral power plots for three normal subjects (A, B, and C) and three abnormal subjects are shown (D, E, and F). The abnormal spectrograms include diplophonia with two vocal folds oscillating at different frequencies (F), unilateral stiffness with loss of power spectra from one vocal fold (E), and rough voice with chaotic vibration resulting in high interharmonic and low frequency energy (D). Such analysis gives the investigator direct insight on the vocal fold oscillatory abnormalities and can be the basis for objective measures of vocal fold vibratory capability.

Laryngeal Electromyography

The initial report of LEMG was documented in the thesis by Faaborg-Andersen.[36] LEMG has been used in the clinic for investigation of vocal fold motion abnormalities since the 1970s.[37] The indications for LEMG are listed in **Table 7.2**. The standard EMG of the laryngeal muscles tests four different muscles that are innervated by the four nerves of interest. The four muscles are the right and left cricothyroid muscles and the right and left thyroarytenoid muscles. These correspond to the right and left superior laryngeal nerves and the right and left recurrent laryngeal nerves. The insertional technique and the testing parameters have been well described.[37–40] While some authors have used bipolar hook wire electrodes to sample the laryngeal muscles,[41] such studies are not common as compared with needle electrodes. The preferred use of monopolar or bipolar concentric needles for sampling is also controversial but not of critical importance as the interpretation. Many authors have cited the value of LEMG in the workup of the patient with immobile vocal folds (see **Table 7.2**).[42–45]

The normal EMG signal is inherently a composite of many motor units. Together they make up the interference pattern

Table 7.2 Clinical Application of Laryngeal Electromyography

- Immobile vocal fold
  - Traumatic ankylosis versus paralysis
  - Prognosis for return of function
  - Site of lesion testing
- Laryngeal dystonia
- Myopathy versus neuropathy
- Motor neuron (MN) disease—upper MN versus lower MN
- ALS, Parkinson, PSA, bulbar palsy
- Stroke functional voice disorders
- Investigation of laryngeal spasm and vocal fold dysfunction
- Investigation of aberrant innervations
- Kinesiology of function in voice and swallow

ALS, amyotrophic lateral sclerosis; PSA, progressive (spinal) muscle atrophy.

(IP). Patient movement and swallow sometimes complicate the technical aspect of validating the needle insertion. The motor unit territory is small as is the size of the muscle to be sampled. The interpretation of the LEMG presents a challenge, as all LEMG examinations are currently interpreted by subjective interpretation. This can result in interpretative bias. Although subjective in nature, interpretation has strict guidelines as to what is considered hard versus soft evidence of neural dysfunction. The interpretation of LEMG is divided into evidence of denervation potentials (fibrillation potentials, complex repetitive discharges, and spontaneous irritability), reinnervation potentials (polyphasic potentials, giant potentials, and nascent units), and insertional irritability. Voluntary motor unit firing and recruitment pattern is also analyzed for the recruitment of larger motor units and unit firing rate according to the size principle. While identification of the denervation potentials and units associated with reinnervation is not difficult, interpretation of loss of recruitment and motor unit firing rate may be subjective. This is further complicated by the fact that the laryngeal muscle is neither a sphincter muscle nor a single pulley muscle with well-defined motor unit end plate territory. Another complication in the evaluation of supramaximal effort to test recruitment is the fact that patients with the needle in the intrinsic laryngeal muscle often exhibit guarding and do not give supramaximal effort on the token asked for. This can result in situations where the motor unit recruitment pattern is highly variable. An approach to overcome the subjective bias and reduce variability is quantitative LEMG. Quantitative electromyography has been used in other areas of electrophysiology for the analysis of nerve disorders but is relatively uncommon in the larynx.[46–48]

The simplest method of automated analysis of the complex IP is by integration analysis. The computer takes the complex AC signal, rectifies the signal, and then integrates the rectified signal. This measures the amplitude of the IP area. This is the oldest method for quantitative EMG. The integrated surface EMG has a rough correlation to the force output of the muscle. Simple integration is used to compare activation patterns in different muscles but does not have diagnostic value in interpretation of reduced recruitment or prognostication. It is mostly used in surface EMG kinesiology studies.

The IP, like any other signal, can be analyzed using frequency analysis using fast Fourier transformation. This mathematical analysis of complex signals divides the complex waveform signal into sine waves of different frequencies. The transformation of time-based signal into frequency-based analysis results in a power spectrum plot with the frequency plot on the x-axis and the power or density at each frequency on the y-axis. The amplitude of the frequency gives some information on the firing rate of the EMG signal. For example, in myopathic disorders, the IP spectrum contains relatively more power in the higher frequencies, reflecting shorter mean motor unit action potential (MUAP) duration. The opposite seems to hold in neurogenic disorders. This can be explained by increased MUAP duration as motor unit territory is increased in denervation and reinnervation. Spectral analysis and power spectrum analysis have also been shown to be useful in the study of muscle fatigue. With increased muscle fatigue, there is a shift to lower frequency spectral power. This may be due to increased MUAP duration resulting from slowing of muscle fiber conduction velocity.[49,50]

Turns and amplitude analysis is by far the best studied and most widely used method of automatic analysis. The concept of a turn is a change in signal direction of at least 100 PV. A comparable definition of amplitude is defined as the potential difference between successive turns. The turn and amplitude analysis was able to detect increased numbers of turns per second and reduced amplitude in myopathy, while the converse has been found in chronic denervation with compensatory reinnervation. In studies of patients with vocal fold paralysis, turn analysis and quantitative EMG were found to be helpful in predicting return of function.[51] Whether this technique can be used instead of qualitative analysis is controversial. It has been found to be complementary to combine both qualitative and quantitative methods for clinical diagnosis.[52]

Automatic measurements made on the IP have the advantage of incorporating signals from more of the muscle under study than just the very lowest threshold MUAPs. The meaning of this analysis is not clear. The parameters measured generally cannot be related directly to the properties of the constituent MUAPs.

At the minimal threshold of activation, single motor units are recruited and the lowest threshold small motor unit potentials may be analyzed. Because only the smallest units at the threshold of initial muscle activation are able to be isolated and subject to analysis, the motor units must be identified as being identical in morphology and size. Measurements of the size and amplitude of the individual motor units have been gathered for limb muscles but have not been done for laryngeal muscles.

Attempts to decompose the IP into individual motor units for analysis can be done but continues to be labor intensive.

Early report of quantification has not been used routinely in the clinic. Over the past 40 years, sporadic reports have appeared in the otolaryngology and neurological literature describing techniques and applications of LEMG. Despite considerable refinements in methodology and instrumentation over that time, LEMG has not been widely adopted in routine clinical practice. With increased familiarity with this technique, the usefulness of the information obtained by this examination has become more accepted.[53]

A few articles in the literature have looked at quantitative LEMG and its role. This is done primarily to overcome the deficiencies of qualitative examination. Twenty-one control patients and 16 patients with vocal fold paralysis were studied. A standardized protocol used a concentric needle electrode with subjects performing variable force thyroarytenoid-lateral cricoarytenoid muscle contraction. The IP was quantified by turns and mean amplitude per turn.

In controls performing variable contraction, median turns per second were significantly higher compared with those for patients. Patients with unilateral vocal fold paralysis had significantly reduced turns when compared with controls.[51]

Patients with swallow dysfunction have had their neck EMG activation patterns assessed using quantitative EMG methods. These have been done using quantitative surface EMG methods.[54] It is not clear whether this represents the pharyngeal muscles or the extrinsic laryngeal elevators. Its use is largely investigational and its clinical role is not yet routine.

In summary, although quantitative methods for LEMG present with many methods for analysis, its clinical application has not yet been demonstrated to be superior to that of qualitative analysis for general clinical applications. Despite the cumbersome issues associated with qualitative analysis, it represents the best method for analysis in the clinical arena. Future clinical trials may demonstrate the clinical utility of automated analysis of the LEMG signal.

References

1. Schönharl E. Die Stroboskopie in der praktischen Laryngologie. Stuttgart: Georg Thieme Verlag; 1960
2. Colton RH, Woo P, Brewer DW, Griffin B, Casper J. Stroboscopic signs associated with benign lesions of the vocal folds. J Voice 1995;9(3):312–325
3. Rihkanen H, Reijonen P, Lehikoinen-Söderlund S, Lauri ER. Videostroboscopic assessment of unilateral vocal fold paralysis after augmentation with autologous fascia. Eur Arch Otorhinolaryngol 2004;261(4):177–183
4. Moore P, von Leden H. Dynamic variation of the vibratory pattern in normal larynx. Folia Phoniatr (Basel) 1958;10(4):205–238
5. Timcke R, von Leden H, Moore P. Laryngeal vibrations: measurements of the glottic wave. Part 1. The normal vibratory cycle. Arch Otolaryngol 1958;68:1–19
6. Timcke R, von Leden H, Moore P. Laryngeal vibrations: measurements of the glottic wave. II. Physiologic variations. Arch Otolaryngol 1959;69(4):438–444
7. von Leden HV, Moore P, Timcke R. Laryngeal vibrations: Ill. The pathologic larynx. Archives of Otology. Rhinol Laryngol 1960;71:1232–1250
8. Verikas A, Uloza V, Bacauskiene M, Gelzinis A, Kelertas E. Advances in laryngeal imaging. Eur Arch Otorhinolaryngol 2009;266(10):1509–1520
9. Deliyski DD, Hillman RE. State of the art laryngeal imaging: research and clinical implications. Curr Opin Otolaryngol Head Neck Surg 2010;18(3):147–152
10. Blitzer A, Crumley RL, Dailey SH, et al. Recommendations of the Neurolaryngology Study Group on laryngeal electromyography. Otolaryngol Head Neck Surg 2009;140(6):782–793
11. Dorfman LJ, McGill KC. AAEE minimonograph #29: automatic quantitative electromyography. Muscle Nerve 1988;11(8):804–818
12. Hirano M. Clinical Examination of Voice. New York, NY: Springer-Verlag; 1981
13. Woo P, Colton R, Casper J, Brewer D. Diagnostic value of stroboscopy examination in hoarse patient's. J Voice 1991;5(3):231–238
14. Woo P, Casper J, Colton R, Brewer D. Aerodynamic and stroboscopic findings before and after microlaryngeal phonosurgery. J Voice 1994;8(2):186–194
15. Hibi SR, Bless DM, Hirano M, Yoshida T. Distortions of videofiberoscopy imaging: reconsideration and correction. J Voice 1988;2(2):168–175
16. Peppard R, Bless DM. A method for improving measurement reliability in laryngeal videostroboscopy. J Voice 1990;4(3):280–285
17. Lee JS, Kim E, Sung MW, Kim KH, Sung MY, Park KS. A method for assessing the regional vibratory pattern of vocal folds by analysing the video recording of stroboscopy. Med Biol Eng Comput 2001;39(3):273–278
18. Olthoff A, Woywod C, Kruse E. Stroboscopy versus high-speed glottography: a comparative study. Laryngoscope 2007;117(6):1123–1126
19. Omori K, Slavit DH, Kacker A, Blaugrund SM. Influence of size and etiology of glottal gap in glottic incompetence dysphonia. Laryngoscope 1998;108(4, Pt 1):514–518
20. Fang TJ, Li HY, Tsai FC, Chen IH. The role of glottal gap in predicting aspiration in patients with unilateral vocal paralysis. Clin Otolaryngol Allied Sci 2004;29(6):709–712
21. Farnsworth DW. High Speed Motion Pictures of Human Vocal Cords. Bell Labs Record 1940; 18:203–208
22. Woo P. Quantification of videostrobolaryngoscopic findings—measurements of the normal glottal cycle. Laryngoscope 1996; 106(3, Pt 2; Suppl 79): 1–27
23. Yumoto E. Aerodynamics, voice quality, and laryngeal image analysis of normal and pathologic voices. Curr Opin Otolaryngol Head Neck Surg 2004;12(3):166–173
24. Hirose H. High-speed digital imaging of vocal fold vibration. Acta Otolaryngol Suppl 1988;458:151–153
25. Kiritani S, Hirose H, Imagawa H. High-speed digital image analysis of vocal cord vibration in diplophonia. Speech Commun 1993;139(1–2):23–32
26. Eysholdt U, Rosanowski F, Hoppe U. [Measurement and interpretation of irregular vocal cord fold vibrations]. HNO 2003;51(9):710–716
27. Schade G, Müller F. [High speed glottographic diagnostics in laryngology]. HNO 2005;53(12):1085–1086, 1088–1091
28. Hertegård S, Larsson H, Wittenberg T. High-speed imaging: applications and development. Logoped Phoniatr Vocol 2003;28(3):133–139
29. Hertegård S. What have we learned about laryngeal physiology from high-speed digital videoendoscopy? Curr Opin Otolaryngol Head Neck Surg 2005;13(3):152–156
30. Mortensen M, Woo P. High-speed imaging used to detect vocal fold paresis: a case report. Ann Otol Rhinol Laryngol 2008;117(9): 684–687
31. Svec JG, Schutte HK. Videokymography: high-speed line scanning of vocal fold vibration. J Voice 1996;10(2):201–205
32. Schutte HK, Svec JG, Sram F. First results of clinical application of videokymography. Laryngoscope 1998;108(8, Pt 1):1206–1210
33. Schade G, Hess M, Müller F, et al. [Physical and technical elements of short-interval, color-filtered double strobe flash-stroboscopy]. HNO 2002;50(12):1079–1083
34. Tigges M, Wittenberg T, Mergell P, Eysholdt U. Imaging of vocal fold vibration by digital multi-plane kymography. Comput Med Imaging Graph 1999;23(6):323–330
35. Wittenberg T, Tigges M, Mergell P, Eysholdt U. Functional imaging of vocal fold vibration: digital multislice high-speed kymography. J Voice 2000;14(3):422–442
36. Faaborg-Andersen K, Edfeldt AW. Electromyography of intrinsic and extrinsic laryngeal muscles during silent speech: correlation with reading activity. Acta Otolaryngol 1958;49(6):478–482

37. Bevan K, Morgan MH, Griffiths MV. The role and techniques of laryngeal electromyography. Clin Otolaryngol Allied Sci 1988;13(4):299–305

38. Buchthal F, Faaborg-Andersen K. Electromyography of laryngeal and respiratory muscles: correlation with phonation and respiration. Ann Otol Rhinol Laryngol 1964;73:118–123

39. Cathala HP, Chouard CH, Le Guérinel J, Verdy MF. [Critical study of various technics of laryngeal electromyography]. Ann Otolaryngol Chir Cervicofac 1968;85(4):283–291

40. Kotby MN, Haugen LK. Clinical application of electromyography in vocal fold mobility disorders. Acta Otolaryngol 1970;70(5):428–437

41. Thumfart WF. Electromyography of the larynx and related technics. Acta Otorhinolaryngol Belg 1986;40(2):358–376

42. Elez F, Celik M. The value of laryngeal electromyography in vocal cord paralysis. Muscle Nerve 1998;21(4):552–553

43. Munin MC, Murry T, Rosen CA. Laryngeal electromyography: diagnostic and prognostic applications. Otolaryngol Clin North Am 2000;33(4):759–770

44. Kimaid PA, Crespo AN, Quagliato EM, Wolf A, Viana MA, Resende LA. Laryngeal electromyography: contribution to vocal fold immobility diagnosis. Electromyogr Clin Neurophysiol 2004;44(6):371–374

45. Xu W, Han D, Hou L, Zhang L, Zhao G. Value of laryngeal electromyography in diagnosis of vocal fold immobility. Ann Otol Rhinol Laryngol 2007;116(8):576–581

46. Fuglsang-Frederiksen A. Quantitative electromyography. I. Comparison of different methods. Electromyogr Clin Neurophysiol 1987;27(6–7):327–333

47. Fuglsang-Frederiksen A. Quantitative electromyography. II. Modifications of the turns analysis. Electromyogr Clin Neurophysiol 1987;27(6–7):335–338

48. Farkas C, Hamilton-Wright A, Parsaei H, Stashuk DW. A review of clinical quantitative electromyography. Crit Rev Biomed Eng 2010;38(5):467–485

49. Xu W, Han D, Hou L, Hu R, Wang L. Clinical and electrophysiological characteristics of larynx in myasthenia gravis. Ann Otol Rhinol Laryngol 2009;118(9):656–661

50. Boucher VJ, Ayad T. Physiological attributes of vocal fatigue and their acoustic effects: a synthesis of findings for a criterion-based prevention of acquired voice disorders. J Voice 2010;24(3):324–336

51. Statham MM, Rosen CA, Nandedkar SD, Munin MC. Quantitative laryngeal electromyography: turns and amplitude analysis. Laryngoscope 2010;120(10):2036–2041

52. Chan KM, Brown WF. Quantitation in EMG. Can J Neurol Sci 1998;25(1):S27–S31

53. Blair RL. Laryngeal electromyography. Arch Otorhinolaryngol 1989;246(5):395–396

54. Vaiman M, Segal S, Eviatar E. Surface electromyographic studies of swallowing in normal children, age 4-12 years. Int J Pediatr Otorhinolaryngol 2004;68(1):65–73

8 Laryngeal Photography and Documentation

Michael M. Johns and Taryn Davids

Laryngeal photodocumentation is an essential component of patient assessment, treatment planning, and facilitation of communication between physicians, therapists, patients, and students. Photodocumentation reduces ambiguity of subjective descriptions of laryngeal pathology. This establishes baseline findings, simplifies secondary assessments, outcome reviews, medicolegal proceedings, and permits objective comparison between visits.

Clinical Pearls

Benefits of laryngeal photodocumentation
- Communication
- Teaching
- Preoperative planning
- Medicolegal documentation
- Comparison/follow-up

Principles of Photography

Photography

Photography is the art or science of creating durable images by recording light on an image sensor (digitally) or a light-sensitive material (photographic film).

To capture a photographic image, light passes through or is reflected by the subject medium into a glass lens, which bends it into a focused image that is captured and recorded on a grid of microscopic-sized light-sensitive elements during a timed exposure. Photographers control the camera lens to expose the light recording material by shutter speed (duration of exposure) and diameter of light (aperture).

The medium on which light is recorded can be a film or an electronic image sensor. In digital cameras, exposed light falls onto a solid-state image sensor known as a charge-coupled device (CCD). The CCD is a solid silicon chip comprising a tightly packed grid of photocell receptors (photosites) that each record the intensity of exposed light after it has passed through red-, blue-, and green-colored filters. Each photosite generates a single pixel. The greater the number of pixels on a chip, the higher the resolution and greater the detail and quality of the image. Each pixel is converted into a numeric value determined by the color and intensity of light sensed during the photographic exposure. Internal software then converts the numeric data into an image storage format (e.g., JPEG, TIFF). Image files are compressed via mathematical algorithms to facilitate storage on a memory chip, internal hard drive, USB, or other storage devices. The resulting image is stored electronically but can be reproduced on paper or film. A triple-chip camera has three separate image sensors that record three sequential exposures of one CCD with a rotating filter and maximizes color depth, intensity, and clarity.

Videography

Videography is the process of capturing images on a film medium such as videotape, disk, and digital media. It records horizontal and vertical synchronization signals that are interlaced to form a video frame[1] and then are presented quickly enough for the viewer to perceive motion. As with digital cameras, video cameras also incorporate a CCD as the analog device for detecting the image. The image is then digitized using an analog-to-digital converter. Every field is captured and stored in real time. Given the massive number of images required to represent motion accurately, the video information is compressed via compression–decompression (CODEC) algorithms into media files, for example, MPEG. Once created, the files can be stored on a variety of media devices such as personal computer's hard drive, digital video disk (DVD), and USB. A media player is then required to load and control playback of digitized media (audio and video).

History of Laryngeal Imaging

Laryngeal Photography

The first laryngeal images were rendered by detailed artistic illustrations. This was the standard approach of documentation for 25 years until the first successful photographs of the human larynx were recorded by Lennox Browne in 1883,[2] followed a year later by Thomas French of New York[3,4] using a laryngeal mirror, sunlight reflected off a head mirror, and a single lens camera. The photographic devices used to obtain these images were innovative, yet cumbersome to use, and lacking in resolution and color. Further contributions came from Garel[5] and Clerf[6] who described their methods for recording stereoscopic laryngeal pictures. In the 1940s, Holinger and Brubaker published a series of articles on the use of the Holinger-Brubaker endoscopic camera for obtaining color photographs using an open-tube system with proximal illumination and a proximal optical system[7,8]; this was a major advancement in laryngeal photodocumentation.

In 1993, a technique of laryngeal photography using rigid telescopes was described by Benjamin,[9] which was then extrapolated to indirect laryngoscopy in the clinical setting.[10] Traditionally, a 35-mm single-lens reflex (SLR) camera was used to collect images in conjunction with a laryngeal mirror, a laryngoscope (flexible and rigid), and an operating microscope; however, the advancement of technology has transitioned practice to include the use of digital imaging.

The National Aeronautics and Space Administration (NASA) initially used digital imaging in the 1960s to map the surface of the moon, but it was not until the early 1990s that the first commercial digital camera became available. Initial comparisons between 35-mm and digital camera images yielded conflicting results; however, image quality for diagnostic purposes is comparable and the benefits of digital imaging far outweigh any limitations that might exist.[11]

The benefits of digital photography include rapid image production, quick and easy assessment of images for quality, deletion of poor images and capture of improved images, image quality longevity, improved ease of editing and storage, ease of publication, record sharing, communication, comparison, and rapid advancement of telemedicine. Its limitations include lower image resolution, limited depth of field (affected by distance of camera from endoscope and shutter size) detail, continuously evolving technology, and image backup files.

Clinical Pearls

Advantages of digital imaging
- Immediate image quality assessment
- Image sharing (communication, publication, patient information, medicolegal)
- Image editing
- Storage (archiving, organization, longevity)
- Cost

Videography

Dynamic videography of the larynx was developed in 1937, but it was much later adopted in the clinical setting because of its high cost. Farnsworth was the first to use high-speed motion picture to capture the vocal folds in motion.[12] This was further developed by Holinger and Brubaker in the 1940s[7,8] with their open-tube system with proximal illumination, but continued to remain in use primarily as a research tool until the 1980s when Yanagisawa began to advocate the use of commercially available analog video recorders, tape-based video systems, and color printers for the education of peers, learners, patients, and treatment planning.[13–15] Similar to the replacement of film with digital imaging, analog video has been replaced by digital video.

Office-Based Photo/Video Documentation

Photodocumentation begins in the office setting. It is at this time that the initial images/video will be obtained that will establish the diagnosis and provide baseline characteristics of a patient's presenting complaint. Setup and optimization of laryngeal imaging is thus crucial and is detailed below.

The room and equipment should be arranged such that it is convenient for the clinician and comfortable for the patient. An upright examining chair that can be adjusted by height and angle is ideal for the positioning of the patient. Positioning of the clinician's equipment should be within reach of the examining chair with easy access to shutter controls (often in the form of a foot pedal).

- Laryngoscope selection: Laryngeal visualization can be performed with either a rigid telescope or a flexible endoscope. Rigid laryngoscopy is typically performed using a 10-mm telescopic laryngeal endoscope with a 70-degree forward angle. The rigid laryngoscope has greater built-in magnification that provides superior image quality to flexible fiberoptic endoscopes.[16] The flexible endoscope permits the clinician to evaluate the larynx while performing a greater range of dynamic phonatory behaviors. Traditional flexible laryngoscopes transmit the visual image via fiberoptic channels to the camera positioned at the eyepiece; newer "chip-tip" cameras have the CCD camera positioned at the distal aspect of the flexible laryngoscope allowing a more magnified view with greater resolution than provided by the traditional flexible laryngoscope, thus narrowing the gap between rigid and flexible endoscopy.
- Camera selection: Available camera options include attaching a stand-alone 35-mm or digital camera to the head of an endoscope; however, this can be bulky and difficult to maneuver. In addition, the standard digital screen is small and difficult to appreciate the details of focus and resolution. A more convenient option is the use of a camera head attached to an endoscopic tower. Camera shutter can be controlled at the head of the camera or from a remote control such as a foot pedal.
- Light source: Typically available light sources include halogen (constant) and xenon (strobe) light sources. Ideally, halogen lighting is used to establish static parameters, while stroboscopic lighting is used to evaluate dynamic parameters such as mucosal wave. The hazards of illumination on the interpretation of the examination have been well described[17]; therefore, the choice of light source should result in a natural looking image that remains consistent from patient to patient and from examination to examination.

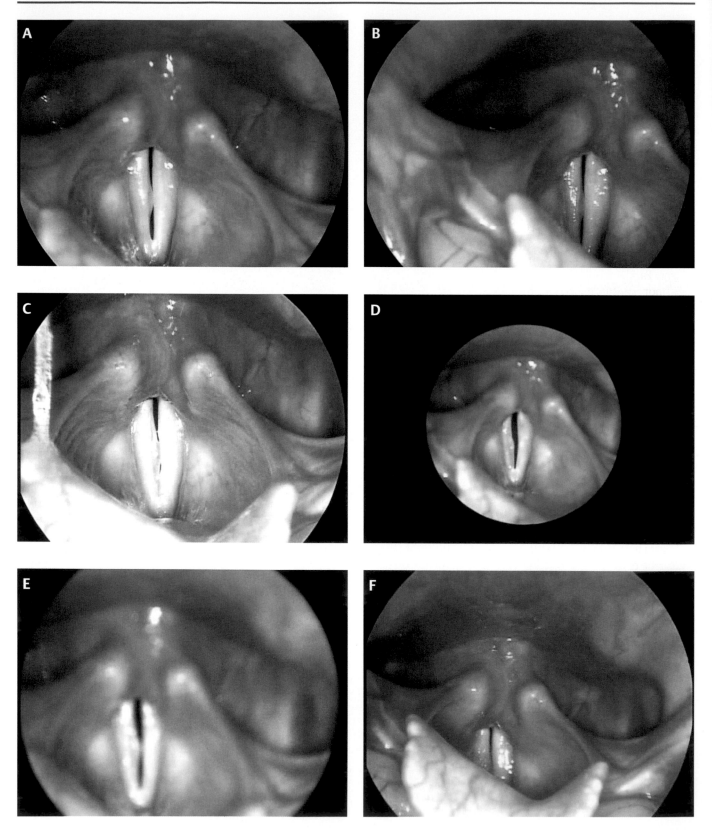

Figure 8.1   Clinical photodocumentation. (A) Good-quality image; (B) camera head misaligned with the head of the endoscope; (C) white balance not adjusted; (D) standard magnification, zoom unadjusted; (E) focus unadjusted; and (F) anterior commissure not visualized.

Endoscope–Camera Optimization

Once the choice of flexible versus rigid laryngoscope has been established, the camera head is coupled onto the eyepiece of the laryngoscope using a lens adapter. Care should be taken to ensure that the head of the endoscope and the camera are aligned. Misalignment can alter the appearance of vocal fold symmetry and motion (**Fig. 8.1A, B**). A reference point such as an article of text or the unit keyboard can be used to confirm the alignment. Ensure that the camera unit is correctly oriented with the laryngoscope such that posterior will be up and anterior will be down.

The light source is attached to the endoscope and brightness is adjusted as needed to achieve reasonable true-to-life color accuracy. The camera is white balanced to enhance color contrast and maintain consistency between images. Failure to white balance can result in dim pictures and poor resolution of subtle findings (**Fig. 8.1C**). The technique of white balance will vary with the systems used.

Camera zoom is maximized for the laryngoscope being used to achieve maximal magnification of the vocal folds (**Fig. 8.1D**). Rigid laryngoscopes allow for high optical magnification, while flexible laryngoscopes are limited by the number of fiberoptic bundles contained within the sheath. That is, greater magnification results in pixelation of the image.

Camera focus is optimized next. With the camera coupled to the laryngoscope, position the tip of the laryngoscope to a fixed point (e.g., article of text) at a distance approximating the depth of the vocal folds (approximately 2 or 3 inches for a rigid laryngoscope) and adjust the focus dial on the camera head until maximum sharpness and clarity is achieved (**Fig. 8.1E**). Flexible laryngoscopes have a separate focus that should be adjusted before being coupled to the camera head.

Before insertion of the laryngoscope into the nasal or oral cavity, the distal tip is dipped in a defog solution or warmed to prevent misting that occurs from using a cold scope in a warm environment (body temperature).

The laryngoscope is then positioned above the laryngeal introitus and centered such that the full length of the membranous vocal fold is visualized including the anterior commissure and the arytenoids posteriorly. Failure to visualize the full length of the vocal folds may result in the omission of a visible lesion (**Fig. 8.1F**). Failure to center the camera may result in an inappropriate diagnosis of the vocal fold asymmetry due to camera angle and optical skew.

Photodocumentation and Storage

Still photographs can be acquired at any point in the examination; in our practice, we recommend at minimum images from the vocal cycle that include full abduction and open and closed phases during adduction.

More commonly, dynamic examination of the larynx is performed first and video files are created from which still frame selections can be made and converted into individual image files. Video or image files can then be exported, stored, or printed in a secure database. In archiving photodocuments, it is important to develop a consistent filing system such that images can be recalled easily in future searches by key word searches.

It is important to remember that photodocumentation is a part of an individual's medical health record and should be secured and stored as such. In many cases, digital images exist in a separate database from the medical record, resulting in an increased risk of accessibility. It is the responsibility of the institution and individual collecting the photographic and video footage to protect the individuals' privacy as defined by their governing health laws. Consent should be obtained before photodocumentation and strict confidentiality should be maintained by secure data storage facilities.

Video Documentation and Storage

A variety of digital video recording systems are available for recording examinations that can be interfaced to the camera. A recording trigger can be controlled by a foot pedal, allowing the user to alternate between illumination sources and control stroboscopy modes. Camera optimization techniques are similar to those suggested earlier for laryngeal photography. The importance of endoscopic technique is emphasized. Keeping the camera centered above the laryngeal introitus, without angulation, and full visualization of the vocal folds are essential. Dynamic examination should highlight the full range of laryngeal and pharyngeal tasks and focus on problematic areas (**Table 8.1**).

Table 8.1 Dynamic Features of Laryngoscopy

Rigid	Flexible	Stroboscopic Examination
Anatomic panorama	Anatomic panorama	Anatomic panorama
Sustained /i/	Sustained /i/	Sustained modal and high /i/
Repeated /i-i-i/	/i/-sniff repeated	(comfortable loudness, soft, loud)
Glissando (up, down)	Glissando (up, down)	Repeated /i-i-i/
Quiet respiration	Connected speech	Glissando (up, down)
	Sing (happy birthday)	Inhalation phonation
	Whistle	Quiet respiration
	Phonetic loading	Focused examination around
	(for spasmodic dysphonia)	patient's difficulties
	"whee" and "hey"	
	(pharyngeal examination)	
	Quiet respiration	

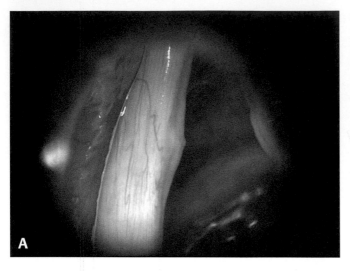

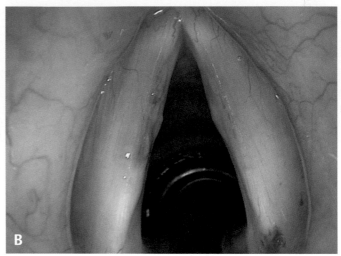

Figure 8.2   Intraoperative photography with (A) working arm of microscope versus (B) Hopkins rod.

Digital videos can be stored in several formats. Files can be stored and/or exported onto an external storage device such as DVD, USB, and external hard drive. Several archive and data storage programs are available for backup of data.

Clinical Pearls

Steps for in-office photodocumentation
- Obtain consent
- Check equipment
- Select laryngoscope
- Adjust laryngoscope focus if needed
- Align and couple camera and laryngoscope scope securely
- Illuminate
- Optimize camera zoom and focus
- Warm/defog distal laryngoscope tip
- Position over laryngeal introitus
- Record/store/archive images on secure server

Operating Room-Based Photodocumentation

Photodocumentation is of particular importance in the operative setting in medicolegal proceedings. Clear photodocumentation can eliminate ambiguity in incomplete or poor-quality medical records.

Optimization of laryngeal photography begins with the insertion and suspension of the laryngoscope. On insertion of the laryngoscope, care should be taken not to invert the epiglottis and to obtain a clear view that includes the full length of the vocal folds from the anterior commissure to the vocal processes posteriorly without distortion and asymmetry of the laryngeal anatomy.

The choice is then made to obtain images using a camera coupled either to a Hopkins rod system or directly to the microscope itself.

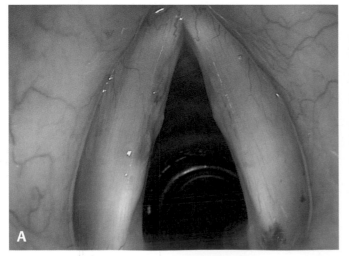

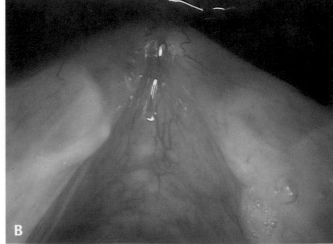

Figure 8.3   Laryngeal views with (A) 0-degree and (B) 30-degree telescope.

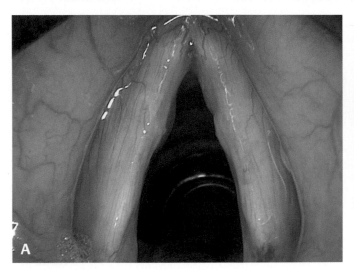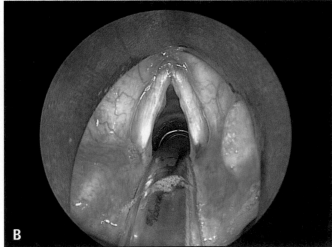

Figure 8.4 View of the larynx with Hopkins rod at (A) maximal magnification versus (B) unmagnified.

Microscope

The microscope is brought into the field of view and a 400-mm focal length objective lens is used. Magnification is maximized and the microscope is focused on the larynx at a 400-mm focal length. The camera head is directly coupled to an operating arm of the microscope (**Fig. 8.2A**).

Telescope

While the microscope provides excellent detail of the superior surfaces of the larynx, difficult areas such as the laryngeal ventricles, anterior commissure, subglottis, vallecula, and laryngeal surface of the epiglottis can often be better visualized with a Hopkins rod (**Fig. 8.2B**) system. A variety of telescopic angles such as 0, 30, 70, and 120 degree are available. Telescope diameters range from 1.9 to 10 mm. The authors routinely use a 0- and 30-degree, 10-mm telescope for the majority of laryngeal photodocumentation (**Fig. 8.3A**).

The telescope is attached to the light source and coupled to the camera using a standard lens adapter. The camera is white balanced, magnification is maximized (**Fig. 8.4**), and focus is adjusted using the camera dials. The telescope is warmed or dipped into a commercially available defog solution before entering the airway. The 0-degree telescope is centered above the laryngeal introitus; care must be taken to include the full length of the vocal folds from the anterior commissure to the posterior vocal processes. A consistent distance from the superior surface of the vocal folds should be maintained for comparison purposes. The 30-degree telescope is then used to assess the anterior commissure and laryngeal ventricles (**Fig. 8.3B**). Preoperative and postoperative images are recommended for ideal communication.

Camera

As in the clinical setting, several camera options exist. A digital camera or camera head coupled to an endoscopy tower can be used to collect photo- or video documentation.

The files can be printed, stored, or exported directly from the system.

Limitations of Laryngeal Photography/Videography

As with any diagnostic tool, one should be aware of the limitations of the equipment being used. The first limitation is depth of the field; laryngeal photography provides a two-dimensional view of the vocal folds, thereby limiting our appreciation of the three-dimensional nature of the tissue. The second limitation is the choice of endoscope used for the examination.[17] Fiberoptic endoscopes have a "fish-eye" lens that permits wide-angle visualization of the laryngopharynx, but may distort the image as we get further from the center of the image. The third limitation is optimization of the equipment. Depending on the equipment, magnification, or operator settings, illumination can vary from examination to examination, thus affecting interpretation and reliability between examinations.[17] Focus and zoom are approximated before introduction of the laryngoscope to the laryngeal introitus; however, fine adjustments may be needed during laryngoscopy. Finally, skill and technique of the clinician should not be underestimated in laryngeal imaging[18,19] as any angulation of the endoscope may alter the appearance of the vocal folds.

References

1. Crump JM, Deutsch T. Exchanging digital video of laryngeal examinations. J Voice 2004;18(1):13–23
2. Browne L. On photography of the larynx and soft palate. BMJ 1883;2(1191):811–816
3. French TR. Photographing the larynx. Arch Laryngol 1882;3:221–222
4. French TR. On a perfected method of photographing the larynx. N Y State J Med 1884;40:653–656
5. Garel J. Nouvelappareilperfectionne pour la photographiestereoscopique du larynx sur le vivant. Rev Laryng 1919;40:249–253
6. Clerf LH. Photography of the larynx. Ann Otol Rhinol 1925;34:101–107
7. Holinger PA, Brubaker JD, Brubaker JE. Open tube, proximal illumination mirror and direct laryngeal photography. Can J Otolaryngol 1975;4(5):781–785

8. Holinger PA. Photography of the larynx, trachea, bronchi, and esophagus. Trans Am Broncho-Esophagol Assoc 1984:123

9. Benjamin B. Technique of laryngeal photography. Ann Otol Rhinol Laryngol Suppl 1984;109(109):1–11

10. Benjamin B. Indirect laryngeal photography using rigid telescopes. Laryngoscope 1998;108(2):158–161

11. Melder PC, Mair EA. Endoscopic photography: digital or 35 mm? Arch Otolaryngol Head Neck Surg 2003;129(5):570–575

12. Farnsworth D. High-speed motion pictures of the human vocal cords. Bell Lab Rec 1940;18:203–208

13. Yanagisawa E. Videolaryngoscopy using a low cost home video system color camera. J Biol Photogr 1984;52(2):9–14

14. Yanagisawa K, Shi JM, Yanagisawa E. Color photography of video images of otolaryngological structures using a 35 mm SLR camera. Laryngoscope 1987;97(8 Pt 1):992–993

15. Yanagisawa E, Yanagisawa R. Laryngeal photography. Otolaryngol Clin North Am 1991;24(5):999–1022

16. Yanagisawa E, Yanagisawa K. Stroboscopic videolaryngoscopy: a comparison of fiberscopic and telescopic documentation. Ann Otol Rhinol Laryngol 1993;102(4 Pt 1):255–265

17. Milstein CF, Charbel S, Hicks DM, Abelson TI, Richter JE, Vaezi MF. Prevalence of laryngeal irritation signs associated with reflux in asymptomatic volunteers: impact of endoscopic technique (rigid vs. flexible laryngoscope). Laryngoscope 2005;115(12):2256–2261

18. Low C, Young P, Webb CJ, et al. A simple and reliable predictor for an adequate laryngeal view with rigid endoscopic laryngoscopy. Otolaryngol Head Neck Surg 2005;132(2):244–246

19. Poburka BJ, Bless DM. A multi-media, computer-based method for stroboscopy rating training. J Voice 1998;12(4):513–526

9 Office Procedures in Laryngology: Office-Based Laryngeal Laser Surgery with Local Anesthesia

Steven M. Zeitels, James A. Burns, and Anca M. Barbu

Office-based transoral laryngeal surgery was performed initially and routinely in surgeons' offices in the 19th century. Migration to the operating room in the early 20th century occurred with direct laryngoscopic surgery, which was optimized by assistants administering anesthesia and procedural support. Improvements in imaging provided by the surgical microscope, along with hemostatic cutting facilitated by the carbon dioxide laser, anchored precise endolaryngeal surgery to the operating theater. Recent advancements in distal-chip flexible endoscopic technology and fiber-based lasers have allowed for the creation of office-based laryngeal laser surgery, which was first instituted in 2001 and first presented at the American Laryngological Association in 2003.[1] **Fig. 9.1** shows a patient undergoing office-based flexible laryngoscopic laser surgery with topical local anesthesia. In this minimally invasive approach, an assistant holds the laser fiber as it courses from the laser to the side-port working channel of the flexible laryngoscope and the surgeon observes the surgical field on the monitor. Our current treatment strategies using office-based laryngeal laser surgery are primarily limited to treatment of benign epithelial proliferative disorders such as dysplasia and papilloma. Precise microsurgery of phonatory mucosa (nodules, polyps, cysts, ectasias, and varices) is optimally managed by means of general anesthesia with stereoscopic magnification and bimanual dissection to maximally preserve the normal overlying epithelium and underlying

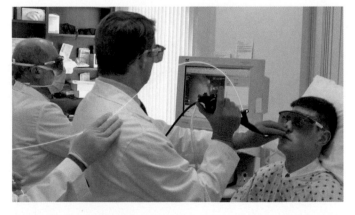

Figure 9.1 Office-based treatment of a patient with glottic papillomatosis, using pulsed potassium-titanyl-phosphate laser. The laser fiber (green due to a pulse of 532-nm laser energy) is passed through the side-port working channel of a flexible laryngoscope.

superficial lamina propria (SLP). Fiber-based lasers currently widely utilized in office-based laryngeal laser surgery include the selective photoangiolytic 532-nm potassium-titanyl-phosphate (KTP) pulsed laser[2] and the ablative 2013-nm continuous-wave thulium laser.[3]

Selective Photoangiolysis and the 532-nm KTP Laser

In the 1980s, Anderson et al[4-6] proposed concepts of selective photothermolysis that allowed for specific targeted damage to cells by "suitably brief pulses" of optical radiation based on properties of the target tissue. Anderson, a dermatologist, applied selective photothermolysis to the development of yellow light (585 to 600 nm) pulsed-dye laser (PDL) for the treatment of vascular malformations by targeting oxyhemoglobin.[6] This concept eventually evolved into two angiolytic lasers: the 585-nm PDL and the 532-nm pulsed KTP laser. These wavelengths are precisely selected to target absorbance peaks of oxyhemoglobin (~571 nm and ~541 nm) and can fully penetrate intraluminal blood and deposit heat uniformly into the vessel, thereby causing intravascular coagulation and "photoangiolysis" of the subepithelial microcirculation. The short pulse width is precisely selected to contain the heat to the vessel without causing collateral damage to the extravascular soft tissue from heat conduction. The output of these lasers is transmitted through a thin flexible glass fiber (≤ 0.6 mm).

When applied to vocal folds, the precise coagulation of subepithelial microcirculation within the layered microstructure of the phonatory mucosa has since been shown to be an effective strategy to treat papillomatosis,[2,7-12] dysplasia,[13-15] and microvascular angiomata.[16-18] The KTP laser has also been demonstrated to be effective for treating early glottic cancer.[19,20] Photoangiolytic lasers, which were originally used by our group over 10 years ago to facilitate microflap resection of vocal fold dysplasia, are now used routinely in office-based laryngeal surgery to involute premalignant laryngeal disease and papilloma without resection.[2,15] **Fig. 9.2** shows vocal folds with diffuse dysplasia (**Fig. 9.2A**) being treated in the office setting with pulsed KTP laser photoangiolysis (**Fig. 9.2B**). The selectivity of photoangiolytic lasers leads to improved vocal outcomes by allowing for aggressive treatment of dysplasia and papilloma

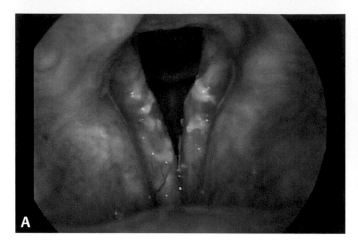

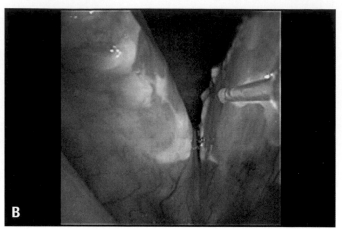

Figure 9.2 (A) Rigid transoral examination showing diffuse bilateral vocal fold dysplasia with keratosis (white) and erythematous (red) regions. (B) This same patient is undergoing office-based pulsed potassium-titanyl-phosphate laser photoangiolysis via transnasal endoscopy. Note the laser fiber (right side of image) treating disease on the medial surface of the left vocal fold.

with maximum preservation of the layered microstructure of the vocal fold including the SLP.

Our current treatment strategies using office-based laryngeal laser surgery are limited to the treatment of dysplasia and papilloma, and we do not favor the use of office-based techniques in the management of malignancy, microvascular angiomata, benign phonotraumatic lesions such as polyps, or chronic inflammatory conditions such as polypoid corditis unless the patient's medical comorbidities prohibit general anesthesia.[21,22] Office-based laryngeal laser surgery sacrifices a certain degree of precision due to the loss of binocular visualization, high-powered magnification, and an immobile and insensate operative field that exists when surgery is performed in patients who are under general anesthesia. Office-based laryngeal laser surgery is advantageous in cases of recurrent dysplasia and papilloma due to the avoidance of multiple general anesthetics and the ability to treat regrowth of disease more often with less recovery time.

Dysplasia and papillomatosis are the two most common indications for photoangiolysis using pulsed KTP laser, both in the operating room and in the office.[23] Our current strategy is to treat patients initially in the operating room where the extent of epithelial disease and the prior surgically induced soft-tissue changes can be adequately assessed. The KTP laser has proven its utility in ablating disease with maximum preservation of the underlying SLP, and this laser is used in almost every patient with dysplasia or papilloma. **Fig. 9.3** shows a patient with recurrent laryngeal papilloma (**Fig. 9.3A**) who presents for office-based pulsed KTP laser photoangiolysis (**Fig. 9.3B**) after previously undergoing surgery in the operating room under general anesthesia. Subsequent treatments are done in the office depending on patient tolerance and preference, extent of disease, and location of the disease. Office-based KTP laser use for dysplasia and papilloma is primarily for disease on the superior and medial glottic surfaces as well as in the supraglottis. Disease on the inferior surface of the vocal folds

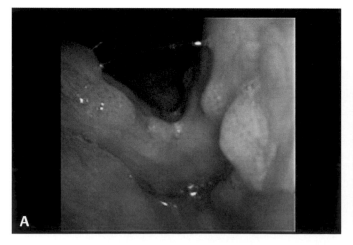

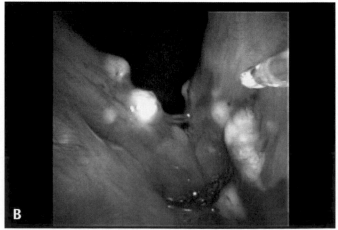

Figure 9.3 (A) Transnasal distal-chip scope endoscopy of a patient with diffuse vocal fold and supraglottic recurrent papilloma. (B) This same patient is undergoing office-based pulsed potassium-titanyl-phosphate laser photoangiolysis of papilloma. Note the characteristic white blanching of the disease that has already been treated. The laser fiber (right side of image) is being withdrawn after treating supraglottic papilloma.

and subglottis is harder to treat in the office setting. These patients require extended follow-up to detect recurrent disease. Even though office-based pulsed KTP laser ablation is sometimes less effective than similar photoangiolytic treatment in the operating room, due to time constraints associated with topical anesthesia, posttreatment dysphonia is often diminished as well. Although this treatment strategy often results in more frequent procedures (and therefore more total cases) due to limitations of the therapeutic window provided by topical anesthesia, patients are able to avoid the risks of multiple general anesthetics.

Ablation and the 2013-nm Continuous-Wave Thulium Laser

Recently, a 2013-nm continuous-wave laser was developed to simulate the cutting properties of the carbon dioxide laser.[3] The RevoLix laser (LISA Laser Products, Katlenburg-Lindau, Germany) is a diode-pumped solid-state laser that has a thulium-doped yttrium-aluminum-garnet laser rod that produces a continuous-wave beam with a wavelength of 2013 nm. This wavelength has a target chromophore of water, making it an effective laser for hemostatic cutting. A distinct advantage of the thulium laser is its glass fiber delivery system, which allows for tangential endoscopic dissection as well as office-based use through a flexible fiberoptic laryngoscope. Our preliminary use with the thulium laser during endoscopic partial laryngectomy procedures in both the glottis and the supraglottis[3,24] revealed that this laser created effective hemostasis with increased thermal damage on the soft tissues at the margin of the cancerous section as compared with the carbon dioxide laser, although this degree of thermal damage did not seem excessive.

While there is not a significant need for nonselective ablation of laryngeal lesions in the office-based setting, there are occasional indications where patients would benefit from this technique. We have used the thulium laser through the flexible laryngoscope to perform ablation of diffuse recurrent respiratory papillomatosis and lesions of the larynx apart from the phonatory membranes.[3] Often these are patients who require multiple procedures for severe, extensive disease or who are poor candidates for general anesthesia and require ablation of a lesion where precise preservation of the vocal fold layered microstructure is not of major concern.

Anesthetic Considerations

Patients undergoing office-based laryngeal laser surgery require optimal anesthesia of the entire upper aerodigestive tract. Timing is important during delivery of topical anesthesia to ensure that treatment commences shortly after maximum anesthesia is achieved. There is generally a small therapeutic time period during which patients can be treated before they start to react to the lasering with increased secretions and discomfort. In some cases, it is helpful to have patients take Valium (diazepam, 5 mg, taken orally 30 minutes before the procedure) or the equivalent antianxiolytic before beginning office-based surgery. Most patients tolerate office-based laryngeal laser surgery quite well, and it is unusual to have the patient undergo general anesthesia solely on the basis of tolerance of the procedure.[25]

The nasal passage is decongested and anesthetized by spraying a mixture of Neo-Synephrine (phenylephrine) and Topicaine (lidocaine) transnasally. Butamben (cetacaine) spray is judiciously applied to the tongue base and soft palate. Patients are then asked to inhale an atomized solution of 4% lidocaine to begin to directly numb the glottis. Final anesthesia at the target treatment site or sites within the larynx is achieved by directly dripping up to an additional 4 mL (in adult patients) of 4% lidocaine onto the treatment site under direct visualization of the transnasal scope. Treatment should begin within 5 to 10 minutes of application of the topical anesthetic to ensure a maximum period of time for lasering before secretions accumulate and patients' tolerance for the procedure diminishes.

Surgical Steps

For office-based surgery, a flexible laryngoscope with suction and a side-port working channel is necessary to deliver the laser fiber to the target tissue. A small fiber size is desirable because the fiber lies within the suction port, and large fibers can make suctioning of thick secretions difficult (**Fig. 9.4A, B**). Basic surgical principles are the maximum reduction of disease with preservation of the vocal fold with little or no scarring. In adults, surgical intervention is often done solely for voice-related symptoms, unlike the concern for airway obstruction that is the predominate reason for surgical management of pediatric patients. **Fig. 9.1** depicts the typical office-based setup for the treatment of laryngeal papilloma in an awakened patient with topical anesthesia.

1. Patients are seated in a standard otolaryngologic examination chair and the optimal height is adjusted for the operating surgeon. It is helpful to place a pillow behind the patient's back to provide comfortable padding against which they may brace themselves.
2. After adequate topical anesthesia is achieved, transnasal flexible laryngoscopy is performed with a scope that contains both suction and a side-port working channel.
3. The laser fiber is delivered through the side-port working channel of the flexible scope and used to treat the disease in both contact and noncontact modes. Treating laryngeal papilloma in an awakened patient is less precise than when the patient is under general anesthesia due to the patient's respiration and occasional swallowing. However, when using the KTP laser, the selectivity of this laser to be preferentially absorbed by the more vascular papilloma ensures optimal treatment of disease.

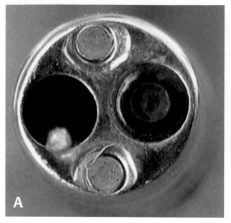
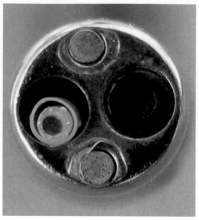
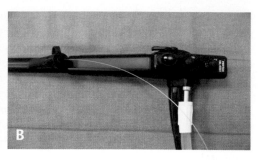

Figure 9.4   (A) The distal flexible laryngoscope revealing the 2-mm working channel with laser fibers and sheaths. Note that the 0.4-mm potassium-titanyl-phosphate laser fiber (left) with its sheath allows for substantially more area to suction secretions and blood than the larger (0.6-mm) pulsed-dye laser fiber (right) with sheath. (B) The image shows a typical flexible laryngoscope with suction attached (white tubing) and laser fiber being inserted into the side-port working channel.

4. Disease is treated to the endpoint of white blanching (indicating that the intralesional vasculature has been coagulated). Bulky exophytic disease can be suctioned away. The base of the treatment site can then be treated again with laser energy.
5. Lasering continues until all visible disease has been adequately treated or until patients' tolerance and increased secretions prohibit further lasering.

Complications

Scarring of the vocal fold can occur if treatment is too aggressive or if there is excessive thermal trauma from the laser. Even the highly selective photoangiolytic KTP laser can cause thermal trauma to the layered microstructure of vocal folds with resulting scarring and dysphonia. Unfortunately, there is no optimal solution for the formation of vocal fold scarring currently, so this complication is best avoided with meticulous technique and careful use of the laser. It is sometimes advantageous to leave the disease rather than risk excessive scarring.

Even though office-based procedures are less precise, careful laser technique can avoid excessive scar formation. Care must be taken to avoid lasering if blood has extravasated outside of the microvasculature during vessel rupture. If this happens, KTP laser energy will be absorbed nonselectively with potential vocal fold scarring.

Conclusion

Since their introduction in laryngology nearly 40 years ago, lasers have facilitated critically important innovations that have now evolved into office-based surgery. These advancements accommodated well to our specialty, which has been the leader in designing minimally invasive surgical approaches since mirror-guided interventions in the 19th century. Lasers discussed herein are providing technologies that will likely lead to enhanced treatment of several benign and malignant laryngeal disorders. In an expanding group of centers, fiber-based technologies have already caused many procedures to be performed by means of local anesthesia in the clinic or office, especially for chronic diseases such as papillomatosis and dysplasia. This approach is likely to expand significantly due to diminished patient morbidity along with socioeconomic pressures of health care delivery. One of the substantial roadblocks to the dissemination of these clinical advancements is the cost required to install laser technology in institutions and surgeons' offices. Furthermore, critical development of these new lasers is limited by the relatively small numbers of patients with laryngeal disorders, which discourages industry from investing substantially in research and development. To solve this problem, our hope is that laryngeal surgery will continue to serve as a model for high-performance minimally invasive surgery that can be translated to other mucosal diseases of the upper and lower aerodigestive tract, genitourinary organs, and the cervix. Broader use of these new lasers in other surgical disciplines should diminish costs for all surgeons and their associated institutions.

Vocal Fold Injections

One of the most common indications for office-based vocal fold injection is unilateral vocal cord paralysis (UVCP). This condition leads to glottic insufficiency, which can result in dysphonia, weakened cough, aspiration, and pneumonia. Vocal fold medialization by injecting an absorbable gel into the paraglottic space can be helpful for temporarily restoring glottic competence, thereby improving voice and potentially reducing aspiration.[26,27] Patients with delayed glottic onset during phonation due to Parkinson disease can benefit from bilateral deep paraglottic space injections.[28] Recent retrospective studies[29,30] suggest an association between early vocal cord medialization injection and a reduced need for open neck laryngeal framework surgery in patients with persistent UVCP. Injection medialization procedures can be performed with topical anesthesia either at the hospital bedside or in the clinic, using either transoral[31] or transcervical[32] methods.

Transoral Techniques

Transoral injection techniques commonly use rigid transoral laryngoscopes for visualization. After topically anesthetizing the oropharynx with cetacaine spray, patients are asked to inhale an atomized solution of 4% lidocaine to begin to directly numb the glottis. Final anesthesia at the target treatment site or sites within the larynx is achieved by directly dripping up to an additional 4 mL of 4% lidocaine (in adult patients) onto the treatment site under direct visualization of the transnasal scope. A transoral Ford injection catheter (Xomed, Minneapolis, Minnesota, United States) fitted with a 25-gauge needle is used to deliver the desired material to the larynx. Temporary space-filling gels are directed more deeply into the paraglottic space (**Fig. 9.5A, B**), and medications for the adjuvant treatment of epithelial proliferative disorders are injected more superficially in the immediate subepithelial plane (**Fig. 9.6A**).

Paraglottic Space (Deep) Injections

Some form of temporary gel is typically utilized for deep paraglottic injections when vocal fold medialization to improve glottic efficiency is desired. Materials such as cymetra,[33] calcium hydroxylapatite,[34] carboxymethylcellulose,[35] and cross-linked hyaluronic acid[36]—to name a few—have been popularized recently. Our group favors any material that offers easy "off-the-shelf" administration with no preinjection preparation

and a predictable *temporary* effect. Patients may hold their own tongue or an assistant can be employed to hold the patient's tongue extended as the surgeon uses both hands during injection by holding the scope and injection catheter. Glottic insufficiency due to unilateral vocal fold immobility (**Fig. 9.5A**) can be corrected by augmenting the paraglottic space (**Fig. 9.5B**) to achieve medialization of the immobile vocal fold and better glottic sufficiency.

Subepithelial (Superficial) Injections

Superficial injections in the immediate subepithelial plane (**Fig. 9.6A**) are commonly given to map areas of vocal fold scar with saline or to deliver a therapeutic drug such as a steroid[37] or Avastin (bevacizumab).[38] The technique of vocal fold infusion was first reported in the 1890s as a means of understanding aerodigestive tract infectious disease and defining connective tissue compartments of the larynx.[39,40] Similar infusion studies were repeated to better understand patterns of glottic lymphatic spread[41–43] and to determine the effect of hydrodissection in facilitating preservation of SLP and epithelium during phonomicrosurgery for malignant[44] and benign[45] lesions. Broader applications of this technique have emerged to assist during office-based laryngeal procedures so that saline infusion can provide real-time information to the surgeon about vocal fold lesions and deliver medication to a specific vocal fold location.

A recent prospective open-label investigation in 20 adult patients with bilateral vocal fold papillomatosis provided preliminary evidence that bevacizumab injections enhanced photoangiolytic laser treatment of glottal papillomatosis with associated improvements in phonatory function.[38] The use of bevacizumab is based on the possible role of vascular endothelial growth factor (VEGF) in the neoplastic progression of recurrent respiratory papillomatosis.[46] Bevacizumab is a recombinant humanized

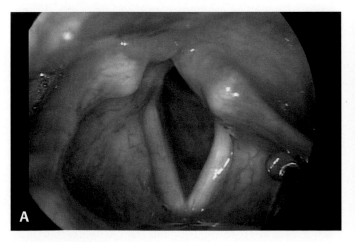
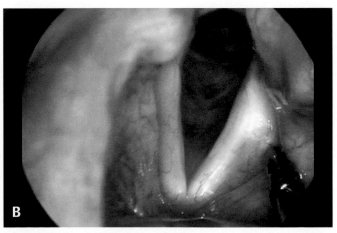

Figure 9.5 (A) Transoral endoscopic view of glottic insufficiency due to an immobile left vocal fold. Note the "bowing" of the left vocal fold posteriorly. A catheter (far right side of image) is used to apply topical anesthesia at the injection site. (B) This same patient undergoing transoral injection of Restylane into the left paraglottic space. Note the increased fullness at the injection site.

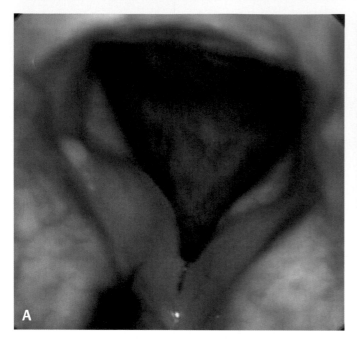 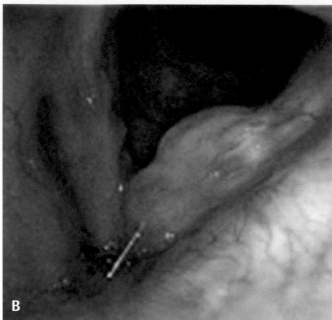

Figure 9.6 (A) Transoral injection of bevacizumab into the subepithelial plane with volume expansion of the superficial lamina propria (SLP) layer as the drug is administered. Note that the needle tip is visible under the epithelium indicating a superficial placement. (B) Transcervical injection of bevacizumab into the subepithelial plane with expansion of the SLP layer. The needle enters the laryngeal introitus above the anterior commissure (bottom of image) and is directed into the patient's left vocal fold. The needle tip is visible under the epithelium.

monoclonal immunoglobulin G1 antibody that binds to and inhibits the biologic activity of human VEGF. The drug is formulated as a clear to slightly opalescent, colorless sterile solution and is supplied in 100-mg preservative-free single-use vials at a concentration of 25 mg/mL. Our current treatment strategy for the delivery of this drug is either to inject 0.5 to 1.0 mL into the subepithelial plane of a vocal fold or supraglottic location following ablation of the disease with a pulsed KTP laser or to inject a similar volume intralesionally without lasering. The optimal treatment strategy may vary between patients and is still being determined with ongoing study. **Fig. 9.6A** shows the transoral injection of bevacizumab in the subepithelial plane.

Transcervical Techniques

Surgeon's preference or patient tolerance may dictate a transcervical injection either for deep paraglottic placement of material or for superficial subepithelial injections. The technique for this approach was first described by Amin[32] and involves placement of the needle through the thyrohyoid membrane just superior to the thyroid notch. Once identified within the lumen of the airway just superior to the vocal folds, the needle can be directed laterally for injection into the superficial or deep plane of the vocal fold under direct visualization of the flexible laryngoscope. **Fig. 9.6B** shows an endoscopic view of the needle being inserted transcervically and directed into the left vocal fold in the immediate subepithelial plane. This technique has proven to be well tolerated by patients given local anesthesia in the

office setting. Alternatively, injections into the paraglottic space can be given with a puncture through the ala of the thyroid cartilage at the presumed level of the vocal fold.[36]

Botox Injections for Laryngeal Dystonia and Arytenoid Granuloma

Injection of botulinum toxin has gained widespread acceptance in the management of symptoms associated with spasmodic dysphonia (SD), a focal dystonia involving laryngeal muscles that interferes with normal phonation.[47–49] Temporary relief from the characteristic strained/strangulated speech pattern of adductor SD and breathiness of abductor SD is achieved with office-based botox injections. After reconstituting the toxin in saline, the mixture is drawn into a 1.0-mL tuberculin syringe fitted into an electrode needle for transcervical electromyography (EMG)-guided injection. A specialized monopolar 25-gauge concentric hollow-bore needle is used to deliver the toxin, and EMG signals help confirm proper needle placement.[50] For the adductor type of SD, the needle is inserted just superior to the cricoid cartilage in the midline, through the cricothyroid membrane, then directed superolaterally into the thyroarytenoid (TA) muscle. Vocalization of a high-pitched /E/ adducts the vocal folds and localizes the TA muscle for delivery of botox. For the abductor type of SD, the needle is inserted into the posterior cricoarytenoid (PCA) muscle after rotating the larynx to expose the posterolateral edge. The PCA muscle is localized by having the patient sniff, which creates abduction of the vocal folds by activating the PCA muscle. Most patients tolerate this in the office setting without the use of topical anesthesia or sedation. Alternatively, transnasal flexible laryngoscopy can be performed to visually guide the needle into each TA muscle,[51] and this technique can be used instead of EMG confirmation or as an additional means of confirming needle placement. Arytenoid granulomas that are refractory to conservative treatments such as optimal reflux management and speech and language therapy can be managed with office-based injection of botox.[52] The muscle weakness created by injecting botox into both the TA and lateral cricothyroid muscles reduces or eliminates collision forces between the arytenoid cartilages during phonation and allows for healing of the granuloma. Patients are warned about a potentially lengthy (>2 weeks) period of extreme breathiness shortly after botox injection due to profound muscle weakness.

Conclusions: Office Procedures in Laryngology

Office-based laryngeal surgery with topical anesthesia is proving to be a safe and effective treatment option for many patients with upper aerodigestive tract pathology. Recent advancements in distal-chip flexible endoscopic technology and fiber-based lasers that allowed for the creation of office-based laryngeal laser surgery will undoubtedly continue to evolve. The development of new drugs to inhibit angiogenesis via transoral injection into vocal folds will offer the surgeon new options in treating epithelial proliferative disorders. Future biomaterials that re-establish vocal fold pliability and restore vocal function will be delivered to patients in an office setting with topical anesthesia. The laryngeal procedures described herein provide a solid foundation upon which future advances will continue to improve patient care and provide the option of office-based treatment without the need for general anesthesia.

References

1. Zeitels SM, Franco RA Jr, Dailey SH, Burns JA, Hillman RE, Anderson RR. Office-based treatment of glottal dysplasia and papillomatosis with the 585-nm pulsed dye laser and local anesthesia. Ann Otol Rhinol Laryngol 2004;113(4):265–276
2. Zeitels SM, Akst LM, Burns JA, Hillman RE, Broadhurst MS, Anderson RR. Office-based 532-nm pulsed KTP laser treatment of glottal papillomatosis and dysplasia. Ann Otol Rhinol Laryngol 2006;115(9):679–685
3. Zeitels SM, Burns JA, Akst LM, Hillman RE, Broadhurst MS, Anderson RR. Office-based and microlaryngeal applications of a fiber-based thulium laser. Ann Otol Rhinol Laryngol 2006;115(12):891–896
4. Anderson RR, Parrish JA. Selective photothermolysis: precise microsurgery by selective absorption of pulsed radiation. Science 1983;220(4596):524–527
5. Anderson RR, Parrish JA. Microvasculature can be selectively damaged using dye lasers: a basic theory and experimental evidence in human skin. Lasers Surg Med 1981;1(3):263–276

6. Anderson RR, Jaenicke KF, Parrish JA. Mechanisms of selective vascular changes caused by dye lasers. Lasers Surg Med 1983;3(3):211–215
7. Bower CM, Waner M, Flock S, Schaeffer R. Flash pump dye laser treatment of laryngeal papillomas. Ann Otol Rhinol Laryngol 1998;107(12):1001–1005
8. McMillan K, Shapshay SM, McGilligan JA, Wang Z, Rebeiz EE. A 585-nanometer pulsed dye laser treatment of laryngeal papillomas: preliminary report. Laryngoscope 1998;108(7):968–972
9. Valdez TA, McMillan K, Shapshay SM. A new laser treatment for vocal cord papilloma—585-nm pulsed dye. Otolaryngol Head Neck Surg 2001;124(4):421–425
10. Franco RA Jr, Zeitels SM, Farinelli WA, Anderson RR. 585-nm pulsed dye laser treatment of glottal papillomatosis. Ann Otol Rhinol Laryngol 2002;111(6):486–492
11. Burns JA, Zeitels SM, Akst LM, Broadhurst MS, Hillman RE, Anderson R. 532 nm pulsed potassium-titanyl-phosphate laser treatment of laryngeal papillomatosis under general anesthesia. Laryngoscope 2007;117(8):1500–1504
12. Zeitels SM. Papillomatosis. Atlas of Phonomicrosurgery and Other Endolaryngeal Procedures for Benign and Malignant Disease. San Diego, CA: Singular; 2001:119–131
13. Zeitels SM. Vocal Fold Atypia/Dysplasia and Carcinoma. Atlas of Phonomicrosurgery and Other Endolaryngeal Procedures for Benign and Malignant Disease. San Diego, CA: Singular; 2001:177–218
14. Franco RA Jr, Zeitels SM, Farinelli WA, Faquin W, Anderson RR. 585-nm pulsed dye laser treatment of glottal dysplasia. Ann Otol Rhinol Laryngol 2003;112(9 Pt 1):751–758
15. Zeitels SM, Franco RA Jr, Dailey SH, Burns JA, Hillman RE, Anderson RR. Office-based treatment of glottal dysplasia and papillomatosis with the 585-nm pulsed dye laser and local anesthesia. Ann Otol Rhinol Laryngol 2004;113(4):265–276
16. Zeitels SM, Hillman RE, Desloge R, Mauri M, Doyle PB. Phonomicrosurgery in singers and performing artists: treatment outcomes, management theories, and future directions. Ann Otol Rhinol Laryngol Suppl 2002;190:21–40
17. Hsiung MW, Kang BH, Su WF, Pai L, Wang HW. Clearing microvascular lesions of the true vocal fold with the KTP/532 laser. Ann Otol Rhinol Laryngol 2003;112(6):534–539
18. Zeitels SM, Akst LM, Bums JA, Hillman RE, Broadhurst MS, Anderson RR. Pulsed angiolytic laser treatment of ectasias and varices in singers. Ann Otol Rhinol Laryngol 2006;115(8):571–580
19. Zeitels SM, Burns JA, Lopez-Guerra G, Anderson RR, Hillman RE. Photoangiolytic laser treatment of early glottic cancer: a new management strategy. Ann Otol Rhinol Laryngol Suppl 2008;199:3–24
20. Friedman AD, Hillman RE, Landau-Zemer T, Burns JA, Zeitels SM. Voice outcomes for photoangiolytic laser treatment of early glottic cancer. Ann Otol Rhinol Laryngol 2013;122(3):151–158
21. Zeitels SM, Burns JA. Office-based laryngeal laser surgery with local anesthesia. Curr Opin Otolaryngol Head Neck Surg 2007;15(3):141–147
22. Zeitels SM, Burns JA. Office-based laryngeal laser surgery with the 532-nm pulsed-potassium-titanyl-phosphate laser. Curr Opin Otolaryngol Head Neck Surg 2007;15(6):394–400
23. Burns JA, Friedman AD, Lutch MJ, Hillman RE, Zeitels SM. Value and utility of 532 nanometre pulsed potassium-titanyl-phosphate laser in endoscopic laryngeal surgery. J Laryngol Otol 2010;124(4):407–411

24. Stansel F, Raasch P, Haeussinger K. A New 2 micron Laser in Airway Disobliteration: A Feasibility and Safety Study. Presented at the European Respiratory Society: Copenhagen, Denmark; 2005

25. Rees CJ, Halum SL, Wijewickrama RC, Koufman JA, Postma GN. Patient tolerance of in-office pulsed dye laser treatments to the upper aerodigestive tract. Otolaryngol Head Neck Surg 2006;134(6):1023–1027

26. Anderson TD, Mirza N. Immediate percutaneous medialization for acute vocal fold immobility with aspiration. Laryngoscope 2001;111(8):1318–1321

27. Grant JR, Hartemink DA, Patel N, Merati AL. Acute and subacute awake injection laryngoplasty for thoracic surgery patients. J Voice 2008;22(2):245–250

28. Berke GS, Gerratt B, Kreiman J, Jackson K. Treatment of Parkinson hypophonia with percutaneous collagen augmentation. Laryngoscope 1999;109(8):1295–1299

29. Friedman AD, Burns JA, Heaton JT, Zeitels SM. Early versus late injection medialization for unilateral vocal cord paralysis. Laryngoscope 2010;120(10):2042–2046

30. Arviso LC, Johns MM III, Mathison CC, Klein AM. Long-term outcomes of injection laryngoplasty in patients with potentially recoverable vocal fold paralysis. Laryngoscope 2010;120(11):2237–2240

31. Ford CN. A multipurpose laryngeal injector device. Otolaryngol Head Neck Surg 1990;103(1):135–137

32. Amin MR. Thyrohyoid approach for vocal fold augmentation. Ann Otol Rhinol Laryngol 2006;115(9):699–702

33. Karpenko AN, Dworkin JP, Meleca RJ, Stachler RJ. Cymetra injection for unilateral vocal fold paralysis. Ann Otol Rhinol Laryngol 2003;112(11):927–934

34. Belafsky PC, Postma GN. Vocal fold augmentation with calcium hydroxylapatite. Otolaryngol Head Neck Surg 2004;131(4):351–354

35. Mallur PS, Morrison MP, Postma GN, Amin MR, Rosen CA. Safety and efficacy of carboxymethylcellulose in the treatment of glottic insufficiency. Laryngoscope 2012;122(2):322–326

36. Sulica L, Rosen CA, Postma GN, et al. Current practice in injection augmentation of the vocal folds: indications, treatment principles, techniques, and complications. Laryngoscope 2010;120(2):319–325

37. Mortensen M, Woo P. Office steroid injections of the larynx. Laryngoscope 2006;116(10):1735–1739

38. Zeitels SM, Barbu AM, Landau-Zemer T, et al. Local injection of bevacizumab (Avastin) and angiolytic KTP laser treatment of recurrent respiratory papillomatosis of the vocal folds: a prospective study. Ann Otol Rhinol Laryngol 2011;120(10):627–634

39. Hajek M. Anatmische Untersuchungen uber das Larynxodem. Arch Klin Chir 1891;42:46–93

40. Reinke F. Uber die Funktionelle Struktur der Menschlichen Stimmlippe mit Besonderer Berucksichtigung des Elastischen Gewebes. Anat Heft 1897;9:103–117

41. Pressman JJ, Dowdy A, Libby R, Fields M. Further studies upon the submucosal compartments and lymphatics of the larynx by the injection of dyes and radioisotopes. Ann Otol Rhinol Laryngol 1956;65(4):963–980

42. Pressman JJ, Simon MB, Monell C. Anatomical studies related to the dissemination of cancer of the larynx. Trans Am Acad Ophthalmol Otolaryngol 1960;64:628–638

43. Welsh LW, Welsh JJ, Rizzo TA Jr. Laryngeal spaces and lymphatics: current anatomic concepts. Ann Otol Rhinol Laryngol Suppl 1983;105:19–31

44. Zeitels SM. Premalignant epithelium and microinvasive cancer of the vocal fold: the evolution of phonomicrosurgical management. Laryngoscope 1995; 105(3 Pt 2, Suppl 67):1–51

45. Kass ES, Hillman RE, Zeitels SM. Vocal fold submucosal infusion technique in phonomicrosurgery. Ann Otol Rhinol Laryngol 1996;105(5):341–347

46. Rahbar R, Vargas SO, Folkman J, et al. Role of vascular endothelial growth factor-A in recurrent respiratory papillomatosis. Ann Otol Rhinol Laryngol 2005;114(4):289–295

47. Blitzer A, Brin MF, Fahn S, Lovelace RE. Localized injections of botulinum toxin for the treatment of focal laryngeal dystonia (spastic dysphonia). Laryngoscope 1988;98(2):193–197

48. Blitzer A, Brin MF, Stewart C, Aviv JE, Fahn S. Abductor laryngeal dystonia: a series treated with botulinum toxin. Laryngoscope 1992;102(2):163–167

49. Ford CN, Bless DM, Patel NY. Botulinum treatment of spasmodic dysphonia: techniques, indications, efficacy. J Voice 1992;6:370–376

50. Blitzer A, Lovelace RE, Brin MF, Fahn S, Fink ME. Electromyographic findings in focal laryngeal dystonia (spastic dysphonia). Ann Otol Rhinol Laryngol 1985;94(6 Pt 1):591–594

51. Ford CN, Bless DM, Lowery JD. Indirect laryngoscopic approach for injection of botulinum toxin in spasmodic dysphonia. Otolaryngol Head Neck Surg 1990;103(5 Pt 1):752–758

52. Nasri S, Sercarz JA, McAlpin T, Berke GS. Treatment of vocal fold granuloma using botulinum toxin type A. Laryngoscope 1995;105(6):585–588

10 Evaluation of Voice Outcome and Quality-of-Life Measures

Declan Costello and Nicholas Gibbins

The evaluation of voice is an area with few high-quality studies to inform and lead the clinician. In part, this is due to the fact that assessment of the voice and of the dysphonic patient can be a vague area. A grossly dysphonic patient may be entirely at ease with the quality of his or her voice and not consider it abnormal, whereas a small loss of range in a professional singer may be a great cause for concern. The assessment of the voice begins with a comprehensive and detailed history.

History

The history should be divided into case history, general medical history, and the general framework of the patient's life. This last category has a greater significance than a general medical history as it includes the patient's job, the vocal demands, and any factors that may be affecting these.

Case History

As with any medical history, a detailed description of the problem at hand is needed and a good history often gives the diagnosis.

The nature and time frame of the problem may often hint at the diagnosis and may lead the questioning. The time of day at which it is worse, whether the problem is constant or intermittent, and any exacerbating or relieving factors should be examined.

Beginning the consultation with an open question such as "tell me what is the problem with your voice" will allow patients to explain the problem in their own words and will allow the clinician to pick up on aspects of the problem that are important to the patient. It is also important to watch and listen closely to patients while they explain their problems in the way in which they comport themselves, the words they use in describing their ailments, and the emotions with which they speak.[1] This may also aid in judging the perceived severity of the problem for the patient and may help the clinician explain the problem to the patient in appropriate language. Highly stressed or emotional patients may need far more reassurance and a simplistic plan than those patients who present in a more considered manner when an explanation of the anatomy and physiology of

their condition will allow them to feel that they have some measure of control and understanding of the problem.

Vocal Hygiene

The health of the vocal tract relies on maintenance of the pliability of the mucosal surfaces. Hydration is key to this, and it is recommended that patients should drink around 2 L of water per day to ensure adequate hydration of the vocal tract. Avoiding caffeine intake (tea, coffee, and soft drinks) is also important in this regard. The use of steam inhalations can help maintain laryngeal hydration. Smoking cessation is imperative as is the avoidance of excessive alcohol intake. Throat clearing is profoundly irritating to the laryngeal mucosa and should be avoided. Vocal behaviors that are considered "abusive", including screaming and yelling and talking above background noise for prolonged periods, should be avoided..

Reflux History

There is often a degree of laryngopharyngeal reflux (LPR) present in patients who present with dysphonia. Although there is still debate about whether silent reflux is a quantifiable diagnosis, what is certain is that the presence of gastric fluid will cause dehydration in the hypopharynx and larynx. To this end, a reflux scoring system is often used. "The two most popular evaluation scales LPR are the Reflux Symptom Index (RSI)[2] and the Reflux Finding Score (RFS) (**Table 10.1**).[3] Both these scales are brief questionnaires that may help assess whether the treatment of LPR has been beneficial.

LPR can be limited with some lifestyle modifications: these include the avoiding eating meals late in the evening, avoiding spicy foods, and eating and drinking nothing (except water) for 3 hours before going to sleep.

General Medical History

Laryngeal dysfunction may be caused by an intrinsic laryngeal problem. However, it may be due to surrounding structures affecting the larynx indirectly. Problems with the lower respiratory tract, stomach and oesophagus, and nose

Table 10.1 Evaluation Scales for Laryngopharyngeal Reflux

Reflux Symptom Index	RSI
Reflux Finding Score	RFS

and paranasal sinuses may all cause extraneous material to bathe the larynx, affecting its function.

Lower respiratory tract pathology may cause chronic cough (asthma, bronchitis) or may include the expectoration of infected mucus (emphysema). Bacterially infected material is acidic and may directly damage the vocal tract or indirectly cause dysphonia due to drying of the laryngeal epithelium. Treatment of chronic lower respiratory tract problems often includes steroid inhalers that may dry and thin the laryngeal mucosa.

Acute, chronic, or acute-on-chronic rhinosinusitis may cause infected pus or thick mucus to run down into the oropharynx as a postnasal drip. This may cause cough, irritation of the vocal folds, or drying of the oropharyngeal mucosa.

Gastric problems range greatly and are not confined solely to the esophageal reflux. Vomiting, dysphagia, and bowel habit changes may indicate the presence of a sinister pathology. However, nausea and vomiting may also cause dehydration and inflammation of the oropharyngeal and laryngeal lining. Young singers who are being trained to become performers and who present with dysphonia should be asked about eating habits to exclude anorexia or bulimia.

In addition to these specific areas, a systematic review of systems including a brief assessment of the patient's psychological well-being will uncover any systemic pathology that may be relevant. This should include a gynecological history (vocal fold cycle related to menstruation) and a musculoskeletal history (osteoarthritis or rheumatoid arthritis).

Smoking and drinking history must be obtained. When patients deny either, do not forget to ask whether they ever did in the past—they may have given up last week before coming to your clinic! Spirits are especially irritating to the oropharyngeal mucosa and may overspill into the larynx.

Professional Voice Users

Professional voice users can be divided into performers (singers, actors) and those with professions that demand voice use (lecturers, teachers, call center workers), and the common theme being that voices are crucial to their careers. As such, changes in the voice can be seen as a catastrophic event even if the cause is fairly benign such as an upper respiratory tract infection.[4]

Specific questions concerning the role they are currently performing, the range of the role, how often and for how long they are performing, and the environment in which they practice and perform should be asked. Many theaters have dusty wings scenery and curtains, and artificial smoke can be an irritant.

At the end of taking a history, one should ascertain what the patient wishes to get from the consultation and possible treatment. This will ensure that both patient and clinician are aiming for the same goals and have realistic aims.

Subjective Evaluation of Voice

Evaluation of the voice is divided into subjective and objective measures. Under the umbrella term of subjective measures lie both perceptual evaluation and patient questionnaires measuring quality of life. In the modern voice clinic, both of these should be routinely used. In the authors' practice, the patients are asked to fill in a questionnaire in the waiting room before the appointment—a patient-centered evaluation. This is followed by the doctor's assessment while listening to the patient—a clinician-centered evaluation. Often these two evaluations give similar overall pictures. However, if there is a large discrepancy, for example, if the clinician hears very little wrong with the voice but the patient questionnaire suggests a terrible condition impinging on the patient's life, the aims of the appointment and treatment must be carefully addressed and any psychological overlay should be examined.

There are several scoring systems for the clinician to assess the voice (**Table 10.2**). One of the most widely used is the Grade, Roughness, Breathiness, Asthenia, Strain (GRBAS) scale that marks the overall grade, the roughness, the breathiness, the asthenia (weakness), and the strain of the voice. First described by Hirano,[5] it is easy to be trained to use, has good inter-user reliability,[6] and remains one of the most important, reliable, and valid methods of voice evaluation.[7] Each of the five categories is graded from 0 (no perceived abnormality) to 3 (severe abnormality). Studies have suggested that the GRBAS has a strong inter-user reliability for the grade, roughness, and breathiness but less so for asthenia (weakness) and strain.[8]

The Grade, Roughness, Breathiness, Asthenia, Strain, Instability (GRBASI)[9] scale is essentially the same but includes an instability score, allowing a score for vocal breaks in an otherwise normal voice.

The Consensus Auditory Perceptual Evaluation of Voice (CAPE V)[10] is a visual analogue score on a 10-cm line and includes measures of pitch and loudness. It was developed as a consensus statement in 2003 by the American Speech-Language-Hearing Association (ASHA).

Table 10.2 Grading Schemes for Evaluation of the Voice

Grade, Roughness, Breathiness, Asthenia, Strain	GRBAS
Grade, Roughness, Breathiness, Asthenia, Strain, Instability	GRBASI
Consensus Auditory Perceptual Evaluation of Voice	CAPE V
Vocal Profile Analysis	VPA

The Vocal Profile Analysis (VPA)[11] is a detailed descriptor; however, it is considered by many to be too complex for regular use and its outcomes are not, at the time of going to press, validated.

Patient Questionnaires (Quality-of-Life Measures)

The role of patient-centered questionnaires is to determine the impact of the perceived vocal abnormality on the day-to-day life of the patient (**Table 10.3**). If there is no sinister cause for their dysphonia, treatment can be based on the perceived impairment or handicap.[12] To determine the level of disability, several patient-centered questionnaires have been developed.

- The Voice Handicap Index: The Voice Handicap Index (VHI)[13] is probably the most widely used. It has 30 questions that determine the physical, functional, and emotional impairment that the patient's dysphonia causes. Each is scored between 0 (never) and 4 (always), giving a maximum total score of 120. It is useful for the clinician and psychologically for the patient to see the change in scores before and after treatment. Such changes have been well documented[14] and are important to record to both justify the treatments used and to be able to assess changes in technique or treatment methods.

- The Voice Handicap Index 10: The Voice Handicap Index 10 (VHI-10)[15] is an adaptation of the VHI (**Appendix 10.1**). It has been reduced from 30 to 10 questions and has been validated. The personal preference of the authors is to use the VHI-10 questionnaire as it is quick and easy to fill in and patients seem to prefer a shorter questionnaire.

- The Voice Symptom Scale: The Voice Symptom Scale (VoiSS)[16] is also a 30-item questionnaire that examines three main parameters: impairment (15 items), emotional symptoms (8 items), and related physical symptoms (7 items). It has been subject to rigorous psychometric evaluation and is the most extensively validated self-report voice measure available.[17] However, it is not yet widely used.

- The Voice-Related Quality of Life: The Voice-Related Quality of Life (V-RQOL)[18] is a 10-item questionnaire that

Table 10.3   Patient Quality-of-Life Questionnaires

Voice Handicap Index	VHI
Voice Handicap Index 10	VHI-10
Voice Symptom Scale	VoiSS
Voice-Related Quality of Life	V-RQOL

Appendix 10.1   Voice Handicap Index 10

Instructions: These are statements that many people have used to describe their voices and the effects of their voices on their lives. Circle the response that indicates how frequently you have the same experience.

0 = Never	
1 = Almost never	
2 = Sometimes	
3 = Almost always	
4 = Always	
1. My voice makes it difficult for people to hear me.	0 1 2 3 4
2. People have difficulty understanding me in a noisy room.	0 1 2 3 4
3. People ask, "What's wrong with your voice?"	0 1 2 3 4
4. I feel as though I have to strain to produce voice.	0 1 2 3 4
5. My voice difficulties restrict my personal and social life.	0 1 2 3 4
6. The clarity of my voice is unpredictable.	0 1 2 3 4
7. I feel left out of conversation because of my voice.	0 1 2 3 4
8. My voice problem causes me to lose income.	0 1 2 3 4
9. My voice problem upsets me.	0 1 2 3 4
10. My voice problem makes me feel handicapped.	0 1 2 3 4

Adapted from Deary, IJ, Webb A, Mackenzie K, Wilson JA, Carding PN. Short, Self-Report Voice Symptom Scales: Psychometric Characteristics of the Voice Handicap Index-10 and the Vocal Performance Questionnaire. *Otolaryngology - Head and Neck Surgery.* 2004;131(3):232–235.

measures well in validity, reliability, and responsiveness tests. It has not been through the same rigorous validation as the VoiSS but is an easy-to-use questionnaire.

Each of the above is validated and has its exponents and its detractors. Other than the level of validation, none of these have proven benefit over any of the others and so it is, in large part, the personal preference of the clinician to use any of these. The reason that none of these has any benefit over any of the others is probably in part due to the fact that they measure the patient's perception of their own voice that may or may not correlate with the clinician's perception of the patient's voice. As long as the questionnaire used has good reliability and can be used pre- and post-treatment, any of these may be used.

Whichever of the various scoring systems are used (remembering that patient- and clinician-rated systems should both be employed), it is imperative that quantification of the progress of treatment is recorded. This provides a valuable research tool and allows for audit and comparison of treatments.

Clinical Pearls

A patient who presents with a significantly elevated VHI, or in whom the VHI seems inappropriately high given the clinician's evaluation of their voice, may have significant psychological overlay. This should be addressed.

Evaluation of the voice continues with a comprehensive laryngeal examination including videostroboscopy. This is covered Chapter 7. Beyond that there are additional measures that can be undertaken to further quantify the extent of the patient's vocal difficulties. Numerous objective measures of voice exist, and the choice of which to use is largely a matter of personal preference and the availability of specialist equipment. Indeed, many of the tests outlined below are (relatively) time-consuming and require recording equipment, computer analysis software, and the time of a trained clinician or technician.

Objective Acoustic Analysis

Under standardized conditions, voice recordings are made and software algorithms are used to analyze a variety of aspects of the acoustic waveform. It is important that the recordings are repeatable (in other words, performed in the same way each time) and that a quiet recording environment (ideally a soundproofed booth) is used. The most widely used measures are jitter, shimmer, and noise-to-harmonic ratio. These three measures are known as *perturbation* measures, because they measure the variation of the sound signal (the perturbation) from one cycle to the next.

Jitter refers to cycle-to-cycle variation in frequency. *Shimmer* refers to cycle-to-cycle variation in amplitude. *Noise-to-harmonic ratio* refers to the amount of extraneous "noise" in the waveform. In a nondysphonic voice, one would expect the cycle-to-cycle vibrations of the vocal folds to be periodic (regular) or almost periodic. In many forms of dysphonia, this periodicity is deranged, and this results in variations in frequency and amplitude from one vibratory cycle to the next. These result in an increase in *jitter* and *shimmer*, respectively.

One of the difficulties in interpreting perturbation measures is that they all rely, to a certain extent, on a degree of periodicity in the acoustic waveform. If the waveform is markedly aperiodic (as one would expect to see in a very dysphonic patient), the mathematical algorithms (based on linear mathematical principles) are unable to make any calculations. For this reason, researchers have focused their attention on *nonlinear* measures that are repeatable and applicable to even the most dysphonic voices. This newer approach recognizes that voice signals in severe dysphonia can be chaotic and markedly aperiodic.

A further problem in the use of classical perturbation measures is that the patient's mode of phonation is not a natural or physiological one. For a voice recording to be analyzed, the patient is required to sustain a vowel (usually /ɑ/—"aaah"). This is not, therefore, a good reflection of the normal phonation used for speech or singing. Furthermore, many voice disorders occur at onset and offset of phonation, which is not captured when sustaining a vowel.

Nonetheless, perturbation measures are widely used in clinical practice and are extensively employed in voice research.

Fundamental Frequency

The fundamental frequency (F_0) refers to the frequency with which the vocal folds vibrate. The perceptual correlate of this measure is pitch. A doubling of the frequency of vibration corresponds to an increase in musical pitch of one octave. Traditionally, fundamental frequency is measured over a period of continuous speech. To allow for meaningful comparisons, a standard text is presented to the patient and the voice is recorded. The choice of text passage varies from institution to institution, but it is important that the text be phonetically balanced. It is also important to choose a text that is relatively neutral in emotional content (or the reader will naturally raise the pitch of the spoken word) and, if possible, avoids quotations (again, because the natural tendency when reading between quotation marks is to raise the pitch of the voice). Standard texts in widespread use include "Arthur the rat," "The north wind and the sun," and "The rainbow passage."

F_0 can be measured in two principal ways: with a microphone directly recording the voice or with electrodes on the patient's neck recording vocal fold contact (electroglottography [EGG], see explanation below).

F_0 may be interpreted in several ways. The average F_0 gives a measure of the patient's overall pitch. For men, this is roughly 110 Hz and for women, it averages 190 Hz. The range of frequencies employed when reading gives a measure of the degree of variability in pitch that the patient can achieve. In patients with Parkinson disease, for example, who can sometimes have voices perceived as monotonous, the variability in F_0 will be relatively small. Conversely, an actor with a very declamatory and dramatic style may achieve a wide range of F_0 over a passage of text.

Aerodynamic Measures

Many different parameters can be measured when considering airflow through the airways. These include the following:

Lung Function Tests (Pulmonary Function Tests)

Figure 10.1 shows lung function tests.

- Tidal volume (TV) is the volume of air inhaled and exhaled in normal quiet respiration.
- Vital capacity (VC) is the total volume of air that can be exhaled after a maximum inspiration.
- Functional residual capacity (FRC) is the volume of air remaining in the lungs at the end of a quiet exhalation.
- Inspiratory capacity (IC) is the maximal volume of air that can be inhaled starting at the functional residual capacity.
- Total lung capacity (TLC) is the total volume of air in the lungs following maximal inspiration.
- FEV_1 is the forced expiratory volume that can be exhaled in 1 second.

These tests are typically performed in patients in whom lower airway disease (e.g., asthma and chronic obstructive pulmonary disease) is suspected. Notwithstanding lung pathology, these parameters will vary according to the patient's age, gender, and size and the general health of the individual.

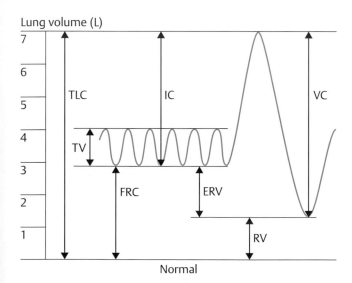

Figure 10.1 Spirogram showing lung function volumes and capacities. ERV, expiratory reserve volume; FRC, functional residual capacity; IC, inspiratory capacity; RV, residual volume; TLC, total lung capacity; TV, tidal volume; VC, vital capacity.

Furthermore, combinations of these tests have been found to correlate with the degree of subglottic stenosis.

Lung function testing requires a laboratory setup and technical staff to perform the testing. It is certainly not required for the vast majority of patients presenting to the voice clinic. In the context of laryngeal pathology, pulmonary function tests are principally of use in patients with airway compromise (e.g., subglottic stenosis, bilateral vocal fold paralysis). Changes in lung function parameters can then be measured pre- and postintervention.

Maximum Phonation Time and s/z Ratio

The sphincter ability of the larynx can be simply measured in the clinic with the maximum phonation time (MPT). The patient is asked to inhale maximally and then sustain the vowel /ɑ/ ("ah") for as long as possible, vocalizing at a comfortable pitch and loudness. This is performed three times and the best of the three times is recorded. This is a very useful measure in patients with glottal insufficiency: a patient with a vocal fold paralysis, for example, will have a reduced MPT, and one would hope to achieve a lengthening of this after a clinical intervention. Thus, the MPT can be seen as a proxy measure of glottal sphincter efficiency. However, it must be borne in mind that patients with pulmonary pathology, and a reduced capacity to inhale maximally, will also have a shortened MPT.

The s/z ratio compares the maximum duration of a sustained /s/ consonant with a maximum duration of /z/. As this is a comparison of the patient's performance against himself/herself, the variable of lung function is removed. In principle, maximal glottal efficiency will result in an equal duration of the /s/ and /z/ fricatives, giving a ratio of 1.0. An elevated s/z ratio implies glottal insufficiency.

Further Aerodynamic Measures

Further and more complex measures of laryngeal efficiency exist, but are not in widespread use in voice clinics. Direct measurement of subglottal air pressure involves invasive testing, but an accurate estimate can be achieved by measuring the intraoral air pressure measured with a pressure transducer in the mouth.

Electroglottography

EGG provides information about the degree of closure of the vocal folds during the vibratory cycle. An electrical current is passed across the larynx (between electrodes on the skin over each thyroid lamina) and the electrical resistance (impedance) is measured. During complete vocal fold closure, the electrical impedance is small, and during the open phase, the impedance is relatively high. During normal phonation, the waveform seen is as shown in **Fig. 10.2**. The peaks represent minimal impedance (or maximal closure) and the troughs represent the open phase of the vibratory cycle.

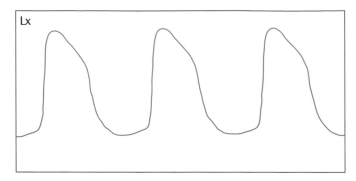

Figure 10.2 Waveform during normal phonation. (*Image courtesy* of Julian McGlashan, F.R.C.S. [Otol].)

By contrast, breathy phonation (e.g., muscle tension dysphonia, with a posterior glottic gap) may result in a waveform as shown in **Fig. 10.3**. It can be seen that the peak amplitude (closure) is shorter and the open phase (trough) is much longer.

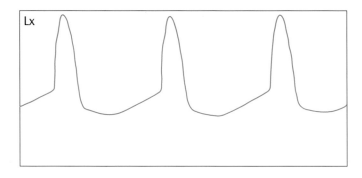

Figure 10.3 Waveform during breathy phonation. (*Image courtesy* of Julian McGlashan, F.R.C.S. [Otol].)

Using EGG data, the *contact quotient* can be calculated. This is the proportion of the vibratory cycle for which the vocal folds are closed. A typical value is 0.4 to 0.6. This is elevated with increasing vocal training and is further elevated in certain styles of singing, such as musical theater. The contact quotient is decreased in conditions characterized by breathy dysphonia such as vocal fold paralysis and muscle tension dysphonia.

Clinical Pearls

In addition to a detailed clinical history and examination of the larynx, voice evaluation should include, at the very least, the following:
- A patient-completed evaluation of the voice (e.g., VHI-10, see below).
- A clinician-rated evaluation of the voice (e.g., GRBAS).
- Further tests are available, but can be time-consuming and expensive.

References

1. Harris T, Harris S, Rubin JS, Howard DM. The Voice Clinic Handbook. 3rd ed. London: Whurr Publishers Ltd.; 2002
2. Belafsky PC, Postma GN, Koufman JA. Validity and reliability of the reflux symptom index (RSI). J Voice 2002;16(2):274–277
3. Belafsky PC, Postma GN, Koufman JA. The validity and reliability of the reflux finding score (RFS). Laryngoscope 2001;111(8): 1313–1317
4. Harries M. The professional voice. In: Gleeson M et al, eds. Scott-Brown's Otorhinolaryngology, Head and Neck Surgery. 7th ed. London: Hodder Arnold; 2008:Chapter 168
5. Hirano M. Clinical Examination of the Voice. Vienna: Springer-Verlag; 1981
6. Dejonckere PH, Obbens C, de Moor GM, Wieneke GH. Perceptual evaluation of dysphonia: reliability and relevance. Folia Phoniatr (Basel) 1993;45(2):76–83
7. McGlashan J, Fourcin A. Objective evaluation of the voice. In: Gleeson M et al, eds. Scott-Brown's Otorhinolaryngology, Head and Neck Surgery. 7th ed. London: Hodder Arnold; 2008:Chapter 166
8. De Bodt MS, Wuyts FL, Van de Hayning PH, Croux C. Test-retest study of the GRBAS scale: influence of experience and professional background on perceptual rating of voice quality. J Voice 1997;11:74–80
9. De Bodt MS, Van de Heyning PH, Wuyts FL, Lambrechts L. The perceptual evaluation of voice disorders. Acta Otorhinolaryngol Belg 1996;50:283–291
10. Consensus Auditory-Perceptual Evaluation of Voice (CAPE V). 2003. Available at: http://www.asha.org/uploadedFiles/members/divs/D3CAPEVprocedures.pdf
11. Pindzola RH. A Voice Assessment Protocol for Children and Adults. Austin, TX: Pro-Ed; 1987
12. Wilson JA, Deary IJ, Millar A, MacKenzie K. The quality of life impact of dysphonia. Clin Otolaryngol 2002;27:179–182
13. Jacobsen BH, Johnson A, Grywalski C, Silbergleit A, Benninger MS. The Voice Handicap Index (VHI): development and validation. Am J Speech Lang Pathol 1997;6:66–70
14. Rosen CA, Murray T, Zinn A, Zullo T, Sonbolian M. Voice handicap index change following treatment of voice disorders. J Voice 2000;14:619–623
15. Rosen CA, Lee AS, Osborne J, Zullo T, Murray T. Development and validation of the voice handicap index-10. Laryngoscope 2004;114:1549–1556
16. Deary IJ, Wilson JA, Carding PN, MacKenzie K, Voi SS. A patient-derived Voice Symptom Scale. J Psychosom Res 2003;54:483–489
17. Wilson JA, Webb A, Carding PN, Steen IN, MacKenzie K, Deary IJ. The Voice Symptom Scale (VoiSS) and the Vocal Handicap Index (VHI): a comparison of structure and content. Clin Otolaryngol Allied Sci 2004;29(2):169–174
18. Hogikyan ND, Sethuraman G. Validation of an instrument to measure voice-related quality of life (V-RQOL). J Voice 1999;13: 557–569

11 Assessment of Swallowing: Clinical Assessment and Diagnostic Procedures

Katherine Young and Sharat Mohan

Identification and assessment of the signs and symptoms of dysphagia is a multidisciplinary responsibility. Dysphagia poses significant risks to health through impact of aspiration on the pulmonary system, and therefore assessments performed need to be able to identify risks to better plan management for patients. Assessment protocols should be chosen for accuracy, efficiency, cost-effectiveness, and repeatability for the conditions being investigated.

Screening

Dysphagia screening assessments efficiently identify at-risk patients and appropriately prioritize high-risk patients. Screening assessments provide information identifying whether a patient is dysphagic or not. This is different from a diagnostic swallow assessment such as videofluoroscopy (VF; modified barium swallow) that provides information regarding physiology of the patient's dysphagia. Screening may consist of observations of patients while eating, observing signs of dysphagia (coughing, food left in the mouth, rejection of food, aspirated food being coughed out of a tracheostomy tube), or review of medical notes.[1] Patients often experience psychological and social stresses due to their dysphagia impacting on their quality of life. Standardized patient questionnaires have been developed, for example, SWAL-QOL. SWAL-QOL is a standardized 93-item questionnaire used both in clinical and research settings for measuring dysphagia outcome for 10 quality-of-life concepts, quality of care, and patient satisfaction.[1]

Bedside/Office

The bedside/office assessment of dysphagia is a familiar process within the role of the speech language pathologist (SLP). Typically bedside/office swallowing assessment involves gathering preparatory information regarding patients' case history and symptoms and should identify medical diagnosis, medical and swallowing history nutritional status, tube feeding, and patient's awareness of swallowing difficulties. Respiratory function during swallowing is important to note.[1] Bedside/office assessment should consider oromotor function and anatomy, oral sensation and sensitivity, dentition, and oral health.

Clinical Pearls

The presence of oral mucosal bacterial infections linked with gingivitis has been shown to increase bacterial pneumonia in patients who aspirate oral secretions.

Oromotor assessment determines age-appropriate oral reflexes and the presence or absence of the gag reflex. In general practice when introducing food and fluid boluses the following sequence is used in the author's practice:

- Teaspoon (5 mL) syrup consistency fluid
- Sip syrup-consistency fluid
- Teaspoon normal fluid
- Sip normal fluid, larger bolus normal fluid
- Sip custard-consistency fluid
- Teaspoon pudding/puree (e.g., sieved kiwi fruit)
- Fork-mashable consistency (e.g., mashed vegetables)
- Soft diet (e.g., banana or soft cake)
- Normal food (e.g., biscuit)

Observations are made of swallowing behaviors and can be monitored by cervical auscultation (CA, described later), palpation of oral and laryngeal movements for example laryngeal elevation, and forward movement of the hyoid by placing fingertips at these locations on the patient's neck.

Successful oral phase of swallow should demonstrate no oral residue in the mouth or around teeth, adequate lip seal to prevent oral escape, and one or two swallows to clear each bolus. The oral phase of swallow should complete as the swallow reflex is triggered. Late-onset swallow may present as a patient with a clear mouth but incomplete or no laryngeal elevation.

Pharyngeal phase of swallow requires complete clearance of the bolus with one swallow. Observations of multiple swallows, struggle to clear the bolus, altered respiratory patterns, and head or postural changes during swallowing are made. Most importantly, coughing/choking before or after swallowing and "wet" voice are important indicators of airway penetration or true aspiration.

During assessment, different consistencies are trialed along with modified swallowing techniques such as supraglottic swallow or Mendelsohn maneuver to determine the safest consistencies and swallowing techniques for the patient to avoid the complications of dysphagia. Clear reporting and communicating with the patient, staff, and carers is of utmost importance.

Cervical Auscultation

CA is experiencing a renewed interest as an addition to the bedside/office swallowing assessment. CA provides audible cues that can enable reliable classification of swallowing problems when incorporated in a comprehensive bedside/office swallowing assessment and is used as such by the author. CA is a controversial technique with a relatively small evidence base. CA requires a stethoscope or microphone to be placed on the thyroid cartilage (lamina) while the patient swallows. Cervical swallowing sounds, "clicks," are associated with the opening of the pharyngotympanic tube and "clunks" are associated with the opening of the upper esophageal sphincter (UES). The "click" and "clunk" are the most reliable sounds described.[1,2] In patients with swallowing difficulties, these sounds may be weaker, absent, or out of sequence.

Videofluoroscopy

VF or "modified barium swallow" is often viewed as the "gold standard" of dysphagia assessment. VF is proficient in imaging swallowing physiology and enables accurate measurement of the sequence and timing of swallowing events, opening of the UES, and identification of physiological causes for aspiration.

VF is useful to determine management and therapeutic strategies and monitor progress of therapy. VF is limited in being able to identify the quantity of material aspirated and the completeness of bolus clearance from the oral and pharyngeal cavities. VF is normally performed by an SLP and radiologist.

During VF, patients are positioned in the lateral view initially to gain best view of aspiration that may occur. Anterior–posterior (AP) view is used later in the assessment to view symmetry of anatomy and function. The patient is seated as upright as possible.

Many clinical settings have facilities to assess patients sitting, standing, or reclined in bed. A specialized chair for VF is used with a radio-transparent back support to allow fluoroscopy imaging in the seated AP position. VF field of view should include the lips to the posterior pharyngeal wall, larynx, and upper and mid-esophagus. In the author's practice, the SLP requests the radiologist routinely to view one or more boluses traveling down the esophagus to identify any indications of esophageal problems that may require further investigation by the appropriate clinician.

Bedside or office assessment is normally completed in the author's practice before VF, enabling appropriate planning of bolus consistencies and volumes presented during VF. Clinical judgment is needed to determine modifications to the procedure if the patient appears unable to protect their airway.

During VF assessment, it is essential to keep fluoroscopy time to minimum (< 3 minutes). The fluoroscopy images are observed on a monitor during the procedure and in some cases stills are taken. The assessment is recorded for further review. It is noninvasive and can accommodate patients of all ages in most feeding positions.

Magnetic Resonance Imaging

Magnetic resonance imaging (MRI) is recognized as an emerging tool in the assessment of dysphagia.[3] MRI is able to visualize soft tissues and individual muscles in detail and complements other assessments, for example, VF or fiberoptic endoscopic examination of swallowing (FEES; described later). The extent of movement of oropharyngeal structures during swallowing can be seen in detail, particularly in patients with soft-tissue deficits or abnormalities, following oropharyngeal surgery to detect soft-tissue gaps or assessing esophageal stricture in laryngectomy patients.

MRI assessment of swallowing has been studied with the patient reclined and the patient sitting in open MRI. Images are taken in the sagittal, coronal, and axial planes providing additional detail without moving the patient. Information achieved through MRI is applicable to surgery planning to minimize impact on function, therapy planning, and evaluation. Limitations include lost information between each picture, altered anatomy in reclined position, and patients with implants or inappropriate dental material.

Electromyography

Electromyography (EMG) provides measurements of the timing and amplitude of contractions of selected muscles involved in the swallowing process. Surface electrodes are used to measure muscles usually in the floor of the mouth and muscles involved in laryngeal elevation. Electrical energy is created by muscle activity. It is therefore possible to measure when the electrical activity occurs and how much. When the muscle(s) begin to contract in the sequence of swallowing, the extent of muscle contraction can be appreciated.[4]

Surface EMG is a simple, reliable, and noninvasive evaluation of some swallowing parameters with low level of discomfort during the assessment. Normative data for the timing of swallowing events can be used for the evaluation of dysphagia symptoms, for comparison in preoperative and postoperative stages, and in EMG monitoring before, during, or after treatment.

Electroglottography

Electroglottography (EGG), sometimes referred to as a "laryngograph," tracks closure of vocal folds by measuring electrical resistance between two electrodes placed on the thyroid lamina.[5] EGG allows measurement of time variations of degree of contact between the vibrating vocal folds during phonation. EGG can be altered to measure larynx elevation to determine onset and completion of pharyngeal swallow and biofeedback on distance and duration of laryngeal elevation during swallowing, for example, when patients are trying to improve swallow function. EGG signal is composed of a high-frequency component related to vocal fold vibration (voice) and a low-frequency component related to slow movement of the larynx (swallowing). For analysis of swallowing, the system filters high frequencies leaving the low-frequency component for swallowing measurement.[6]

Manometry (Pharyngeal)

Pharyngeal manometry evaluates pharyngeal and UES pressures occurring during swallowing. Pharyngeal and upper sphincter manometry detects insufficient relaxation of the UES and coordination between the contractions of the pharynx in relation to the relaxation of the UES. Swallowing is a very rapid activity (< 1 second onset to completion). In VF alone, it can be difficult to determine the degree of pharyngeal impairment, sequence of pressure changes, or cause of residue in a patient with dysphagia. For example, is residue in pyriform sinuses the result of weak pharyngeal contraction and/or reduced UES opening?[7]

Pharyngeal manometry is performed by passing a small manometric catheter containing one or more pressure sensors via the nose to the level of the base of the tongue, the cricopharyngeal sphincter, and/or the cervical esophagus. Pressures are measured locally while swallowing different consistencies and volumes. Pharyngeal manometry is usually combined with VF (manofluorography) or FEES to determine physiology causing pressure changes measured during the test. For example, if decreased UES relaxation/opening is suspected, the SLP may choose to use the Mendelsohn maneuver compensatory technique or the Shaker exercise.[8] However, if weak pharyngeal contraction is identified, the SLP can use effortful swallow.[9] Manometry is also useful in patients following total laryngectomy where the normal pressures in swallowing are disrupted by surgery and reconstruction.

Scintigraphy

Scintigraphy is a nuclear medicine test that enables the measurement of swallow clearance and oropharyngeal function. The main advantage of scintigraphy is the ability to accurately quantify the amount of radionuclide in any structure (e.g., aspirated into lungs) and timing of bolus transit.[10] Patients swallow a measured bolus containing a radionuclide. During the swallow, the bolus transit is imaged and recorded by a gamma camera and computer. Results of scintigraphy demonstrate presence and quantity of aspirated bolus and residue and also the esophageal effects of dysphagia, particularly gastroesophageal reflux disease. Scintigraphy does not, however, enable assessment of physiology of the mouth and pharynx; therefore, it is not possible to diagnose dysfunction causing the dysphagia. The test is most useful when combined with VF to enable diagnosis of the causes of the dysphagia.[11]

Videoendoscopy (FEES, FEES/ST)

FEES allows indirect visualization of the soft palate, base of the tongue, oropharynx, hypopharynx, larynx, and subglottis. FEES enables the assessment and observation of anatomy, secretions, and function before and after swallowing. It can be performed during bedside/office assessment and can incorporate Laryngeal Sensory Testing (LST) or FEES with Sensory Testing (FEES/ST) (described later) and is complementary to other assessments. Normally, FEES is performed by the otolaryngologist and the SLP trained in nasendoscopy. FEES is used in the author's practice to assess in detail patients with pharyngeal-stage swallowing difficulties, for example, posttransoral laser resection of laryngeal and hypopharyngeal carcinomas, at day 2 postsurgery. It is repeatable, does not involve radiation, and can include using any foods the patient finds difficult in addition to the assessment protocol.[12]

During FEES, a nasendoscope is passed into the patient's nose to the level of the soft palate or just over the velum. When assessing the laryngopharyngeal structures and function, the position of the scope tip is normally positioned just beyond the tip of the velum.

Clinical Pearls

If assessing velopharyngeal closure, the scope tip is positioned just superior to the nasopharyngeal port and observations made during swallowing such as presence of nasal regurgitation or soft palate lift.

The presentation of bolus consistencies and volumes is determined by initial case history, screening assessment, and oromotor and bedside/office assessment findings. If the patient is nil by mouth and aspiration of saliva is being evaluated, the patient's tongue is colored with blue/green food dye to color secretions. The patient's ability to manage their secretions can then be observed easily using FEES. When introducing food or liquid boluses, the sequence used is the same as described in "bedside/office assessment" and any particular consistencies brought by the patient.

Clinical Pearls

The scope can be in the pathway of the bolus and therefore coat the scope tip. During the swallow, the scope tip can be drawn back slightly out of the pathway of the bolus to avoid blurring the view.

Observations made during FEES:

- Health of mucosa
- Level of the bolus at onset of swallow
- Laryngeal elevation
- Pharyngeal clearance
- Preswallow/postswallow aspiration risk
- Residue on vocal folds
- Closure of vocal folds (cough and voicing)
- Subjective laryngeal sensation (i.e., "Does the patient cough when laryngeal penetration or aspiration occurs?")
- Safe consistencies and any swallowing strategies to improve swallow success/safety

Comparison studies of VF have shown that FEES is more sensitive at detecting risk in swallowing. FEES was found to be more efficient and sensitive than VF in evaluating swallowing safety when detecting reduced pharyngeal transit, laryngeal penetration, aspiration, effective cough reflex, and velopharyngeal incompetence. VF was more successful in demonstrating overspill of the bolus during the oral phase of swallow in the pharynx.[13]

In the authors' practice, FEES is often used to understand pharyngeal difficulties and risk of aspiration in more detail following identification in VF. Videonasendoscopy can be used for biofeedback in swallowing therapy. FEES is limited by the inability to see the oral stage of swallow and the actual swallow as laryngeal elevation causes the view to be obscured.

Laryngeal Sensory Testing

Laryngeal sensory capacity provides information about the neurological status of the larynx and can be assessed subjectively and more recently objectively using LST. LST is the only calibrated instrumental assessment of swallowing-related sensation.

LST was initially described as a component of FEES/ST.[14] It tests the integrity of the brainstem-mediated laryngeal adductor reflex (LAR) by endoscopically administrating pulsed air onto the arytenoid mucosa immediately lateral to the arytenoid to elicit the LAR (**Fig. 11.1**). In normal individuals, this results in adduction of the vocal folds. The pressure of air required to elicit the LAR indicates the degree of sensory impairment.[15]

LST is performed by using a sensory stimulator calibrated to administer a 50-ms air pulse of varying pressures (2 to 10 mm Hg).

Patients presenting with an LAR less than 4 mm Hg rarely had episodes of laryngeal penetration or aspiration. Those with an LAR of 4 to 10 mm Hg had variable amounts of aspiration and laryngeal penetration. If the LAR could not be elicited at the maximum level of intensity (10 mm Hg), severe laryngeal penetration and/or aspiration is a high risk. LST in children is feasible and correlative.[16]

Transnasal Esophagoscopy

Transnasal esophagoscopy (TNE) is a technology allowing visualization of the nose, nasopharynx, hypopharynx, larynx, postcricoid area, esophagus, gastroesophageal junction, and the gastric cardia by using a small diameter (3.6 mm) fiberoptic/distal chip flexible endoscope.[17,18]

In 1994, Shaker reported unsedated TNE 4. The first live procedure or TNE was performed at the American Broncho-Esophageal Association Annual Meeting in 1998 by Aviv[15,19] and is now widely undertaken as a diagnostic tool for patients with symptoms of LPR or dysphagia.

TNE assessment of dysphagia symptoms is indicated in patients reporting unexplained upper digestive tract dysphagia. TNE enables the clinician to rule out lower esophageal causes, for example, stenosis, laryngospasm, globus, suspected reflux, unexplained dry cough, Barrett's, chronic cough.[19] It allows a direct view of the esophageal mucosa and esophagogastric junction (Z-line) in patients with LPR symptoms such as chronic cough, globus, and dysphagia (**Fig. 11.2**). Patients with these symptoms tend to present to the otolaryngologist rather than the gastroenterologist.

TNE is a well-tolerated, safe office procedure while not missing important pathology. The procedure is performed during a relatively short outpatient appointment by a trained otolaryngologist avoiding a visit to the endoscopy suite or operating theater requiring sedation or general anesthetic. The authors have introduced TNE to clinical practice in their hospital setting. Patient tolerance is high and reduced need for panendoscopy and barium swallow has been found in this patient group.

Digital video recording allows review of important anatomical areas such as the postcricoid area, which may only be seen for a fraction of a second. If a gastroenterology problem is found, the patient is referred to a gastroenterologist. Early esophageal adenocarcinoma can present with LPR symptoms. TNE can detect esophageal abnormalities including Barrett's esophagus and esophageal adenocarcinoma and can be used

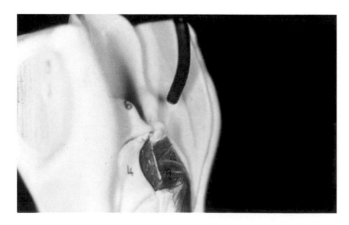

Figure 11.1 Position of scope tip in laryngeal sensory testing.

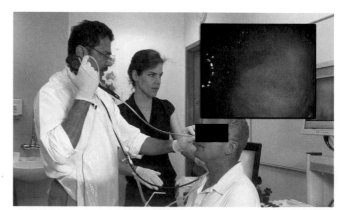

Figure 11.2 Transnasal esophagoscopy assessment clinic setup. Inset image showing Barrett's at the Z-line at the 2-o'clock position. The otolaryngologist is passing the scope and the speech–language pathologist is jointly assessing the assessment findings.

to diagnose conditions such as LPR; therefore, the need for further investigations may be reduced.

For description of TNE, we refer the reader to Aviv and Murray.[14]

Tracheostomy

Assessment of patients with tracheostomy or ventilator dependency often involves similar assessment techniques as those patients without, but involves consideration of altered respiratory features of swallowing. The comprehensive discussion of dysphagia assessment in patients who are tracheostomized or ventilator dependent is beyond the capacity of this chapter. Key issues to consider in dysphagia assessment are only outlined.

During swallowing, respiration stops briefly. Swallowing in most normal individuals (80%) occurs in the exhalatory phase of respiration. Age, chronic obstructive pulmonary disease, decreased respiratory volume, reduced respiratory defenses, and increased respiratory rate have been shown to effect timing of the swallowing in the respiratory cycle, increasing the risk of aspiration.[20] In a tracheostomized and ventilator-dependent patient, these features are further compromised, making the consequences of aspiration more serious.

History-taking before assessing a dysphagic tracheostomy patient must include the type and size of tracheostomy tube present and different tubes used earlier in the patient's care. It is important to note fenestration, cuff/cuffless tubes and cuff inflation decisions, frequency and quantity of suctioning, ventilator settings, and patterns of use. Some patients may use speaking valves that have also been shown to assist swallowing by sealing the airway and producing breath-hold on exhalation during the swallow otherwise lost due to the airway being open.[1]

Impact of a tracheostomy or ventilator equipment includes the following:

- Anchoring larynx elevation due to surgical incision, weight of equipment, or cuff over inflation.
- Reduced larynx elevation and base of tongue movement.
- Increased secretion due to altered filtering and humidity of lung air.
- Reduced laryngeal clearance due to exhalatory airflow directed away from the larynx.
- Reduced cough reflex due to reduced laryngeal sensation resulting from limited/no airflow through the larynx.
- Poor coordination of glottic closure response during swallow.
- Patients being unable to time inhalation or exhalation with ventilator.

The blue dye test can be used to color food and secretions to assist detection of aspirated material in the tracheostomy tube, which can be monitored when the patient coughs, when cleaning the tube, or suction is given. The blue dye test is used in the author's practice but only in a comprehensive assessment process and interpreted with caution.

Conclusion

Dysphagia can be a serious threat to patients' health due to the risks associated with aspiration pneumonia, malnutrition, dehydration, weight loss, and airway obstruction. Accurate, timely, evidence-based and efficient assessment of dysphagia is essential to create a clinical practice that is invested in by all professionals associated with dysphagia assessment and management. Patients and carers are very much a part of the process and should understand what information the assessment is providing and what this means in their diagnosis and management. Valid and reliable techniques should be chosen to quantify the efficiency of the oropharyngeal phase of swallowing and to measure objectively the causes and severity of dysphagia along with changes in swallowing following intervention.

References

1. Logemann J. Evaluation and Treatment of Swallowing Disorders. 2nd ed. Austin, TX: Pro-Ed; 1998
2. Leslie P, Drinnan MJ, Finn P, Ford GA, Wilson JA. Reliability and validity of cervical auscultation: a controlled comparison using videofluoroscopy. Dysphagia 2004;19(4):231–240
3. Panebianco V, Ruoppolo G, Pelle G, et al. Morpho-functional patterns of physiologic oropharyngeal swallowing evaluated with dynamic fast MRI. Eur Arch Otorhinolaryngol 2010;267(9):1461–1466
4. Vaiman M, Eviatar E, Segal S. Surface electromyographic studies of swallowing in normal subjects: a review of 440 adults. Report 1. Quantitative data: timing measures. Otolaryngol Head Neck Surg 2004;131(4):548–555
5. Fourcin AJ, Abberton E. First applications of a new laryngograph. Med Biol Illus 1971;21(3):172–182
6. Baken RJ. Clinical Measurement of Speech and Voice. Boston, MA: College Hill Press; 1987
7. Butler SG. The Role of Pharyngeal and Upper Esophageal Manometry in Swallowing Assessment. The ASHA Leader. 2009
8. Shaker R, Easterling C, Kern M, et al. Rehabilitation of swallowing by exercise in tube-fed patients with pharyngeal dysphagia secondary to abnormal UES opening. Gastroenterology 2002;122(5):1314–1321
9. Crary MA, Baldwin BO. Surface electromyographic characteristics of swallowing in dysphagia secondary to brainstem stroke. Dysphagia 1997;12(4):180–187
10. Kazem I, Wagemakers G, Verbeeten E. A new scintigraphic technique for the study of the oesophagus. Am J Roentgenol Radium Ther Nucl Med 1972;15:681–688
11. Argon M, Secil Y, Duygun U, et al. The value of scintigraphy in the evaluation of oropharyngeal dysphagia. Eur J Nucl Med Mol Imaging 2004;31(1):94–98
12. Langmore SE, Schatz K, Olsen N. Fiberoptic endoscopic examination of swallowing safety: a new procedure. Dysphagia 1988;2(4):216–219
13. Wu CH, Hsiao TY, Chen JC, Chang YC, Lee SY. Evaluation of swallowing safety with fiberoptic endoscope: comparison with videofluoroscopic technique. Laryngoscope 1997;107(3):396–401

14. Aviv J, Murray T. FEES/ST: Fiberoptic Evaluation of Swallowing with Sensory Testing. San Diego, CA: Plural Publishing; 2005

15. Dale O, Alhamarneh O, Young K, Mohan S. The role of laryngeal sensory testing (LST) in neurological voice disorders and laryngopharyngeal reflux disease (LPR). J Laryngol Otol 2010;124(3):330–332

16. Link DT, Willging JP, Miller CK, Cotton RT, Rudolph CD. Pediatric laryngopharyngeal sensory testing during flexible endoscopic evaluation of swallowing: feasible and correlative. Ann Otol Rhinol Laryngol 2000;109(10 Pt 1):899–905

17. Amin MR, Postma GN, Setzen M, Koufman JA. Transnasal oesophagoscopy: a position statement from the American Bronchoesophagological Association (ABEA). Otolaryngol Head Neck Surg 2008;138:411–414

18. Shaker R. Unsedated trans-nasal pharyngoesophagogastroduodeno-scopy (T-EGD): technique. Gastrointest Endosc 1994;40(3):346–348

19. Aviv JE, Takoudes TG, Ma G, Close LG. Office-based esophagoscopy: a preliminary report. Otolaryngol Head Neck Surg 2001;125(3): 170–175

20. Dikeman KJ, Kazandjian MS. Pathophysiology: interrelationship of tracheostomy, ventilator dependence, and swallowing. In: Dikeman KJ, Kazandjian MS, eds. Communication and Swallowing Management of Tracheotomised and Ventilator Dependent Adults. 2nd ed. Canada: Singular; 2003:261–286

12 Imaging of the Larynx

Curtis Offiah

The evolution of modern imaging techniques, particularly over the past decade, has significantly improved the ability of the radiologist to visualize and assess laryngeal anatomy and disease. While the laryngologist is able to use modern endoscopy to evaluate mucosal surfaces, it is the radiologist's role to elucidate the depth of submucosal disease extension through imaging as well as characterize the imaging appearances of such lesions. What is paramount, however, is that the findings of both clinical and radiological examinations are discussed and correlated together in an interdisciplinary setting to optimize benefit to the patient; it is also imperative that the radiologist has a good working knowledge of the descriptive anatomy used by the laryngologist.

Imaging Techniques

Historical Perspectives

Historically, imaging techniques such as plain film tomography, laryngography, and barium swallow were the methods used for radiological depiction of laryngeal anatomy and disease. The majority of these techniques have fallen out of use, largely because of the development of computed tomography (CT) and magnetic resonance imaging (MRI).

Plain Film Radiography

This was the first technique used to image the larynx. Soft-tissue lateral projections of the neck are still used in current modern-day practice as an overview to look for ingested, penetrated, or aspirated radiopaque foreign bodies (but usually as an adjunct to flexible nasendoscopy) and to assess gross airway patency.

Conventional tomography was in routine use until toward the end of the 1980s but is now obsolete, superseded by CT and MRI.

Cross-Sectional Imaging

Cross-sectional imaging, either CT or MRI, has become essential for optimal pretreatment assessment of laryngeal disease, in particular neoplastic laryngeal pathology.

Clinical evaluation allows the mucosal layer of the larynx to be defined; however, the deep extent of potentially infiltrating lesions can be assessed indirectly by clinical evaluation alone. Objective assessment of submucosal disease extension, disease volume, and involvement of the laryngeal cartilaginous skeleton can be achieved with CT and MRI cross-sectional imaging in cases of neoplastic

and inflammatory disease.[1-3] In acute traumatic and posttraumatic pathology, cross-sectional imaging, in particular CT, is useful in the evaluation of the laryngeal cartilaginous framework and soft tissues[4-6]; laryngeal and tracheal stenoses can be objectively documented with a view to planning of appropriate reconstructive surgery.[7-11]

Computed Tomography

Modern CT involves, in simplistic terms, the simultaneous translatory movement of a patient through a rotating X-ray source. If the CT scanner consists of multiple small X-ray sources with multiple detectors for the X-ray sources, this is termed multidetector helical CT. This multidetector helical technology is the current CT imaging technology of choice. Multidetector technology allows acquisition of faster scans of higher resolution. Probably the key consideration in CT is the fact that this imaging technology uses radiation. The patient undergoing CT assessment is exposed to a radiation dose (so are the radiation-sensitive tissues such as the thyroid gland)—this should always be borne in mind when request for CT assessment of the neck is made. To justify the radiation exposure to the patient, the benefit of the information yielded by the CT assessment must always outweigh the risks posed by the inherent radiation exposure. This is particularly the case if imaging assessment of the larynx is required in the pediatric population. There are several advantages of CT (relative to MRI) in imaging assessment of the larynx. CT is a faster technique—the imaging acquisition of the entire neck is of much shorter duration than MRI assessment of the larynx (the CT acquisition takes less than 30 seconds compared with 20 to 30 minutes for comprehensive MRI assessment of the soft tissues of the neck and larynx). Because the CT acquisition is a shorter scan time, the resultant images are less affected by motion degradation caused by swallowing or respiration, particularly in those patients who may already have labored breathing because of laryngeal airway pathology. CT is a *relatively* cheaper technology compared with MRI and, as such, is a more widely available imaging modality. Multidetector CT allows postprocessing generation of high-resolution multiplanar (coronal and sagittal) image reconstructions. Modern-day (multidetector helical) CT not only provides good soft-tissue contrast but also offers excellent depiction of osseous and calcific structures, which is particularly useful for demonstration of the ossified laryngeal cartilaginous skeleton. For many of the reasons outlined, CT is the first-line imaging modality of choice for assessing laryngeal pathology. An important nonsequitur to this is imaging assessment of the larynx in the nonsequitur pediatric population, where MRI may be an appropriate alternative for first-line imaging to avoid radiation exposure. Such considerations are best taken by the specialist radiologist.

Technique

The majority of CT assessments of the larynx are best performed with the administration of intravenous contrast material (in those patients where renal function permits and there is no past history of allergic reaction to iodinated contrast material). Intravenous contrast medium increases the conspicuity of lesions of the larynx as well as allows better differentiation between lymph nodes and vessels in the extralaryngeal soft tissues of the neck. Multidetector CT images can be reconstructed to high quality along any plane, including a true axial orientation through the true and false vocal cords (**Fig. 12.1**). Although CT acquisitions can be obtained during specific dynamic maneuvers to enhance visualization of particular anatomical subsites (e.g., scan acquisition during a modified Valsalva maneuver distends the hypopharynx including the pyriform fossae and postcricoid region), acquisitions should generally be performed during quiet respiration by the patient to avoid adduction and approximation of the true vocal cords that hinders identification and delineation of superficial mucosal abnormalities.

Magnetic Resonance Imaging

The basic principle of MRI employs the application of pulses of radiofrequency energy within a magnetic field. The nuclei of hydrogen atoms in water and fat (the predominant constituents of the human body) absorb and re-emit the radiofrequency energy. It is the re-emitted radiofrequency energy that is eventually translated into a contrast image of each particular tissue component. By varying the nature of the radiofrequency pulses applied, different sequences that highlight different tissue contrast characteristics can be obtained (**Fig. 12.1**).

As an imaging modality, as with CT, there are several relatively advantageous and disadvantageous features of MRI. MRI scanners as well as the requisite hardware and software (in addition to the long-term maintenance) are expensive, far more so than CT. MRI is also a slower technique with comprehensive scan times of particular body regions lasting anything from 20 minutes to 45 minutes or more. As such, the quality of MR images is particularly prone to patient movement degradation and artifact. For anatomical regions where motion artifact may be an issue, this can be problematic. The laryngopharynx can be one such region. Inherent in the MRI technique is susceptibility to significant image artifact created by ferromagnetic material, which can have a major deleterious effect on image quality. Because of the nature of the strong magnetic fields related to MRI scanners (at present, 1.5 T and 3 T are routinely used clinically), there exist relative and absolute contraindications to MRI of particular patients; for example, patients with cardiac pacemakers cannot undergo an MRI (although the first generation of MR-"compatible" cardiac pacemakers may soon be available) and patients with ferromagnetic (typically steel) intraorbital foreign

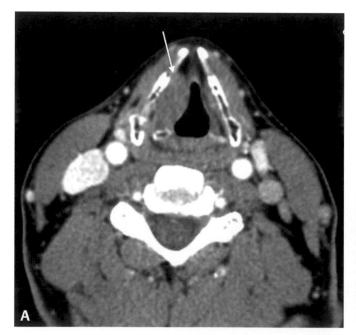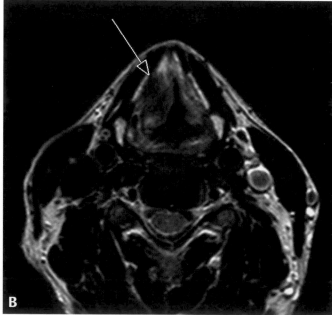

Figure 12.1 (A) Axial contrast-enhanced computed tomography image through the larynx of a 60-year-old man with hoarseness. There is a submucosal lesion in the right true and false cords (arrow) but no laryngeal cartilage destruction. The radiological features are not entirely typical of a neoplastic carcinoma. (B) Axial T2-weighted magnetic resonance (MR) sequence through the larynx of the same patient as in (A). The submucosal lesion in the right false and true cords (arrow) demonstrates MR signal characteristics and appearances consistent with amyloidosis. Microlaryngoscopy and biopsy confirmed amyloidosis.

bodies, such as might occur as a frequent occupational hazard in metal workers, cannot undergo MR scan as such foreign bodies may be subject to movement in the strong magnetic field of the scanner. For those patients who have never had to endure an MRI scan of the head or neck region, the bore of the majority of current standard 1.5 T and 3 T MRI scanners is relatively small to maximize image quality. This can pose a very claustrophobic environment for even the most stoic individuals (let alone those prone to claustrophobia) required to lie in such a position for scan times of 30 minutes or more and, therefore, should not be underestimated; not infrequently, patients are unable to endure such scans even with oral sedation administered an hour before the MRI examination. One of the most salient advantages of MRI is that the technique does not involve the use of ionizing radiation, a particular advantage in the pediatric population. Other relative advantages of MRI include the relatively superior soft-tissue contrast detail of MRI over CT (although the detail of ossified structures such as bone and ossified cartilage is relatively less well served by MRI); the inherent orthogonal multiplanar capability of MRI (axial, sagittal, and coronal planes) is also advantageous.

Technique

Swallowing and respiratory movement artifacts may seriously degrade the MRI study. The patient is therefore instructed to breathe quietly, in particular, without moving the neck. Patients are encouraged to use "abdominal" instead of "thoracic" respiration and to swallow as seldom as possible during individual scan sequence acquisitions.

Axial and coronal planes are used in MRI of the larynx (**Fig. 12.2**). The axial planes should be angled in a plane parallel to the true vocal cords (equivalent to a plane parallel to the C4/5 and C5/6 cervical spine intervertebral disks). Where midline pathology is a consideration, sagittal plane MRI sequences should also be performed. The choice of sequences can be variable and will not be discussed in detail because it is beyond the scope of this discourse but will routinely incorporate the use of contrast-enhanced sequences where intravenous paramagnetic contrast material (gadolinium) is administered. In cases of malignant neoplastic pathology, this can increase the conspicuity of primary tumors as well as prove essential for the evaluation of cervical lymph nodes. Gadolinium is very rarely associated with allergic reaction and this is therefore rarely a consideration in contradistinction to iodinated contrast material used in CT. However, intravenous gadolinium contrast material is contraindicated in patients with renal impairment (because of the risk of nephrogenic systemic fibrosis).[12-16]

Ultrasound

Primarily, ultrasonography has no role in the radiological assessment of the larynx for local pathology. This is largely because ossification of the laryngeal cartilages prevents adequate insonation and detailed visualization of the endolaryngeal soft tissues. This, therefore, is particularly the case in the adult larynx. However, in large T3 and T4 laryngeal tumors, particularly where extralaryngeal tumor extension is identified on ultrasound assessment, the author has, on occasion, utilized the facility of ultrasound to guide fine-needle aspiration of such tumors for cytological diagnosis where microlaryngoscopy and biopsy has yielded repeatedly indeterminate histology.

The false and true vocal cords can sometimes be identified on ultrasound assessment of the neck in the adult (and routinely in the pediatric patient), and it is the author's routine practice to attempt such limited assessment when undertaking ultrasound examination of the neck, particularly with a view to confirming satisfactory and symmetrical vocal cord mobility on quiet respiration and phonation.

Positron Emission Tomography

Positron emission tomography (PET) is a functional nuclear medicine imaging modality that is a very sensitive and specific technique for in vivo imaging of metabolic pathways. For this reason, it is sometimes referred to as a form of metabolic imaging. PET utilizes positron-emitting short-living radioisotopes of natural elements such as fluorine-18, carbon-11, and nitrogen-13. Depending on the selected radiopharmaceutical, PET can provide quantitative information on several tissue metabolism variables including blood flow, DNA metabolism, glucose metabolism, or amino acid metabolism.

The radiopharmaceutical tracer most commonly used in clinical practice throughout the world at the present time is fluorine-18-labeled 2-fluoro-2-deoxy-D-glucose (FDG). The use of FDG for in vivo imaging of malignant neoplastic disease is based on the higher rate of glucose metabolism in

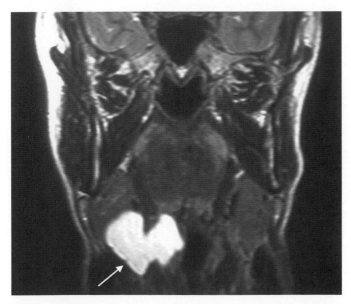

Figure 12.2 Coronal T2-weighted magnetic resonance sequence through the larynx in a 33-year-old female professional orchestral trumpet player demonstrates typical appearances of a right internal–external laryngocele (arrow).

most malignant tumors.[17] PET is usually combined with CT in one scanner facility, allowing simultaneous acquisition of a whole-body CT and PET study. In this way, the two image modalities can be co-registered to create a whole-body PET–CT assessment integrating the metabolic (functional) characteristics with the structural and morphological (CT) characteristics of the pathological process.[17,18] More recently, co-registration of PET with MRI scanning has been attempted, but, given the relatively slow acquisition times of MRI, this has limited value in current oncological radiological practice.[19,20]

One of the limitations of FDG-PET is that, being a functional metabolic modality, it is not the only malignant disease in which significantly raised glucose metabolism occurs. Infective and inflammatory processes will also exhibit "FDG-PET positive" increased metabolic activity[20]; as an example, this includes sites of recent surgical biopsy where normal active tissue repair processes will have been initiated by the inherent tissue-traumatizing effect biopsy procedure. For this reason, wherever possible, PET should be performed before any surgical (or radiological) biopsy procedure. Benign processes such as laryngitis and radiotherapy-related mucositis can also be a major source of false-positive PET diagnoses.[17,20–22] For this reason, it is imperative that requests for PET imaging are discussed with the appropriate radiologist with full clinical information made available if the potentially negative impact of false-positive FDG-PET results on patient management is to be avoided.

In his current practice, the author, largely, limits the use of FDG-PET in the assessment of laryngeal neoplastic pathology to cases where there is potential for PET to upstage disease burden (i.e., where the likelihood of distant metastases or synchronous second primary malignancy is high) or for the detection and staging of recurrent disease in the post-treatment neck where detection of such recurrent disease can prove difficult radiologically with CT and MRI if the normal morphological anatomy of the upper aerodigestive tract and neck has been significantly distorted by previous surgery and radiotherapy. True-positive FDG-PET diagnosis requires an adequate volume of tumor to be present: very low volume (and microscopic) neoplastic disease is unlikely to yield a positive result.[20–22]

The radiation burden to the patient (and the environment) posed by PET is far higher than CT alone and the risk–benefit must always be considered. Also, the high cost of PET imaging provision should not be discounted, both in terms of the entire facility and also in the cost relating to individual examinations.

Examples of Imaging of Pathological Entities

The choice of imaging modalities will be discussed in brief in relation to radiological assessment of very broad pathology categories to provide a flavor of the ways in which imaging may assist the laryngologist in the evaluation of laryngeal

pathology. The following discussions and recommendations are neither exhaustive nor inflexible as such more detailed narrative is beyond the scope of this chapter; nevertheless, it is hoped that the examples may highlight a few of the important considerations when recommending imaging modalities.

- Congenital: Congenital lesions of the larynx are rare and are usually diagnosed in childhood because of the association with respiratory distress. Where imaging is required for these pathologies, such as laryngomalacia, subglottic stenosis, and subglottic hemangioma, CT assessment is a valuable imaging modality.[7–9] It not only provides a global assessment of the upper aerodigestive tract including, in particular, all of the subsites of the larynx but is also a fast imaging technique in the pediatric population where respiratory distress may be an issue. Nevertheless, consideration of the ionization radiation exposure to the pediatric population should always be borne in mind.
- Trauma: Acute laryngeal trauma has many diverse causes. Penetrating and blunt mechanisms are examples. CT remains the imaging modality of choice in acute trauma (**Fig. 12.3**). It is fast, widely available, and can easily provide simultaneous assessment of other regions of the body that may have also been injured by the traumatic mechanism; the intubated and ventilated patient can be accommodated by this modality without the need for specialized instruments (such as MR-compatible anesthetic and monitoring equipment). The exquisite demonstration of ossified structures also recommends CT to identification of

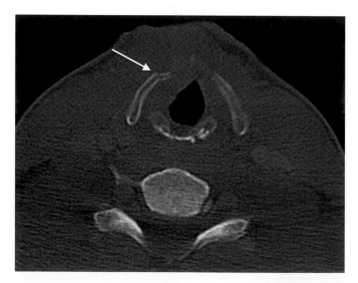

Figure 12.3 Axial contrast-enhanced computed tomography (CT) image of the larynx on bone windows in a 26-year-old man who sustained a "glassing" injury to the anterior neck with a broken bottle. There is a fracture of the right thyroid cartilage lamina (arrow) and right endolaryngeal hematoma and laceration. (Widespread soft-tissue emphysema, laceration, and perforation of the posterior wall of the contralateral left pyriform fossa were present as well as a glass fragment in the retropharyngeal space [CT images not shown].)

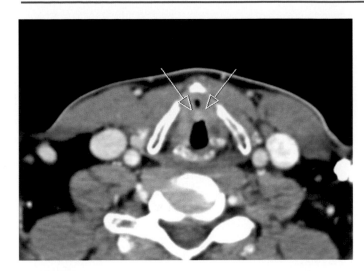

Figure 12.4 Axial contrast-enhanced computed tomography image through the true vocal cords of a 47-year-old male nonsmoker with a 3-week history of a hoarse voice. There are symmetrical "kissing" mucosal nodules (arrows) affecting the anterior one-third of the true vocal cords consistent with "singer's nodules." The diagnosis was confirmed at microlaryngoscopy.

fractures of the laryngeal skeleton as well as outlining hematomas and soft-tissue disruption. Granulation and scar tissue, webs, and abnormalities of the cricoarytenoid joint representing chronic laryngeal trauma can be well demonstrated on CT assessment.

- Infection/inflammation: Acute and chronic laryngitis and their associated features such as mucositis, mucosal and submucosal edema, and vocal cord nodules related to voice abuse (**Fig. 12.4**) are demonstrated on CT assessment of the larynx. Systemic inflammatory conditions affecting the larynx can also be highlighted

on appropriate CT assessment of the larynx. Erosive joint changes related to rheumatoid arthritis can affect the synovial cricoarytenoid joint, the abnormal appearances of which can be identified on CT. Soft-tissue inflammatory changes of the endolarynx as might occur in pathologies such as sarcoidosis and Wegener's granulomatosis will be evident on CT or MRI assessment of the larynx. Given the faster scan time offered by CT, it is usually the first-line imaging modality of choice.

- Malignancy: The value of CT in the assessment and staging of malignant disease of the larynx, which is most commonly squamous cell carcinoma, is recognized and has already been alluded to in previous discussions (**Fig. 12.5**). Laryngeal cartilaginous invasion can be evaluated with relative ease in the well-ossified laryngeal cartilage. Difficulty can arise however, given that a variable heterogeneous pattern of the thyroid cartilage ossification is a normal and frequent occurrence. Accurate delineation of such thyroid cartilage invasion upstages associated squamous cell carcinoma from T3 to T4a by current tumor-node-metastasis (TNM) criteria.[23] MRI of the larynx can assist such delineation, although it can also yield false-positive findings because reactive inflammation, edema, and fibrosis in cartilage in the vicinity of the tumor may display diagnostic features similar to those of cartilage infiltrated by tumor (**Fig. 12.6**).[24–27]

- Posttreatment changes: Imaging evaluation of the postradiotherapy and postsurgical larynx is best served, in the first instance, by CT, particularly where altered ossified laryngeal cartilaginous assessment due to surgery may need to be distinguished from posttreatment complications

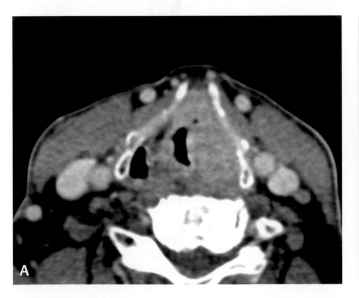

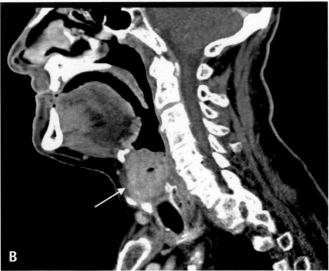

Figure 12.5 (A) Axial contrast-enhanced computed tomography (CT) of the larynx in a 74-year-old male smoker demonstrates a large T3 squamous cell carcinoma of predominantly the left hemilarynx invading paraglottic fat but not causing any through–through erosion of the thyroid cartilage. (B) Sagittal reconstruction of the CT of the larynx performed on the same patient as in (A). The large tumor (arrow) has also invaded the pre-epiglottic fat space.

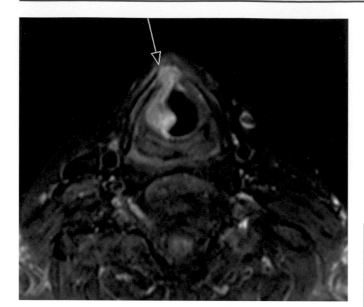

Figure 12.6 Axial postcontrast fat-saturated T1-weighted image through the larynx of a 66-year-old male smoker with a T4a squamous cell carcinoma of the glottis with focal through-and-through invasion of the anterior aspect of the right thyroid cartilage lamina (arrow). The patient subsequently underwent total laryngectomy and tumor invasion of the thyroid cartilage was confirmed on postoperative histopathology.

such as chondroradionecrosis of the larynx. MRI can serve as a useful secondary imaging modality where low-volume coexistent tumor recurrence on a background of markedly iatrogenically altered laryngeal morphology is a consideration. Where imaging findings are complicated by posttreatment anatomical distortion, functional metabolic imaging with FDG-PET may identify tumor recurrence (**Fig. 12.7**), although a false-negative finding is likely if the volume of recurrent disease is very low; additionally, chondroradionecrosis is one cause of false-positive FDG-PET assessment.[21,28]

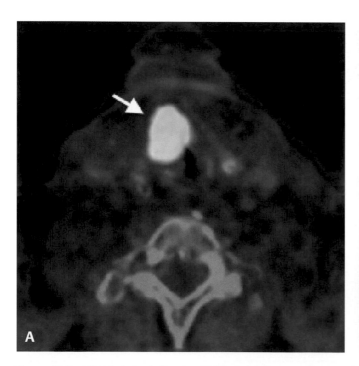

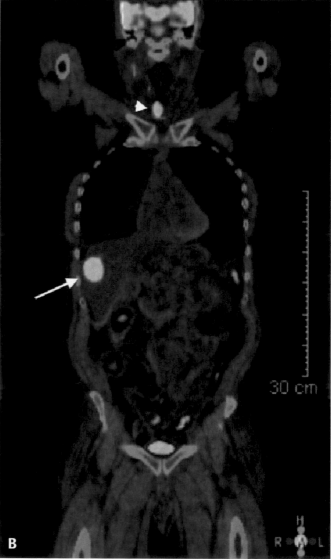

Figure 12.7 (A) Whole-body fluorine-18-labeled 2-fluoro-2-deoxy-D-glucose (18-FDG) computed tomography-positron emission tomography (CT-PET) coregistered images through the larynx in a 71-year-old male smoker and chronic alcohol user who had previously received radiotherapy for a T3 squamous cell carcinoma of the larynx. CT-PET was performed because of difficulty differentiating postradiotherapy change from possible recurrent disease on surveillance CT and MR assessments despite suspicious features on both imaging modalities. Clinical examination including flexible nasendoscopy was indeterminate. The significantly increased metabolic activity in the right true vocal cord and anterior commissure extending into thyroid cartilage on the CT-PET confirmed recurrent T4a disease. (B) Whole-body 18-FDG CT-PET coregistered images of the same patient as in (A) identified an incidental hepatocellular carcinoma of the liver (arrow) in addition to the recurrent squamous cell carcinoma in the right hemilarynx (arrowhead).

Conclusion

Imaging is an invaluable assist to the clinical evaluation of laryngeal pathology allowing assessment of the submucosal soft tissues and laryngeal cartilaginous skeleton. The imaging modalities at the disposal of the radiologist that are used most commonly for laryngeal disease are CT and MRI. PET and ultrasound also play a more limited role in imaging assessment of the larynx.

CT is typically the first-line imaging modality of choice for the larynx because it is fast (ameliorating deleterious motion artifact on the images), relatively widely available, and provides good soft-tissue detail but also excellent characterization of ossified cartilaginous structures. However, the use and request for CT should be tempered in the pediatric population because of the associated ionizing radiation burden. MRI may be an appropriate substitute where nonemergency cross-sectional imaging of the larynx is a prerequisite for appropriate diagnosis and treatment planning.

PET can provide a useful third-line diagnostic imaging modality in assessment of the posttreatment larynx that has sustained distorting postsurgical and/or postradiotherapy changes where there is significant clinical and radiological concern for recurrent malignant disease, particularly if CT or MRI findings are indeterminate.

As a final consideration, multidisciplinary dialogue between the laryngologist and the radiologist can maximize the efficiency of the patient-management pathway.

References

1. Becker M, Burkhardt K, Dulguerov P, Allal A. Imaging of the larynx and hypopharynx. Eur J Radiol 2008;66(3):460–479

2. Hermans R. Staging of laryngeal and hypopharyngeal cancer: value of imaging studies. Eur Radiol 2006;16(11):2386–2400

3. Glastonbury CM. Non-oncologic imaging of the larynx. Otolaryngol Clin North Am 2008;41(1):139–156, vi

4. Robinson S, Juutilainen M, Suomalainen A, Mäkitie AA. Multidetector row computed tomography of the injured larynx after trauma. Semin Ultrasound CT MR 2009;30(3):188–194

5. Bell RB, Verschueren DS, Dierks EJ. Management of laryngeal trauma. Oral Maxillofac Surg Clin North Am 2008;20(3):415–430

6. Schaefer SD. The treatment of acute external laryngeal injuries. "State of the art". Arch Otolaryngol Head Neck Surg 1991;117(1):35–39

7. Parida PK, Gupta AK. Role of spiral computed tomography with 3-dimensional reconstruction in cases with laryngeal stenosis—a radioclinical correlation. Am J Otolaryngol 2008;29(5):305–311

8. Chung CJ, Fordham LA, Mukherji SK. The pediatric airway: a review of differential diagnosis by anatomy and pathology. Neuroimaging Clin N Am 2000;10(1):161–180, ix

9. Hermans R, Verschakelen JA, Baert AL. Imaging of laryngeal and tracheal stenosis. Acta Otorhinolaryngol Belg 1995;49(4):323–329

10. Lev S, Lev MH. Imaging of cystic lesions. Radiol Clin North Am 2000;38(5):1013–1027

11. Vazquez E, Enriquez G, Castellote A, et al. US, CT, and MR imaging of neck lesions in children. Radiographics 1995;15(1):105–122

12. Prince MR, Zhang H, Zou Z, Staron RB, Brill PW. Incidence of immediate gadolinium contrast media reactions. AJR Am J Roentgenol 2011;196(2):W138-43

13. Leiner T, Kucharczyk W. Special issue: nephrogenic systemic fibrosis. J Magn Reson Imaging 2009;30(6):1233–1235

14. Mayr M, Burkhalter F, Bongartz G. Nephrogenic systemic fibrosis: clinical spectrum of disease. J Magn Reson Imaging 2009;30(6):1289–1297

15. Rees O, Agarwal SK. Nephrogenic systemic fibrosis: UK survey of the use of gadolinium-based contrast media. Clin Radiol 2010;65(8):636–641

16. Altun E, Semelka RC, Cakit C. Nephrogenic systemic fibrosis and management of high-risk patients. Acad Radiol 2009;16(7):897–905

17. Blodgett TM, Fukui MB, Snyderman CH, et al. Combined PET-CT in the head and neck: part 1. Physiologic, altered physiologic, and artifactual FDG uptake. Radiographics 2005;25(4):897–912

18. Gordin A, Golz A, Keidar Z, Daitzchman M, Bar-Shalom R, Israel O. The role of FDG-PET/CT imaging in head and neck malignant conditions: impact on diagnostic accuracy and patient care. Otolaryngol Head Neck Surg 2007;137(1):130–137

19. Castelijns JA. PET-MRI in the head and neck area: challenges and new directions. Eur Radiol 2011;21(11):2425–2426

20. Boss A, Stegger L, Bisdas S, et al. Feasibility of simultaneous PET/MR imaging in the head and upper neck area. Eur Radiol 2011;21(7):1439–1446

21. Fukui MB, Blodgett TM, Snyderman CH, et al. Combined PET-CT in the head and neck: part 2. Diagnostic uses and pitfalls of oncologic imaging. Radiographics 2005;25(4):913–930

22. Chisin R, Macapinlac HA. The indications of FDG-PET in neck oncology. Radiol Clin North Am 2000;38(5):999–1012

23. Edge SB, Byrd DR, Compton CC, Fritz AG, Greene FL, Trotti A, eds. American Joint Committee on Cancer. In: Cancer Staging Handbook. 7th ed. New York, NY: Springer; 2010:57–62

24. Becker M, Zbären P, Casselman JW, Kohler R, Dulguerov P, Becker CD. Neoplastic invasion of laryngeal cartilage: reassessment of criteria for diagnosis at MR imaging. Radiology 2008;249(2):551–559

25. Ljumanovic R, Langendijk JA, van Wattingen M, et al. MR imaging predictors of local control of glottic squamous cell carcinoma treated with radiation alone. Radiology 2007;244(1):205–212

26. Becker M. Neoplastic invasion of laryngeal cartilage: radiologic diagnosis and therapeutic implications. Eur J Radiol 2000;33(3):216–229

27. Blitz AM, Aygun N. Radiologic evaluation of larynx cancer. Otolaryngol Clin North Am 2008;41(4):697–713, vi

28. Offiah C, Hall E. Post-treatment imaging appearances in head and neck cancer patients. Clin Radiol 2011;66(1):13–24

Section D

Therapeutic Principles

13 Principles of Phonomicrosurgery

Abir K. Bhattacharyya, Nupur Kapoor Nerurkar, and Sonna Njideka Ifeacho

Phonomicrosurgery is performed endoscopically using a microscope on the vocal folds to restore, improve, or alter a person's voice and may also be performed in both benign and select malignant laryngeal pathology. A successful surgery is underpinned by a sound knowledge of the anatomy, particularly microanatomy of the vocal folds and understanding of the physiological principles of phonation.

Key Principle: Understanding the Microanatomy of the Vocal Folds

Hirano has described the vocal folds as a multilayered structure comprising stratified squamous epithelium overlying a gelatinous superficial lamina propria (SLP) and together comprising the vocal fold cover. This is followed by the intermediate and deep layers of the lamina propria, which constitute the vocal ligament. This vocal ligament serves as a transition layer to the body of the vocal fold composed of the most medial part of the thyroarytenoid muscle, i.e., vocalis muscle.[1] The epithelium is secured to the lamina propria by the basement membrane zone (BMZ), which is a collection of protein and nonprotein structures. The basal cells of the BMZ have anchorage filaments and fibers that attach themselves to the lamellar proteins in the lamina propria. Thus, the cellular epidermis is attached to gelatinous lamina propria. Interestingly, fewer anchoring fibers per unit area predispose to vocal nodules.[2,3] When cancer has not infiltrated into the BMZ, it is referred to as carcinoma in situ, and chances of local or distal metastasis are highly unlikely. It is consequently essential to dissect below the BMZ when performing a biopsy of a suspicious vocal fold lesion to enable the histopathology experts to make a correct diagnosis regarding depth of invasion of the cancer.

The SLP is composed of a loose fibrous tissue network in an extracellular matrix of hyaluronic acid, mucopolysaccharides, decorin, and other proteins. Although the SLP is also known as Reinke space, it is not a space, but a potential space due to the loose arrangement of its integral components. This structure affords the flexibility required for complex vibrations by the vocal fold during vocalization. The intermediate lamina propria acts as a shock-absorbing layer, especially at its anterior and posterior condensation referred to as anterior and posterior macula flava, hence its structure is predominantly made of elastin and hyaluronic acid arranged in a regular longitudinal manner. The deep layer of the lamina propria comprises fibroblasts and collagen.

Key Principle: Preservation of the Superficial Lamina Propria Layer

Respect for these different layers and an appreciation of their contribution to the vocal fold function is essential before undertaking phonomicrosurgery. Not only is the SLP integral to the vibratory characteristics of the vocal fold, but it also has a poor propensity toward regeneration following excision or thermal damage and therefore must be handled with care and preserved to ensure optimal healing with minimal scarring and distortion to the mucosal wave.

Clinical Insight

The superficial lamina propria (SLP) layer is vital for production of the mucosal wave and cannot regenerate; therefore, handle this layer with care while preserving as much normal epithelium as possible.

Key Principle: Appropriate Dissection Techniques—Subepithelial Infiltration Technique and Microflap Dissection

Infiltration of the subepithelial space with 1 to 2 cc of 1 : 10,000 of adrenaline in saline before surgery permits expansion of the SLP, although temporarily, allowing for dissection in the most superficial part of the SLP. Subepithelial infiltration technique (SEIT) also helps achieve hemostasis, lesion demarcation, and estimation of depth penetration of the vocal fold lesion.[4] A safe approach during vocal fold surgery is to use mini-micro flaps with clean incisions through the epithelium and a gentle dissection through the SLP to excise the pathological lesion.[5] Removal of the lesion is then performed by staying in the SLP as superficial as possible.

Key Principle: Avoiding Collateral Damage and Minimizing Trauma to Vocal Ligament

It is important to avoid trauma to the vocal ligament whenever possible because the vocal ligament is a source of fibroblasts that are activated during the postoperative recovery phase. The vocalis muscle should not be routinely instrumented during phonomicrosurgery, as benign lesions are mostly located in the most superficial layers of the vocal fold.

Key Principle: Why Operate, When to Operate, and When not to Operate

Before operating on the vocal folds, it must be established that there is a pathological lesion causing a change in voice. Conservative management, when indicated, must be instituted before planning for surgery.

Phonomicrosurgery is indicated when a lesion is present on the vocal folds, which has a detrimental effect on the voice. Lesions such as large hemorrhagic polyps, Reinke edema, and intracordal cysts are most amenable to surgery. However, some lesions may not present such a clear case for excision, such as vocal fold sulci where surgical results are unpredictable and soft vocal nodules before exposure to the benefit of speech therapy. The potential risk of scarring and causing more damage to the voice must be borne in mind during the decision-making process before phonomicrosurgery. Lesions that will not respond, have not responded, or indeed have worsened in response to voice therapy make a strong case for surgery, as do cases of suspected malignancy. A decision-making algorithm highlighting the key steps in the management of vocal pathology is outlined in **Fig. 13.1**.

A patient's goals and desires must be considered before surgery. A patient with hoarseness may be anxious to exclude a cancer diagnosis with no desire for surgery once there is reassurance that the lesion is benign. Conversely, a patient who is a professional voice user may wish for expedient surgery with the best possible outcome to restore normal voice characteristics.

Preoperative Evaluation

Treatment planning before surgery necessitates thorough history analysis and clinical examination. A voice history must be taken and include details of symptoms impacting the voice and laryngeal function, vocal hygiene, vocal use, and ascertaining the presence of known risk factors for voice pathology. Further questioning with regards to the patients general medical history is important as this may affect their fitness for surgery and specifically impact measured outcomes after phonomicrosurgery. For further details on aspects of history-taking and clinical assessment, refer to Chapter 6.

Clinical examination should include fiberoptic evaluation of the vocal folds and larynx. Videostroboscopy is essential to assess the vocal fold in more detail and the mucosal wave during phonation. Videostroboscopy is performed using a rigid endoscope or a flexible laryngoscope with distal chip technology for a clearer picture than previously provided by older flexible laryngoscopes. Objective assessment of voice is dealt with in Chapter 7.

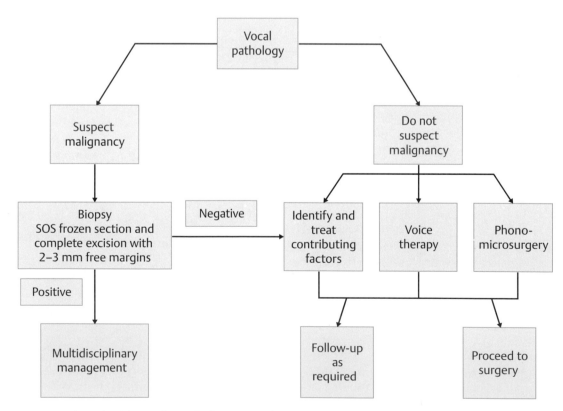

Figure 13.1 Decision-making algorithm outlining the key steps in the management of vocal pathology.

Both objective and subjective voice assessments before surgery set a baseline for comparison of future assessments. The former can be recorded using the Grade, Roughness, Breathiness, Asthenia, Strain rating scale.[6] The latter can be achieved using several quality of life instruments, such as the voice handicap index.[7] The evaluation of voice outcome and quality of life measures are described in Chapter 10.

Preoperative assessment permits the acquisition of informed consent. Informed consent mandates a clear explanation of the procedure and its benefits, all alternatives, and the risks and complications. These include a risk of trauma to the orofacial soft tissues, chipping/loosening the dentition, and scarring of the vocal folds with potential worsening of their presenting complaint. The latter is a rare complication in the hands of a voice specialist using the appropriate equipment and instruments.

Role of Preoperative Speech and Language Therapy

Preoperative voice therapy is essential in the management of voice pathology and is important in establishing rapport between patient and therapist, thereby laying the foundation for a strong therapeutic alliance. In some instances, lesions and voice changes may be reversed by this conservative approach alone, for example, vocal nodules. In other instances, it provides a vital opportunity for patient education that serves to enhance the beneficial outcomes of surgery. During voice therapy, adverse patient-specific habits can be identified, vocal technique can be developed, and postoperative advice disseminated. In those cases where there is ambiguity as to the exact nature of the lesion, for example, early small vocal nodules, its response to voice therapy can indicate whether surgical excision is warranted.[8,9]

Timing of Surgery

Phonomicrosurgery is one step in the management of voice pathology. Factors specific to the patient and the etiology of the vocal fold pathology must be considered before surgery. Patients must be willing and able to attend preoperative evaluations that may include voice therapy sessions, undergo surgery, and adhere to the postoperative regime to ensure a successful outcome.

Surgery may need to be delayed or rescheduled, for example, in the professional voice users where a mandatory performance must be given. Or, for example, patients who are unlikely to follow postoperative voice rest instructions due to family commitments. Patients who have systemic factors prohibiting the provision of safe general anesthesia need those factors to be controlled or corrected before contemplating surgery. Medical conditions that impact the larynx and/or the vocal folds must be optimized before surgery, for example, laryngopharyngeal reflux. For specific vocal fold pathology, as mentioned earlier, vocal fold nodules and small polyps may respond to voice therapy; therefore, the indication for surgery is explored after voice therapy.[10]

Intraoperative Factors

Access and Exposure

Adequate visualization of the vocal folds is imperative when performing vocal fold surgery. Good access is achieved by correct positioning and exposure of the structures of the larynx. The ideal patient position is to lie in the "sniffing the morning air" position. The patient is placed supine on the table, the head is extended at the atlanto-occipital joint, and the neck is flexed on the chest. One must have prior knowledge of any cervical pathology likely to impact on neck movement and bear this in mind when positioning the patient.

Clinical Pearls and Pitfalls

Use of cold adrenaline-soaked neurosurgical patties improves visualization manifold. This along with the subepithelial infusion technique minimizes blood loss and avoids trauma underlying structures, for example, vocal ligament—this technique is particularly useful with the subepithelial cysts.

The largest laryngoscope that can comfortably fit is inserted into the larynx, and the degree of exposure of the vocal folds and laryngeal structures is checked. The laryngoscope can now be attached to a laryngeal suspension system, of which there are several. Some suspension systems allow a degree of flexibility in viewing the larynx. When a chest piece is being used, placing it on a Mayo's trolley placed just above the patient's chest provides extension with no movement of the system during ventilation (**Fig. 13.2**). Measures to improve visualization of the anterior commissure include the application of "sticky tape" or a cotton bandage across the larynx at the level of the cricothyroid membrane and attaching both ends to the

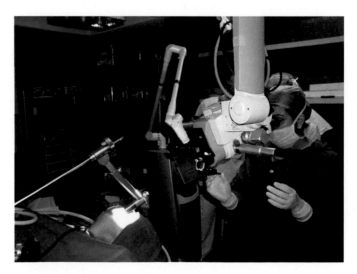

Figure 13.2 Operation theater setup for microlaryngeal surgery.

sides of the operating table. In a very anteriorly placed larynx, the flexion–flexion position may prove to be useful for both intubation and laryngeal exposure. Magnification is an essential step during phonomicrosurgery; the operating microscope is now positioned ready for surgery to commence. A 400-mm lens is the ideal lens for laryngeal surgery, as it provides optimum magnification at a reasonable distance from the operating field permitting easy passage of instruments down the laryngoscope. Some phonosurgeons prefer to operate using a laryngoscope that has an inbuilt channel for an endoscope that is attached to a camera. In this situation, the surgeon is operating off the monitor and not through the microscope. Before commencing surgery, a preoperative photo of the lesion is taken using a zero-degree Hopkins telescope.

Most instrumentation in phonomicrosurgery has the tips of the forceps and scissors to be around 1 mm in contrast to 3 mm of the conventional microlaryngeal instruments. Special microflap elevators, both blunt and sharp, of various degrees, a "27" number infiltration needle, vocal fold retractor, and thin microflap suction all form part of the armamentarium of a phonosurgeon's operating trolley.

There is a dichotomy in opinion among phonosurgeons regarding the use of lasers in different vocal fold pathology. The primary concern is the heat dissipation that may cause irreversible thermal damage to the SLP. The advent of highly specialized laser delivery systems has made it possible to operate accurately using the laser especially with the SEIT that serves as a heat sink. Vascular lesions are more amenable to laser excision as are malignancies. However, the final decision to perform laser or cold-steel surgery lies with the surgeon.

Due to the presence of anchoring fibrils between the BMZ and the SLP, every effort should be made to elevate the minimum amount of epithelium, as even though epithelium regenerates with time, these anchoring fibrils do not re-anchor. It is recommended that mini-microflap surgery is undertaken with the incision (epithelial cordotomy) being made precisely on the lateral edge of the lesion. The SEIT does not appear to disturb these anchoring fibrils. A study investigating the microflap technique for similar benign glottic lesions operated on with and without SEIT showed better vocal outcome measures in the group on whom SEIT had been used.[10,11]

Specific Considerations

Hemorrhagic Polyps and Varices

Mucosal ectasia, including dilated and tortuous capillaries, can alter vocal fold function. Blood vessels can be found running the length of the true vocal folds. When vocal folds are subjected to trauma from chronic over-talking, high-volume talking, screaming, a cough, or aggressive singing, blood vessels may tear with blood seeping out into the vocal fold. The result is a red vocal fold at the time of injury

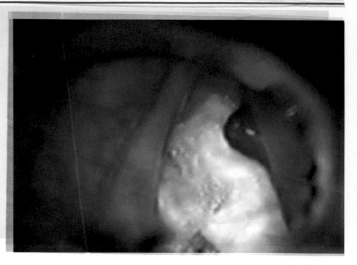

Figure 13.3   Right hemorrhagic polyp.

with the subsequent healing phase in keeping with a bruise occurring anywhere else in the body. Once the blood vessels heal, they tend to take on a more dilated and tortuous form probably due to thinner vessel walls. As most trauma affects the midportion of the vocal folds, this is the site of most ectatic vessels. If dilated vessels are located on the vibratory edge of the vocal fold, then they can interfere with voice quality; the vessels may become engorged during phonation with the risk of subsequent rupture leading to subepithelial hemorrhage. In this situation, conservative management with voice rest and steroids is recommended. Episodes of frequent bleeding validate the need for surgical excision of these varices during a quiescent period. In earlier times, surgeons would dissect and excise the varices with cold steel instruments; however, the more current approach is to use a laser with an extremely small Acuspot and SEIT.

Polyps (**Fig. 13.3**) may also be managed conservatively initially, but usually require surgical excision using the mini-microflap technique with maximum preservation of the SLP and minimum elevation of the epithelium. Following subepithelial infiltration, an incision is made using a sickle knife or upward-angulated scissors on the lateral edge of the polyp following which a microflap elevator is used to separate the overlying epithelium from the polyp (**Fig. 13.4**). The polyp is then separated from the underlying SLP and excised (**Fig. 13.5**). All redundant epithelium is then excised (**Fig. 13.6**). The postoperative appearance should ideally reveal a precise edge-to-edge approximation of the epithelium (**Fig. 13.7**).

Clinical Insights

The anterior commissure must be given due respect during surgery and should only be operated on when absolutely necessary. It is imperative to have a plan ready for tackling the almost certain postoperative complication of synechiae formation.

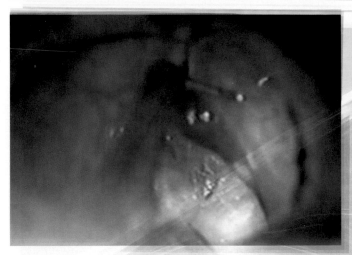

Figure 13.4   Right subepithelial infusion techniques using "27" number needle.

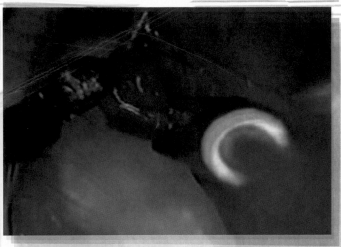

Figure 13.5   Right mini-microflap excision of right hemorrhagic polyp.

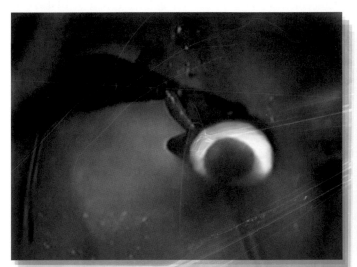

Figure 13.6   Trimming of redundant epithelium.

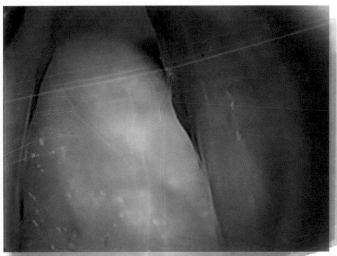

Figure 13.7   Postoperative view with reposition of epithelium.

Vocal Fold Nodules

These are paired firm lesions located in the center of the membranous vocal fold, which is the junction of the anterior and posterior two-thirds of the true vocal fold (**Fig. 13.8**). These lesions affect voice production in several ways. Patients complain of breaks, where there is sudden loss of voice midsentence and there may be variation in the pitch. The underlying etiology is vocal overuse and misuse, and is mostly seen in those who use their voices excessively particularly in relation to their careers and professions, the so-called professional voice user. Careful endoscopic examination is required to clearly identify small nodules that can have significant effects on the voice. Management includes moderation of their voice use, best achieved by voice therapy targeted to poor habits and reduced vocal use. It is important to exhaust voice therapy as the treatment modality before considering surgery.

Clinical Insights

Occasionally, vocal nodules and other benign lesions are responsible for the characteristic voice of a professional voice user. It is vital to discuss that a change in this characteristic voice should be expected in the case of surgical intervention.

Vocal Fold Cysts

Vocal fold cysts may be mucous retention or epidermoid. Histopathology of the former reveals thin respiratory mucosa and that of the latter, thick stratified squamous epithelium. Epidermoid cysts are filled with a cheesy material unlike the clear fluid of the mucous retention cysts. The management of both involves complete excision, which is challenging, due to the tendency of these tense cysts to rupture during mini-microflap surgery. SEIT helps in hydrodissection

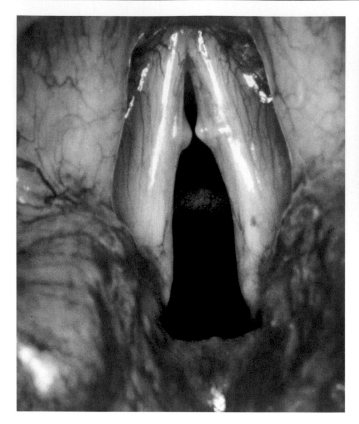

Figure 13.8 Bilateral vocal fold nodules.

following which repeat palpation helps delineate the exact site for the epithelial cordotomy (**Fig. 13.9**). Both blunt and sharp dissection is needed to deliver the cyst (**Fig. 13.10**), and the cyst should not be held as far as possible, to prevent rupture. In the second author's experience, thick fibrotic bands are almost always found anteriorly and posteriorly giving the appearance of a pearl (cyst) on a string (fibrotic bands). Sharp dissection of these bands is recommended. If

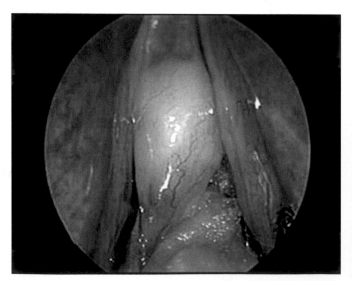

Figure 13.9 Epithelial cordotomy just lateral to left subepithelial cyst being performed with a sickle knife, following subepithelial infiltration technique.

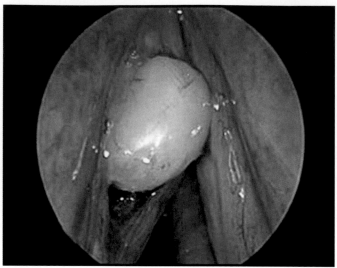

Figure 13.10 Left subepithelial cyst being delivered preserving the superficial lamina propria layer.

the cyst ruptures during excision, then all effort to completely dissect out the capsule should be made.

Reinke Edema

Reinke edema is due to inflammation within the SLP, also known as Reinke space (**Fig. 13.11**). It is most commonly seen in smokers, hence its alias smoker's polyps. Reinke edema is usually precipitated by a combination of vocal overuse on a background of smoking. Patients usually present with a

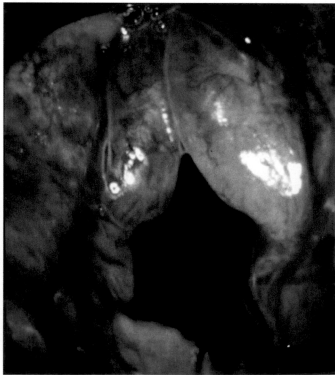

Figure 13.11 Bilateral Reinke edema.

rough voice and experience pitch variation. The latter occurs because of excessive adduction in an attempt to bring the true vocal cords together in spite of the significant overlying edema, the resultant false vocal cord phonation causes the altered voice characteristics. Smoking cessation advice is an important component of the management of Reinke edema. Surgical excision may be undertaken with cold steel instrumentation or the laser. The presence of abundant SLP works in the patients favors, however, excessive removal and the resultant thinning of vocal folds may dramatically raise the pitch of postoperative voice, which is especially unacceptable to the male patient. Respecting the integrity of the anterior commissure is of paramount importance to prevent postoperative synechiae and web formation.

Vocal Process Granulomas/Contact Granuloma

Vocal process granulomas arise as a result of the inflammatory healing process that takes place after a vocal cord has been subjected to trauma (**Fig. 13.12**). Granulomas are most commonly located on the vocal process of the arytenoid cartilage (**Fig. 13.13**), although they may occur on the arytenoid cartilage too. The most usual source of trauma is from endotracheal intubation. The friction between the endotracheal tube and the mucosa of the larynx and vocal cords causes ulceration of the mucosa with exposure of the underlying cartilage. The other main cause is chronic trauma from vocal overuse, chronic cough, or vocal cords weakened by innervation injury or lack of use with a resultant atrophied thyroarytenoid muscle. In the latter case, the vocal cords are thinned and bowed, and require forceful adduction to compensate for the bowing, causing repeated trauma to the arytenoid and arytenoid process of the vocal cord. Management consists of removing the causative factor and voice rest. Small granulomas may be treated effectively with office injection of Botulinum toxin in the thyroarytenoid muscle along with protein pump inhibitors.

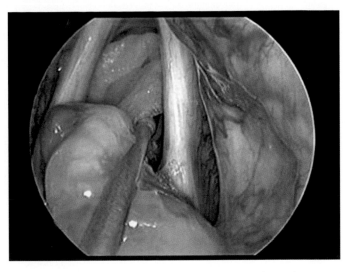

Figure 13.13 Granuloma being retracted to reveal attachment to vocal process.

Large granulomas may be excised in the operating theater with simultaneous Botulinum toxin injection directly in the thyroarytenoid muscle. The vocal fold paresis created by the action of the Botulinum toxin allows for forced voice rest with adequate time for healing over the vocal process. Simple excision is associated with very high rates of recurrence of the granuloma, often larger than the one treated.

Recurrent Respiratory Papillomas

Recurrent respiratory papillomas (**Fig. 13.14**) may be juvenile-onset or adult-onset, both caused by the human papilloma virus (HPV). The aim of management is maintaining an airway, preventing tracheostomy, and giving the patient a serviceable voice. Despite the surgeon's best efforts, recurrence is rampant due to the presence of the virus in the neighboring normal tissue. Laryngeal microdebrider debulking and carbon dioxide laser excision

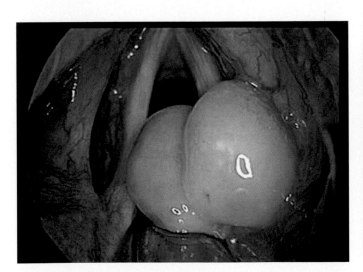

Figure 13.12   Right contact granuloma.

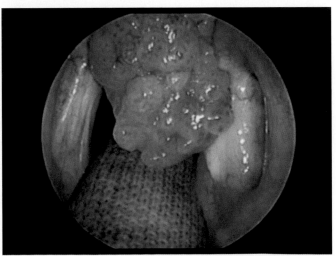

Figure 13.14   Recurrent respiratory papillomas in the adult larynx.

is a standard of treatment. Hemoangiolytic lasers such as 585-nm pulse dye laser and potassium titanyl phosphate (KTP) laser are especially useful in the management of this vascular lesion. Antivirals such as cidofovir have shown good results; however, concern regarding possible dysplastic conversion exists. Intralesional Avastin injections along with pulsed KTP laser have also been used recently in a bid to control RRP.[12]

Keratosis

Microflap excision of keratosis (**Fig. 13.15**) may be performed with cold steel or lasers. Histopathology of the lesions determines the degree of aggressiveness of the excision. Initial benign lesions may recur and undergo malignant transformation necessitating biopsy and histopathology studies with every recurrence.

Sulcus Vocalis

A congenital absence or idiopathic loss of lamina propria results in a sulcus vocalis (**Figs. 13.15** and **13.16**). Most sulci are congenital and run through the entire length of the membranous vocal fold, referred to as linear vergeture (grade 2 sulcus). On stroboscopy, an absent or markedly decreased mucosal wave is observed with a spindle-shaped phonatory gap. The voice is hoarse, breathy, and often high pitched. When performing stroboscopy, occasionally, normal mucosal wave pattern may be seen in the presence of a sulcus. This is suggestive of a physiologic sulcus vocalis (grade 1 sulcus). Following the surgery, especially when performed for malignant lesions, a postoperative focal pit may develop where there is an absence of lamina propria and vocalis.

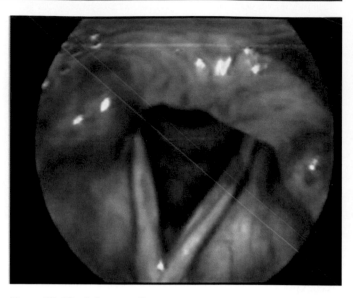

Figure 13.16   Sulcus vocalis.

Management of sulcus vocalis remains a challenge. The results of both voice therapy and surgery leave much to be desired, even in the most experienced hands. Numerous approaches to surgery have been described, as no one particular approach provides a consistently excellent outcome. A small epithelial cordotomy with elevation of epithelium over the sulcus with fat implantation is the preferred surgery of the second author. This is followed by a long course of voice therapy with the patient counseled regarding postoperative voice improvement expected at 6 to 8 weeks.

It is not unusual to find a subepithelial cyst coexisting with sulci. One of the proposed etiology of a sulcus is a ruptured cyst. Almost 25 to 30% of patients with sulcus are seen to have a mucosal bridge overlying it (**Fig. 13.17**). This is more easily appreciated on the operating table.

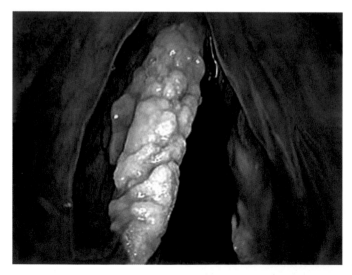

Figure 13.15   Keratosis of left vocal fold and right vocal fold posteriorly.
Printed with permission from Jaypee. Nerurkar N, Kapre G. Leukoplakia of the vocal folds. In: Hathiram BT, Khattar VS, eds. *Atlas of Operative Otorhinolaryngology and Head & Neck Surgery.* Vol. 2. New Delhi, India: Jaypee Brothers Medical Publishers; 2013:Chapter 113.

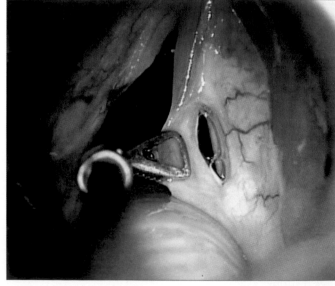

Figure 13.17   Mucosal bridge with sulcus vocalis on right vocal fold.

Postoperative Care

Postoperative care is essential for optimizing surgical outcomes. The aim is to reduce the incidence of inflammation and scarring.

Voice Rest—How Long

There is great variability and controversy with regards to the duration of postoperative voice rest. The main aim of voice rest is to prevent further injury to the vocal folds while they are most vulnerable during the healing phase.[13,14] At a cellular level, myofibroblasts, which are cells of repair, are present in high concentration in the SLP layer and have a turnover of 48 to 72 hours. The primary repair occurs within the first 72 h of any surgical intervention, the initial repair "cycle" lasting 48 to 72 hours would equate to a period of approximately 2 or 3 days absolute voice rest.

Voice rest may be absolute or relative; various regimes are reported in the literature as ranging from no voice rest up to 14 days for absolute rest and up to 21 days for relative voice rest. The most common advice was for a 7-day voice rest period. The most commonly given advice is a 7-day period of voice rest.[15,16] Using the outcome of postoperative dysphonia, a study investigated the effect of various voice rest regimes versus patient compliance and found that the type of voice rest did not influence postoperative dysphonia, but patient compliance did. This makes a case for the more practical option of relative rather than for absolute voice rest; it is also more likely that patients will adhere to the former.

Regeneration of the epithelial layer and SLP is well underway in the first 2 days postoperatively; therefore, at a minimum, patients should be advised to rest their voices for 48 h. The only permitted voice use in this period is in an emergency, for example, to shout out for help and to alert others of an emergency. Whispering inflicts even greater trauma to healing vocal folds than everyday speech and patients must be advised against this accordingly.

Patients are seen typically on the seventh postoperative day and are permitted gradual increasing use of voice such that by 3 to 4 weeks full use of speaking voice is permitted. Using voice for singing is not recommended up to from 6 to 8 weeks when a stroboscopic confirmation of return of mucosal wave is performed. Postoperative videostroboscopic evaluation of the vocal folds will determine the speed with which a patient can progress to full voice use; this is usually guided by the return of the mucosal wave.

Medication: Steroids/Proton Pump Inhibitors

Analgesia is a universal postoperative medication; however, there is great variability in the use of other medicines following vocal surgery. Antibiotics may be given prophylactically to prevent infection. Surgery on the vocal folds will result in a degree of postoperative swelling with some impact on the airway. Hence, short courses of oral preparations of steroids may be prescribed. Patients with a history of gastroesophageal or laryngopharyngeal reflux must be treated to ensure the larynx is not subject to further insult during the recovery phase. The authors treat most patients with a month of postoperative proton pump inhibitors and do not routinely use postoperative steroids. A short course of antibiotics is used by the second author.

Speech and Language Therapy

Postoperative voice therapy is a continuum of the preoperative input. Postoperatively, the speech therapist can reiterate essential vocal hygiene advice.

Conclusion

Phonomicrosurgery for vocal lesions is a vitally important, but nevertheless just one cog in the multidisciplinary approach to the management of vocal fold pathology. Understanding and applying the key principles outlined earlier assist the laryngologist in achieving maximal voice improvement in patients subjected to phonomicrosurgery. The postoperative care and subsequent speech therapy are as important in the voice care pathway as preoperative planning and performing the procedure meticulously with attention to detail.

References

1. Hirano M. Phonosurgery. Basic and clinical investigations. Otoliga (Fukuoka) 1975;21:239–442

2. Gray SD. Cellular physiology of the vocal folds. Otolaryngol Clin North Am 2000;33(4):679–698

3. Gray SD, Pignatari SS, Harding P. Morphology and ultrastructure of the anchoring fibers in normal vocal fold basement membrane zone. J Voice 1994;8(1):48–52

4. Zeitels SM, Hillman RE, Franco RA, Bunting GW. Voice and treatment outcome from phonosurgical management of early glottic cancer. Ann Otol Rhinol Laryngol Suppl 2002;190:3–20

5. Courey MS, Gardner GM, Stone RE, Ossoff RH. Endoscopic vocal fold microflap: a three-year experience. Ann Otol Rhinol Laryngol 1995;104(4, Pt 1):267–273

6. Hirano M. Clinical Examination of Voice, 1st ed. Vienna, Austria: Springer; 1981

7. Jacobson BH, Johnson A, Grywalski C, Silbergleit A, Benninger MS. The voice handicap index (VHI): development and validation. Am J Speech Lang Pathol 1997;6:66–70

8. Rosen CA, Lee AS, Osborne J, Zullo T, Murry T. Development and validation of the voice handicap index-10. Laryngoscope 2004;114(9):1549–1556

9. Leonard R. Voice therapy and vocal nodules in adults. Curr Opin Otolaryngol Head Neck Surg 2009;17(6):453–457

10. Yun YS, Kim MB, Son YI. The effect of vocal hygiene education for patients with vocal polyp. Otolaryngol Head Neck Surg 2007;137(4):569–575

11. Nerurkar N, Narkar N, Joshi A, Kalel K, Bradoo R. Vocal outcomes following subepithelial infiltration technique in microflap surgery: a review of 30 cases. J Laryngol Otol 2007;121(8):768–771

12. Zeitels SM, Lopez-Guerra G, Burns JA, Lutch M, Friedman AM, Hillman RE. Microlaryngoscopic and office-based injection of bevacizumab (Avastin) to enhance 532-nm pulsed KTP laser treatment of glottal papillomatosis. Ann Otol Rhinol Laryngol Suppl 2009;201:1–13

13. Cho KJ, Nam IC, Hwang YS, et al Analysis of factors influencing voice quality and therapeutic approaches in vocal polyp patients. Eur Arch Otorhinolaryngol 2011;268(9):1321–1327

14. Cho SH, Kim HT, Lee IJ, Kim MS, Park HJ. Influence of phonation on basement membrane zone recovery after phonomicrosurgery: a canine model. Ann Otol Rhinol Laryngol 2000;109(7):658–666

15. Thibeault SL, Gray SD, Bless DM, Chan RW, Ford CN. Histologic and rheologic characterization of vocal fold scarring. J Voice 2002;16(1):96–104

16. Behrman A, Sulica L. Voice rest after microlaryngoscopy: current opinion and practice. Laryngoscope 2003;113(12):2182–2186

14 Injection Medialization Procedures for the Vocal Fold

Paul Stimpson and Abir K. Bhattacharyya

Injection medialization aims to establish vocal fold approximation to achieve airway protection and to improve the voice quality in patients suffering from inadequate glottic closure.

In small defects (typically <1 mm), the opposite vocal fold may adequately compensate following speech therapy, and surgical intervention can be avoided. For larger defects or for those patients refractory to speech therapy, vocal fold injection or formal laryngeal framework surgery may be considered.

Aims

The ultimate goal of treatment is to bring the edge of the nonfunctioning vocal fold closer to the midline to facilitate glottal closure during phonation and swallowing by allowing the functioning vocal fold to approximate to the nonfunctioning side more easily.

Laryngeal framework surgery has been discussed elsewhere. In this section, the alternative use of injection laryngoplasty to achieve vocal fold medialization will be discussed.

Indications

Conditions for which vocal fold injection procedures may be considered include

- Vocal fold paralysis and paresis
- Vocal fold atrophy
- To augment laryngeal framework surgery
- Presbylarynx

Background

The first report of the procedure was published by Brunings in 1911. He described using paraffin via a direct laryngoscopic approach under local anesthetic.[1] Over the last century, the procedure has evolved and now provides a safe, effective, and reliable method for providing voice improvement in certain patients with defective glottic closure.

Injection techniques offer anterior glottic approximation for small-to-medium-sized defects (up to 3 mm) and have the potential advantage of straightening small irregularities in the free edge of the vocal fold depending on the material used. The procedure is generally quick and provides immediate results.

Potential disadvantages include airway compromise secondary to over-injection, migration, and foreign body reaction with granuloma formation. In this section, we will address the options for treatment and describe the various injectable materials that may be considered. For each option, the specific advantages and disadvantages will be discussed.

Patient Selection

As always, each patient presents a unique set of circumstances that must be considered when contemplating injection laryngoplasty. Patient selection will depend on numerous factors, including comorbidities, surgical access issues, and patient expectations. A thorough history and examination is paramount to establish an accurate diagnosis, and the injectable material used will differ depending on the underlying cause of glottic insufficiency. The tolerance to procedures under local anesthetic is also very important when considering local versus general anesthetic techniques.

Some patients may benefit from a "trial" injection with a short-term, absorbable material before considering more permanent treatments.

Techniques

Several techniques are available and must be tailored to suit the individual patient requirements and the experience of the surgeon.

In general, operative methods may be subdivided into endoscopic and percutaneous techniques. The choice of injectable material used will depend on the desire for a temporary or permanent treatment, diagnosis, availability of materials, experience, and cost.

Where possible, injections should be performed under *local anesthetic* as this allows immediate auditory feedback and may avoid airway compromise from over-injection. However, endoscopic treatment under general anesthetic will be required for patients who are unable to tolerate the procedure while awake.

The site of injection is dependent on the clinical indication. Superficial injection of a substance into the lamina propria may be indicated for vocal fold scarring and lamina propria defects, with the aim of correcting vibratory defects. More commonly, the injection will be directed deeper and more laterally into the thyroarytenoid/lateral cricoarytenoid complex to achieve vocal fold augmentation. This method results in medialization of the affected fold in

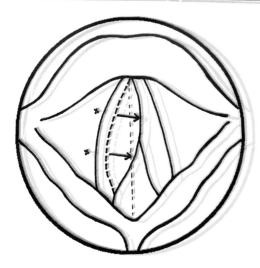

Figure 14.1   A schematic diagram demonstrating the site of injection (thyroarytenoid/lateral cricoarytenoid complex) to medialize anterior vocal fold.

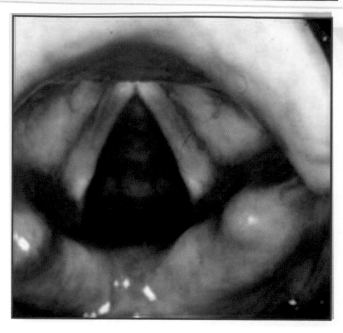

Figure 14.2   Photograph demonstrating the site of injection to achieve right vocal fold medialization.

a similar way to type 1 thyroplasty (**Figs. 14.1 and 14.2**). Lateral injection may be used to correct mild-to-moderate glottal insufficiency (1 to 3 mm glottal gaps).[2]

Approaches

Endoscopic Injection

Direct Laryngoscopy

Most commonly, endoscopic procedures are performed under *general anesthetic* via formal suspension laryngoscopy with a small tube or jet ventilation. This allows a controlled setting with a full array of microsurgical instruments and high-definition endoscopic visualization of static vocal folds (**Fig. 14.3**). It is also possible to perform a direct laryngoscopy in an awake, *sedated* patient with a small laryngoscope using telescopic visualization without the need for formal general anesthetic.

The volume of injection may be difficult to judge due to lack of patient feedback via phonation under general anesthesia.[3] Over-injection may lead to airway compromise and this may only become apparent when the patient is extubated. Underinjection risks an inadequate result and the need for a repeat procedure. In addition to the usual anesthetic risks, access may prove difficult using this technique due to anatomical factors and cervical spine problems.

A common error when performing this technique is unintentional superficial injection into the superficial lamina propria of the vocal fold. This results in scarring and

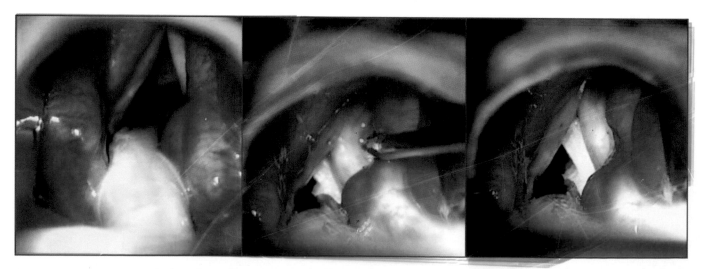

Figure 14.3   Intraoperative photographs to demonstrate successful endoscopic medialization.

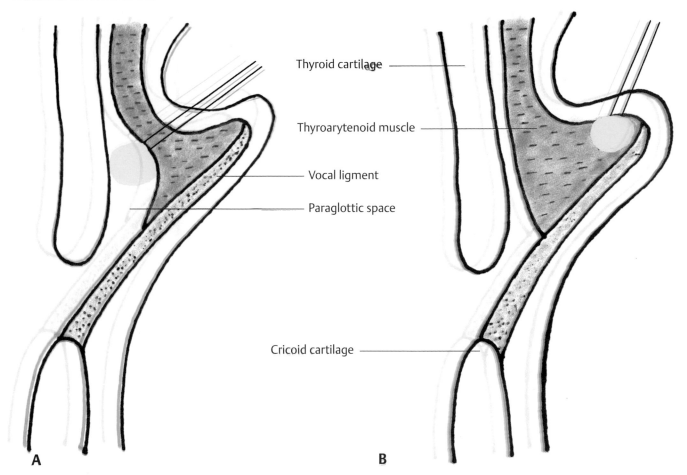

Thyroid cartilage

Thyroarytenoid muscle

Vocal ligment

Paraglottic space

Cricoid cartilage

A

B

Figure 14.4 Site of injection for direct laryngoscopy. (A) Correct position (deep) into paraglottic space used for medialization. (B) Superficial injection may be used to map scarring and deliver therapeutic drugs, this is unsuitable for medialization as it distorts the mucosal wave.

may adversely affect the mucosal wave with consequent compromise of vocal outcomes (**Fig. 14.4**).

> ### Clinical Pearls and Tips
>
> Ensure that the injection needle is fully loaded with the implant material till the needle tip to prevent any false medialization with air.
>
> Stabilization of the vocal folds with neurosurgical patties placing the patties under the affected fold is helpful in preventing the "hammock effect." The implant material is optimally distributed to achieve medialization in the stabilized position. The patties also prevent any accidental spill and inhalation of the implant material in the airways.

Vocal fold injections can be performed as "office procedures". Please refer to Section C, Chapter 4 for a detailed description of the techniques.

Per-Oral Injection

In an *awake patient*, under topical local anesthesia, per-oral injection may be performed with a curved needle under flexible

endoscopic guidance. The patient adopts a "sniffing the morning air" position (neck flexed, head slightly extended) and protrudes their tongue. The needle (typically 220 to 250 mm length) is inserted via the mouth and passed into the vocal fold following retraction of the false vocal fold with the needle shaft.[2]

Flexible Endoscopic Injection

Flexible endoscopic injections may be performed under *local anesthesia* and recently, some surgeons have described using flexible endoscopes (e.g., via transnasal esophagoscopy setup) through the mouth or nose with a side port from which injection may be performed following appropriate topical anesthetic. This method is technically demanding in an awake patient and requires specialist experience and advanced equipment. Large amounts of the injectable material may be required to account for the dead space in the long injection catheters, further increasing potential costs.

Percutaneous Injection

This technique uses a transcutaneous injection under direct visualization with a flexible nasoendoscope in an *awake* patient. The use of modern chip-tip endoscopes provides excellent image resolution to allow accurate placement of the injection. With experience, outcomes of percutaneous techniques match those of direct laryngoscopic approaches.[4,5]

There are several advantages in using this technique, in particular, the opportunity for direct auditory feedback from the patient during the injection. This technique may also be preferred for patients too frail or elderly to tolerate general anesthesia. Patient selection is crucial, and a calm, cooperative patient without a strong gag reflex is required. A concern with percutaneous approaches is a lack of accuracy in needle placement when compared with direct laryngoscopic methods.

The injection needle may be inserted *trans-cricothyroid*, *trans-thyrohyoid membrane*, or *trans-thyroid cartilage*.[2,6–8] For each approach, the injection effect can be directly monitored by the operating surgeon both visually via a transnasal endoscope and also by monitoring auditory changes during phonation. This also lessens the risk of over-injection as airway compromise can be immediately detected (**Fig. 14.5**).

Trans-Cricothyroid

A needle is inserted below the inferior border of the thyroid cartilage, from 3 to 7 mm lateral to the midline and the directed superolaterally in the submucosal tissues. Alternatively, the needle may be inserted in the midline below the vocal folds and aimed superolaterally across the tracheal lumen to penetrate the deep vocal fold (**Fig. 14.6**).

Trans-Thyroid

The injection needle is inserted at right angles to the thyroid ala 3 to 5 mm above the inferior border. Gentle pressure medially is assessed endoscopically to confirm needle position before injection. This approach may be difficult with heavily calcified cartilages in older patients.

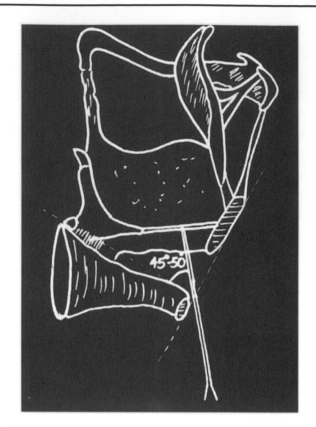

Figure 14.6 Injection technique via transcricothyroid approach.

Trans-Thyrohyoid

The needle is inserted immediately above the thyroid notch to penetrate the thyrohyoid membrane and then aimed inferiorly to enter the vocal fold on its superior surface. The injection proceeds under endoscopic guidance.

Materials

A wide variety of injectable materials have been described (see **Table 14.1**). The choice will depend on surgical aims, experience, availability, and cost.

Ideal Injection Material

The ideal injectable material would have the following properties:

- Lack of antigenic response
- Resist migration and resorption
- Have similar viscoelastic and biomechanical properties as the vocal fold itself
- Require minimal preparation
- Be easy to inject with precise control of location and volume of injection via easy delivery system
- Have low cost

Currently available materials can be broadly grouped into those providing temporary or more permanent effects.[2]

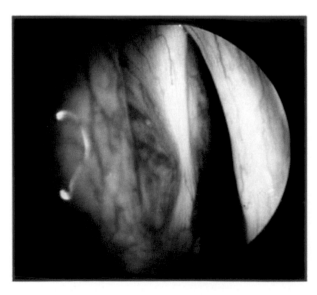

Figure 14.5 Over-injection of left vocal fold causing medial bowing.

Table 14.1 Injectable Materials

Material	Ease of Use	Duration	Comments
Gelfoam	++	1–2 mo	Large bore needle
Collagen—bovine	+++	4–6 mo	Requires pretesting
Collagen—human	++	4–6 mo	Short shelf life, cross-infection risk
Collagen—human autologous	+	Variable	Perfect biocompatibility, requires skin harvest, expensive
Fat	+	6+ mo	GA, donor site, superficial or deep use
Radiesse voice gel	+++	2–3 mo	Inert, low allergy risk, supplied ready to use
Hyaluronic acid	+++	6–12 mo	Good rheology, superficial or deep use
Glycerine	++	2–6 wk	Safe, short-term use only
Calcium hydroxylapatite	+++	Up to 2 y	Bony defects, nonvibratory, over-injection required
Silicone—polydimethylsiloxane	+++	Permanent	Long-term studies awaited, extrusion
Teflon	+++	Permanent	Granuloma, extrusion, rarely used

mo, months; wk, weeks; y, years.

Temporary Agents

Temporary agents may be used as short-term treatment where recovery of function is expected, for example following neuropraxia of the recurrent laryngeal nerve with resultant vocal fold palsy with favorable results on EMG studies. In addition, these agents may provide a useful treatment trial before considering a more permanent surgical solution.

Fat—6 Months or More (Variable)
Autologous fat is popular and has multiple advantages, including no antigenicity, availability and lack of foreign body reaction. It is easy to prepare and inject but requires a separate incision at the donor site. Fat has similar viscoelastic properties to the vocal fold but may be rapidly absorbed, requiring multiple repeat injections.[9] Fat may be used for deep augmentation or superficially for vocal scar and atrophy.[10,11]

Hyaluronic Acid—Up To 6 Months
Hyaluronic acid (e.g., Restylane [Q-Med, Watford, United Kingdom], and Rofilan [Rofil Aesthetics, Cyprus]) is a natural polysaccharide residing in the extracellular space of all mammalian connective tissue. It creates viscoelasticity, hydration, lubrication, and matrix stabilization.[12] This material has similar physical properties to the superficial layer of lamina propria and gives excellent biocompatibility. For this reason, hyaluronic acids offer potential for superficial injections for vocal fold scars and sulcus. However, clinical results have been disappointing, and injection may worsen vibratory function in some cases.

Over time, it is entirely resorbed, and no foreign body reactions have been described in long-term follow-up studies.[13] Hyaluronic acid is embedded in biogels to improve durability and effects may last for up to 6 months.[14]

Bovine-Based Gelatin Products—4 to 8 Weeks
Bovine gelatin agents such as Gelfoam and Surgifoam have the advantage of proven safety, efficacy, and predictability. Despite recent popularity, Gelfoam does have disadvantages such as a large (18-gauge) needle requirement and a short duration of effect.

Collagen—4 to 6 Months
Autologous human collagen preparations offer perfect biocompatibility but take many weeks to prepare and are very expensive. Bovine collagen offers a useful alternative and following cross-linking with glutaraldehyde is less immunogenic. A disadvantage is that skin testing should be performed ~4 to 6 weeks before laryngeal injection. An alternative is human cadaveric micronized acellular dermis (Cymetra; Lifecell, Bridgewater, United States) which is freeze-dried into a powder and then reconstituted when required. Although well-tolerated and effective, there are potential cross infection risks. Collagen preparations are typically effective for 3 to 6 months.

Carboxymethylcellulose—2 to 3 Months
Carboxymethylcellulose (Radiesse Voice Gel; Merz Aesthetics, Germany) is inert with a very low allergy risk. It has the advantage of being supplied in a ready to use injectable form and is commonly used for temporary defects.

Glycerine—2 to 6 Weeks
Glycerine offers a short-term, safe, and completely reversible option. It is well suited for management of temporary vocal fold palsy in conjunction with laryngeal EMG studies suggesting imminent recovery of function.

Permanent/Longer Term Agents

Calcium Hydroxylapatite—up to 2 Years
Calcium hydroxylapatite (Radiesse Voice; Merz Aesthetics, Germany) consists of hydroxylapatite spheres suspended in a gel carrier consisting of glycerine and water. Following injection, the glycerine component is absorbed, and is in part replaced by soft tissue in-growth that may be variable in its

extent. Hydroxylapatite has been used for many years in other specialties such as orthopedics and dentistry with a good safety record. Results may last up to 2 years or longer but re-absorption may be difficult to predict and varies between individuals.[14]

Bioplastique (Vox)—Permanent

Bioplastique is a polydimethylsiloxane elastomer (particulate silicone) and is considered an "injectable implant."[14] It has high particle size and therefore resists phagocytosis and it not absorbed. Due to its high density, it requires a large needle for injection (20 G) and a pressure gun device and is therefore not suitable for percutaneous use. Bioplastique should be injected far laterally into the paraglottic space to avoid irregularity over the free edge of the vocal fold. Cases of extrusion and foreign body reactions have been reported and may require implant removal in some instances.

Teflon—Rarely Used

Although popular during the latter part of the 20th century, Teflon (a tetrafluoroethylene derivative) has fallen out of favor due to the unpredictability of its effect and high incidence of migration of the implant and local granuloma formation. It may rarely be used for terminally ill patients to give vocal improvement and airway protection where life expectancy is short (**Table 14.1**).[15]

Use of Injection "Trials"

A trial injection may be indicated for patients in whom the clinical outcome is unpredictable or the benefits are unclear. Trial injections are useful to give an indication of potential outcome following more permanent interventions. This aids both the surgeon and patient to plan future therapy and manage outcomes.

Treatment of Patients with Limited Life Expectancy

The treatments described in this section may be of great use in the management of terminally ill patients suffering with glottic incompetence. Given the safety and relative ease of the procedures described, all options should be considered. In very unwell patients, an injection of a temporary agent may offer enough improvement in laryngeal function to offer a dramatic improvement in quality of life by improving voice, cough, and swallowing ability. As described, the procedures may be safely repeated as required as part of palliative care management.

Summary

Injection medialization offers good results for patients with small phonatory gaps (< 3 mm). It may be used as a trial to assess the potential outcome from more permanent procedures. Ideally, injections should be performed under local anesthesia to allow direct acoustic feedback and to prevent complications related to over-injection. The perfect injectable material does not exist, and therefore several substances are available with different characteristics and length of treatment effect. Materials may be broadly grouped into temporary and permanent. The choice of material and injection technique will depend on multiple factors, including patient comorbidities, required length of treatment, experience of surgeon, availability, and cost. Patient expectations must be appropriately managed from the outset to establish realistic treatment goals.

Acknowledgment

The authors are grateful to Mr P. Sen for the line drawings used in this chapter and acknowledge his contribution.

References

1. Brünings W. Uber eine neue bahandlungs methode der Rekurhenslahmung. Verhandlungen des Vereins Deutscher Laryngologen 1911;8:93–151
2. Mallur PS, Rosen CA. Vocal fold injection: review of indications, techniques, and materials for augmentation. Clin Exp Otorhinolaryngol 2010;3(4):177–182
3. Hartl DM, Hans S, Crevier-Buchman L, Vaissière J, Brasnu DF. Long-term acoustic comparison of thyroplasty versus autologous fat injection. Ann Otol Rhinol Laryngol 2009;118(12):827–832
4. Bové MJ, Jabbour N, Krishna P, et al. Operating room versus office-based injection laryngoplasty: a comparative analysis of reimbursement. Laryngoscope 2007;117(2):226–230
5. Mathison CC, Villari CR, Klein AM, Johns MM III. Comparison of outcomes and complications between awake and asleep injection laryngoplasty: a case–control study. Laryngoscope 2009;119(7):1417–1423
6. Jin SM, Park CY, Lee JK, Ban JH, Lee SH, Lee KC. Transcutaneous injection laryngoplasty through the cricothyroid space in the sitting position: anatomical information and technique. Eur Arch Otorhinolaryngol 2008;265(3):313–319
7. Zeitler DM, Amin MR. The thyrohyoid approach to in-office injection augmentation of the vocal fold. Curr Opin Otolaryngol Head Neck Surg 2007;15(6):412–416
8. Amin MR. Thyrohyoid approach for vocal fold augmentation. Ann Otol Rhinol Laryngol 2006;115(9):699–702
9. Shaw GY, Szewczyk MA, Searle J, Woodroof J. Autologous fat injection into the vocal folds: technical considerations and long-term follow-up. Laryngoscope 1997;107(2):177–186
10. Laccourreye O, Papon JF, Kania R, Crevier-Buchman L, Brasnu D, Hans S. Intracordal injection of autologous fat in patients with unilateral laryngeal nerve paralysis: long-term results from the patient's perspective. Laryngoscope 2003;113(3):541–545
11. Hsiung MW, Woo P, Minasian A, Schaefer Mojica J. Fat augmentation for glottic insufficiency. Laryngoscope 2000;110(6):1026–1033
12. Lee SW, Oh JW, Lee HJ, et al. Cross-linked hyaluronic acid gel injection for patients with unilateral vocal cord paralysis. Korean J Otolaryngol–Head Neck Surg 2005;48(10):1248–1253
13. Borzacchiello A, Mayol L, Gärskog O, Dahlqvist A, Ambrosio L. Evaluation of injection augmentation treatment of hyaluronic acid based materials on rabbit vocal folds viscoelasticity. J Mater Sci Mater Med 2005;16(6):553–557
14. Sittel C. Larynx: implants and stents. GMS Curr Top Otorhinolaryngol Head Neck Surg 2009;8:Doc04
15. Costello D. Current surgical management of unilateral vocal fold paralysis. J ENT Masterclass 2009;2(1):26–29

15 Laryngeal Framework Surgery

Meredydd Harries and Nicholas Gibbins

History

Payr,[1] a German surgeon, is credited with the first description of a laryngoplasty via a transthyroidal approach, but it was Isshiki in 1974,[2] who first classified the main techniques that alter the skeleton of the larynx (and therefore the vibrational properties of the vocal folds) rather than operating directly on the vocal folds themselves. His research and elegant classification prompted others to adopt this approach, and several surgeons, including Koufman,[3] published case series of patients who had undergone successful vocal fold implantation. Until this time, intracordal injection was the cornerstone of surgical therapy for symptomatic vocal fold paralysis (VFP), but laryngoplasty has many advantages over this as shown in **Table 15.1**.

Definition

In 2001, the Phonosurgery Committee of the European Laryngological Society (ELS)[4] proposed the collective term "laryngeal framework surgery" as synonymous with laryngoplasty or glottoplasty. For ease of use and syntax, the term laryngoplasty will be used throughout in this chapter. These procedures are performed open, as opposed to the majority of operations performed on the vocal folds that are performed either perorally or transcutaneously. They involve an external approach to the laryngeal skeleton and a change in its shape or position. This causes vocal fold repositioning and subsequent vocal alteration. They are used to change the quality of the voice rather than for removal of disease.

Table 15.2 shows the classification of laryngoplasty, but it is mainly the approximation type that is performed and that will be described in detail in this chapter. Expansion and relaxation laryngoplasty are rarely performed, many centers preferring the use of repeated Botulinum injections, and tension laryngoplasty has a role not only for the transsexual voice, but also for patients with superior laryngeal nerve paralysis.[5]

Approximation Laryngoplasty

Indications

The primary aim of this procedure is to approximate the vocal folds, so that glottic closure is achieved and voice restored. In addition, this will ensure competence of the larynx and allow protection of the lower respiratory tree.

A unilateral VFP, with the fold in the lateralized position, results in a breathy, quiet voice due to the inability of the vocal folds to meet. As well as VFP, vocal fold immobility caused by scars, atrophy, and Grade III sulcus can also be treated with approximation.[6] As well as symptoms of the voice, glottal insufficiency may lead to aspiration and dysphagia that can also be an indication for approximation of a paralyzed vocal fold.[7] In these cases, it is usually a high vagal lesion affecting both superior and recurrent laryngeal nerves and having both sensory and motor laryngeal deficits.

Most patients with unilateral VFP have a synkinetic cord where there has been some reinnervation but this has been nonselective, resulting in uncoordinated movement but they do have muscle tone.[8] Reinnervation procedures now focus

Table 15.1 Comparison of Closed (Injection) versus Open (Laryngoplasty) Medialization Thyroplasty

Technique	Injection	Laryngoplasty
Anesthetic	Local and/or general	Local and/or general
Glottic closure	Small to medium—can straighten small irregularities in medial edge	Small, medium, and large—not good for small irregularities in medial edge
Mucosal wave	Can be reduced if there is migration or placement too superficial	Lies lateral to muscle and does not reduce mucosal wave
Time for procedure	Around 30 min	Around 60 min
Alters tension	No	Yes
Alters position	Yes	Yes
Alters vibrational mass	Yes	No
Morbidity	Minimum with endoscopic or transcutaneous approach	Open wound
Level of skill required	Moderate	Moderate to high

Table 15.2 European Laryngological Society Classification of Laryngoplasty

Approximation laryngoplasty		
Medialization thyroplasty	Thyroplasty I	Isshiki et al[2,21]
Arytenoid adduction	Rotation techniques	Isshiki et al[16]
	LCA pull technique	Iwamura[22]
	Fixation techniques	Morrison[23]
		Maragos[24]
	Adduction arytenopexy	Zeitels et al[17]
Expansion laryngoplasty		
Lateralization thyroplasty	Lateral approach	
	Thyroplasty IIa	Isshiki et al[2,25]
	Medial approach	
	Thyroplasty IIb	Isshiki et al[2,25,26]
Vocal fold abduction	Suture technique	Isshiki[25]
	Resection technique	Woo and Genack[27]
Relaxation laryngoplasty		
Shortening thyroplasty	Lateral approach	
	Thyroplasty III	Isshiki[25]
	Medial approach	
	Anterior commissure retrusion	Tucker[28–30]
Tensioning laryngoplasty		
Cricothyroid approximation	Thyroplasty IVa	Isshiki et al[2]
	Cricothyroid subluxation	Zeitels et al[31]
Elongation thyroplasty	Lateral approach	
	Thyroplasty IVb	Isshiki et al[17,32,33]
	Medial approach	
	Springboard advancement	LeJeune et al[34]
	Anterior commissure advancement	Tucker[35]

LCA, lateral cricoarytenoid muscle.

on selective neural anastomosis, identifying the adductor and abductor branches separately with theoretically better functional outcomes.[9,10]

Less than 10% of cases have complete denervation and atrophic muscles, but these are important to identify preoperatively as there is an increased risk of perforating the laryngeal mucosa when forming the pocket for the implant.

Patient Selection

The investigations of a patient with a unilateral immobile vocal cord will not be discussed in this chapter, but thorough assessment and investigations are important and must be performed for every case preoperatively.[11]

Symptomatic glottic insufficiency can be due to numerous causes, but approximation laryngoplasty (medialization thyroplasty) is our operation of choice for:

- Unilateral vocal cord immobility with a small-to-medium glottic gap.
- Severe presbylaryngeal changes with bilateral bowing and a glottic gap greater than 2 mm.

Perhaps, more importantly, it is useful to know who is NOT a good candidate and why?

- Patients who have had laser resection of the vocal cords and are left with mainly scar tissue lying on the inner surface of the cartilage. Although medialization of this tissue is possible, the implant needed is usually large, and pitfalls include implant extrusion through the thin tissue into the airway and poor vibration of the medialized tissue. Inserting a local muscle flap to lie between the implant and the scar tissue can be done but this can shrink with time, and long-term results are variable.

- Very small glottic gaps due to scarring/sulcus have an irregular edge, and laryngoplasty will not give a smooth vibrating straight edge to the vocal fold. This is better achieved in our practice with either a local injection or tunneling and insertion of a strip of fascia or alloplastic material.
- Large glottic gaps, especially posteriorly, will need the addition of an arytenoid adduction procedure and are unlikely to get good closure with laryngoplasty alone.
- Patients with neuromuscular diseases such as multiple sclerosis do not do well as although glottic closure can be achieved, there is a lack of power to achieve this regularly as well as the secondary effect of poor respiratory function.
- Patients with widespread malignancy and a short life expectancy can be treated quickly and efficiently with a transcutaneous injection under local anesthesia in the clinic. Although the long-term results in our hands are not as good as with laryngoplasty, the priority here is a competent larynx for voice and swallowing, and this can be achieved immediately in clinic rather than waiting for theater time, etc.

Technique

All laryngeal framework surgical procedures must be performed in theater under aseptic conditions and ideally local anesthesia with sedation.

Anesthesia

Always try to do this under local anesthesia. The main advantages are auditory feedback from the patient to fine-tune the size and placement of the implant and to prevent over medialization and airway compromise. Reported cases of airway compromise are usually performed under general anesthesia, and the problem is only identified in recovery as the patient awakes. It is essential to work with the same anesthetist regularly and to develop a team approach. Levels of consciousness need to be fairly low during the exposure phase of the procedure, but then higher when the patient is asked to speak.

A variety of agents have been used to sedate patients, including benzodiazepine/opioid combinations, with flumazenil administered when patient cooperation is required. However, with the availability of the short-acting opioid remifentanil, this has become the preferred agent, often in combination with a target-controlled infusion of propofol. Bispectral Index (Bis) monitoring can be used to aid the anesthetist in ensuring the patient remains comfortable and relatively motionless without suppressing respiratory drive, and avoid dramatic fluctuations in conscious level during the procedure. In certain instances, the patient may not be able to tolerate local and general anesthesia may be required. An endotracheal tube can alter the endolaryngeal

anatomy, so it is suggested that a laryngeal mask airway is used. This will also allow a fiberscope to be passed through it to visualize the glottis intraoperatively, but there will not be any auditory feedback hence the superiority of using local anesthesia.

Positioning

Use a headlight and magnifying loupes. Initially, stand on the opposite side of the table to the side of surgery. It is easier to get under the strap muscles and onto the thyroid cartilage from the opposite side. Current trials are looking at the role of preserving the strap muscles, including the cricothyroid muscle on postoperative voice results but it often comes down to access and the deeper lying, less acutely angled thyroid cartilages may need more extensive dissection for adequate exposure. When the cartilage has been exposed, it can be easier to be on the same side of the table especially if using a drill. Leave the patient's head completely exposed—this allows access for the anesthetist and for insertion of the flexible nasoendoscope later.

Placement of the Window

The technique is well described[12] but essentially involves removing a cartilaginous window from the thyroid alar on the affected side overlying the vocal fold (**Fig 15.1**). In contrast to absolute measurements, the relative proportions are more constant,[13,14] and one should start by identifying the superior and inferior thyroid cartilage notches and the midpoint in the midline. This is the point of insertion of Broyles tendon and is at the horizontal level of the vocal folds. From this point, the vocal fold, within the endolarynx, runs posteriorly and inferiorly at an angle of approximately 15 degree. Due to the variability of laryngeal rotation and anterior projection, it is easier to think of the vocal fold running parallel to the inferior border of the thyroid cartilage.[14]

With this in mind, the rectangular window excised from the thyroid cartilage must run also run parallel to the inferior border of the thyroid cartilage so as to have the body of the implant running in the same axis as the vocal fold. There

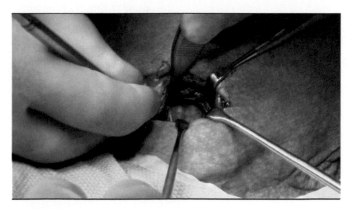

Figure 15.1 Exposing left thyroid lamina.

is debate as to where the most anteriorly based vertical incision should be made; Isshiki suggested 5 to 7 mm from the midline, however, Friedrich has postulated that it should be made in the area of the oblique line.[13] The authors prefer to make their anterior incision approximately 7 mm (female) or 9 mm (male) from the midline but this does vary with the size of the thyroid cartilage. We remove a 12 × 5 mm window for men (10 × 4 mm for women) but one size does not fit all, and the size of the window needs to be tailored to the patient's dimensions.

The most common problem found at revision procedures is a high window with the implant medializing the false cord or entering the ventricle. We now always use a flexible scope during the procedure for two main reasons. First, it allows us to see that the window has been made at the level of the vocal cords and, if not, then this can be rectified at the time with a larger or differently shaped window. Second, it gives visual feedback before cutting the shape of the bespoke Silastic (TM Dow Corning Corporation, Midland, Michigan, United States) implant, which can be adjusted accordingly. The thyroid cartilage will have variability in its anterior angle. This means that the dimensions, and more specifically the width, of the implant will need to be judged intraoperatively. An acute anterior thyroid cartilage angle will need a thinner implant, the converse being true for a more obtuse angle. This is another reason why the authors prefer a bespoke Silastic implant that can be cut to shape at the time of surgery.

Inner Perichondrium

We always try to create an anteriorly based flap and elevate using an otological elevator (aka spud, first incision knife, round black knife; **Figs. 15.2** and **15.3**). Inserting a cotton wool pledget soaked in local anesthetic mixed with adrenaline helps free the pocket and reduce local bleeding. Troublesome bleeding from the cartilage can be stopped with bipolar diathermy. Bone wax placed in the marrow space has also been useful. The perichondrium may tear, especially when using a drill to remove the cartilage window, but preserving the perichondrium helps keep the implant lateral to the thyroarytenoid muscle and produce a better mucosal

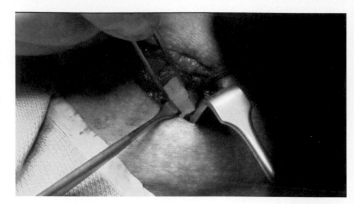

Figure 15.3 Inserting prosthesis.

wave. This is also very important if the muscle is atrophic where it is easier to perforate the mucosa. What to do if this happens? Previously, we would abandon the procedure and return in 4 weeks after the tear had healed. We now suture the Silastic implant to the thyroid cartilage so that it will not fall medially. In the past, we have also inserted a thin Silastic sheet or muscle flap to lie between the implant and the tear and, if the tear is large, then we would still attempt this to give a soft tissue vibrating edge. Antibiotic cover would be advised here but is not used in routine cases. Steroids are also not used routinely, neither is a drain in the wound, and 96% of cases are done as day case procedures going home within 4 hours of the surgery.[15]

Materials

Many implant materials for medialization can be found in the literature. Alloplastic (silicone, Gore-Tex, titanium, and hydroxyapatite) and autogenic materials (cartilage and fascia) are widely used. None appears to confer an advantage over another, so before choosing one implant material over another, one must examine the safety of each and any possible negative effects. This is very much an individual choice with the range from Gore-Tex ribbon and Silastic that can be modified at the time of the operation (**Fig 15.4**; insertion of Silastic prosthesis) to preformed implants in different materials, including Silastic or titanium that are sized to the degree of medialization needed. Other factors that may influence choice include cost and personal experience and training.

Postoperative Advice

It is important to warn the patient that the voice may deteriorate in 12 to 24 hours due to local edema and not to be worried if this happens. After 5 days, this should settle, and the voice returns to its quality immediately after surgery. The voice will continue to improve up to 9 months after surgery as the patient gets used to the new position of the vocal cord, and we have only needed to use postoperative speech therapy in under 10% of cases.

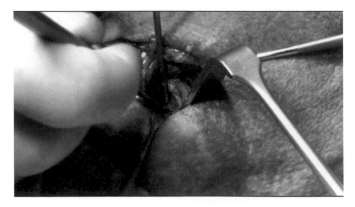

Figure 15.2 Elevating perichondrium.

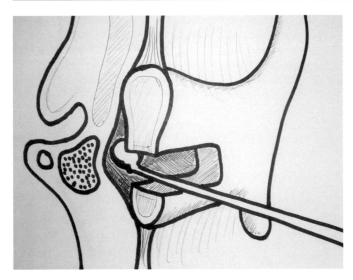

Figure 15.4 Diagrammatic representation of inner perichondrial elevation through a thyroid cartilage window.

Arytenoid Adduction

Isshiki described this procedure for patients in which there is a large posterior glottic gap, and the paralyzed vocal fold is at a different level to the functioning one.[16] Good results have been reported in both short- and long-term outcomes, but the technique does require considerable surgical skill especially when performed under local anesthesia.

Zeitels et al described a modification of this technique with arytenoid adduction and cricothyroid subluxation.[17] With an extended incision, the arytenoid cartilage is exposed, its attached muscles divided, and the arytenoid cartilage is fixed in a midline position. Tension of the paralyzed cord is obtained by a suture between the inferior horn of the thyroid cartilage and the anterior part of the cricoid cartilage. This is usually combined with a medialization thyroplasty and allows correct positioning of the arytenoid cartilage and gives bulk to the affected vocal cord. Again, this requires a high level of skill but to the authors seems to give a better result than Isshiki's original procedure.

Complications

These are rare and are mainly limited to bleeding, infection, implant extrusion, and undermedialization. Bleeding is usually in patients who are on anticoagulants or have had previous surgery that should be identified preoperatively with consideration of a drain and possible overnight stay. Infection is rare as is extrusion especially if atrophic or scarring has been identified preoperatively.

Undermedialization is apparent in the first few weeks and is due to inserting too small an implant that is usually avoidable with a combination of flexible scope and local anesthetic technique to give both visual and auditory feedback. If apparent after more than a year, it can be due to muscle atrophy or shrinkage of the implant if cartilage used.

In both cases, revision is usually required, but again this is a rare occurrence.

Outcomes

It is important to be able to document how interventions benefit the patient and are cost-effective. The easiest way to demonstrate this for laryngoplasty is with a subjective voice questionnaire pre and postsurgery. Our preference is to use the VHI 10, as it is quick to fill in and effective in demonstrating change but there are others that can be more extensive, and we would suggest that the voice team trial these and come to their own choice of preference.

There is a role for more extensive measurements, including maximum phonation time, S/Z ratio, other acoustic and quantitative parameters, but these can be harder to interpret and ideally have a voice-recording laboratory with relatively expensive equipment beyond most departments' budgets.

Perceptual voice analysis—GRBAS is the main tool in the UK and is used by the speech therapists in our voice clinic—can also give useful information but for research or audit purposes, there should be blinding of the observers, which is not always practical.

Approximation laryngoplasty is generally a very successful procedure, and there are good published results supporting its use in clinical practice today.[18-20]

This chapter gives an overview of laryngeal framework surgery, specifically approximation laryngoplasty, and although mainly reflecting our personal experiences and ideas, we hope it will help others in their selection of patients and our tips on surgical technique are useful.

References

1. Payr E. Plastikamschildknorpelzur Behebung der Folgeneinseitiger Stimmbandlahmung. Dtsch Med Wochenschr 1915;43:1265–1270
2. Isshiki N, Morita H, Okamura H, Hiramoto M. Thyroplasty as a new phonosurgical technique. Acta Otolaryngol 1974;78(5–6):451–457
3. Koufman JA. Laryngoplasty for vocal cord medialization: an alternative to Teflon. Laryngoscope 1986;96(7):726–731
4. Friedrich G, de Jong FI, Mahieu HF, Benninger MS, Isshiki N. Laryngeal framework surgery: a proposal for classification and nomenclature by the Phonosurgery Committee of the European Laryngological Society. Eur Arch Otorhinolaryngol 2001;258(8):389–396
5. Gibbins N, Bray D, Harries ML. Long-term quantitative results of an Isshiki type 4 thyroplasty—a case study. J Voice 2011;25(3): 283–287
6. Su CY, Tsai SS, Chiu JF, Cheng CA. Medialization laryngoplasty with strap muscle transposition for vocal fold atrophy with or without sulcus vocalis. Laryngoscope 2004;114(6):1106–1112
7. Carrau RL, Pou A, Eibling DE, Murry T, Ferguson BJ. Laryngeal framework surgery for the management of aspiration. Head Neck 1999;21(2):139–145
8. Crumley RL. Laryngeal synkinesis: its significance to the laryngologist. Ann Otol Rhinol Laryngol 1989;98(2):87–92
9. Kwak PE, Friedman AD, Lamarre ED, Lorenz RR. Selective reinnervation of the posterior cricoarytenoid and interarytenoid muscles: an anatomical study. Laryngoscope 2010;120(3):463–467

10. Marie JP, Dehesdin D, Ducastelle T, Senant J. Selective reinnervation of the abductor and adductor muscles of the canine larynx after recurrent nerve paralysis. Ann Otol Rhinol Laryngol 1989;98(7, Pt 1): 530–536

11. Stimpson P, Patel R, Vaz F, et al. Imaging strategies for investigating unilateral vocal cord palsy: how we do it. Clin Otolaryngol 2011;36(3):266–271

12. Harries M, Morrison M. Phonosurgery and microlaryngeal surgery. In: Bleach N, Milford C, Van Hasselt A. eds. Operative Otorhinolaryngology. Oxford, UK: Blackwell Science; 1997:315–325, Chapter 45

13. Friedrich G. Laryngeal framework surgery. In: Remacle M, Heckel HE. eds. Surgery of Larynx and Trachea. Berlin, Germany: Springer; 2010, Chapter 5

14. Friedrich G, Lichtenegger R. Surgical anatomy of the larynx. J Voice 1997;11(3):345–355

15. Bray D, Young JP, Harries ML. Complications after type one thyroplasty: is day-case surgery feasible? J Laryngol Otol 2008;122(7):715–718

16. Isshiki N, Taira T, Tanabe M. Surgical alteration of the vocal pitch. J Otolaryngol 1983;12(5):335–340

17. Zeitels SM, Hochman I, Hillman RE. Adduction arytenopexy: a new procedure for paralytic dysphonia with implications for implant medialization. Ann Otol Rhinol Laryngol Suppl 1998;173: 2–24

18. Dursun G, Boynukalin S, Ozgursoy OB, Coruh I. Long-term results of different treatment modalities for glottic insufficiency. Am J Otolaryngol 2008;29(1):7–12

19. Vinson KN, Zraick RI, Ragland FJ. Injection versus medialization laryngoplasty for the treatment of unilateral vocal fold paralysis: follow-up at six months. Laryngoscope 2010;120(9):1802–1807

20. Hartl DM, Hans S, Crevier-Buchman L, Vaissière J, Brasnu DF. Long-term acoustic comparison of thyroplasty versus autologous fat injection. Ann Otol Rhinol Laryngol 2009;118(12):827–832

21. Isshiki N, Okamura H, Ishikawa T. Thyroplasty type I (lateral compression) for dysphonia due to vocal cord paralysis or atrophy. Acta Otolaryngol 1975;80(5–6):465–473

22. Iwamura S. A newer surgical treatment of one vocal fold paralysis—lateral cricoarytenoid muscle pull technique—methods and results.

Abstract: the Second International Symposium on Laryngeal and Tracheal Reconstruction, Monte Carlo. 1996;182:26

23. Morrison LF. The reverse King operation; a surgical procedure for restoration of phonation in cases of aphonia due to unilateral vocal cord paralysis. Ann Otol Rhinol Laryngol 1948;57(4):945–956

24. Maragos NE. Arytenoid fixation surgery for the treatment of arytenoid fractures and dislocations. Laryngoscope 1999;109(5): 834–837

25. Isshiki N. Phonosurgery—Theory and Practice. 1989. Tokyo: Springer.

26. Isshiki N. Progress in laryngeal framework surgery. Acta Otolaryngol 2000;120(2):120–127

27. Woo P, Genack S. Thyroarytenoid myectomy: a new surgical alternative for intractable spasmodic dysphonia. Trans Am Broncho-Esophagol Assoc 1995;95:187–192

28. Tucker HM. Laryngeal framework surgery in the management of spasmodic dysphonia. Preliminary report. Ann Otol Rhinol Laryngol 1989;98(1, Pt 1):52–54

29. Tucker HM. Combined laryngeal framework medialization and reinnervation for unilateral vocal fold paralysis. Ann Otol Rhinol Laryngol 1990;99(10, Pt 1):778–781

30. Tucker HM. Anterior commissure repositioning for adjustment of tension in the vocal cords. Oper Tech Otolaryngol Head Neck Surg 1993;4(3):232–235

31. Zeitels SM, Hillman RE, Desloge RB, Bunting GA. Cricothyroid subluxation: a new innovation for enhancing the voice with laryngoplastic phonosurgery. Ann Otol Rhinol Laryngol 1999; 108(12):1126–1131

32. Isshiki N, Taira T, Tanabe M. Surgical alteration of the vocal pitch. J Otolaryngol 1983;12(5):335–340

33. Isshiki N, Ohkawa M, Goto M. Stiffness of the vocal cord in dysphonia-its assessment and treatment. Acta Otolaryngol Suppl 1984;419:167–174

34. LeJeune FE, Guice CE, Samuels PM. Early experiences with vocal ligament tightening. Ann Otol Rhinol Laryngol 1983;92(5, Pt 1): 475–477

35. Tucker HM. Anterior commissure laryngoplasty for adjustment of vocal fold tension. Ann Otol Rhinol Laryngol 1985;94(6, Pt 1): 547–549

16 Lasers in Laryngology

Sachin Gandhi and Marc Remacle

LASER is an acronym for light amplification by the stimulated emission of radiation.

- Light: Light beam has four fundamental characteristics, namely intensity, coherence, high collimation, and monochromaticity. Depending on the hydration, temperature, color, and thickness of the human tissue, lights of different wavelength are absorbed.
- Amplification: The medium of laser has more stable than unstable atoms. During amplification this produces a tremendous source of energy. The electromagnetic emission released by stimulated emission is amplified by an external power source to produce an intense beam that will excite the atoms. The resultant excited state permits the emission of photons from the atoms. Thus, this creates a chain reaction in the laser.
- Stimulated emission of radiation: Radiation emitted from a laser consists of a spectrum of wavelengths ranging from 200 (ultraviolet) to 10,000 nm (infrared). The most common types of lasers used in surgery are listed below with their corresponding wavelengths:
  - 500 nm: Argon laser
  - 532 nm: Potassium-titanyl-phosphate (KTP) laser
  - 585 nm: Dye laser
  - 1060 nm: Neodymium yttrium-aluminum-garnet (Nd-YAG) laser
  - 10,600 nm: Carbon dioxide (CO_2) laser

Components of Surgical Laser

There are three components of surgical laser:

1. Active medium of laser
2. A power source to pump energy
3. Optical chamber

Laser and Interaction with Tissue

Four possible interactions may occur when a laser beam makes a contact with tissue. A single reaction or multiple reactions may occur upon contact with tissue.

1. Reflection: The laser beam is neither absorbed nor does it pass through the tissue.
2. Transmission: The laser beam is not absorbed and it passes directly through the tissue.
3. Absorption: The laser beam is fully absorbed by the tissue.
4. Scatter/dispersion: The laser beam is partially absorbed, transmitted, and scattered by the tissue.

Each type of laser has a specific mechanism by which it reacts with tissue in a specific way producing characteristic patterns of heat conduction, coagulation, ablation, and charring. Knowledge of laser physics and typical tissue interactions allows the surgeon to select the best laser for the respective pathology in the larynx. The CO_2 laser produces a cone-shaped impact that has three characteristic levels from the center of impact to the outer layer; these are areas of charring, a region of tissue desiccation, and an outer layer of edema.

Besides wavelength, laser tissue interaction depends on the mode of impact of the CO_2 laser. The CO_2 laser operates in either a continuous firing or pulsed mode.

- Continuous mode: Photons are emitted in a constant and stable manner, enabling the stable delivery of energy and intensity. A constant power source to keep the active medium in an excited state, which is essential to maintain stimulated emission.
- Repeat mode: An intermittent power source such as flash lamp is used to provide short bursts of energy to the active medium. A pulsed-mode laser delivers high energy in a very short time frame which produces deeper tissue cutting with less associated thermal damage.

Lasers Used in Otolaryngology

Lasers are named according to the lasing material within them that can be solid, gas, liquid, or semiconductors. Nd-YAG is a solid-state laser that has a yttrium-aluminum-garnet crystal acting as host for neodymium ions. Gas lasers use either a single gas or a combination of gases. The CO_2, argon, and krypton lasers are examples of gas-based lasers. Semiconductor lasers have two layers of a semiconducting medium. Though they are of a low power, they provide sufficient power for clinical use. The diode laser is an example of a semiconductor laser.

Carbon Dioxide Laser

The CO_2 laser was the first laser to be used in otolaryngology and remains the workhorse laser to this day.[1] It can be used for incision, excision, and vaporization of tissue. It was first used in laryngology by Strong and Jako.[2]

Its wavelength of 10.6 μm is best suited for absorption by water. This characteristic is of importance because absorption of this wavelength into soft tissue (90% water content) will concentrate the energy, permitting little heat to dissipate to adjacent tissues. The laser light is transformed within the tissue to thermal energy, raising the tissue temperature to 100°C and hence vaporizes the tissue's water content. This wavelength makes the CO_2 laser a precise cutting tool, ideal for excision of small lesions located on delicate structures, such as the vocal cords. It also gives depth of penetration with minimal damage to adjacent tissue.

The rapid thermal drop of laser energy in the tissue surrounding an incision results in shallow and predictable tissue penetration with minimal edema. It has good hemostatic capability, but this is limited to blood vessels not larger than capillaries (0.5 mm). Its beam can be focused to create a precise cut and also defocused to coagulate small blood vessels.

A traditional CO_2 laser has the disadvantage that it cannot be transmitted through flexible fibers but requires an articulated mirror system though the newer ones can deliver CO_2 laser by a flexible fiberoptic cable.

Neodymium:Yttrium-Aluminum-Garnet Laser

The Nd:YAG laser has a wavelength of 1.06 μm that is poorly absorbed by water, and, therefore, penetrates tissue deeply. The energy is not dissipated at the surface but scatters within the tissue dependent on the degree of tissue pigmentation.

The Nd:YAG laser can be transmitted through flexible fibers, thus it can be used in the tracheobronchial tree. The wavelength is well absorbed by pigmented and vascular tissue, which along with its deep penetration into most tissues gives it good coagulation properties. Care must be taken while using the Nd:YAG laser to apply it to tissues in brief exposures of 1 second or less at a power setting below 50 W. Continuous application of this laser at high power settings may result in explosion of the tissue caused by the concentration of high energy below the tissue surface causing an expanding cavity. The thermal effect of the Nd:YAG laser goes beyond its immediate area of visible impact.

Diode Laser

The diode laser is a semiconductor laser. It is a sturdy and compact laser that requires minimal maintenance. The energy is transmitted through an optical fiber and can be used in contact mode and noncontact mode.

Hemoangiolytic Lasers

The 532-nm KTP and 585-nm pulse dye laser are both hemoangiolytic lasers which are best absorbed by oxyhemoglobin. Due to this property, these fiber delivery laser systems are useful in vascular lesions such as papillomas and dysplasias. Both these lasers are noncontact laser systems. They can be used via the working channel of the flexible bronchoscope as an office procedure.

Clinical Pearls

- All clinicians using lasers must undergo laser safety training.
- Each department using lasers must have a named laser protection supervisor.
- The laser unit must remain switched off and locked with an identifiable key when not in use.
- Lasers must be used in an appropriate theater, with clear notification when in use and an audible alarm if the notification is not heeded.
- All personnel in theater must wear designated eye protection when the laser is in use.
- When the laser is in use, but not actively firing, it must be kept in standby mode.
- The surrounding tissues such as subglottic mucosa should be protected with wet cottonoid from inadvertent damage by the laser beam.
- Wet swabs are placed over the eyes and around the field of use of the laser, for example, around the mouth and face.
- A jug of water should be kept close by to quench an inadvertent airway fire.

Laryngology is one of the specialty areas in which lasers are most often used. As a result of its precise cutting, superficial well-delineated effect with minimal lateral thermal damage, the CO_2 is widely used in laryngology.

Benign Lesions

The endoscopic use of the CO_2 laser with a micromanipulator permits excellent precision and good hemostasis. This may not be possible with cold instruments. With the advancement of technology and a refinement of surgical techniques, good functional results have followed. The development of a microspot micromanipulator, as described by Shapshay et al, facilitated tissue excision with precise cutting and minimal damage to the surrounding mucosa and underlying vocalis muscle.[3] The CO_2 laser has been used to excise benign laryngeal lesions and is especially effective for excising vascular polyps, large sessile nodules, cysts, and the evacuation of polyps. The technique of excising benign laryngeal lesions by the CO_2 laser is simple and is well described in the literature.[4]

The key to successful laryngoscopic excision is good exposure. A Kleinsasser anterior commissure laryngoscope with or without suspension system can be used for this purpose. Some benign conditions in which the laser may be used effectively are discussed below (**Table 16.1**).

Vocal Cord Nodules

These are commonly located at the junction of anterior third and posterior two-thirds of the vocal cords which is the site of maximum mucosal vibration. These are generally superior to the free margin of vocal cords.

Table 16.1 Classification of Airway Lesions

	Congenital	Acquired
Supraglottis	Laryngomalacia Vallecular cysts	Chemical trauma Vallecular cyst Epiglottic neoplasm Aryepiglottic fold cyst Ventricular fold fibrosis Laryngopharyngeal angioma
Glottis	Glottic web Bilateral vocal cord palsy	Glottic web: Anterior, midglottic, posterior Neoplasm Bilateral fixed vocal cord
Subglottic and tracheal	Stenosis Hemangioma	Stenosis Granulomatous lesion Hemangioma

Surgical excision with the CO_2 laser scanning technology (Acublade, Lumenis, Israel) and the high-power pulsed mode (super or ultrapulse) in single pulse mode is the treatment for hard organized nodules (line of 1.5 mm, depth of incision of 200 μm—two passes, power of 10 to 12 W). Voice rest for 10 days followed by voice therapy is advised after excision.

Cysts

A large variety of cystic lesions occur in the larynx. In the newborn it can form from an epithelial rest, in adults it may be a retention cyst of salivary gland and rarely can be associated with neoplasm. Intracordal cysts appear as small spheres on the margin of the vocal fold. The CO_2 laser is a good tool for managing these lesions as achieving complete excision with cold instruments may be difficult.

The CO_2 laser is a useful tool to surgically treat vocal fold cysts. It is important that cysts are completely excised to prevent any chance of recurrence. CO_2 laser provides a better precision in dealing with such delicate lesion and the Acublade is a better alternative.[5]

Vocal Cord Polyps

These are pedunculated or broad-based lesions developing on the vocal fold. They present in a variety of shapes and sizes. Microsurgery and CO_2 laser excision is, in the surgeon's view, the appropriate treatment for the same. **Fig. 16.1A, B** shows the pre- and postoperative photographs of a vocal fold polyp excised using CO_2 laser. Voice rest for 10 days after the surgery is advised, followed by a course of voice therapy.

Granuloma

These are benign lesions induced by healing granulomatous tissue secondarily epithelialized overlying the vocal process and medial aspect of arytenoids. If a granuloma persists, excision with a CO_2 laser, especially the base of the granuloma, at low wattage with minimum lateral damage, should be the treatment. Recurrence is common while healing and many studies have shown a remarkable decrease in postoperative recurrence rates following injection of botulinum toxin in the thyroarytenoid muscle to prevent the slamming together of both the vocal processes, thus permitting perichondrial healing over the vocal process of the arytenoids.

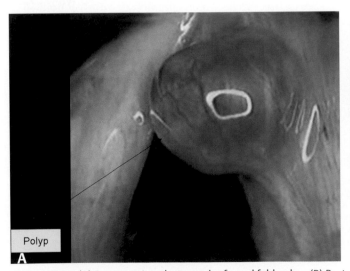

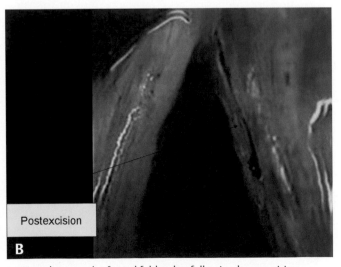

Figure 16.1 (A) Preoperative photograph of vocal fold polyp. (B) Postoperative photograph of vocal fold polyp following laser excision.

Vascular Pathology

Capillary ectasia is a varicose dilation of the capillaries of the vocal fold. Hemangiomas and hemorrhage of the vocal fold are other vascular pathologies commonly seen. These lesions are most often located on the superior surface of the vocal folds and close to the free edge. Surgery should not be performed during the acute phase of bleeding, and sufficient time should be allowed until the blood is reabsorbed and the ectasia are clearly seen.

Neuromuscular Disorders

Spasmodic Dysphonia (Focal Laryngeal Dystonia)

Spasmodic dysphonia (SD) is a voice disorder characterized by involuntary movements of one or more intrinsic muscles of the larynx during speech. All three types of SD such as (1) adductor SD, (2) abductor SD, and (3) mixed SD, are amenable to treatment.

Treatment

Botulinum toxin A injection of the laryngeal hyperfunctional muscles has been found to be the treatment of choice to control the dystonic symptoms in most patients with SD. The botulinum toxin injections generally improve the voice for a period of 3 to 4 months after which the symptoms gradually return.

Surgical treatment options suggested for this are section of the recurrent laryngeal nerve, selective bilateral denervation, external framework surgery (Isshiki type 2 thyroplasty), and bipolar radiofrequency-induced thermotherapy.

Carbon dioxide Laser-Assisted Myoneurectomy
CO_2 laser-assisted myoneurectomy is a feasible alternative to current methods to treat SD. This was initially proposed via open approach through thyroplasty, but this is more easily performed transorally with proven long-term positive results.[6,7]

The technique is mainly based on a partial CO_2 laser-assisted myomectomy of the inferior thyroarytenoid muscle (vocal fold muscle). Only the lateral part of the muscle involved in the adduction and tension activity of the vocal fold must be ablated. The medial part, more involved in the regulation of the vibration during phonation, must be spared. Bilateral surgery in one or two sessions is recommended.

Bilateral Abductor Palsy

For long, surgeons have been searching for techniques to safely widen the glottic airway in patients with bilateral vocal cord paralysis without detracting from vocal quality and/or causing aspiration. Surgical methods were designed to attain good respiration, phonation, and swallowing. For the past 15 years the CO_2 laser endoscopic arytenoidectomy has become perhaps the most commonly used method for attaining these goals.

Subtotal Arytenoidectomy

The initial incision is made between the vocal process and the membranous part of the vocal fold. It is then extended laterally onto the ventricular fold and posteriorly to encircle the anteromedial part of the arytenoid cartilage. The posterior third of the vocal fold, a 2 or 3 mm strip of the ventricular fold and the anteromedial aspect of the body of the arytenoid are removed with the laser in super pulse mode.

The Acublade with settings of 0.5 to 0.7 mm in length, 0.2 mm in depth, and 5 to 8 W of power is ideal for this surgical procedure. Laser application is performed in the continuous mode. Flash scanner mode with 0.7 mm diameter and 2 to 2.5 W of power was used in continuous mode for vaporization and reduction of the posterior shelf of the arytenoids to minimize and prevent aspiration.

The sectioning is more easily performed in super-pulse mode because of its superior sectioning effect with less carbonization that can mask the limits of the tissues which ideally are to be spared. If necessary, hemostasis of the arytenoid artery is achieved by electrocoagulation via the monopolar cautery attachment of microforceps.

Unilateral Posterior Cordectomy

The CO_2 laser with Acublade 0.5 to 0.7 mm in length, 0.2 mm in depth, and 5 W of power was used. A 3.5 or 4 mm c-shaped wedge of posterior vocal cord is excised from the free border of the membranous cord, anterior to the vocal process, extending 4 mm laterally over the ventricular band. The excision begins anterior to the vocal process without exposing cartilage. This excision creates a 6 to 7 mm transverse opening at the posterior larynx as shown in **Fig. 16.2A, B**.

Glottic Web

Glottic stenosis is narrowing of the larynx at the level of vocal cords, usually involving the anterior or posterior commissure. **Fig. 16.3** depicts the classification and the management of glottic webs.[8]

Management

The transoral CO_2 laser is used for the surgical management of extensive webs causing airway obstruction. The expanding laryngoscope provides the best exposure, but where its introduction is not possible due to the anatomical configuration of the larynx, an anterior commissure laryngoscope is a suitable substitute. A thin anesthetic boogie is used to palpate for fibrosis of the anterior or posterior commissure. The mobility of the cricoarytenoid joints are checked with a probe. For excision of a web, the CO_2 laser is used with an Acublade. The CO_2 laser settings are Acublade mode, 5 W, 0.5 mm length, linear shape, and single pass.

Glottic Web Involving Commissures

These webs involve anterior or posterior commissure along with a variable degree of the free edge of the vocal fold. Each condition warrants a specific surgical approach:

- Glottic web involving anterior commissure: Many of these webs involve the anterior commissure and

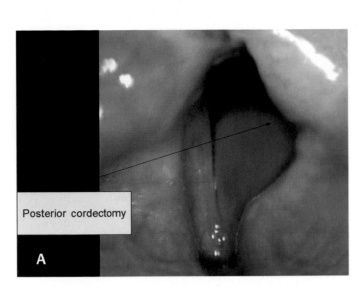

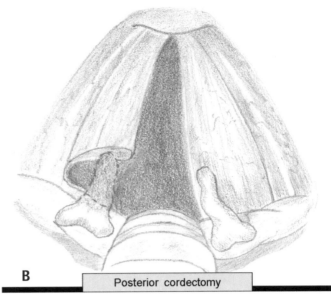

Figure 16.2 (A) Healed posterior cordectomy. (B) Line diagram outlining posterior cordectomy.

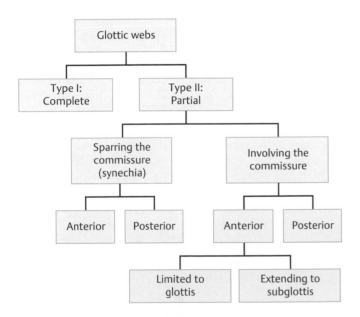

Figure 16.3 Classification of glottic webs.

extend posteriorly along the free edge of the vocal cord up to the junction of anterior two-thirds and posterior one-third. They may be limited to the glottis or in a few cases may extend to the subglottis. For these webs, posterior cordectomy is performed on one side with the CO_2 laser.

- Glottic web involving posterior commissure: These cases present as a thick band stretching between the medial surface of the arytenoids. In most cases, clinically, the arytenoids are immobile indicating ankylosis of the cricoarytenoid joint. The band is severed in the midline. Particular care is taken to avoid inadvertent laser strikes or transmission of heat to the interarytenoid muscle.

- Glottic webs sparing the commissures: These webs are synechia and involve predominantly the anterior or posterior part of the glottis, sparing the commissures. In most cases the cricoarytenoid joint is not involved. The synechia are easily excised with the CO_2 laser in scanning mode.

Recurrent Respiratory Papillomatosis

Recurrent respiratory papillomatosis (RRP) is the most common laryngeal neoplasm in children but can occur in adults too. Endoscopic excision is the standard treatment, but the rapid recurrence and need for repeated surgical removal has been a matter of discussion.

Laser Principles

In the authors' opinion the CO_2 laser is the laser of choice for management of RRP. The use of the CO_2 laser Acublade in ablation mode (diameter of 0.5 to 2 mm, super or ultrapulse, repeat mode of 0.1 second and a power of 10 W is favorable). The location of the papillomata is an important consideration to avoid inadvertent collateral damage. Initially, debulking of the papilloma is achieved by using the laser in continuous mode and as vital areas are approached, a systematic and precise method is to be followed by switching between the repeat and single pulse mode. These vital areas are the free margin of the vocal cord, anterior commissure, posterior commissure, subglottis, and cricoarytenoid joint. Viral presence has not been demonstrated in subepithelial tissues, so the laser is used with utmost care in such areas to minimize thermal damage. Papillomata on the free margin of the vocal cords are dissected rather than being vaporized. For tracheal application, the CO_2 laser can be connected to a bronchoscope through a micromanipulator. In the author's view, the diode laser may also be used if the area is inaccessible for CO_2 laser. In the treatment of RRP, care should be taken to evacuate smoke safely. In a published study, higher rates of remission were achieved when RRP was excised using a CO_2 laser.[9]

Reinke Edema

This is edema occurring in the Reinke space. It has been classified into three stages.[10] Stages II and III may be treated with laser surgery and combined speech therapy.

Chronic Laryngitis

Chronic laryngitis is a common pathology in adults. Laryngitis is an acute or chronic inflammation of the vocal folds and larynx causing dysphonia. Tobacco, alcohol, drugs intoxication, environmental agents, upper respiratory tract infections, and vocal abuse are known factors responsible for chronic laryngitis.

If left untreated it may result in serious complication. It may become a premalignant lesion. Besides the laser biopsy with the microspot by microlaryngoscopy, smear testing is a technique of choice to follow-up these patients.

Laser phonosurgery needs an excellent pathologist to study the frozen section during the operation.

Endoscopic Excision of Laryngeal Cancer

Transoral laser surgery is now a widely used surgical approach in the management of small glottic and supraglottic carcinoma. Though commonly used for early malignancies, successful treatment of stage II through stage IV lesions of the glottic and supraglottic larynx and hypopharynx have also been reported in the literature.[11,12]

The Nomenclature Committee of the European Laryngological Society (ELS) has proposed a classification for the endoscopic excision of glottic cancer.[13] **Table 16.2** describes the ELS classification of endoscopic cordectomy.

Table 16.2 ELS Classification of Endoscopic Cordectomy

Type	Description
I	Subepithelial cordectomy or decortications
II	Subligamentous cordectomy
III	Transmuscular cordectomy
IV	Total or complete cordectomy
V	Extended cordectomy Va: contralateral vocal fold and anterior commissure Vb: arytenoidectomy Vc: ventricle Vd: subglottis
VI	Anterior commissurotomy

Documentation of cases along the lines approved by the Nomenclature Committee of the ELS will allow comparison of results obtained by endoscopic and external surgery, as well as by radiotherapy. Only then will it be possible to rationalize the endoscopic use of lasers for selected lesions, with an equitable outcome.

Laser-assisted surgery for supraglottic carcinoma now plays a prominent role with the main advantage being that the resection can be tailored to the extent of the tumor. As in case of the glottic tumors, ELS has recently proposed a classification for the endoscopic excision of supraglottic lesion.[14]

The literature reports the use of lasers in the management of hypopharyngeal malignancy (Steiner 1994, Zeitels 1994).[14,15] Laser-assisted surgery for hypopharyngeal cancer can also be used as salvage surgery.

- Laryngomalacia: Laryngomalacia is the most common congenital anomaly presenting with stridor in the first year of life.
  - Laser management: CO_2 laser aryepiglottopexy is used for the management of laryngomalacia. In this procedure, redundant mucosa over the arytenoids is vaporized with CO_2 laser scanner mode. Aryepiglottic and pharyngoepiglottic folds are severed to enlarge the introitus. If epiglottis is deemed to be the cause of obstruction, the edges are trimmed (epiglottopexy).
- Vallecular cysts: Vallecular cysts are actually mucus retention cysts of either epiglottis or from base of the tongue. In infants and children this may present with stridor and feeding difficulty. In adults these may be asymptomatic or may present with globus, voice change, dysphagia, and rarely dyspnea. These are cause for difficult intubation. Management consists of initial aspiration of the fluid so that airway becomes patent. Then intubation takes place followed by CO_2 laser marsupialization of the cyst wall.
- Corrosive injury: Caustic and thermal injuries do cause laryngeal and tracheal airway strictures. Inhalation injury to the larynx due to burns and direct caustic ingestion are common form of injuries which can cause complication compromising the airway. Laser excision of fibrous tissue usually restores the airway and the swallowing. In severe cases a staged procedure may be required to achieve desired results and patency.
- Supraglottic fibrosis
  - Epiglottis and aryepiglottic fold fibrosis
  - Ventricular fold fibrosis (complete partial)

These may occur following caustic injury, inhalation injury, or idiopathic, but may lead to airway compromise. Management requires excision of the fibrosis from both the sides with CO_2 laser. Long-term follow-up and flexible laryngoscopy is essential, especially in children where restenosis is common.

- Glottic webs: These have been discussed in section "Benign Lesions."

- Bilateral abductor palsy: Discussed earlier.
- Intubation granuloma: Discussed earlier.
- Laryngeal malignancy: The main purpose of use of laser in malignant lesionscausing airway obstruction is to create airway avoiding tracheostomy. In terminal cases of malignancy, it is used to debulk the tumour and improve the airway. Mainly diode and KTP lasers are used for this purpose.
- Subglottic hemangioma: Subglottic hemangiomata are benign vascular neoplasms. Propranolol is the currenttreatmentofchoiceforsubglottichemangiomas; however, surgery remains a valid treatment option especially in propranolol nonresponders. Treatment with laser surgery involves using the diode or KTP laser in noncontact mode to ablate the hemangioma.
- Laryngopharyngeal hemangioma: These are relatively rare and usually arise in the supraglottis. The treatment remains tumor ablation same as in form of subglottic hemangioma. The diode or KTP Laser is used in noncontact mode.
- Subglottic stenosis: Infants will require tracheostomy before any definitive management in cases of severe stridor. Trauma remains the most common cause of subglottic stenosis in both children and adults. In stage I through III, laser can be a useful tool for management. Radial cuts to the stenotic mucosa are made using the laser followed by balloon dilatation of the stenotic segment. It is essential to have a follow-up of these patients. During follow-up, laryngoscopy is performed to remove slough if any and repeat dilatation may be required.
- Lymphedema following radiotherapy: Radiotherapy may lead to gross lymphatic obstruction with lymphedema of the arytenoids mounds. Dysphonia, difficulty in breathing, and dysphagia can be helped by laser vaporization of the solid tissue covering the arytenoids.
- Laryngeal trauma: This results in airway problems.

External Trauma

A common cause of external laryngeal injury is involvement in motor vehicle accidents and clothes line injury. Punch-up fights, manual strangulation, and sports injuries are other rare causes.

These may result in injuries to the laryngeal framework and intraluminal structures, the extent of which depends on the severity and anatomical location of injury. Within the lumen of the larynx, damage ranges from bruising, hematomas, mucosal tears, and detachment of the epiglottis and the vocal folds. A degree of airway obstruction is inevitable. Symptoms may vary from stridor and dyspnea, which needs emergency management to that of just hoarseness, odynophobia, and odynophagia.

- Supraglottis: Mucosal injury may cause supraglottic stenosis. In cases of dislocation of arytenoids, the aryepiglottic folds may collapse during inspiration.
- Glottis: Tear and loss of vocal fold may lead to aspiration and dysphonia. Vocal cord hematoma may form and its resorption may lead to sulcus vocalis.
- Subglottis: Stenosis may result due to persistent hematoma for more than 3 weeks due to slough and granulation.

Conservative Management of Laryngeal Trauma

Patients found to have minimal endolaryngeal injury on flexible endoscopy and a stable laryngeal framework with a patent airway can be managed conservatively with close observation, repeated flexible endoscopy, corticosteroids, broad-spectrum antibiotics, and proton pump inhibitors.

Follow-Up

Delayed finding may be in the form of fibrosis and stenosis.

Endoscopic Laser Management

Cases presenting with compromised airway require conventional management. Endoscopic evaluation is done under general anesthesia to assess the damage, carry out wound toilet, remove hematoma, and any mucosal tags within the airway. For sequelae in the form of adhesions, stenosis, webs, and fibrous bands detected at ongoing follow-up, endoscopic laser management is beneficial.

For cricoarytenoid dislocation intruding the airway, management is by excising or vaporizing the intruding portion of the arytenoid or other cartilages. Unilateral paralysis of the cord may require augmentation to restore phonation.

Bilateral abductor paralysis needs lateralization of vocal fold or unilateral cordectomy. Laser surgery is similar to that described for various benign lesions. The management depends on the findings. Generally, for stenosed ventricular bands, transoral CO_2 laser excision, undertaken in two stages, is the treatment of choice. Mitomycin-C is used topically following resection. Restenosis is not uncommon in the supraglottis. Follow-up laryngoscopy and removal of slough within a week discourages restenosis.

Circumferential narrowing of the supraglottis poses a challenge. Partial epiglottectomy may help in these cases. Aryepiglottopexy as in cases of laryngomalacia is useful for patients presenting with a lax supraglottis and collapsing aryepiglottic tissues.

Endolaryngeal Trauma

Endolaryngeal trauma occurs in a variety of ways. The most common trauma being iatrogenic: intubation injury. Improper use of the laser in the larynx is another iatrogenic cause. Accidental or suicidal ingestion of corrosives leads to superficial or deep chemical burns of the mucosa.

Intubation Injury and Its Laser Management

Prolonged tracheal intubation causes mucosal damage due to pressure necrosis and perichondritis. Intubation granuloma is a well-recognized entity following prolonged intubation. It usually forms on the medial side of the arytenoid and may be bilateral. The granuloma can be removed with cold instruments or laser.

In the subglottis, inflated cuff leads to pressure necrosis and loss of mucosa is replaced by fibrotic tissue encircling the lumen to a variable degree. Management depends on the type of pathology that gets formed for stage I and II laser excision with radial cuts, followed by serial dilatation or balloon dilatation works, while for severe grade stenosis open surgery may be required.

Conclusion

Adopting safe laser practice as standard has enabled lasers to become a well-established part of the armamentarium in laryngeal surgery. Several types of lasers are available for use in the larynx; the clinicians' challenge is to choose the appropriate laser for each pathology and keep abreast of new developments for early implementation into clinical use.

Acknowledgment
The editors would like to thank Miss Sonna Ifeacho for her help with the editing of the chapter and providing inputs with the clinical insight boxes.

References

1. Remacle M, Hassan F, Cohen D, Lawson G, Delos M. New computer-guided scanner for improving CO_2 laser-assisted microincision. Eur Arch Otorhinolaryngol 2005;262(2):113–119
2. Strong MS, Jako GJ. Laser surgery in the larynx. Early clinical experience with continuous CO_2 laser. Ann Otol Rhinol Laryngol 1972;81(6):791–798
3. Shapshay SM, Wallace RA, Kveton JF, Hybels RL, Bohigian RK, Setzer SE. New microspot micromanipulator for carbon dioxide laser surgery in otolaryngology. Early clinical results. Arch Otolaryngol Head Neck Surg 1988;114(9):1012–1015
4. Shapshay SM, Rebeiz EE, Bohigian RK, Hybels RL. Benign lesions of the larynx: should the laser be used? Laryngoscope 1990;100(9):953–957
5. Matar N, Amoussa K, Verduyckt I, et al. CO_2 laser-assisted microsurgery for intracordal cysts: technique and results of 49 patients. Eur Arch Otorhinolaryngol 2010;267(12):1905–1909
6. Woo P. Carbon dioxide laser-assisted thyroarytenoid myomectomy. Lasers Surg Med 1990;10(5):438–443
7. Tsuji DH, Chrispim FS, Imamura R, Sennes LU, Hachiya A. Impact in vocal quality in partial myectomy and neurectomy endoscopic of thyroarytenoid muscle in patients with adductor spasmodic dysphonia. Braz J Otorhinolaryngol 2006;72(2):261–266
8. Gandhi S. Transoral laser surgery for glottic stenosis caused by webs. Oper Tech Otolaryngol-Head Neck Surg 2011;22(2):146–151
9. Gandhi S, Jacob R. Remission in juvenile-onset recurrent respiratory papillomatosis. J Laryngol Voice 2012;2(1):30–34
10. Yonekawa H. A clinical study of Reinke's edema. Auris Nasus Larynx 1988;15(1):57–78
11. Eckel HE, Staar S, Volling P, Sittel C, Damm M, Jungehuelsing M. Surgical treatment for hypopharynx carcinoma: feasibility, mortality, and results. Otolaryngol Head Neck Surg 2001;124(5):561–569
12. Vilaseca I, Bernal-Sprekelsen M, Luis Blanch J. Transoral laser microsurgery for T3 laryngeal tumors: Prognostic factors. Head Neck 2010;32(7):929–938
13. Remacle M, Hantzakos A, Eckel H, et al. Endoscopic supraglottic laryngectomy: a proposal for a classification by the working committee on nomenclature, European Laryngological Society. Eur Arch Otorhinolaryngol 2009;266(7):993–998
14. Steiner W. [Therapy of hypopharyngeal carcinoma. Part V: Discussion of long-term results of transoral laser microsurgery of hypopharyngeal carcinoma]. HNO 1994;42(3):157–165
15. Zeitels SM, Koufman JA, Davis RK, Vaughan CW. Endoscopic treatment of supraglottic and hypopharynx cancer. Laryngoscope 1994;104(1 Pt 1):71–78

17 Management of Voice Disorders: Key Principles of Speech–Language Therapy

Ruth Epstein

The practice of speech–language therapy includes the application of procedures and principles for measurement, testing, identification, counseling, or instruction related to the development and disorders of communication, voice, and swallowing. Speech–language counseling therapists (SLTs) follow an undergraduate or postgraduate courses and graduate with a science-based qualification. The courses and clinicians are regulated by a professional body, for example, American Speech-Hearing-Language Association in the United States or the Royal College of Speech and Language Therapists and the Health Professions Council in the United Kingdom. Clinicians who specialize in the treatment of voice disorders do not undergo specific training to become voice specialists. There are a few postgraduate courses that offer training in voice pathology to ENT surgeons and SLTs, but most clinicians acquire their experience "on the job."

SLTs who specialize in the treatment of individuals with voice disorders work in collaboration with the laryngologist. They are concerned with understanding, assessing, and modifying vocal behaviors. SLTs do not provide medical diagnosis or treatment; neither do they provide vocal training that would enhance the aesthetic quality of voice. Rather, they are primarily concerned with the "pathological" aspect of a voice problem in one or more physical, perceptual, or behavioral components.

Initial Referral

In most countries, the general family doctor is the first "port of call" available to an individual with a voice problem. The family medical practitioner may prescribe a course of antibiotics, and if the problem persists, he may refer the patient to an ENT specialist. The current preferred practice is to assess voice disorders in voice clinics, based on a constructive partnership between ENT specialists and SLTs.

The Voice Clinic

Voice clinics provide more detailed and accurate information on the vocal tract and vocal function,[1] which is very useful to the treating SLT. The ENT surgeon has the prime responsibility for examining the larynx and for making the appropriate diagnosis; however, increasingly, SLTs undertake special training that enables them to visualize the larynx in parallel or therapy clinic.[2] This enables them to examine the

impact of voice therapy on vocal function and to consider how they may alter their therapeutic approach on the basis of "live" evidence.[3]

Voice Evaluation

The goal of the voice assessment is to establish a set of parameters that describe voice quality and voice use, and to relate these parameters to a well-designed treatment.[4] Voice therapy aims to assist the dysphonic patient to return to a realistically achieved voice quality that will satisfy his or her emotional, occupational, and vocational needs. Achieving this objective depends on the patient's anatomic, physiological, and psychological capabilities that may require the involvement of the multidisciplinary voice team and, of course, the patient's ability to understand his or her vocal limitations.

Case History

The initial voice therapy session usually consists of case history taking. The aim of this initial clinical interview is to explore the history of the patient's presenting symptoms. This session often determines the success of the speech therapy intervention, which depends on the clinician's skill to put the patient at ease and to manage their expectations, emotions, and understanding of their problem.[5] During the case history taking, the clinician aims to explore the patient's perspective on the nature of their voice problem and how it affects their life. We seek to learn about the onset of the current episode and how it developed over time, the consistency of voice quality and other associated symptoms, for example, vocal fatigue or laryngeal discomfort. Questions are asked about voice use/vocal load and about the manner/intensity of voice use in a professional/vocational, social, and recreational context.

Armed with this information, the clinician may carry out the following assessments:

Perceptual Assessment

Auditory perceptual assessment is a primary tool for voice clinicians. Similarly, the effectiveness of voice therapy is judged by patients and their families on the basis of their auditory perception.[6] The GRBAS scheme developed by Hirano[7] is the most commonly used rating scheme in voice disorders. The listener is required to rate the severity of five parameters using a four-point scale: 0 (normal); 1 (mild); 2 (moderate); and 3 (severe). The vocal attributes rated are as follows: G—grade, which represents the overall severity of the voice disorder; R—roughness, which represents the overall degree of irregularity of vocal fold vibrations, heard as harshness; b—Breathiness, which corresponds to the "air leakage" heard on phonation; A—asthenia, perceived as vocal weakness; and S—strain heard as hyperfunctional or effortful quality. GRBAS is considered a useful tool for clinicians working with voice disorders; it is simple to use, easy to learn, and yields high inter-rater reliability.[8]

Another scheme, used particularly in the United States, is the CAPE-V (consensus auditory-perceptual evaluation of voice), proposed by the American Speech-Language and Hearing Consensus Conference. The CAPE-V rates six vocal attributes: overall severity, roughness, breathiness, strain, pitch, and loudness. It uses a visual analogue scale on which the parameters are scored on a continuous scale, rather than the discrete four-point scale used in GRBAS. Evidence showed that this adaptation enables the scorer to note small differences within and among subjects.[9] It also makes this scheme a useful tool in research.

Both informal and formal auditory perceptual evaluations provide the SLT with valuable information about the quality and severity of the voice disorder, as well the way in which the patient uses the voice. The British Voice Association recommended the use of GRBAS for any clinician working with voice disorders.[10] While it is difficult to find an "ideal" auditory perceptual clinical tool, it is important to stress that any voice clinician is expected to use a formal perceptual voice assessment scheme as it facilitates the recording of changes over time and it contributes to standardization of communication among colleagues.

Laboratory Testing: Instrumental Assessment/Acoustic Analysis

The current approach to the assessment of voice disorders involves instrumental assessment.[4] Many hardware and software packages (e.g., KayPentax Computerized Speech Laboratory [KayPENTAX, New Jersey, United States] or Laryngograph Speech Studio [Laryngograph Ltd., Greater London, United Kingdom]) offer acoustic analysis and visual feedback of various aspects of speech and voice, which are used by SLTs in their voice therapy work. The acoustic analysis can yield aspects of voicing that may not be detected by the human ear, which would impact voice therapy.[11] The visual display can help patients gain further insight into the nature of their voice and helps them adjust their vocal behavior on the basis of what they see on the screen.

Instrumentation is also available for the analysis of the interaction between respiration and phonation. This is used by the SLT as part of the diagnostic evaluation, providing measures such as mean airflow rate, estimated subglottic air pressure, and laryngeal valving efficiency.

On the whole, there is agreement among clinicians and researchers that there is currently no single acoustic measurement that correlates best to perceived impression, but a combination of acoustic values. So clinicians will have to rely on a combination of assessments until an easy, accurate, and meaningful way of measuring voice quality is evolved.

Noninstrumental Voice Evaluation

The SLT may carry out other forms of noninstrumental assessments, for example, maximum phonation time, which provides information about the individual's respiratory function and glottal efficiency on the basis of his or her ability to sustain.[12] S/z ratio is used as another test among other tests to sustain a vowel sound.[13]

Patients Rating Scales

SLTs often ask patients to complete health-related questionnaire, exploring the impact of the voice disorder on their life. These questionnaires enable the clinician to identify particular issues related to voice use at work and in social interaction. They may be completed before and after intervention and can be used by the clinician as an outcome measure, demonstrating the effectiveness of intervention. The Voice Handicap Index (VHI)[14] is one of the most widely used questionnaires, offering insight into the perceived impact of the voice disorder on the person's life, and its severity. The shortened modified version of the VHI makes it easy and practical clinical and research tool, with strong reliability and validity.

Voice Therapy

Once the diagnosis and treatment plan have been established, the role of the SLT is to provide the course of voice therapy. The goal of therapy is to restore the best voice possible that would satisfy the individual's communication, vocational and social needs. The course of therapy would vary in accordance with the laryngeal diagnosis and with patient's ability to comply with the treatment program. Voice therapy may be conducted in conjunction with other treatment modalities such as physical therapy, for example, in the case of muscle tension dysphonia. If the patient is due to undergo phonosurgery, the SLT should ideally see him or her preoperatively for case history taking and advice regarding the postoperative course of treatment.

The first step in voice therapy is patient's education.[4] Helping patients familiarize themselves with normal voice production and understanding the outcome of their laryngeal examination would help them understand their problem and engage them in the treatment process.

Vocal Hygiene

Vocal hygiene or voice care is one of the principles that is a routine part of every voice therapy program. It includes ideas about the do's and don'ts of voice care such as limiting talking time and vocal loudness, avoiding speaking against background noise, reducing vocally abusive behaviors such as throat clearing, coughing, and maintaining an adequate level of hydration. Vocal hygiene focuses on healthy use of the vocal apparatus.[4] It may include antireflux advice in terms of diet and lifestyle, and voice rest/conservation program, to assist healing.

Vocal Rehabilitation Techniques

Direct voice therapy consists of exercises targeting specific faulty vocal behaviors that contribute to the dysphonia. Voice therapy moves gradually from one activity to the next while allowing the patient sufficient time for mastering and practicing the technique. As stated by Aronson and Bless,[15] "no introduction to voice therapy approaches would be complete without a concomitant discussion of evidence-based medicine." Although increasingly clinicians are requested to define estimated length of treatment and to provide information about its effectiveness, many treatment approaches used by voice clinicians do not have an evidence base.[16]

In nonorganic voice disorders involving excess musculoskeletal tension, treatment is based on the principle that reduction in muscle tension allows the larynx to return to its normal phonatory ability. This is achieved by mechanical relaxation of musculature and psychological release of any anxiety causing or associated with the tension. Progression from abnormal to normal voice occurs as a product of the patient's conscious, voluntary response to the clinician's instruction and encouragement. In organic disorders, the main principle of therapy is either muscle strengthening

> **Symptomatic Voice Therapy**
> - Education and explanation
> - Vocal tract care, diet, and lifestyle advice
> - Posture and body alignment
> - Laryngeal manual therapy
> - Body awareness to identify, facilitate, and maintain physical change
> - Ear training to identify, facilitate, and maintain auditory change
> - Breathing techniques, including semi-occlusion exercises
> - Vocal exercises (specific to the patient's needs)
> - Resonance and forward vocal focus

Figure 17.1 Symptomatic voice therapy.

or adaptation to the mechanical problems through compensatory phonatory and respiratory maneuvers[17] (**Fig. 17.1**).

Manual therapies are increasingly used by voice clinicians in treating patients with muscle tension dysphonia, which is a feature of most voice disorders of both organic and behavioral etiology. Manual therapy involves the use of direct manual intervention, or kneading the laryngeal muscles, to reduce excess musculoskeletal tension in the perilaryngeal muscles. A variety of methods used by clinicians have been reported in the literature.[18-21] The technique was first described by Aronson.[18] Mathieson[22] conducted a recent review of the evidence for laryngeal manual therapies in the treatment of muscle tension dysphonia. She concluded that "there is evidence that laryngeal manual therapy in various forms can be a useful primary intervention" although the evidence base remains very small.

A variety of other techniques can be used in the treatment of voice disorders. Relaxation is applied to reduce musculoskeletal tension in the laryngeal area.[18] Breathing exercises are employed to optimize breath support for the voice. Various phonation exercises are used to promote soft

Table 17.1 Commonly Used Voice Therapy Techniques

Voice Therapy Technique	Benefit
Auditory training	• Instant auditory feedback
Respiratory control	• Increasing expiratory air volume • Providing sufficient breath support for optimum voice
Accent method[24]	• Facilitating easy phonation with appropriate resonance balance
Yawn-sigh[25]	• Opening inlet to the larynx • Promoting relaxation of the pharynx
Tone focus[26]	• Optimizing pitch
Resonant voice therapy[27]	• Promoting forward vocal focus
Semi-occluded vocal tract techniques[28]	• Improving vocal efficiency
Lip trills	• Facilitating balanced resonance
Voice rest	• Promoting tissue healing and reducing vocal fatigue
Lee Silverman technique[29]	• Improving loudness, pronunciation, inflection, and facial animation in individuals with neurologic disorders

initiation of vocalization, rather than hard glottal attack. Attention is paid to pitch, volume, and rate of speech to ensure that these are used appropriately. Voice therapy also aims to reduce stress factors that drive the individual into patterns of vocal misuse. **Table 17.1** provides a summary of various facilitation techniques commonly used by SLTs as part of the course of voice therapy.

Voice therapy techniques are continuously evolving.[15] Some techniques are evaluated through clinical research, but on the whole, there is limited evidence base available. Voice problems are mostly multifactorial. As such, therapy focuses on the restoration of the mechanical and acoustic properties of the vocal mechanism and aims to restore the normal biomechanics to the vocal apparatus. Commonly, however, dealing with this aspect alone does not provide optimal results and the experienced clinician would therefore be mindful of emotional aspects and personality. These in fact are common principles that form the basis for voice therapy.

Evidence-based voice therapy literature is still lacking. A higher level of evidence, including randomized controlled studies, is required to prove the efficacy of voice therapy interventions, determined by clinical, functional, and patient-defined outcomes. Future research should also demonstrate that treatment approaches can be replicated effectively by other clinicians.[23]

References

1. Phillips PS, Carlson E, Chevretton EB. Does a specialist voice clinic change ENT clinic diagnosis? Logoped Phoniatr Vocol 2005;30(2):90–93
2. Shewell C. Voice Work: Art and Science in Changing Voices. Chichester, UK: Wiley-Blackwell; 2009
3. Casper JK. Voice therapy constructs: their physiological bases. Voice 1995;4:61–69
4. Murry T, Rosen CA. The role of the speech-language pathologist in the treatment of voice disorders. In: Rubin JS, Sataloff RT, Korovin GS, eds. Diagnosis and Treatment of Voice Disorders. 3rd ed. San Diego, CA: Plural Publishing; 2006:575-584
5. Hersen M, Turner SM. Diagnosis Interviewing. New York: Plenum Press; 1985
6. Kreiman J, Gerratt BR, Kempster GB, Erman A, Berke GS. Perceptual evaluation of voice quality: review, tutorial, and a framework for future research. J Speech Hear Res 1993;36(1):21–40
7. Hirano M. Clinical Examination of Voice. New York: Springer-Verlag; 1981
8. Webb AL, Carding PN, Deary IJ, MacKenzie K, Steen N, Wilson JA. The reliability of three perceptual evaluation scales for dysphonia. Eur Arch Otorhinolaryngol 2004;261(8):429–434
9. Karnell MP, Melton SD, Childes JM, Coleman TC, Dailey SA, Hoffman HT. Reliability of clinician-based (GRBAS and CAPE-V) and patient-based (V-RQOL and IPVI) documentation of voice disorders. J Voice 2007;21(5):576–590
10. Carding PN, Carlson E, Epstein R, Mathieson L, Shewell C. Re: Evaluation of voice quality. Int J Lang Commun Disord 2001;36(1):127–134
11. Baken RJ, Orlikoff RF. Clinical Measurement of Speech and Voice. San Diego, CA: Singular Publishing Group; 2000
12. Colton RH, Casper JK. Understanding Voice Problems: A Physiological Perspective for Diagnosis and Treatment. 2nd ed. Baltimore, MD: Lippincott Williams & Williams; 1996
13. Boone DR. The Voice and Voice Therapy. Englewood Cliffs, NJ: Prentice-Hall; 1977
14. Jacobson BH, Johnson A, Grywalski C, et al. The Voice Handicap Index (VHI): development and validation. Am J Speech Lang Pathol 1997;6:66–70
15. Aronson AE, Bless DM. Clinical Voice Disorders. 4th ed. New York, NY: Thieme Medical Publishers; 2009
16. Frattali CM, ed. Measuring Outcomes in Speech–Language Pathology. New York, NY: Thieme Medical Publishers; 1998
17. Epstein R, Rubin JS. Voice disorders. In: de Souza C, ed. Head and Neck Surgery. New Delhi, India: Jaypee Brothers Medical Publishers (P) Ltd.; 2009:1600–1605
18. Aronson AE. Clinical Voice Disorders. 3rd ed. New York, NY: Thieme Medical Publishers; 1990:314–315
19. Roy N, Nissen SL, Dromey C, Sapir S. Articulatory changes in muscle tension dysphonia: evidence of vowel space expansion following manual circum laryngeal therapy. J Commun Disord 2009;42(2):124–135
20. Mathieson L, Hirani SP, Epstein R, Baken RJ, Wood G, Rubin JS. Laryngeal manual therapy: a preliminary study to examine its treatment effects in the management of muscle tension dysphonia. J Voice 2009;23(3):353–366
21. Van Houtte E, Van Lierde K, Claeys S. Pathophysiology and treatment of muscle tension dysphonia: a review of the current knowledge. J Voice 2011; 25(2):202–207
22. Mathieson L. The evidence for laryngeal manual therapies in the treatment of muscle tension dysphonia. Curr Opin Otolaryngol Head Neck Surg 2011;19(3):171–176
23. Bos-Clark M, Carding P. Effectiveness of voice therapy in functional dysphonia: where are we now? Curr Opin Otolaryngol Head Neck Surg 2011;19:160–164
24. Smith S, Thyme K. Statistic research on changes in speech due to pedagogic treatment (the accent method). Folia Phoniatr (Basel) 1976;28(2):98–103
25. Boone DR, McFarlane SC. A critical view of the yawn-sigh as a voice therapy technique. J Voice 1993;7(1):75–80
26. Cooper M. Modern Techniques of Vocal Rehabilitation. Springfield, IL: Charles C Thomas; 1973
27. Verdolini K, Druker DG, Palmer PM, Samawi H. Laryngeal adduction in resonant voice. J Voice 1998;12(3):315–327
28. Titze IR. Voice training and therapy with a semi-occluded vocal tract: rationale and scientific underpinnings. J Speech Lang Hear Res 2006;49(2):448–459
29. Ramig LO, Sapir S, Fox C, Countryman S. Changes in vocal loudness following intensive voice treatment (LSVT) in individuals with Parkinson's disease: a comparison with untreated patients and normal age-matched controls. Mov Disord 2001;16(1):79–83

Section E

Disorders of the Larynx

18 Vocal Fold Paralysis

Abir K. Bhattacharyya, Paul Stimpson, and Purushotam Sen

The principal function of the larynx is to protect the lower respiratory tract. In addition, the larynx facilitates Valsalva maneuver and phonation. These functions are maintained by coordinated action of intrinsic and extrinsic laryngeal muscles and are dependent on an intact neural supply. The term vocal fold paralysis (VFP) is often used to describe the immobile fold; however, an immobile vocal fold is not always paralyzed and may be fixed due to separate pathological process. Historically, no distinction has been made in the literature between neurogenic VFP and mechanical fixation, but their evaluation and management are very different. Until proven otherwise, VFP must be regarded as a sign of underlying disease and not simply as a diagnosis unto itself.

Advances in diagnostic techniques, improved clinical assessments, and broadening treatment options have aided in understanding the etiopathogenesis and management of unilateral VFP. By contrast, advances in the treatment of bilateral VFP have been slow to follow.

Etiology

A wide range of disorders can cause VFP (**Table 18.1**). There is significant bias in the reported incidence of major causes of impaired vocal fold function. Incidence varies with geographical location[1] and reporting institution. Traditionally, the etiology is divided into thirds, with one third due to tumor, one third traumatic (surgery), and one third idiopathic.[2] This trend is changing, with extralaryngeal malignancy now taking a greater proportion and other surgical causes gradually replacing thyroidectomy as the leading cause of surgical trauma.[3] This could be either due to improved diagnostics such as computed tomography (CT) and magnetic resonance imaging (MRI) or due to an increase in oncological skull base, neck, and chest surgeries.[4] It is important to note that the laryngoscopic appearance of VFP does not reflect the site of lesion, type of injury, or prognosis.

Etiology of Unilateral Vocal Fold Paralysis

- Malignancy (20 to 40%): Tumors anywhere along the course of the RLN from the skull base to the larynx may lead to vocal fold palsy.[3,5] Local tumors of the laryngopharynx can also fix the vocal fold or compress the laryngeal nerve. It is important to be aware that occult tumors in the thyroid, neck, chest, or mediastinum may also lead to VFP.

- Surgical trauma (22 to 44%): Surgical trauma accounts for the largest proportion of unilateral lesions. Most are due to purposeful resection of the nerve, though a significant number result from accidental injury.[4] Although incidence of recurrent laryngeal nerve (RLN) injury during thyroid surgery is decreasing, it remains the principal cause of iatrogenic injury.[3,5]

- Nonsurgical trauma (9 to 10%): Blunt and penetrating trauma to the neck and chest can result in nerve injury. Endotracheal intubation injury accounts for 7 to 11% of unilateral vocal cord paralysis[3,6] and is the result of excessive cuff pressure, laryngeal mask injury, or hyperextension of the neck. The RLN is usually compressed between the lateralized arytenoid cartilage, thyroid cartilage, and the inflated cuff. The compression injury resulting in paralysis must be distinguished from the immobile vocal fold due to traumatic arytenoid dislocation.

- Neurological causes (2 to 3%): Lesions of the cortex rarely give rise to isolated paralysis, whereas lesions involving the medulla or extending to the peripheral nerve produce a flaccid unilateral paralysis. Some of the common central neurological causes are cerebrovascular accidents, syringobulbia, multiple sclerosis, and parkinsonism.[5,7] In children, neurological abnormalities such as Arnold-Chiari malformation, meningomyelocele, and hydrocephalus should be considered.[8] Other rare conditions such as myasthenia gravis and Eaton-Lambert syndrome may give rise to VFP due to disorders of the neuromuscular junction. Many primary muscle disorders may present with laryngeal dysfunction such as polymyositis and dermatomyositis.[9]

- Inflammatory and infectious causes (2 to 3%): Laryngeal neuropathy leading to RLN paralysis can be caused by diabetes, rheumatoid arthritis, polyarteritis nodosa, gout, collagen vascular disease, mumps, and other viral diseases. Besides resulting in laryngeal neuropathy, it is important to understand that inflammatory disorders can also affect the cricoarytenoid joint or the larynx as a whole. For example, granulomatous diseases such as tuberculosis, syphilis, and sarcoidosis can affect the larynx locally or affect the laryngeal nerve in its course in the chest. Fibrotic lesions such as cicatricial pemphigoid, granulomatosis with polyangiitis (GPA + Wegener granulomatosis), and relapsing polychondritis can also affect vocal fold function. In young children presenting with a fluctuating polyneuropathy of the IX, X, and XII nerves, sarcoidosis may be an important cause.[5]

Table 18.1 Etiology of Unilateral Vocal Cord Paralysis

Surgical trauma
- Head and neck
  - Thyroid, parathyroid
  - Esophageal
  - Carotid end-arterectomy
  - Cervical spine fusion
  - Malignant resections
  - Skull base surgery
  - Posterior fossa surgery
- Thoracic
  - Thyroid
  - Tracheal
  - Cardiac surgery
  - Mediastinal

Nonsurgical trauma
- Blunt/penetrating Injuries
- Anesthetic intubation: excessive cuff pressure, laryngeal mask
- Injury, hyperextension neck
- Aortic aneurysm
- Cardiomegaly

Neurological causes
- Amyotrophic lateral sclerosis
- Bulbar/pseudo-bulbar palsy
- Multiple sclerosis
- Stroke
- Poliomyelitis
- Parkinsonism
- Wallenberg syndrome

Neoplastic
- Thyroid/lung
- Esophageal
- Mediastinal
- Vagal neoplasms

Inflammatory and infections
- Viral
- Sarcoidosis
- Diabetes
- Systemic lupus erythematosus
- Rheumatoid arthritis
- Tuberculosis
- Drug toxicity, e.g., vincristine, taxol, and organophosphates
- Radiation

Idiopathic

Congenital

- Idiopathic (12 to 22%): Improved assessment techniques, in particular, advances in the contemporary cross-sectional imaging, have enabled more accurate diagnosis.[5,10] This has resulted in the decrease of "idiopathic" causes from around 50 to around 20%.

Patient Evaluation and Assessment

The evaluation and assessment of VFP has evolved in the past few decades. Simpler protocols have now emerged replacing previous exhaustive ones. These are based on clinical evidence provided by extensive analysis of data in patients with VFP.[3,5]

History

As always, a thorough history of a patient is essential. Evaluation and assessment of the voice begins when the patient enters the physician's office. It is of utmost importance to obtain a detailed history of the onset, duration, and severity of the dysphonia. Taking a history provides ample time to the physician to make a detailed assessment of the patient's voice. Qualities such glottic fry, hard glottal attacks, breathiness, diplophonia, pitch breaks, phonation breaks, and tense phonation can be assessed.

Not only is the larynx involved in voice production, but it is also crucial in protecting the lower respiratory tract. Hence, the patient may also present with coughing and choking episodes, aspiration, stridor, dyspnea, dysphagia, or odynophagia. A history of intubation, head and neck surgery, or trauma is very important. Other pertinent medical questions include the presence of seasonal allergies, history of reflux disease, life stress, diabetes, and medications.

A specific vocal history is also important. Many patients who present for an initial evaluation of voice complaints are unfamiliar with questions of vocal use and hygiene. It is important for the physician to explain these concepts to the patient during the questioning to facilitate accurate responses and educate the patient. Questions should include voice demands at home and at work, recreational singing, and episodes of abuse such as shouting at sporting events. Smoking, water intake, caffeine intake, and environmental irritants should be documented. An occupational history is essential. The effect of voice change may be significant for professional voice users and may cause significant distress for the patient.

A patient with unilateral VFP typically presents with a hoarse or weak voice. Attempts to speak loudly will lead to rapid laryngeal and respiratory muscle fatigue and vocal endurance is diminished. The voice cannot be projected easily when there is background noise. Some may complain of an inability to sing. Others may have subclinical symptoms. A compensated VFP may come to light when there is a respiratory infection leading to delayed recovery of hoarseness, or even breathing difficulties. Sometimes, patients may complain of shortness of breath and inability to perform daily routine work. Some may complain of aspiration, especially to liquids. These complaints are due to incomplete glottic closure. Physical activity such as lifting, pulling, or pushing requires extra effort due to lack of Valsalva ability.

The mode of onset can also influence the presenting symptoms. Sudden onset may follow viral illness or following surgery, whereas gradual onset of symptoms may be due to tumor involving the path of the RLN. Tumor may arise anywhere from the posterior fossa to the mediastinum and questions should aim to elicit important clinical signs and symptoms to guide further investigation.

Physical Examination

A thorough physical examination is performed including a full and detailed cranial nerve examination. Inspection and palpation of the neck for masses, with particular attention to the thyroid gland, restriction of movement, excess muscle tension, and scars from previous surgery or trauma should be performed. Normal laryngeal vertical mobility and abnormal laryngeal tilt and fixity, if any, should be noted. During palpation of the neck, the laryngeal framework should be assessed. The "manual compression test" is an easy, noninvasive clinical procedure that can evaluate several voice disorders. The lateral manual compression test may be useful in determining whether a patient with a wide glottic gap from unilateral VFP or vocal bowing will benefit from a medialization thyroplasty.[11]

Dynamic and static laryngeal assessment is performed using flexible laryngoscopy, and ideally videostroboscopy. The laryngoscopic findings in a patient with unilateral VFP due to RLN involvement will reveal the paramedian position of the ipsilateral vocal fold with the opposite cord active on abduction and adduction. Complete immobility is usually seen. Rarely, decreased range of motion may be seen due to the pull of the interarytenoid, incomplete paralysis, or due to reinnervation of the RLN. The vocal fold may appear atrophic or "noodle-like." The ventricle may look more capacious and the conus may demonstrate some loss of tissue fullness.

The arytenoid cartilage on the paralyzed side may have a prolapsed appearance tipping anteriorly into the airway, but this rarely causes airway obstruction in practice. This abnormal position of the cartilage may be mistaken for dislocation. Sometimes, the lax-infolded aryepiglottic fold may be drawn into the airway causing obstruction. All these features may give the paralyzed fold a shortened or bowed appearance. The paralyzed fold may also be at a lower vertical level compared with the functioning fold during phonation.[12]

The opposite mobile fold tends to adjust its length to match the paralyzed fold by shortening, so that the vocal processes

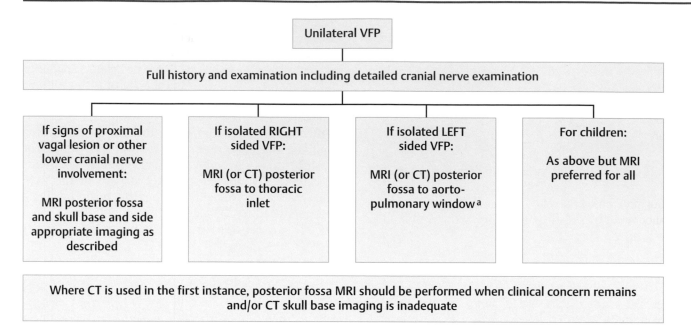

Figure 18.1 Suggested imaging guidelines for investigating unilateral vocal fold paralysis. CT, computed tomography; MRI, magnetic resonance imaging; VFP, vocal fold paralysis. *Modified* from Stimpson P, Patel R, Vaz F, et al. Imaging strategies for investigating unilateral vocal cord palsy: how we do it. *Clin Otolaryngol* 2011;36(3):266–271.
[a]Proceed to formal chest imaging if any chest abnormality detected on screening scan.

are opposite each other. This compensatory mechanism closes the glottic chink, but abnormal configuration of the posterior glottis persists.

The severity of the paralytic dysphonia is determined by the distance of the vocal folds from the midline, the degree of bowing, the size of the glottic gap, vertical relationships, and compensatory mechanisms.

Stroboscopy is useful in assessing the vibratory pattern of the vocal fold and provides valuable information on the effect of VFP on glottic closure. Vibratory patterns are influenced by the presence or absence of reinnervation, reduction in the mass of the vocal fold, and glottic gap.

Investigations

Over recent decades there has been a dramatic change in the investigation of patients with VFP. Historically, a comprehensive battery of tests was included in an attempt to evaluate all possible causes in a rather broad differential diagnosis. In recent years emphasis has been placed on a more focused approach based on the most probable cause.

Nearly one-third of the causes of VFP can be diagnosed on the basis of history of surgery and trauma alone,[13] with the cause of the paralysis being evident at presentation.[14]

Tests relevant to the etiology or metabolic diseases are performed only if indicated from the history. Routine hematological studies have a low diagnostic yield and are not recommended routinely.

Radiology/Imaging

Modern imaging techniques are highly sensitive and a CT scan will detect masses not seen on a plain chest film. In cases where paralysis is limited to the left vocal fold with no detectable lesion clinically, a contrast CT covering the course of the RLN from the posterior fossa to the aortopulmonary window is indicated. For lesions on the right side, imaging should again include the posterior fossa and extend inferiorly as far as the clavicle. If other branches of the vagus are involved, or other cranial neuropathies are present, or if clinical doubt remains, then a gadolinium-enhanced MRI of the posterior fossa and skull base, neck, and if necessary the brain, is advised. If dysphagia coupled with the suspicion of an esophageal lesion is suspected (not due to aspiration), a contrast esophagogram or an esophagoscopy may be performed (**Fig. 18.1**).

Objective Measures of Voice

A more detailed description of objective measures of voice (**Table 18.2**) may be found in Section C, Chapter 10, "The Evaluation of Voice Outcome and Quality of Life Measures."

Management Principles

The management of VFP requires a multidisciplinary approach from otolaryngologists, speech therapists, voice coaches, and other professionals. Active patient involvement with clear, realistic goals is crucial. The specific

Table 18.2 Objective Measures of Voice That May Be Considered for Patients with VFP

Measure	Description	Effect of VFP on Measure
Phonation airflow	• Airflow rates in speech are measured. • Useful in pre- and postoperative evaluation of thyroplasty or arytenoid adduction procedures.	• Elevated in unilateral VFP due to air escape.
Subglottal air pressure[16]	• Evaluation of the pressure in the subglottis (the opening force for vocal fold oscillations) • Useful in assessing the ability of the vocal fold to close effectively to contain the subglottal pressure and the available air resource.	• Reduced due to air escape.
Maximum phonation time	• Thought to give an index of glottal efficiency. • Refers to the maximum length of time which a patient can sustain a vowel sound on a single breath. • May be difficult to interpret. • Restoration of the glottic closure can dramatically increase the MPT to normal levels[17]	• Reduced due to air escape. • Normal values > 20 s. • In VFP values of < 12 s are typical.
Acoustic assessment	• Objective recording of the salient perceptual characteristics of voice such as the average fundamental frequency (F_0) and intensity, the amount of harmonics noise ratio and the percentage of perturbations (jitters and shimmers) • Integral in the evaluation of the voice in patients with VFP[18]	• Variable. • Useful for baseline analysis and to assess response to treatment.
Laryngeal EMG[19]	• Addresses important questions such as the prognosis of return of vocal fold function.[20] • Allows differentiation of neurogenic paralysis from mechanical vocal fold fixity. • Helps pinpoint the site of a neurological lesion and aids in the identification of incomplete neural injury or synkinesis. • Assists in determining the timing and type of surgery on the paralyzed fold. • In post-reinnervation surgery, the EMG is helpful in demonstrating return of function/innervation of the paralyzed muscles.[21]	• No polyphasic reinnervation potentials at 6–12 wk postinjury suggests good prognosis and observation versus temporary injection augmentation of the fold can be considered. • If by 3 mo reinnervation is not demonstrable on EMG, early medialization surgery may be undertaken, rather than waiting the standard 6 mo to 1 y.

VFP, vocal fold paralysis; s, second(s); EMG, electromyography; wk, week(s); mo, month(s); y, year.

management for a patient has to be tailored to his or her individual needs. An overview of the clinical management algorithm for patients with unilateral vocal fold palsy is shown in **Fig. 18.2**.

The initial assessment in the multidisciplinary voice clinic confirms the presence of a VFP. Objective and subjective voice and laryngeal assessment with particular attention to the glottal chink and level of the vocal folds are performed. Many patients with small glottic defects will benefit from early speech therapy. Subsequent management depends on the initial response to speech therapy intervention, and further therapy is indicated in those cases where the normal vocal fold is attempting to compensate adequately. In this situation, surgical intervention may be avoided.

In those cases where the voice is found to be suboptimal and compensation unlikely to occur, appropriate surgical management is considered. Various surgical techniques have been developed ranging from open thyroplasty to endoscopic injection techniques. Recent evidences suggest a combination of techniques give better results.[22]

Injection Medialization

(Please refer to section "Injection Medialization Procedures for the Vocal Fold," in Chapter 14 for detailed description of technique and materials.)

Injection medialization was introduced in 1911 by Bruenings.[23] The principle is to medialize the paralyzed vocal fold by injecting a substance lateral to the vocal fold. It remains the most common procedure performed for managing VFP. A variety of materials are available and can be broadly grouped into those providing a temporary or more permanent treatment effect. Examples include polytetrafluoroethylene (PTFE) (Teflon) paste, DuPont, United States) (rarely used nowadays), hydroxyapatite, collagens, and silicone, among others. Injections may be performed under general or local anesthesia. Local anesthetic techniques (with or without

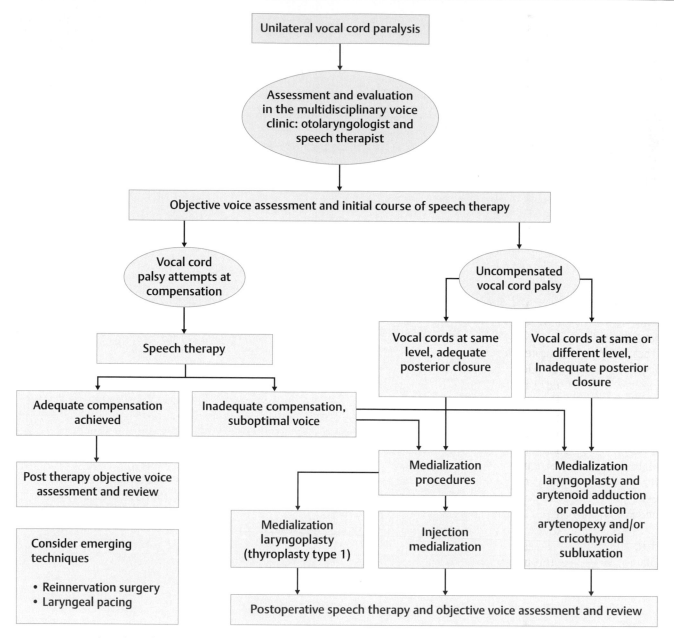

Figure 18.2 Unilateral vocal cord paralysis—a clinical management algorithm.

sedation) offer the advantage of direct auditory feedback and lessen the risk of overinjection with resultant airway compromise. Ultimately, the choice of material and the method of injection depend on expertise of the surgeon, availability of materials, patient factors, and cost.

Medialization Laryngoplasty

The term medialization laryngoplasty was coined in 1986 by Koufman.[24] It describes several surgical manipulations of the laryngeal framework with the principal goal of providing vocal fold medialization and pitch adjustments. Medialization laryngoplasty has evolved to be a dominant treatment modality for the dysphonia associated with

unilateral VFP. The convergence of physiological principles of glottal vibration has enhanced vocal outcomes. Frequently, laryngeal framework surgery also improves the swallowing dysfunction that may accompany an RLN or vagal paralysis.

Medialization Technique (Thyroplasty Type I)

(Please refer to Chapter 15 for detailed description of approaches and technique.)

This procedure may be done alone or combined with other medialization techniques, for example, arytenoid adduction/ adduction arytenopexy, cricothyroid subluxation, and injection medialization.

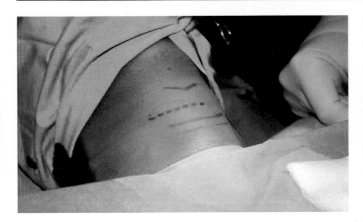

Figure 18.3 Skin incision for thyroplasty.

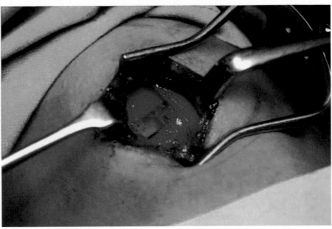

Figure 18.5 The Silastic implant in situ secured with permanent sutures to the laryngeal skeleton.

Local anesthesia permits per-operative monitoring and fine tuning of the voice while the patient phonates. It is important to predetermine the surface marking and level of the vocal cord for accurate positioning of the implant. Following a small skin incision (**Fig. 18.3**), a window is fashioned in the thyroid cartilage to enable insertion of the implant. Several commercially available implant systems made of hydroxyapatite, polymeric silicone, and now expanded polytetrafluoroethylene (ePTFE) (Gore-Tex, W. L. Gore & Associates Inc., Flagstaff, Arizona, United States) are available.[22,25] The Silastic implant (**Fig. 18.4A, B**) offers flexibility, allowing shaping of the implant according to the patient requirement to achieve optimal medialization. Preformed implants come in different sizes and may achieve similar results. Intermittent flexible laryngoscopy may be used to continuously assess the vocal fold position as the implant is inserted through the thyroplasty window

and then secured in place with permanent sutures to the laryngeal skeleton (**Fig. 18.5**).

Arytenoid Adduction

If the posterior glottic chink is not adducted adequately, then air escape is still inevitable and the voice turns out to be breathy. Medializing the posterior one-third of the cord by arytenoid adduction may overcome this problem.[26] The posterior border of the thyroid cartilage is approached either by elevating the outer perichondrium or dissecting lateral to the strap muscles and incising the inferior constrictor. The cricothyroid joint is opened or a small portion of the thyroid cartilage itself is cut at this point. The piriform fossa mucosa is then elevated carefully to palpate the posterior aspect of the arytenoids and the posterior cricoarytenoid muscle is cut. This is done to avoid the counter pulling effect of the muscle. The muscular process is passed through twice with

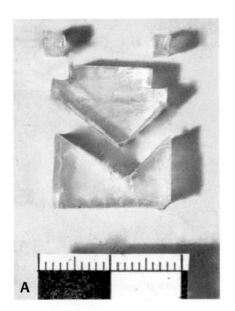

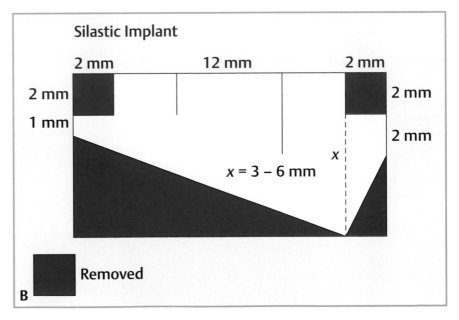

Figure 18.4 (A) Design and (B) size of the Silastic implant.

a 3–0 Prolene suture. It is pulled gently and tied with the anterior aspect of implant itself. Otherwise, it could also be tied with the lower border of thyroid cartilage approximately 6 or 7 mm behind the laryngeal prow. Before tying the knot, the tension in the suture is optimally adjusted through videolaryngoscopic monitoring. This suture renders the pulling effect of the thyroarytenoid muscle. In this process, the cricoarytenoid joint need not be opened unlike that of Isshiki's original description. This avoids overadduction and prolapse of the cartilage into the laryngeal lumen.

A recent advancement is augmentation of the postero-medial aspect of the implant as a tail-like projection. It helps in effective posterior medialization and supplements the arytenoid adduction and potentially substitutes it.

Adduction Arytenopexy

This is a modification of Isshiki's arytenoid adduction procedure developed by Zeitels et al.[27] Arytenoid adduction technique simulates the action of the lateral cricoarytenoid muscles, whereas adduction arytenopexy resembles the synchronous adductor contraction of all the intrinsic musculature. Unlike the classic arytenoid adduction where an anteriorly directed suture is used in adduction arytenopexy, a longer vocal cord is achieved by posteriorly displacing the arytenoids and maintaining its position with a posteriorly based suture.

Cricothyroid Subluxation

This procedure simulates cricothyroid muscle contraction for counter-tension on the thyroarytenoid muscle and for increasing the length of the musculomembranous vocal cord.[28] Cricothyroid subluxation procedure has further enhanced the vocal quality by enabling the ability to adjust the length and tension of the vocal cords. This procedure is performed by placing a nonabsorbable suture around the inferior cornu of the thyroid lamina. The suture is then passed submucosally underneath the cricoid anteriorly, and finer adjustments to the tension are made while the patient performs various phonatory tasks.

Reinnervation Techniques

Restoration of abductor motor function to the paralyzed larynx has interested otolaryngologists for years. Various surgical procedures have been attempted to restore function to one or both posterior cricoarytenoid muscles. Reinnervation techniques include nerve–muscle pedicle transfer,[29] as well as direct implantation of a donor nerve (such as the phrenic root) into the posterior cricoarytenoid.[30] Anatomoses of various donor (phrenic, ansa cervicalis, and hypoglossal) nerves to the RLN or its abductor division as direct neurorrhaphy or as a split graft have been attempted and have shown promising results in expert hands.[31,32] Combinations of adductor and abductor reinnervation techniques to restore "physiological (bidirectional) motion" are being studied. The early successes of reinnervation techniques have not been consistently duplicated. This has led to this technique not gaining widespread popularity among most laryngologists.

> ### Clinical Insight
>
> The assessment of outcome following any form of intervention, surgical or otherwise, to improve the vocal function has moved away from clinician-centered scoring systems to patient-centered quality of life measures. Interestingly, the patient's perception of their own voice may not correlate with the clinician's perception of the patient's voice. It is therefore important to record the pre- and post-"intervention" data in an objective manner to quantify effectiveness of treatment and compare various treatment modalities.

Speech and Language Therapy

Speech therapy plays a major role in improving the quality of life in patients with VFP. The voice becomes weak and breathy due to air escape. Loudness is reduced making it difficult to talk against background noise. Habitual pitch is lowered and pitch becomes unstable, with a reduction in the dynamic range. The cough is weak, making it difficult to clear secretions, and airway protection on swallowing is reduced. This may result in aspiration, especially of liquids. Effort closure, as when bearing down, is also impaired due to lack of Valsalva ability.

The main aims of therapy are to eliminate or prevent the development of inappropriate compensation, maximize glottal competency, provide a consistent subglottic air pressure, increase vocal power, stamina and agility, and provide strategies for airway clearance and minimizing the risk of aspiration.

A typical therapy program involves a full explanation of vocal fold palsy and a discussion of realistic outcomes of therapy. Techniques include relaxation for the head and neck area to prevent hyperfunction, diaphragmatic breathing with abdominal support of exhalation to develop a consistent and controllable subglottic air pressure, and glottal valving to encourage compensation by the healthy fold. Vocal strength and stamina are increased by phonating while varying the subglottic air pressure in a series of pulses using abdominal control, and vocal flexibility is developed by phonating throughout the pitch range. The exercises are aimed at maximizing the function of the impaired vocal mechanism while preventing overcompensation and allowing for spontaneous recovery.

Techniques such as pulling and pushing can be used while coughing to increase the efficiency of airway clearance.[33] Thickening liquids and maneuvers such as a head tilt to the unaffected side or a head turn to the paralyzed side while swallowing can reduce the risk of aspiration.

Bilateral Vocal Fold Paralysis

Etiology

Bilateral VFP in adults is commonly iatrogenic (57%), and its causes include thyroidectomy, pneumonectomy, and posterior fossa surgery, closely followed by trauma to the larynx such as postintubation or whiplash injury. Neurological causes such as encephalitis, syringobulbia, multiple sclerosis, and progressive bulbar palsy also constitute a large group (21%), as do malignancies. Certain infections (thyroiditis, syphilis, and viral diseases) are also thought to cause bilateral vocal cord paralysis, and in a large group of patients the cause remains unknown.[34]

Symptomatology

In the early stages, bilateral VFP presents with breathy or no voice, choking, and poor cough, and with a feeling of being out of breath due to the greatly reduced airway resistance caused by the abducted cords. With return of muscle tone and perhaps with partial reinnervation of adductors (laryngeal synkinesis[35]), the voice improves and choking becomes less problematic. Breathing at rest appears normal but rapidly worsens with any activity.

- Bilateral RLN paralysis: Patients present with stridor and dyspnea on exertion; good phonation.
- Bilateral superior laryngeal nerve paralysis: This is a rare condition. It causes severe aspiration due to reduced supraglottic sensation and subsequent pneumonia.
- Bilateral recurrent and superior laryngeal nerve paralysis: The vocal folds remain in the intermediate position, are flaccid and motionless, and cause complete aphonia and severe aspiration.

Management

Bilaterally paralyzed folds tend to assume the adductor position, therefore affecting the voice only mildly. The vocal folds may also move paradoxically causing more respiratory embarrassment. Therefore, the basic aims of management are as follows:

- Achieve a safe and stable airway.
- Preserve speech and voice quality.
- Allow safe swallowing without aspiration.

Tracheostomy is likely to be a part of the management of most patients with bilateral VFP, even if temporarily. This procedure can be performed under local anesthesia, and immediate relief of airway obstruction is obtained with relatively little reduction in the voice quality. Disadvantages include cosmetic and long-term care problems of the stoma as well as the need to occlude the stoma/use a speaking valve to phonate.

Vocal Fold Lateralization

There are several techniques to widen the glottal opening. However, with airway improvement, the quality of voice suffers. In general, surgical intervention is performed about a year following the paralysis to permit any spontaneous reinnervation to occur. The exception to this is in arytenoid fixation where surgery may be considered sooner.

1. Arytenoidectomy: This entails removing part or whole of the arytenoid cartilage and may be done endoscopically with the laser or microsurgically or externally via a lateral neck approach (Woodman procedure).
2. Arytenoidopexy: This involves displacement of vocal fold and arytenoid by means of suture passed around the vocal process of the arytenoid and secured laterally. This procedure has a relatively high failure rate.
3. Cordectomy: This consists of carbon dioxide laser (or cold steel) removal of a c-shaped wedge from posterior edge of one true vocal fold (posterior partial cordectomy) with or without additional removal of part of the false fold and arytenoidectomy.[36,37]

Bilateral adductor paralysis requires medialization techniques as for unilateral fold paralysis but modified on the contralateral side.

Superior Laryngeal Nerve Paralysis

Although RLN paralysis has received the lion's share of attention, there has been an awareness of superior laryngeal nerve paralysis throughout the history of laryngology. The superior laryngeal nerve is at risk of injury during surgical procedures such as thyroidectomy, neck dissection, cricopharyngeal myotomy, carotid endarterectomy, anterior approach to cervical spine, and supraglottic laryngectomy.

A wavy vocal fold margin was for long considered a hallmark of superior laryngeal nerve paralysis.[38] Different studies have revealed other signs such as glottic rotation, shortened flaccid or bowed vocal fold ipsilateral to the deficiency, height mismatch between the vocal folds, lack of mucosal blanching, and asymmetric mucosal wave.[39] The vocal fold maintains normal position during quiet respiration. Deviation of the posterior commissure to the paralyzed side is noticeable during phonatory effort (posterior commissure points to side of paralysis).[40] At rest, the vocal fold on the paralyzed side is slightly shortened and bowed, and may be depressed below level of normal side.

Loss of sensation to the supraglottic larynx may cause subtle symptoms such as frequent throat clearing, paroxysmal coughing, voice fatigue, and vague foreign body sensation. A slight voice change, which the patient usually interprets as hoarseness, may be induced by loss of motor function to the cricothyroid muscle. A common finding is diplophonia with decreased range of pitch, most noticeable when trying to sing. Other symptoms reported are vocal fatigue, lowered speaking pitch, reduction of vocal range, and monotony of voice.[41,42]

Clinical Insights

The subtle changes following superior laryngeal nerve paralysis can be missed by the untrained "eye" or "ear". The changes may not be that obvious at rest; they become more evident when the larynx is made to work harder and stretched. Diplophonia is pronounced when an attempt is made to reach the higher octaves; the wavy asymmetrical fold is better appreciated in this situation.

Table 18.3 Comparison of Clinical Findings of Recurrent and Superior Laryngeal Nerve Paralysis

	Unilateral	Bilateral
Recurrent laryngeal nerve		
• Incidence	Common	Rare
• Position of vocal cords	Paramedian/phonatory gap	Midline
• Voice	Normal/breathy	Normal/stridulous
• Airway	Adequate	Compromised
Superior laryngeal nerve		
• Incidence	Rare (unrecognized)	Very rare
• Position of vocal cords	Asymmetrical length Apparent shortening	Apparent shortening
• Voice	Diplophonia/unable to attain high pitch	Loss of dynamic range
• Aspiration	Likely	Serious risk

Electromyography (EMG) has emerged as an important tool in providing more information on superior laryngeal nerve dysfunction. A decrease in electrical activity on cricothyroid activation or fibrillations or positive sharp waves suggesting frank denervation are signs of superior laryngeal nerve dysfunction especially if the contralateral exhibits normal findings. However, the potential for errors exists here due to inaccurate needle placement. Some studies have indicated that EMG may not be an entirely reliable test.[21,43]

The clinical features comparing aspects of unilateral and bilateral recurrent and superior laryngeal nerve paralysis are listed in **Table 18.3**.

Pediatric Vocal Fold Paralysis

VFP is a rare disorder in children, differing in cause and management from that in adults. Early detection of pediatric laryngeal paralysis requires a high index of suspicion. The first case of unilateral vocal fold palsy was reported in 1881 by Sommerbrodt.[44] Murty et al[45] estimated the incidence of bilateral VFP at 0.75 cases per million births per year. Among congenital laryngeal anomalies, unilateral, or bilateral paralysis accounts for approximately 10% of all lesions, second only to laryngomalacia as a cause of congenital stridor.[46]

Etiology

The etiology of VFP may be divided according to the age of presentation: neonates (<6 months) and children (>6 months). In neonates, the important causes are congenital and birth trauma. VFP in children has been associated with hydrocephalus, meningomyelocele, meningocele, Arnold-Chiari malformation, and encephalocele.[46] The anatomy of the RLNs makes them vulnerable to injury during birth. Other iatrogenic causes include endotracheal intubations,

surgical correction of thoracic and cardiovascular anomalies such as repair of tracheoesophageal fistulas, Arnold-Chiari malformations, or myelomeningoceles.[46,47]

In older children, the etiological factors could be neurological as in multiple sclerosis, or due to surgical procedure or endotracheal intubation. Antibiotics and vaccinations have greatly reduced infectious causes of VFP due to whooping cough, encephalitis, polio, diphtheria, rabies, tetanus, syphilis, and botulism. Tumors of the larynx, thyroid, and lymphomas may also present with VFP.[48]

Presentation

VFP may affect any of the normal laryngeal functions of voice production, respiration, or deglutition. In neonates, unilateral VFP may cause airway obstruction and inspiratory stridor. In addition, this may lead to weak cry or phonation, poor swallowing coordination, and aspiration or may go undetected in the absence of airway or feeding problems until speech anomalies are detected. In older children, unilateral paralysis may present with soft or breathy voice.

Biphasic stridor is the most common feature of bilateral VFP. More than half of these patients are seen in the first 12 hours after birth. Some may require urgent airway intervention if the posterior glottic chink is inadequate.

Examination

A complete history should be sought, given the association of other systemic disorders with congenital VFP. The patient's respiratory status, feeding ability, weight gain, and vaccination status must be noted. This should be complemented by a thorough physical examination, especially of the neurological and cardiovascular systems.

Awake flexible fiberoptic nasopharyngolaryngoscopy is useful for bedside evaluation of a pediatric patient who is maintaining oxygen saturation with no cardiac anomaly.[49] It provides dynamic and direct visualization of the supraglottis and vocal folds. However, in a crying child, its view may be limited and formal evaluation under anesthesia is often required.

CT and MRI scans of the head and thorax help reveal the associated congenital neurological or cardiovascular anomalies. Electromyography has been found to have limitations in the neonatal larynx.[21]

The method of choice to evaluate vocal fold mobility is laryngoscopy and bronchoscopy with rigid telescopes under anesthesia. The advantage of direct rigid laryngoscopy is that it provides the opportunity to palpate the vocal folds and thereby help differentiate between VFP and conditions that mimic the problem, including interarytenoid web, posterior glottic stenosis, or cricoarytenoid fixation. During anesthesia, the child spontaneously ventilates and vocal fold movement may be directly observed toward the end of anesthesia as the child begins to wake up. Photographic and videodocumentation is extremely helpful for management but also for patient and parent education.

Management

In the absence of airway distress, management of neonates with unilateral VFP should be conservative as there is a possibility of recovery within 6 months of life. Rarely, tracheostomy may be required for airway distress. In the older child with unilateral VFP, surgical intervention may be required following a period of observation for recovery.

Future Research and Conclusion

There have been significant new developments in the past two decades leading to better understanding and improved assessment of patients with VFP.

Treatment options have multiplied and continue to evolve since the initial landmark work by Isshiki et al[50] over four decades ago. Newer techniques including laryngeal pacing may offer restoration of ventilation without surgical morbidity.[51,52] Laryngeal transplantation has already been attempted and as our understanding develops this may become a realistic option for certain patient groups.[53] The future holds further promise as research in gene therapy and tissue engineering has shown promise in facilitating neural regrowth, possibly enabling restoration of function of a paralyzed vocal fold.

References

1. Yumoto E, Minoda R, Hyodo M, Yamagata T. Causes of recurrent laryngeal nerve paralysis. Auris Nasus Larynx 2002;29(1):41–45
2. Myssiorek D. Recurrent laryngeal nerve paralysis: anatomy and etiology. Otolaryngol Clin North Am 2004;37(1):25–44, v
3. Benninger MS, Gillen JB, Altman JS. Changing etiology of vocal fold immobility. Laryngoscope 1998;108(9):1346–1350
4. Netterville JL, Koriwchak MJ, Winkle M, Courey MS, Ossoff RH. Vocal fold paralysis following the anterior approach to the cervical spine. Ann Otol Rhinol Laryngol 1996;105(2):85–91
5. Sulica L, Blitzer A. Vocal fold paresis: evidence and controversies. Curr Opin Otolaryngol Head Neck Surg 2007;15(3):159–162
6. Yamada M, Hirano M, Ohkubo H. Recurrent laryngeal nerve paralysis. A 10-year review of 564 patients. Auris Nasus Larynx 1983;10(Suppl):S1–S15
7. Younger D, Lange DJ, Klasner RE, et al. Neuromuscular disorders of the larynx. In: Blitzer A, et al, eds. Neurological Disorders of the Larynx. New York, NY: Thieme Medical Publishers; 1992
8. Daya H, Hosni A, Bejar-Solar I, Evans JN, Bailey CM. Pediatric vocal fold paralysis: a long-term retrospective study. Arch Otolaryngol Head Neck Surg 2000;126(1):21–25
9. Ertekin C, Seçil Y, Yüceyar N, Aydoğdu I. Oropharyngeal dysphagia in polymyositis/dermatomyositis. Clin Neurol Neurosurg 2004;107(1):32–37
10. Yumoto E, Minoda R, Hyodo M, Yamagata T. Causes of recurrent laryngeal nerve paralysis. Auris Nasus Larynx 2002;29(1):41–45
11. Núñez Batalla F, Suárez Nieto C, Llorente Pendás JL, Rodrigo Tapia JP, del Campo Rodríguez A, López Llames A. Preoperative evaluation in thyroplasty: the laryngeal lateral compression. Acta Otorrinolaringol Esp 2001;52(1):47–51
12. Hong KH, Jung KS. Arytenoid appearance and vertical level difference between the paralyzed and innervated vocal cords. Laryngoscope 2001;111(2):227–232
13. Richardson BE, Bastian RW. Clinical evaluation of vocal fold paralysis. Otolaryngol Clin North Am 2004;37(1):45–58
14. Terris DJ, Arnstein DP, Nguyen HH. Contemporary evaluation of unilateral vocal cord paralysis. Otolaryngol Head Neck Surg 1992;107(1):84–90
15. Stimpson P, Patel R, Vaz F, et al. Imaging strategies for investigating unilateral vocal cord palsy: how we do it. Clin Otolaryngol 2011;36(3):266–271
16. Rothenberg M. Interpolating subglottal pressure from oral pressure. J Speech Hear Disord 1982;47(2):219–223
17. Netterville JL. Rehabilitation of the unilaterally paralyzed larynx. Curr Opin Otolaryngol Head Neck Surg 1997;5:122–128
18. Dejonckere PH. Perceptual and laboratory assessment of dysphonia. Otolaryngol Clin North Am 2000;33(4):731–750
19. Sulica L, Blitzer A. Electromyography and the immobile vocal fold. Otolaryngol Clin North Am 2004;37(1):59–74
20. Munin MC, Rosen CA, Zullo T. Utility of laryngeal electromyography in predicting recovery after vocal fold paralysis. Arch Phys Med Rehabil 2003;84(8):1150–1153
21. Koufman JA, Postma GN, Whang CS, et al. Diagnostic laryngeal electromyography: the Wake Forest experience 1995-1999. Otolaryngol Head Neck Surg 2001;124(6):603–606
22. Jacobs IN, Finkel RS. Laryngeal electromyography in the management of vocal cord mobility problems in children. Laryngoscope 2002;112(7 Pt 1):1243–1248
23. Bruenings W. Uber eine neue Behandlungsmethode der Rekurrenslahmung. Verl Deutsch Laryng 1911;18:93–153
24. Koufman JA. Laryngoplasty for vocal cord medialization: an alternative to Teflon. Laryngoscope 1986;96(7):726–731
25. Cummings CW, Purcell LL, Flint PW. Hydroxylapatite laryngeal implants for medialization. Preliminary report. Ann Otol Rhinol Laryngol 1993;102(11):843–851
26. Slavit DH, Maragos NE. Physiologic assessment of arytenoid adduction. Ann Otol Rhinol Laryngol 1992;101(4):321–327
27. Zeitels SM, Mauri M, Dailey SH. Adduction arytenopexy for vocal fold paralysis: indications and technique. J Laryngol Otol 2004;118(7):508–516

28. Zeitels SM, Hillman RE, Desloge RB, Bunting GA. Cricothyroid subluxation: a new innovation for enhancing the voice with laryngoplastic phonosurgery. Ann Otol Rhinol Laryngol 1999;108(12):1126–1131

29. Tucker HM. Human laryngeal reinnervation: long-term experience with the nerve-muscle pedicle technique. Laryngoscope 1978;88(4):598–604

30. Goding GS Jr, Cummings CW, Bright DA. Extension of neuromuscular pedicles and direct nerve implants in the rabbit. Arch Otolaryngol Head Neck Surg 1989;115(2):217–223

31. Zheng H, Zhou S, Chen S, Li Z, Cuan Y. An experimental comparison of different kinds of laryngeal muscle reinnervation. Otolaryngol Head Neck Surg 1998;119(5):540–547

32. Paniello RC. Laryngeal reinnervation. Otolaryngol Clin North Am 2004;37(1):161–181, vii–viii

33. Stemple JC, Glaze LE, Klaben BG. Clinical Voice Pathology: Theory and Management. 3rd ed. San Diego, CA: Singular Publishing Group; 2000

34. Holinger LD, Holinger PC, Holinger PH. Etiology of bilateral abductor vocal cord paralysis: a review of 389 cases. Ann Otol Rhinol Laryngol 1976;85(4 Pt 1):428–436

35. Crumley RL. Laryngeal synkinesis revisited. Ann Otol Rhinol Laryngol 2000;109(4):365–371

36. Dennis DP, Kashima H. Carbon dioxide laser posterior cordectomy for treatment of bilateral vocal cord paralysis. Ann Otol Rhinol Laryngol 1989;98(12 Pt 1):930–934

37. Motta S, Moscillo L, Imperiali M, Motta G, Motta G. CO_2 laser treatment of bilateral vocal cord paralysis in adduction. ORL J Otorhinolaryngol Relat Spec 2003;65(6):359–365

38. Mackenzie M. Laryngeal paralysis from disease or injury of the superior laryngeal nerve. In: Mackenzie M, ed. Pharynx Larynx, and Trachea, New York, NY: Wood & Co; 1880:316–319

39. Arnold GE. Physiology and pathology of the cricothyroid muscle. Laryngoscope 1961;71:687–753

40. Abelson TI, Tucker HM. Laryngeal findings in superior laryngeal nerve paralysis: a controversy. Otolaryngol Head Neck Surg 1981;89(3 Pt 1):463–470

41. Titze IR. Principles of Voice Production. Englewood Cliffs, NJ: Prentice Hall; 1995

42. Dursun G, Sataloff RT, Spiegel JR, Mandel S, Heuer RJ, Rosen DC. Superior laryngeal nerve paresis and paralysis. J Voice 1996;10(2):206–211

43. Jansson S, Tisell LE, Hagne I, Sanner E, Stenborg R, Svensson P. Partial superior laryngeal nerve (SLN) lesions before and after thyroid surgery. World J Surg 1988;12(4):522–527

44. Cavanagh F. Vocal palsies in children. J Laryngol Otol 1955;69(6):399–418

45. Murty GE, Shinkwin C, Gibbin KP. Bilateral vocal fold paralysis in infants: tracheostomy or not? J Laryngol Otol 1994;108(4):329–331

46. Gentile RD, Miller RH, Woodson GE. Vocal cord paralysis in children 1 year of age and younger. Ann Otol Rhinol Laryngol 1986;95(6 Pt 1):622–625

47. Robertson JR, Birck HG. Laryngeal problems following infant esophageal surgery. Laryngoscope 1976;86(7):965–970

48. Bindlish V, Papsin BC, Gilbert RW. Pediatric laryngeal cancer: case report and review of literature. J Otolaryngol 2001;30(1):55–57

49. Berkowitz RG. Neonatal upper airway assessment by awake flexible laryngoscopy. Ann Otol Rhinol Laryngol 1998;107(1):75–80

50. Isshiki N, Morita H, Okamura H, Hiramoto M. Thyroplasty as a new phonosurgical technique. Acta Otolaryngol 1974;78(5-6):451–457

51. Mueller AH. Laryngeal pacing for bilateral vocal fold immobility. Curr Opin Otolaryngol Head Neck Surg 2011;19(6):439–443

52. Kwak PE, Friedman AD, Lamarre ED, Lorenz RR. Selective reinnervation of the posterior cricoarytenoid and interarytenoid muscles: an anatomical study. Laryngoscope 2010;120(3):463–467

53. Strome M, Stein J, Esclamado R, et al. Laryngeal transplantation and 40-month follow-up. N Engl J Med 2001;344(22):1676–1679

19 Neurological Voice Disorders

John S. Rubin, Ruth Epstein, and Kevin Shields

Anatomical Considerations: Vagus Nerve

The word vagus comes from the Greek "wanderer," and it is indeed the longest of the cranial nerves with the most wandering course. It provides both afferent and efferent fibers. About 80 to 90% of nerve fibers in the vagus nerve are afferent. Afferents include the somatic sensory fibers from the skin of the ear, the posterior ear canal, and the tympanic membrane. General afferent and efferent visceral fibers include those from the heart, pancreas, stomach, esophagus, upper respiratory tract, and pharynx. There are afferent autonomic fibers and afferent taste fibers.[1,2]

Efferent fibers include the somatic motor fibers to the vocal fold, larynx, and pharynx.

The vagal afferent central fibers originate in the nodose and jugular ganglions, which are sensory ganglions. They enter the medulla oblongata and lie in the groove between the olive and inferior peduncle with nerve roots of IX and XI. Rootlets unite to pass beneath the cerebellar flocculus. The vagus nerve leaves the cranial vault with cranial nerves IX and XI in the jugular foramen.[3]

Taste fibers from the epiglottis and larynx pass up the vagus to join the tractus solitarius. They terminate in the nucleus tractus solitarius. There are contacts with motor centers of medulla oblongata, pons, and spinal cord for mastication and deglutition.

Afferent fibers from the supraglottic larynx are transmitted by the internal branch of the superior laryngeal nerve. Those from the glottis and subglottis are transmitted by the recurrent laryngeal nerve. These go proximally to the nodose ganglion and then to the nucleus tractus solitarius, on an unilateral basis. There are then bilateral axonal impulses to the nucleus ambiguus at which time bilateral efferent fibers can, for example, lead to a bilateral glottic closure reflex arc.

A little more information on neural function to the larynx taken from animal research reveals the following: In squirrel monkey and rat, viscerotopic proprioceptive feedback has been demonstrated from the lungs and larynx to the nucleus tractus solitarius.

In squirrel monkey, the periaqueductal gray and lateral tegmentum of the midbrain have been noted to be crucial for vocalization. They appear to collect auditory, visual, and somatosensory input from diverse processing structures, motivation controlling input from limbic structures, and volitional input from anterior cingulate cortex. These are then connected with phonatory motor neurons via single to multiple interneurons. The nucleus retroambiguus has been noted to be a premotor relay station for laryngeal and expiratory vocalization.

Laryngeal receptors have been noted to be denser on the laryngeal surface of the epiglottis than on the true vocal folds and denser on the posterior than on the anterior aspects of the true vocal folds. Chemoreceptors appear to be limited to the supraglottis. They respond to changes in pH and water and appear able to detect chemical nonsaline-like molecules. Chemoreflexes include vocal fold closure, laryngospasm, apnea, bradycardia, hypertension, cough, and bronchoconstriction.

Peripherally, the velocity of axonal transmission of the recurrent laryngeal nerve is approximately 60 m/s. The recurrent laryngeal nerve supplies all intrinsic muscles except the cricothyroid muscle (supplied by the external branch of the superior laryngeal nerve). The posterior cricoarytenoid muscle is said to be the only abductor of the vocal folds. It is supplied by the recurrent laryngeal nerve. The only intrinsic muscle of the larynx said to have bilateral motor innervation is the interarytenoid muscle, supplied by both recurrent laryngeal nerves.

The course of the left recurrent laryngeal nerve is longer than that of the right, but the maximum diameter of fibers and of the myelin sheath of the left is slightly greater than that of the right, thereby allowing for approximately simultaneous activation of bilateral laryngeal muscles.

Extracranially, the cranial nerve XI joins the vagus near the nodose ganglion to supply motor branches. The vagus nerve trunk runs in the carotid sheath deep to and between the internal jugular vein and carotid artery.

The left vagus nerve enters the thorax between the aorta and the left pulmonary artery. It gives off the left recurrent laryngeal nerve that loops over the aortic arch distal to the ligamentum arteriosum and ascends in the tracheoesophageal groove medial to the thyroid gland, under the inferior constrictor muscle. It enters the larynx through the cricothyroid membrane behind the cricothyroid joint. The right vagus nerve crosses superficial to the subclavian artery. It gives off the right recurrent laryngeal nerve that loops under the subclavian artery and ascends in the tracheoesophageal groove in a more angulated course than the left recurrent laryngeal nerve. Approximately 1% of individuals have a nondescending right recurrent laryngeal nerve, due to the anatomical variant of a retroesophageal subclavian artery. Such individuals may also have dysphagia "lusoria" due to this aberrant positioning of the artery.

The superior laryngeal nerve arises below the nodose ganglion. Its internal branch is sensory. It pierces the thyrohyoid membrane in close association with the superior laryngeal artery. It supplies parasympathetic secretory innervation to glands supplying the true vocal folds as well as general sensory innervation to the supraglottic larynx. The external branch supplies motor innervation to the cricothyroid muscle and the inferior constrictor muscle. Terminal branches of the superior laryngeal nerve communicate with the recurrent laryngeal nerve as the ansa galeni.[1-7]

Language and Central Connections for Voicing

The left hemisphere is dominant in 95% of the population; it is said to be more analytic than the right hemisphere and tends to analyze information collected by the right hemisphere. It deals more with language, understanding, and expression. The left temporal and frontal areas are particularly important for language. There are connections with deeper structures processing sensory data, especially touch and hearing. Analysis of word meaning occurs in Wernicke area: it demonstrates activity, for example, when consonants are heard. Broca area abuts on/instructs the motor cortex relating to articulation and speech.[8]

On positron emission tomography scans, word reading activates parts of the visual cortex. Listening to speech causes activity in the auditory cortex. Thinking about words causes Broca area to activate. Thinking about words and speaking generates widespread activity.

The right hemisphere has roughly equivalent areas for environmental noise, prosody, and spatial skills. It tends to deal with visual activities, is more "intuitive," puts information together, and groups it.

As noted above, there are central connections of voicing involving many layers of the brain and brainstem. In the brainstem, the nucleus ambiguus is of particular importance from an effector standpoint and the solitary nucleus as an afferent center. In the midbrain, the periaqueductal gray and "limbic" system have a significant role. There are multiple connections in the subcortex. In the cortex areas such as Broca area, the motor and premotor cortex, the fronto and parietal cortex, and the anterior cingulate gyrus are all important. To look at it from a different perspective, a vocal idea might originate in Broca area, instructions might be sent to the motor nuclei in the cortex and precentral gyrus; coordinated muscular activity will then occur involving the larynx, thorax, abdomen, and articulators. Refinements occur via the extrapyramidal system, the basal ganglion, cerebellum, and the autonomic nervous system. Of course not only sound but also vibratory and tactile sensations are produced, which feed back among other systems through the auditory cortex. And this is vastly oversimplified.

Jürgens has identified in mammals a subcortical network of brain regions dedicated to phonation controlling many species-specific calls. He has postulated that the periaqueductal gray assists or regulates neurons of the lower brainstem via the reticular formation and lateral pontomedullary and limbic regions with cortical laryngeal projections. In humans, he postulates that this visceromotor pathway is exploited during emotive voicing, but that linguistic and paralinguistic speech involves more direct corticobulbar projections to the reticular formation. He emphasizes the temporal lobe activity for auditory self-regulation.[3-7,9]

Neurological Voice Disorders: Overview

The "classic" classification in relation to neurological damage differentiates lower motor from upper motor neuron deficits, working from peripheral to central. Thus, injuries at the level of the muscle, neuromuscular junction, the peripheral nerve, and the brainstem nucleus all lead to a flaccid lower motor neuron deficit. Lesions more proximal to this tend to cause a spastic upper motor neuron deficit.[10]

In this type of classification, there are several other disorders that fall under categories such as dyskinetic/extrapyramidal (Parkinson disease, essential tremor, dystonia, myoclonus, etc.); ataxia/cerebellar (degenerative disorders, hemorrhage, ischemia, etc.); apraxia of the cortex or subcortex (trauma, stroke, tumor, cerebral palsy, etc.); and mixed (amyotrophic lateral sclerosis [ALS], multiple sclerosis, Shy-Drager syndrome, etc.).

In our voice clinic, we prefer to use the Ramig classification[11] which looks at neurological disorders as they effect the voice from the standpoint of hypoadduction/hyperadduction/maladduction/abduction/mixed/miscellaneous. We find this helpful because it focuses on the effect of the disorder at a laryngeal level. (For swallowing issues, we do not find it as advantageous.)

Using the Ramig system, disorders of hypoadduction refer to any component of the motor unit (muscle, neuromuscular junction, peripheral nerve, or nucleus). Thus, they include all lower motor neuron disorders. They also include some cases of central origin including many cases of Parkinson disease, multiple system atrophy, traumatic and/or closed head brain injury, and trauma.

Hyperadduction refers to pseudobulbar issues, Huntington chorea, and adductor spasmodic dysphonia.

Maladduction refers to abductor spasmodic dysphonia and several paradoxical conditions.

Long-term tremor is seen in essential tremor, Parkinson disease, and cerebellar/dystonic tremor. Mixed disorders and miscellaneous include conditions such as multiple sclerosis (MS), ALS, apraxia, and Tourette syndrome.

Hypoadduction

A typical deficit at the muscular level might be a myopathy such as polymyositis or dermatomyositis. These are fairly unusual and are more likely to present with swallowing rather than pure voice issues. Muscular dystrophy and inclusion body myositis may fit into this category especially with oropharyngeal signs of progressive dysphagia and possibly with velopharyngeal insufficiency.[12,13]

The principal example of a disorder of neuromuscular junction transmission is myasthenia gravis. Myasthenia gravis[14,15] is a flaccid, fatigable condition, with a female to male prevalence of 2:1. Although its primary presentation is said to be ocular, approximately 30% will present initially with oropharyngeal symptoms. Thus, they may initially be seen in the voice clinic with symptoms such as vocal fatigue, dysarthria, dysphagia, and/or dysphonia progressing as the day progresses. To complicate matters, anticholinesterase receptor antibodies may be negative. Other investigations such as single-fiber electromyography (EMG) may also be negative and an empiric trial of pyridostigmine may be required. The Tensilon test, previously the main investigative test, is less used by many neurologists due to potential cardiac complications. Immunomodulatory therapy with corticosteroids, immunoglobulin, or plasma exchange in addition to cholinesterase inhibitors is the mainstay of treatment.

A lesion of the peripheral nerve could be caused by disorders such as trauma, tumor, iatrogenic illness, viral infection, collagen vascular disease, and Guillain-Barre syndrome. Terris et al[16] published a review of recent literature in 1992 of over 1000 cases with unilateral vocal fold paralysis. In their series, 35.8% were caused by neoplasm (54.8% lung cancer); a further 24.6% were postsurgical, the majority being post-thyroidectomy. Recently, for several reasons perhaps including more thyroidectomy being performed in major centers and more being performed with nerve stimulators, the likelihood of a peripheral nerve injury involving the recurrent laryngeal nerve being caused by thyroid surgery is decreasing.

By and large, unilateral recurrent laryngeal nerve injury paralysis is easy to identify with an immobile vocal fold typically in the paramedian position. Unilateral superior laryngeal nerve injury has a more complex presentation. Causes are typically surgical trauma, blunt neck trauma, or viral. Clinical presentation is subtle with vocal fatigue and relatively mild voice complaints. We feel that it is likely that this type of injury is going underdiagnosed.

A lesion at the brainstem nucleus is typically caused by infarction, not uncommonly of the posterior inferior cerebellar artery. Typical signs in a "classic" presentation of a Wallenberg syndrome are an ipsilateral Horner syndrome, facial dysesthesia, and limb ataxia with contralateral body pain/temperature impairment and motor weakness. Symptoms from a laryngeal standpoint are dysphagia, dysphonia, and dysarthria. Other causes include Arnold-Chiari malformation, syringobulbia, tumor, or trauma.

It is not uncommon for Parkinson disease to cause a clinical picture of hypoadduction of the larynx.[11,17,18] Parkinson disease is a degenerative disorder of nigrostriatal extrapyramidal neurons which leads to a deficiency in dopamine. It is a rather common disorder affecting approximately 1:100 population over the age of 60 years and 1:1000 population under the age of 60 years. There are approximately 1,500,000 sufferers in the United States. Typical global symptoms include shuffling gait, muscle rigidity, resting "pill-rolling" tremor, flat facial affect, stooped posture, and impaired postural reflexes.

Management is symptomatic with dopaminergic agents. Unfortunately, this has no effect on the underlying neurodegenerative process, and symptom progression (along with potential complications of treatment) will be seen with the passage of time. Nonpharmacological treatments include neurosurgical deep brain stimulation for selected patients.[19,20]

From the standpoint of voice, most individuals affected with Parkinson will develop some type of voice disorder (70 to 90%), and in early stages, voice and swallowing issues may be presenting signs. Symptoms include a soft, monotonous, often breathy voice with reduced volume and range. Vocal tremor may be present. Signs include bowed thin vocal folds with incomplete apposition on phonation. Articulation may also be impaired and sluggish, particularly involving lingual and labial consonants. On EMG, it is stated that there is reduced activation of the thyroarytenoid muscle, due to reduction of the central drive of the laryngeal motor neuron pool or due to loss of reciprocal suppression of the thyroarytenoid during inspiration. The Lee Silverman voice treatment has proven successful in several cases.

Parkinson plus syndromes generally include aspects of autonomic and/or supranuclear failure. These include syndromes such as progressive supranuclear palsy and multiple system atrophy. The voice is often breathy and can occur with unilateral or bilateral posterior cricoarytenoid dysfunction. Stridor and sleep disorder may be a relatively early symptom and must be watched for and managed aggressively—particularly in multiple system atrophy where it may contribute to nocturnal sudden death.[10,21-26]

Hyperadduction of the vocal folds can be present in many neurological disorders. They can often be divided into constant and irregular.[27]

Upper motor neuron deficits, sometimes called pseudobulbar palsy, typically present with fairly constant strained quality to the speaking voice.[11] Pseudobulbar palsy is an inaccurate term. The pathological findings are found bilaterally in the corticobulbar pathways of the pyramidal tracts at sites rostral to the cranial nuclei—especially the internal capsule. The most common cause is stroke, but it can be due to neurodegenerative (such as ALS), metabolic, and inflammatory conditions as well as neoplasms. The clinical picture is one of speech dysarthria (according to Duffy,[11,28] this is seen in 57% of stroke patients) and emotional lability. Other symptoms include dysphonia and dysphagia, while physical findings include a brisk jaw jerk and frontal release signs. The voice symptoms need to be reviewed in the context of the overlying speech dysarthria. The voice is often harsh, hoarse, monopitched and/or low pitched with a strained–strangled quality. There may also be pitch breaks.

Depending on the severity of the underlying condition, the voice may also be hypernasal with air escape into the nose.

Cerebral vascular accident, or stroke, often presents with pseudobulbar palsy type of voice symptoms. Stroke frequently manifests with other more global symptoms such as aphasia, speech apraxia, and dysarthria, as well as dysphagia. The voice clinic and the speech therapist play significant roles, not so much in diagnosis as in rehabilitation. Aspiration may be severe.

Adductor spasmodic dysphonia is another hyperadduction movement disorder.[29-31] It is a focal, slowly progressive dystonia involving certain laryngeal muscles but reflecting central motor processing issues/abnormalities. Present only during certain specific speech vocal tasks, it can be overridden by vegetative phenomena such as laughing or by chanting or singing. It is not present during sleep. There is a background of normal speech overlain by vocal spasms that are not under voluntary control. This leads to a strained and strangled speech pattern. (See Chapter 21 on dystonias for further information on spasmodic dysphonia.)

Incidence estimates vary, with one suggesting an incidence of 1:100,000. The disorder is more common in women than in men. The most common form (in 85 to 90%) is adductor spasmodic dysphonia, although abductor and mixed forms do occur. It is characterized by pitch breaks associated with vowels, in particular words ending with a vowel and being followed on by a word starting with a vowel (for example, "we—eat") and words with two vowels in tandem (for example, eight, year, eels). The vowels /e/ and /a/ are particularly problematic. Most common management is injection of low-dose botulinum toxin into the thyroarytenoid muscles.[32-38]

Tremor is another form of hyperfunctional voice disorder. It is pervasive in neurological disease but also present in the normal neurological system (as physiological tremor). It can occur as part of spasmodic dysphonia. There are also familial forms of tremor, predominantly with autosomal dominant pattern of inheritance. Tremor is the most common form of movement disorder, with an incidence said to be between 4 and 60 per 1000. While hands and feet are most commonly affected, the larynx is affected in between 4 and 20% of cases.[39-41]

Tremor can also be seen in conditions such as Parkinson disease (Logemann et al noted 13.5% of patients with vocal tremulousness), ataxic dysarthria, and palatopharyngeal myoclonus.[17]

Hyperadduction can occur with Huntington chorea. This is an autosomal dominant disorder affecting 4 to 8 per 100,000 population. There is a general loss of neurons in the caudate nucleus. Globally, the affected individual will have choreic movements affecting any part of the body. From a laryngeal perspective, irregular pitch fluctuations and voice arrests are seen. The voice tends to be harsh, with excess loudness, variations, and a strained–strangled quality.[27,42,43]

When examination of the larynx demonstrates hyperfunction of the supraglottic structures and hyperadduction is being considered, it is most important for the examiner to consider the possibility of underlying hypofunction at the level of the true vocal folds, with secondary supraglottic hyperfunction.

A variety of other neurological disorders can manifest with vocal issues.[10,44-48] These include (among others) ataxic dysphonia that is due to cerebellar dysfunction (a broad differential that includes vascular, inflammatory, metabolic, hereditary, and degenerative etiologies); ALS due to progressive degeneration of both upper and lower motor neurons; MS due to demyelination of white matter; Parkinson plus syndromes such as multiple system atrophy and progressive supranuclear palsy; apraxic dysphonia; and Gilles de la Tourette syndrome. In ALS, oropharyngeal symptoms may predominate in up to 25% of patients, making it a disorder that may initially present to the ENT surgeon. In MS, ENT symptoms such as vertigo, dysphagia, slurred speech, and trigeminal neuritis are common, occurring in upward of 50% of patients. Thus, MS may also present initially to the ENT surgeon. MS often affects young individuals aged 20 to 50. Vocal spasticity is not uncommon, and thus MS must be considered in the voice clinic in young people with unexplained dysphonia.

Evaluation and Management of Neurological Voice Disorders

The key to evaluation and management of neurological voice disorders is the development of a multidisciplinary team. The speech-language therapist and the ENT surgeon will be at the heart of the team together with the neurologist and the neurophysiologist. It is helpful to have a good relationship with the psychologist and psychiatrist as well. A careful case history emphasizing the psychosocial aspects is fundamental to diagnosis as well as successful management. Woodson[49] notes that issues such as vocal fatigue, pain when speaking, increased effort relating to speech, glottic tightness, pitch breaks, and tremor should all be looked at. Nasendoscopic visualization and recording with playback to the patient is the gold standard.[50-52] Assessment by the speech-language therapist with a trial of voice therapy generally occurs, and all patients are referred for baseline neurological evaluation.

The speech-language therapist has a crucial contribution to differential diagnosis.[50] His/her role includes perceptual and instrumental assessment that are critical to measurement of baseline status and outcome; patient counseling in all cases; and voice therapy in some cases.

A thorough voice history including onset and progressiveness is necessary. Typical vocal signs and symptoms to watch out for include quality issues such as hoarseness, harshness, and strain/strangle; vocal effort issues such as vocal fatigue and breathy, reduced range; and pitch issues such as pitch breaks, monopitch, and inappropriately high pitch. Tremor and nasality are also common. Speech issues such as unclear, slurred, or unintelligible character are also important. During the history taking, the physician must also look for swallowing and respiratory issues. While many of these issues may occur in functional voice disorders, pronounced vocal fatigue after mild voice use may represent a disorder of the neuromuscular junction, a jerky tight tremulous voice may be due to defective motor control, and vocal weakness with incomplete adduction of the glottis may be secondary to paresis. Woodson[49] reminds us that isolated hoarseness is not usually the only sign of a neurological disorder, while hoarseness and dysphagia likely point to a neurological basis.

The voice (and speech) examination begins with the ears to look for evidence of tympanic membrane retractions, glue ear, or other signs of eustachian tube dysfunction. It is also important to make certain that hearing loss is not an issue as it may impact on the way the individual hears their own or others' voices.

The nasal examination includes a search for allergic rhinitis (as it is identifiable in over 20% of Europeans and can affect the nasality of the voice). Of great importance is to evaluate the closure of the soft palate against Passavant ridge in the postnasal space. Velopharyngeal insufficiency is a significant feature of many neurological disorders and will allow for air (and also fluid) to escape up into the nasal passages. Sounds such as "ah" and "ee" and high-pressure sentences such as "Suzy stayed all summer" will assist in this investigation. During speech, it is useful to pinch and release the nostrils.[11,53]

Examination of the mouth is crucial. The character of the tongue should be looked for; for example, is it scalloped, discolored, or furred? Movement of the tongue is an important feature of the examination. Fasciculations may be an early feature of motor neuron disorders. And subtle or gross movement disorders on protrusion, retraction, and side-to-side tongue movement may be seen in several movement disorders as well as stroke. The integrity of cranial nerve XII should be assessed. Similarly, diminished voluntary soft palatal movement can be a prominent feature of disorders such as Parkinson plus syndromes and stroke. Palatal movement and sensory assessment are important to study as part of the evaluation of the integrity of the cranial nerves IX and X. During the mouth examination, the articulators should be assessed. Dysarthria is an extremely common symptom of stroke and the articulators can be checked with such sounds as /pa/, /ta/, /ga/. The fine control of the tongue against the hard palate, teeth, and lips should be checked.[11]

Flexible nasendoscopy is, perhaps, the crucial evaluation parameter.[52] During this examination, velopharyngeal insufficiency can be assessed for (as noted). The larynx and pharynx can then be examined in some detail. Observation of the larynx at rest for a full 2 minutes can provide important information about spontaneous movement of the larynx or other respiratory features and should be part of this examination. The larynx should be examined for clonic activity, tremor, supraglottic hyperfunction, paradoxical laryngeal movements, and hyperfunction or hypofunction at the level of the true glottis.

As a part of this examination, connected speech should be assayed as well as individual vowel sounds. The patient should be encouraged to repeatedly and rapidly sniff in (posterior cricoarytenoid muscle) alternating with a short /e/ to assess for vocal fatigue (a feature of myasthenia gravis).

Immobility of one or both vocal folds can be noted and the appearance of flaccidity looked for. A rotated larynx with scissoring of the arytenoids is an indication of possible superior laryngeal nerve palsy. Pooling in one piriform together with one vocal fold held in the "cadaveric" position may be indicative of a high vagal lesion. We use a vocal protocol for assessment of laryngeal dystonia (see **Box 19.1**). It is useful for assessment of all patients with suspected neurological disorders affecting the larynx. It must be recalled that identification of an immobile vocal fold on nasendoscopy cannot definitively differentiate paralysis from cricoarytenoid fixation. EMG is required for this.

Stroboscopy is advisable in all of these patients.[54] Assessment should be formalized using criteria such as described by Ford and Bless.[55] Features such as symmetry, synchrony, mucosal wave aberrations, and closure patterns are best assessed using stroboscopy (at the time of this writing videokymography and high-speed photography do not have routine application in our clinic but may in the future).

In the clinic at the first assessment, a general neurological evaluation should be systemically performed. It should include (at least) complete assessment of cranial nerve function; assessment of cerebellar coordination (gait, finger–nose and heel–shin tests, etc.); assessment of Parkinson disease (resting tremor, rigid tone, and bradykinesia); assessment for upper motor neuron signs (spastic increase in tone on passive movements, brisk reflexes, and upgoing plantar responses); chorea and other movements (unintended tremor of the head or extremities, spontaneous facial movements, etc.).[11]

Box 19.1 Laryngoscopy Protocol

> Quiet respiration
> Prolonged /i/; /a/
> Repetitive /i/ /i/ /i/
> /si/ /si/ /si/
> /mi/ /mi/ /mi
> /isi/ /isi/ /isi/
> We eat eel every day
> She speaks pleasingly
> We mow the lawn all year
> Peter will keep at the peak
> The puppy bit the tape
> Harry has a hat; his hat is on his head
> When he comes home we'll feed him
> Taxi, Taxi, Taxi
> Tell me about your voice problem or how did you get here today

The EMG is an enormously valuable tool.[56] It will help identify between neurogenic disorders, myopathies, and neuromuscular junction dysfunction such as myasthenia gravis. Broadly speaking, in the larynx it will allow for identification of normal function (normal recruitment pattern of normal motor units); old stable injury (decreased recruitment, large motor unit potentials firing at high frequencies, no spontaneous activity); reinnervation (decreased recruitment, low-amplitude polyphasic motor unit potentials, no spontaneous activity); and ongoing denervation (spontaneous activity: fibrillation potentials and positive sharp waves). It will assist in differentiation of immobility from fixation versus nerve injury. It is also essential for intraoperative nerve assessment and monitoring during such manipulations as botulinum injection.

All that said, the cardinal examination involves listening to the patient. Breathiness is often associated with incomplete apposition (not uncommonly due to palsy but also possibly due to Parkinson disease and other neurological disorders listed above); acquired articulation resonance or fluency problems are likely neurological in nature. Ten minutes of careful listening may be worth more than an entire battery of psychoacoustic investigations.

Management very much depends on the type and severity of the disorder and the degree of ENT manifestation.

For hypofunctional disorders with incomplete glottal closure, speech therapy is the initial therapy. Techniques emphasizing resonance and semi-occlusion exercises are often of benefit. Intensive work on the respiratory muscles with focused physiotherapy and/or accent method type of training is often also helpful. In parkinsonism the Lee Silverman technique has proven to be clinically useful.[57]

At times, medialization of one or both vocal folds either with external implant or with injection laryngoplasty has proven to be of benefit. Many of these injections can be performed in an augmented outpatient facility, and collagen, hydroxylapatite, and lyophilized dermis have been used in these settings. Fat is a useful substance to inject, but we do so under anesthesia. It is necessary to evaluate the patient's pulmonary function and ability to undergo a procedure under general anesthesia or even under local anesthesia. Case-by-case evaluation is crucial. In Parkinson plus syndromes with bilateral vocal cord paralysis, a tracheotomy may be lifesaving. As these patients are often wheelchair-dependent and have relatively limited activities of daily living, again a case-by-case determination is needed to decide if a limited glottic aperture may be acceptable for their needs without the requirement of tracheotomy and its attendant requirements of local toilet and aftercare, or with lesser surgical intervention such as a posterior cordotomy.

In hyperfunctional voice disorders, botulinum toxin is often a very useful adjunct. It has a long track record in spasmodic dysphonia. A recent Cochrane review[58] only identified one study meeting its inclusion criteria, but it reported significant benefit in terms of several acoustic and patient ratings. Botulinum toxin may be indicated in essential tremor (although in the cases of tremor it is often of less benefit due to the frequent association of vocal fold atrophy; occasionally these patients benefit from injection augmentation). In supranuclear spasticity, it is also often of benefit. Anecdotally, we have found deep brain stimulation to have some benefit in a few patients who underwent it for generalized dystonia, but we have needed to continue with laryngeal botulinum injections concomitantly.

There are several systemic medications that have been used in movement disorders. It has been hypothesized that central nervous system gamma-aminobutyric acid mechanisms may underlie essential tremor. Primidone and β-blockers have been recommended as the mainstay of medical therapy for disabling limb or head tremor. Anecdotally, we have not noted much voice benefit in those in whom we have recommended use of β-blockers.

We are not aware of any controlled studies demonstrating sustained benefit from neuropharmacological management of spasmodic dysphonia. Anticholinergics, muscle relaxants, central nervous system depressants, and β-adrenergic blockers have all been anecdotally trialled.[59] Occasionally, abductor spasmodic dysphonia can be confused with Parkinson disease and a trial of dopamine may be helpful. In hyperadduction disorders, botulinum toxin remains the medical treatment of choice (although it is not Food and Drug Administration approved for this specific application) in spite of it having adverse affects as well as benefits.

Dysphagia

This chapter has focused on neurological voice disorders rather than dysphagia. A few words about dysphagia management is of benefit, however, as the two issues go together often.[60-63] The key to successful dysphagia management is accuracy of assessment. Such assessment needs to review several features. Above the esophagus these include oral and pharyngeal effort and function, hyolaryngeal and epiglottic function, airway protection, frank or silent penetration of materials into the endolarynx, residual materials in the vallecula and/or hypopharynx, etc. Within the esophagus, they include mucosal integrity (evidence of a pouch, web endo- or extra-esophageal lesion impacting on or compressing the esophagus, etc.), manometric evaluation of the upper and lower esophageal sphincters, evidence of dysmotility, peristalsis, etc. Not all of these evaluations may be available to the practitioner. Videofluoroscopy and bedside fiberoptic endoscopic evaluation of swallow are the gold standard for screening. Management follows accordingly. It may vary from recommendations of chin tuck or head turn during swallow, multiple swallows, to recommendation of nil by mouth with alternative feeding. Esophageal dilatation, cricopharyngeal myotomy, and staple of pouch may all be recommended again depending on the magnitude and type of finding. Occasionally, botulinum injection into the cricopharyngeus is of use for primary cricopharyngeal spasm. For intractable aspiration, tracheotomy, epiglottic flap closure of the laryngeal introitus, or even partial or total laryngectomy or laryngotracheal separation may be required.

Several patients with advanced Parkinson disease and ALS note difficulties with drooling. Botulinum toxin injected directly into the submandibular glands (and/or parotid glands) can prove beneficial in these instances. This may not have a direct impact on their voicing, but is an important adjunct in improvement of their quality of life.

Summary

This chapter presents a brief overview of a rather complex subject. It is not meant to be inclusive but rather offers a perspective on a neurological approach to voice disorders. It covers the anatomy of the vagus nerve, some constructs on language, and central connections for voicing. What follows is an overview of neurological voice disorders, in particular looking at them from the standpoint of hyper- and hypoadduction. It ends with some thoughts about the neurological voice assessment in the clinic and its management.

References

1. Boileau Grant JC, Basmajian JV. Grant's Method of Anatomy. 7th ed. Baltimore, MD: Williams and Wilkins Company; 1965
2. Gray H. Gray's Anatomy. 15th ed (facsimile 1995). New York, NY: Barnes &Noble; 1901
3. Benninger MS, Gardner GM, Schwimmer C, et al. Laryngeal neurophysiology. In: Rubin JS, Sataloff RT, Korovin GK, eds. Diagnosis and Treatment of Voice Disorders. 3rd ed. San Diego, CA: Plural Publishers; 2006:109–114
4. Jürgens U, Ploog D. Cerebral representation of vocalization in the squirrel monkey. Exp Brain Res 1970;10(5):532–554
5. Jürgens U. Neural pathways underlying vocal control. Neurosci Biobehav Rev 2002;26(2):235–258
6. Jürgens U. A study of the central control of vocalization using the squirrel monkey. Med Eng Phys 2002;24(7–8):473–477
7. Jürgens U. The neural control of vocalization in mammals: a review. J Voice 2009;23(1):1–10
8. Spain R, Mandel S, Sataloff RT. The neurology of stuttering. In: Rubin JS, Sataloff RT, Korovin GK, eds. Diagnosis and Treatment of Voice Disorders. 3rd ed. San Diego, CA: Plural Publishers; 2006:115–124
9. Kuypers HG. Corticobulbar connexions to the pons and lower brainstem in man: an anatomical study. Brain 1958;81(3):364–388
10. Aronson AE. Clinical Voice Disorders. 3rd ed. New York, NY: Thieme Medical Publishers; 1990
11. Smith ME, Ramig LO. Neurologic disorders and the voice. In: Rubin JS, Sataloff RT, Korovin G, eds. Diagnosis and Treatment of Voice Disorders. 3rd ed. San Diego, CA: Plural Publications; 2006: 447–469
12. Younger DS, Lange DJ, Lovelace RE, et al. Neuromuscular disorders of the larynx. In: Blitzer A, et al, eds. Neurologic Disorders of the Larynx. New York, NY: Thieme Medical Publishers; 1992:246
13. Mastaglia FL. Genetic myopathies. In: Swash M, Oxbury J, eds. Clinical Neurology. New York, NY: Churchill Livingstone; 1991:1286
14. Fenichel GM. Clinical syndromes of myasthenia in infancy and childhood. A review. Arch Neurol 1978;35(2):97–103
15. Scadding GK, Harvard CW. Pathogenesis and treatment of myasthenia gravis. Br Med J (Clin Res Ed) 1981;283:1008–1012
16. Terris DJ, Arnstein DP, Nguyen HH. Contemporary evaluation of unilateral vocal cord paralysis. Otolaryngol Head Neck Surg 1992;107(1):84–90
17. Logemann JA, Fisher HB, Boshes B, Blonsky ER. Frequency and cooccurrence of vocal tract dysfunctions in the speech of a large sample of Parkinson patients. J Speech Hear Disord 1978;43(1): 47–57
18. Hornykiewicz O. Metabolism of brain dopamine in human parkinsonism: neurochemical and clinical aspects. In: Costa E, Cote L, Yahr M, eds. Biochemistry and Pharmacology of the Basal Ganglia. New York, NY: Raven Press; 1966:171–186
19. Klostermann F, Ehlen F, Vesper J, et al. Effects of subthalamic deep brain stimulation on dysarthrophonia in Parkinson's disease. J Neurol Neurosurg Psychiatry 2008;79(5):522–529
20. D'Alatri L, Paludetti G, Contarino MF, Galla S, Marchese MR, Bentivoglio AR. Effects of bilateral subthalamic nucleus stimulation and medication on parkinsonian speech impairment. J Voice 2008;22(3):365–372
21. Ramig LO, Bonitati C, Lemke J, et al. Voice treatment for patients with Parkinson disease: development of an approach and preliminary efficacy data. J Med Speech-Lang Pathol 1994;2(3):191–209
22. Dromey C, Ramig LO, Johnson AB. Phonatory and articulatory changes associated with increased vocal intensity in Parkinson disease: a case study. J Speech Hear Res 1995;38(4):751–764
23. Ramig LO, Dromey C. Aerodynamic mechanisms underlying treatment-related changes in vocal intensity in patients with Parkinson disease. J Speech Hear Res 1996;39(4):798–807
24. Stewart C, Winfield L, Hunt A, et al. Speech dysfunction in early Parkinson's disease. Mov Disord 1995;10(5):562–565
25. Hanson DG, Gerratt BR, Ward PH. Cinegraphic observations of vocal pathology in Parkinson's disease. Laryngoscope 1984;94:348–353
26. Smith ME, Ramig LO, Dromey C, et al. Intensive voice treatment in Parkinson's disease: laryngostroboscopic findings. J Voice 1995;10:354–361
27. Brin MF, Fahn S, Blitzer A, et al. Movement disorders of the larynx. In: Blitzer A, Brin MF, Sasaki CT, et al, eds. Neurologic Disorders of the Larynx. New York, NY: Thieme Medical Publishers; 1992: 248–278
28. Duffy J. Motor Speech Disorders. St. Louis, MO: Mosby; 1995
29. Blitzer A, Brin MF. The dystonic larynx. J Voice 1992;6(4):294–297
30. Hanson DG, Logemann JA, Hain T. Differential diagnosis of spasmodic dysphonia: a kinematic perspective. J Voice 1992;6:325–337
31. Cannito MP, Kondraske GV, Johns DF. Oral-facial sensorimotor function in spasmodic dysphonia. In: Moore CA, Yorkston KM, eds. Dysarthria and Apraxia of Speech: Perspectives on Management. Baltimore, MD: Paul H. Brookes Publishing Co.; 1991:205–225
32. Izdebski K. Symptomatology of adductor spasmodic dysphonia: a physiologic model. J Voice 1992;6:306–319
33. Blitzer A, Brin MF, Fahn S, Lovelace RE. Clinical and laboratory characteristics of focal laryngeal dystonia: study of 110 cases. Laryngoscope 1988;98(6 Pt 1):636–640
34. Blitzer A, Lovelace RE, Brin MF, Fahn S, Fink ME. Electromyographic findings in focal laryngeal dystonia (spastic dysphonia). Ann Otol Rhinol Laryngol 1985;94(6 Pt 1):591–594
35. Blitzer A, Brin MF. Laryngeal dystonia: a series with botulinum toxin therapy. Ann Otol Rhinol Laryngol 1991;100(2):85–89
36. Ludlow CL, Adler CH, Berke GS, et al. Research priorities in spasmodic dysphonia. Otolaryngol Head Neck Surg 2008;139(4):495–505
37. Ludlow CL. Treatment for spasmodic dysphonia: limitations of current approaches. Curr Opin Otolaryngol Head Neck Surg 2009;17(3):160–165
38. Ludlow CL. Spasmodic dysphonia: a laryngeal control disorder specific to speech. J Neurosci 2011;31(3):793–797
39. Elble RJ, Koller WC. Tremor. Baltimore, MD: Johns Hopkins University Press; 1990

40. Gillivan-Murphy P, Miller N. Voice tremor: what we know and what we do not know. Curr Opin Otolaryngol Head Neck Surg 2011;19(3):155–159

41. Sulica L, Louis ED. Clinical characteristics of essential voice tremor: a study of 34 cases. Laryngoscope 2010;120(3):516–528

42. Penney JB Jr, Young AB, Shoulson I, et al. Huntington's disease in Venezuela: 7 years of follow-up on symptomatic and asymptomatic individuals. Mov Disord 1990;5(2):93–99

43. Ramig LA. Acoustic analyses of phonation in patients with Huntington's disease. Preliminary report. Ann Otol Rhinol Laryngol 1986;95(3 Pt 1):288–293

44. Aronson AE, Brown JR, Litin EM, Pearson JS. Spastic dysphonia. II. Comparison with essential (voice) tremor and other neurologic and psychogenic dysphonias. J Speech Hear Disord 1968;33(3):219–231

45. Darley FL, Brown JR, Goldstein NP. Dysarthria in multiple sclerosis. J Speech Hear Res 1972;15(2):229–245

46. Stacy M, Jankovic J. Differential diagnosis of Parkinson's disease and the parkinsonism plus syndromes. Neurol Clin 1992;10(2):341–359

47. Chen A, Garrett CG. Otolaryngologic presentations of amyotrophic lateral sclerosis. Otolaryngol Head Neck Surg 2005;132(3):500–504

48. Bawa R, Ramadan HH, Wetmore SJ. Bilateral vocal cord paralysis with Shy-Drager syndrome. Otolaryngol Head Neck Surg 1993;109(5):911–914

49. Woodson G. Management of neurologic disorders of the larynx. Ann Otol Rhinol Laryngol 2008;117(5):317–326

50. Woodson GE, Zwirner P, Murry T, et al. Functional assessment of patients with spasmodic dysphonia. J Voice 1992;6:338–343

51. Woodson GE, Zwirner P, Murry T, et al. Use of flexible fiberoptic laryngoscopy to assess patient with spasmodic dysphonia. J Voice 1991;5:85–91

52. Koufman JA. Evaluation of laryngeal biomechanics by fiberoptic laryngoscopy. In: Rubin JS, Sataloff RT, Korovin GK, eds. Diagnosis and Treatment of Voice Disorders. 3d ed. San Diego, CA: Plural Publishing; 2006:193–204

53. Yorkston KM, Beukelman DR, Bell KR (eds). Laryngeal function. In: Clinical Management of Dysarthric Speakers. Boston, MA: College-Hill Press, Little, Brown, and Co.; 1988:241–267

54. Sataloff RT. Physical examination. In: Rubin JS, Sataloff RT, Korovin GK, eds. Diagnosis and Treatment of Voice Disorders. 3rd ed. San Diego, CA: Plural Publishers; 2006:179–192

55. Ford C, Bless D. Assessment and Surgical Management of Voice Disorders. New York, NY: Raven Press; 1991

56. Sulica L, Blitzer A, Meyer T. Laryngeal electromyography. In: Rubin JS, Sataloff RT, Korovin GK, eds. Diagnosis and Treatment of Voice Disorders. 3rd ed. San Diego, CA: Plural Publishers; 2006:249–260

57. Ramig LO, Countryman S, Thompson LL, Horii Y. Comparison of two forms of intensive speech treatment for Parkinson disease. J Speech Hear Res 1995;38(6):1232–1251

58. Watts C, Nye C, Whurr R. Botulinum toxin for treating spasmodic dysphonia (laryngeal dystonia): a systematic Cochrane review. Clin Rehabil 2006;20(2):112–122

59. Rincon F, Louis ED. Benefits and risks of pharmacological and surgical treatments for essential tremor: disease mechanisms and current management. Expert Opin Drug Saf 2005;4(5):899–913

60. Bours GJJ, Speyer R, Lemmens J, Limburg M, de Wit R. Bedside screening tests vs. videofluoroscopy or fibreoptic endoscopic evaluation of swallowing to detect dysphagia in patients with neurological disorders: systematic review. J Adv Nurs 2009;65(3):477–493

61. Langmore SE, Schatz K, Olson N. Endoscopic and videofluoroscopic evaluations of swallowing and aspiration. Ann Otol Rhinol Laryngol 1991;100(8):678–681

62. Logemann JA, Veis S, Colangelo L. A screening procedure for oropharyngeal dysphagia. Dysphagia 1999;14(1):44–51

63. Meyer TK. The larynx for neurologists. Neurologist 2009;15(6):313–318

20 Muscle Tension Dysphonia

Matthew S. Clary, Sarah L. Schneider, and Mark S. Courey

Muscle tension dysphonia (MTD) is a condition that is defined by increased tension of the intrinsic and extrinsic muscles of the larynx that results in a pathological disturbance of voice. MTD was originally described by Morrison et al in 1983 in response to the observation of voice changes in response to stress.[1] Since then MTD has evolved considerably in both the use of the term and its clinical definition.

The condition of MTD has been plagued by a lack of standardization in its use. MTD is often incorrectly used interchangeably with the term "functional dysphonia" and has been used to categorize the amalgam of voice conditions that are not considered secondary to a defined lesion. This ambiguity has led to the use of MTD as a catchall diagnosis for dysphonia not otherwise specified by otolaryngologists who are not well versed in the management of voice patients. Further complicating the diagnosis of MTD is the lack of evidence and agreement in the literature describing the epidemiology, etiology, pathophysiology, methods of diagnosis, and management. There is great variability in the clinical presentation of MTD. As a result of this variability, making the diagnosis may be challenging and the condition may be equally challenging to treat. The purpose of this chapter is to provide the otolaryngologist with a better understanding of MTD and provide a practical approach to its diagnosis and management.

Epidemiology/Etiology

There are very few studies existing that attempt to characterize the epidemiology of MTD. The true prevalence is unknown, although estimates of those with "voice disorders" range from 0.65 to 15% of the general population.[2,3] Roy et al found that almost 30% of their study group had a voice disorder sometime during their lives.[3] Several studies report that MTD accounts for at least 10 to 40% of visits to voice centers.[4-6] Yet, true incidence data are difficult to obtain given the aforementioned inconsistency in terminology and the variable nature of the disease. It has been shown that 40% of dysphonic patients do not have an obvious organic cause.[7] The data that exist show a strong correlation with voice use. As a result, singers, teachers, salespeople, and those whose occupation requires daily intensive voice use are much more likely to be diagnosed with MTD. Laryngopharyngeal reflux (LPR), high stress levels, recurrent respiratory illness, exposure to inhaled irritants, female gender, and advanced age have all been associated with greater risk of developing MTD as well.[3,8-10]

MTD is generally divided into two different subtypes, primary and secondary. Primary MTD is characterized by dysphonia with increased laryngeal tension, without any identifiable mass or neurogenic lesions, and in the absence of any psychological disorder.[4] Secondary MTD is characterized by excess muscle contraction that develops in association with or as a presumed response to an identifiable organic lesion, such as a vocal fold mass or nerve paresis which impairs glottal function. The response of the body to the glottal malfunction is to attempt to regain "normal" function through increased activity in the intrinsic and extrinsic laryngeal musculature. Due to this increased activity, patients with long-standing primary MTD may have an increased propensity to develop organic lesions, thus creating a self-reinforcing cycle.[11-13]

Pathophysiology

MTD can be caused by a multitude of inciting events as they relate to the risk factors discussed previously. Most often the clinician is not able to identify the specific cause for the maladaptive voicing pattern. However, regardless of the etiology, the end result of increased laryngeal tension follows a typical physiological pattern. These patients develop into a state of hyperfunction of the tongue base, neck, and laryngeal muscles, often both during phonation and at rest. The muscles affected include two groups: the intrinsic laryngeal muscles and the extrinsic muscles. The intrinsic muscles include the thyroarytenoid, cricothyroid, lateral and posterior cricoarytenoid, and interarytenoid muscles. The extrinsic group is further divided into those in the perilaryngeal region and those more closely related to the tongue base and floor of the mouth. In the perilaryngeal region, these include the sternohyoid, sternothyroid, thyrohyoid, omohyoid, and sternocleidomastoid muscles. In the tongue base region, these include the digastric, mylohyoid, genioglossus, and hyoglossus muscles. The upper esophageal sphincter (UES), comprised of the cricopharyngeus and thyropharyngeus muscles, has also been implicated by some as contributing to laryngeal position and tension. This could in part help explain the association that LPR may have with MTD.[14]

The extrinsic muscles are generally responsible for elevation of the laryngeal complex during swallowing. They are not activated under normal circumstances during voice production. In patients with MTD, however, they are found to be chronically contracted during voicing, and often even at rest. This hyperfunction generally results in elevation in the position and alteration in the tilt of the larynx.[4,13,15] Changes in the position and forces on the larynx then ultimately lead to changes in the intrinsic muscle function. This may lead to abnormal stress within the vocal fold and specifically the superficial lamina propria.[16] The effect of this abnormal and inefficient vibratory pattern on the vocal fold leads to edema within the lamina propria, which can then cause changes in vocal quality.[16,17] The cumulative effect of these vocal stresses can lead to the development of benign vocal fold lesions such as nodules, cysts, polyps, and granulomas.

Patient Evaluation

When evaluating a patient with possible MTD, it is especially important to pay attention to details of the history and physical examination. Rarely does one point of the history or feature of the examinations allow the physician to confirm the suspected diagnosis. There is a significant variability in the way patients present. As a result, it is important to evaluate the entire set of patient data to arrive at the correct conclusion.

History

The patient histories in MTD do, in general, follow a basic pattern. Their symptoms typically include voice changes for a prolonged duration, from months to years. They will state that they have vocal fatigue that is worse at the end of the day and exacerbated by prolonged voice use. Often they complain of throat discomfort and tightness. When probed further, they frequently have chronic throat clearing that is worse with voicing. They can have variable globus sensation as well. Interestingly, Perera et al demonstrated a significant increase in upper esophageal pressure in normal patients during phonation, which could explain in part this phenomenon.[18] Frequently, patients state that they have undergone previous trials of antireflux medications without improvement in their symptoms.

Clinical Pearls

Most common complaints:
- Hoarseness
- Vocal fatigue
- Reduced range when singing
- Globus sensation
- Throat discomfort that is worse with voice use
- Chronic cough and/or throat clearing

It is important to explore potential risk factors for the development of maladaptive voicing patterns. First and foremost, occupational, recreational, and home voice use should be thoroughly explored. Extended telephone use, public speaking, singing, and crowded home environments are found to be recurring themes with this population. They should be questioned about respiratory illness or laryngitis that was temporally related to the initiation of their complaints. Traumatic injury, as well as chronic neck and spine issues, can lead to an alteration in posture and consequently neck muscle activation. LPR symptomatology should be elucidated along with correlation between reflux

and voice symptoms. Lastly, primary spoken language should be considered as some languages require more activation of the tongue base and extrinsic muscles.

Physical Examination

The physical examination for patients with voice disturbances builds upon the standard head and neck in important ways. First, there needs to be a greater focus on the examiner's perception of the patient's voice. Evaluation of the voice should include both spontaneous speech and phonemically balanced reading samples such as the Rainbow Passage, the Zoo Passage, or those sentences used in Consensus Auditory-Perceptual Evaluation of Voice tool. Voicing features can differ greatly between these two activities and help differentiate MTD from other voice disorders such as spasmodic dysphonia (SD) or Parkinson disease. Attention should be paid to the overall grade of the voice, degree of vocal strain, and whether resonance or vocal tone focus is in the throat or ideally in the anterior vocal tract. Perceptually, the typical MTD patient's voice has a rough, strained quality with reduced airflow or a breathy strained quality.

The second aspect of the examination that should receive greater attention is the manifestation of elevated tension in the tongue base and anterior neck. Difficulty in relaxation of the tongue base can be assessed when evaluating the oral cavity with a tongue depressor and more reliably on insertion of a rigid 70-degree endoscope during stroboscopy. Tongue out and lip trills (raspberries) are useful maneuvers that can help elucidate the presence of tongue base tension. The neck should be evaluated for exaggerated movement of the submental muscle groups during phonation, suggesting tongue base activation (**Fig. 20.1**). On palpation, the relative locations of the hyoid bone and thyroid cartilage should be assessed. In individuals without MTD, there is a relaxed nontender space

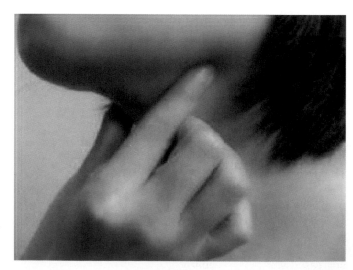

Figure 20.1 Suprahyoid palpation—palpation of this region will help reveal increased tongue base activation.

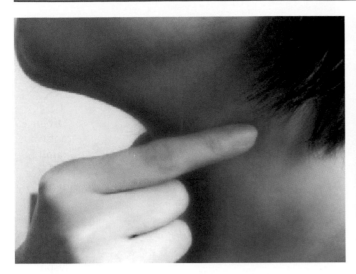

Figure 20.2 Thyrohyoid palpation—firm palpation of this area may reveal a reduction in the thyrohyoid space at rest and during phonation resulting in discomfort in many patients with muscle tension dysphonia.

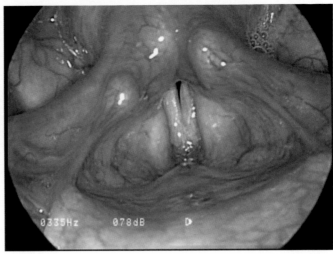

Figure 20.3 Supraglottic constriction—constriction can range from mild lateral compression of the false vocal folds to complete concentric compression that obscures the view of the true vocal folds.

between these structures (thyrohyoid space; **Fig. 20.2**). There is little movement of the hyoid and thyroid cartilage during relaxed voicing, while the thyrohyoid space is maintained in a relatively stable position. In MTD patients, the thyrohyoid space may be reduced or asymmetric at rest and during phonation due to contraction of the extrinsic laryngeal muscles. As a diagnostic maneuver, moderately firm circumlaryngeal palpation can be applied to the region around the larynx and thyrohyoid space. Due to chronic hyperactivity in the strap muscles, patients with MTD will generally report discomfort during this maneuver. Postural asymmetry or an irregular neck position should alert the physician to explore the reason because these can result in increased tension in the perilaryngeal muscles.

The endoscopic portion of the examination is the last component of the patient evaluation and is divided into still-light and stroboscopic findings. Most practitioners have their own preference in using flexible or rigid endoscopy. The rigid endoscope has the benefit of providing tactile feedback on tongue base tension on its insertion, whereas the flexible endoscope provides a more anatomically natural examination. Regardless of the tool that is chosen, the evaluated features are similar. The key elements of the still-light examination are tongue base position, constriction of the supraglottis, rotation of the larynx, and organic causes of glottal incompetence. MTD patients are more likely to retract their tongue base, making the examination more difficult overall. Constriction of the vestibular folds and arytenoids is highly suggestive of increased tension (**Fig. 20.3**). The global appearance of laryngeal rotation can indicate asymmetric muscular activation. Lastly, the examination should focus on identifying glottal incompetence. Potential causes include decreased vocal fold mobility, vocal fold lesions, and vocal fold atrophy. Vocal fold vibration and glottic closure are evaluated during the stroboscopic examination. Asymmetry

in the vibration of the vocal folds and chasing asymmetry during vibration are common findings in MTD patients. Incomplete posterior glottic closure is often present with increased laryngeal tension that is associated with MTD.

It is important to reiterate that the patient examination should be viewed globally. There are many studies demonstrating a high prevalence of muscle tension patterns in asymptomatic patients. As a result, stroboscopic features alone can be misleading and must be considered in conjunction with the collective history, as well as complete physical examination.

Clinical Pearls

There is a clinical variant of MTD that will present with increased laryngeal tension, without voice changes. The primary complaint is typically increased vocal effort and subsequent fatigue. These patients can be managed in the same manner as those with MTD.

Differential Diagnoses

It can be very challenging to evaluate patients with voice disorders. There is considerable overlap in the presenting features of the various disorders affecting the voice. Below is a description of the differentiating factors for some of the diagnoses more commonly confused with the MTD diagnosis.

Laryngopharyngeal Reflux

Reflux is widely used to explain voice changes, especially in the absence of an organic cause. The MTD symptoms in common with reflux include hoarseness, globus, chronic throat clearing, and cough.[19] The impact of refluxate on the vocal folds as an independent cause of hoarseness is likely overstated. Between 35 and 78% of MTD patients are reported to have LPR.[5,20] The prevalence may actually be much lower, as other studies have found.[9] Irrespective of the true prevalence of reflux, causality has not been proven. Reflux may be a cofactor in MTD. Refluxate can exert an effect on the UES leading to increased vocal fold tension.[14] Increased tongue base tension in MTD can cause relaxation of the UES, predisposing the patient to concurrent LPR. Historical features such as correlation of symptoms with voice use, responsiveness to antireflux therapy, and reflux study results are better differentiators. Empirical treatment is a reasonable diagnostic and therapeutic option in patients who are suspected to have symptoms related to LPR.

Spasmodic Dysphonia

SD is a neurogenic focal dystonia of the larynx that typically manifests with sound-specific phonatory breaks. These patients typically use increased tension to compensate for their laryngeal spasm. As a result, their examination can appear very similar to MTD, especially in less severe disease. SD generally has glottal stops on specific sounds, and the patient can often articulate which sounds are particularly troublesome. Improvement in symptoms with whispering, with high pitches, and during emotional voicing can help differentiate the two entities.

Laryngeal Hypersensitivity

Voice disorders included under the umbrella of laryngeal hypersensitivity are irritable larynx, laryngospasm, and paradoxical vocal fold motion. These manifestations can be caused or worsened by MTD. Morrison et al described a significant overlap between these disorders.[21] Laryngeal constriction in MTD is worse during phonation, as opposed to respiration as is the case with the disorders in this group. Whether MTD is a comanifestation or a cause of this group of disorders is uncertain, but there is some evidence to suggest that elevated tension leads to increased hypersensitivity of the larynx.[22,23]

Generalized Neurological Disorders

Frequently, systemic neurological diseases present initially as voice disorders. Amyotrophic lateral sclerosis, Parkinson disease, Meige syndrome, and tremor are examples of generalized neurological disorders that are commonly seen at voice centers. Complete cranial nerve examinations are essential for discerning between MTD and early-stage neurological disorders. Dysphagia should raise the index of suspicion that another disease process is at work other than solely an MTD diagnosis. Upper motor findings on examination, such as an exaggerated gag, can be clues to the underlying etiology of the patient's voice disorder.

Management

Voice therapy by a speech pathologist who is specially trained in voice disorders is the treatment of choice for patients with MTD. This is particularly true for primary MTD. Voice therapy can also serve as an additional diagnostic tool when uncertainty is present. The ultimate treatment of secondary MTD may require addressing the primary cause of the increased laryngeal tension through medical or surgical management. However, efforts by the speech pathologist to optimize the vocal technique of the patient before surgical intervention are generally the accepted first step. This may ameliorate the patient's complaints of pain or discomfort, often leading to their acceptance of a persistent organic cause.

Case

A 52-year-old female preschool teacher presents with a sudden onset of voice change approximately 3 years ago with increased hoarseness, globus sensation, vocal fatigue, and burning sensation in her throat associated with voice use. Her complaints improve during periods of rest, specifically weekends/holidays. She has been evaluated by several otolaryngologists and gastroenterologists. She trialed multiple antireflux medications and eventually underwent a pH study, which was negative. She denies throat clearing, reflux symptoms, and dysphagia. Laryngoscopy with videostroboscopy revealed full vocal fold mobility and intact vibratory parameters with complete vocal fold closure. The patient was treated with four sessions of voice therapy targeting reduced laryngeal tension and improved vocal efficiency with airflow and resonant voice techniques. Her complaints significantly improved over a 3-month period.

The primary goal of voice therapy, whether treating primary or secondary MTD, is to achieve efficient voice production with balanced airflow and appropriate oral/nasal resonance without inappropriate laryngeal tension. Voice therapy can be divided into two main components: indirect and direct voice therapy.

Indirect voice therapy, also referred to as vocal hygiene, has patient education as its underlying objective. It should address management of vocal stressors and promote an optimal environment for improving vocal ease and quality. Furthermore, the voice user must be made aware of vocal habits that contribute to phonotrauma and/or misuse of the vocal mechanism and should be provided with alternatives to these phonotraumatic behaviors. In addition to traditional vocal hygiene recommendations, psychological stressors may be discussed and acknowledged at this time.

Direct voice therapy has the ultimate goal of balancing the three subsystems of voice production: respiration, phonation, and resonance/power-source-filter. Choosing a direct voice therapy technique should be based on a physiological understanding of voice production and guided by knowledge of voice science. Direct voice therapy exercises to address MTD may include circumlaryngeal massage and/or laryngeal reposturing, stretch and flow phonation, resonant voice therapy techniques, and vocal function exercises (VFEs).

Circumlaryngeal massage was first described by Aronson and has been described multiple times in the literature targeting areas of tension that may include the thyrohyoid area, suprahyoid and submental region, and the lateral laryngeal channels.[13,24,25] Laryngeal massage is completed over areas of tension and point tenderness to reduce muscular rigidity and help the patient to increase awareness of holding patterns. Manual laryngeal reposturing maneuvers can also be used during voice production to transiently interrupt the pattern of habituated muscle tension. It is thought that this laryngeal reposturing can provide information with regard to potential vocal improvement and even to causal mechanisms for the resultant voice.[25] Roy and Leeper demonstrated improvement in perceptual and acoustic findings following just one session of manual laryngeal relaxation techniques.[26] Initial gains in the first session may not always be maintained; however, the patient can be instructed in independent massage to be completed outside of the therapy setting.[27]

Stretch and flow phonation, developed by Stone and Casteel, is used to target consistent airflow during phonation without excessive strain. The hand or a tissue is used for tactile or visual feedback for consistent airflow in isolation and then coordinated with voicing on an /u/ vowel. The /u/ is used as a facilitator throughout a hierarchy of increasing complexity (sustained sounds, glides, sirens, words, phrases, etc.). Use of the /u/ is eventually eliminated while maintaining vocal ease and quality. This exercise may be best suited for patients who demonstrate reduced airflow during phonation. This technique does not directly address laryngeal and extralaryngeal tension. It may, however, contribute to reducing laryngeal tension by balancing use of the vocal power source and sound source, which are breath support and vocal fold vibration, respectively.

Resonant voice therapy is another technique employed to reduce tension with the vocal folds and larynx. During resonant voice production, the vocal folds have been found to be in a nearly adducted or slightly abducted position.[28] Resonant voice is achieved by feeling vibration in the mouth and/or lips during "easy" phonation and then practiced through a hierarchy of vocalizations. The patient should be able to identify where they feel their voice and ultimately implement resonant voice therapy techniques in spontaneous conversational speech.

VFEs were first described by Barnes in 1977 and then modified by Stemple to their current form.[29] These exercises were designed to "strengthen and balance the laryngeal musculature and to balance airflow to the muscular effort" through a systematic program of regular exercise.[30] There are four specific exercises to be completed twice each, two times per day for approximately 6 to 8 weeks. Vocal quality is observed and expected to improve as ability to sustain sounds during the exercises increases. VFEs are thought to be helpful for a wide range of voice disorders.[29]

Conclusion

MTD is a condition of increased laryngeal tension with inefficient voicing patterns that result in voice alterations. It can occur primarily or secondarily to any process leading to glottal insufficiency. A comprehensive history and an appropriate physical examination are essential for making the correct diagnosis. MTD can present with symptoms that can overlap with other well-described diseases affecting the voice. Voice therapy is the cornerstone of effective treatment and must be tailored to meet the needs of each individual patient.

References

1. Morrison MD, Rammage LA, Belisle GM, Pullan CB, Nichol H. Muscular tension dysphonia. J Otolaryngol 1983;12(5):302–306
2. Smith E, Lemke J, Taylor M, Kirchner HL, Hoffman H. Frequency of voice problems among teachers and other occupations. J Voice 1998;12(4):480–488
3. Roy N, Merrill RM, Gray SD, Smith EM. Voice disorders in the general population: prevalence, risk factors, and occupational impact. Laryngoscope 2005;115(11):1988–1995
4. Roy N. Functional dysphonia. Curr Opin Otolaryngol Head Neck Surg 2003;11(3):144–148
5. Sama A, Carding PN, Price S, Kelly P, Wilson JA. The clinical features of functional dysphonia. Laryngoscope 2001;111(3):458–463
6. Bridger MW, Epstein R. Functional voice disorders. A review of 109 patients. J Laryngol Otol 1983;97(12):1145–1148
7. Koufman JA, Blalock PD. Functional voice disorders. Otolaryngol Clin North Am 1991;24(5):1059–1073
8. Altman KW, Atkinson C, Lazarus C. Current and emerging concepts in muscle tension dysphonia: a 30-month review. J Voice 2005;19(2):261–267
9. Van Houtte E, Van Lierde K, D'haeseleer E, Van Imschoot B, Claeys S. UES pressure during phonation using high-resolution manometry and 24-h dual-probe pH-metry in patients with muscle tension dysphonia. Dysphagia 2012;27(2):198–209
10. Belafsky PC, Postma GN, Reulbach TR, Holland BW, Koufman JA. Muscle tension dysphonia as a sign of underlying glottal insufficiency. Otolaryngol Head Neck Surg 2002;127(5):448–451
11. Morrison MD, Rammage LA, Belisle GM, Pullan CB, Nichol H. Muscular tension dysphonia. J Otolaryngol 1983;12(5):302–306
12. Hsiung MW, Hsiao YC. The characteristic features of muscle tension dysphonia before and after surgery in benign lesions of the vocal fold. ORL J Otorhinolaryngol Relat Spec 2004;66(5):246–254
13. Mathieson L. The evidence for laryngeal manual therapies in the treatment of muscle tension dysphonia. Curr Opin Otolaryngol Head Neck Surg 2011;19(3):171–176
14. Vilkman E, Sonninen A, Hurme P, Körkkö P. External laryngeal frame function in voice production revisited: a review. J Voice 1996;10(1):78–92
15. Rubin JS, Lieberman J, Harris TM. Laryngeal manipulation. Otolaryngol Clin North Am 2000;33(5):1017–1034
16. Titze IR. Principles of Voice Production. Englewood Cliffs, NJ: Prentice-Hall; 1994

17. Gray S, Titze I. Histologic investigation of hyperphonated canine vocal cords. Ann Otol Rhinol Laryngol 1988;97(4 Pt 1):381–388

18. Perera L, Kern M, Hofmann C, et al. Manometric evidence for a phonation-induced UES contractile reflex. Am J Physiol Gastrointest Liver Physiol 2008;294(4):G885–G891

19. Belafsky PC, Postma GN, Koufman JA. Validity and reliability of the reflux symptom index (RSI). J Voice 2002;16(2):274–277

20. Koufman JA, Amin MR, Panetti M. Prevalence of reflux in 113 consecutive patients with laryngeal and voice disorders. Otolaryngol Head Neck Surg 2000;123(4):385–388

21. Morrison M, Rammage L, Emami AJ. The irritable larynx syndrome. J Voice 1999;13(3):447–455

22. Helliwell PS, Taylor WJ. Repetitive strain injury. Postgrad Med J 2004;80(946):438–443

23. Vertigan AE, Gibson PG, Theodoros DG, Winkworth AL, Borgas T, Reid C. Involuntary glottal closure during inspiration in muscle tension dysphonia. Laryngoscope 2006;116(4):643–649

24. Aronson AE. Clinical Voice Disorders. 3rd ed. New York, NY: Thieme; 1990:314–315

25. Roy N, Nissen SL, Dromey C, Sapir S. Articulatory changes in muscle tension dysphonia: evidence of vowel space expansion following manual circumlaryngeal therapy. J Commun Disord 2009;42(2):124–135

26. Roy N, Leeper HA. Effects of the manual laryngeal musculoskeletal tension reduction technique as a treatment for functional voice disorders: perceptual and acoustic measures. J Voice 1993;7(3):242–249

27. Roy N, Bless DM, Heisey D, Ford CN. Manual circumlaryngeal therapy for functional dysphonia: an evaluation of short- and long-term treatment outcomes. J Voice 1997;11(3):321–331

28. Verdolini K, Druker DG, Palmer PM, Samawi H. Laryngeal adduction in resonant voice. J Voice 1998;12(3):315–327

29. Stemple JC, ed. Holistic voice therapy: vocal function exercises. In: Voice Therapy: Clinical Studies. 2nd ed. San Diego, CA: Singular Publishing; 2000:34–46

30. Stemple JC, Lee L, D'Amico B, Pickup B. Efficacy of vocal function exercises as a method of improving voice production. J Voice 1994;8(3):271–278

21 Spasmodic Dysphonia

Nupur Kapoor Nerurkar

Spasmodic dysphonia (SD) is a focal laryngeal dystonia that is an action-induced laryngeal movement disorder. The action that triggers the spasms in the voice is speaking itself. Only the volitional cortically driven system is affected in SD.

Dystonias are generally classified into two groups, generalized and focal, and may be primary (idiopathic) or secondary to birth injury, hypoxia, infection (encephalitis/meningitis), toxicity (drugs), or stroke. The most common types of focal dystonia are laryngeal dystonia, blepharospasm, torticollis, and writer's cramp. Laryngeal dystonia, also called SD, is a focal, primary dystonia, affecting the muscles of the larynx.

SD patients classically have a spasmodic speech pattern with adductor or abductor spasms. Adductor spasms give a strained and choked quality to the voice and this is referred to as adductor spasmodic dysphonia (ADSD). There is an abrupt initiation and termination of voicing, resulting in short breaks of phonation. In contrast, abductor spasms give a breathy quality to the voice referred to as abductor spasmodic dysphonia (ABSD). It is possible to have a combination of both these types of SD referred to as mixed SD. A study by Cannito and Johnson[1] suggests that all patients have a mixed SD, with one type of an activity predominating the other. Approximately one-third of persons with SD also have voice tremor, which makes the pitch and loudness of the voice waver at 5 Hz during vowels and is most evident when "/a/" as in the word "all" is produced for at least 5 seconds.[2]

Historically, various terminologies have been used to describe SD including spastic dysphonia,[3] spastic aphonia,[4] and coordinated laryngeal spasm.[5] It was Aronson who helped establish SD as an organic disease and also described two distinct types of SD, the adductor and the abductor varieties.[6] Though SD is today thought to be a completely distinct entity to psychogenic dysphonia, there is a worsening of patients' symptoms noticed in the presence of strangers, in crowds, and over the telephone. There is often an improvement of the SD patient's voice with whispering, singing, and shouting or after an alcoholic beverage is consumed. This is in fact one of the mysteries of SD, that it is task specific. Spasms only occur during speaking and not during emotional expressions such as laughter, crying, and shouting. This may be explained by Kuypers' study (1958), which indicates that only humans have a direct corticobulbar pathway from the laryngeal cortex to the nucleus ambiguus.[7] Possibly, neural systems involved in learning speech are likely affected in SD, while those involved in emotional vocalization are not. To identify the neural abnormalities in SD, differences between these two neural systems (one for emotional vocalization and the other for speech) must account for symptoms being absent in the former and present in the latter.[8]

Occasionally, patients with ADSD compensate by producing a breathy voice referred to as compensatory abductor dysphonia. Similarly, ABSD patients may try to tightly contract the vocal folds producing compensatory adductor dysphonia, though this is more uncommon.[9,10]

Historical Anecdotes

- Traube used the term *spastic dysphonia* in 1871 while describing a patient with nervous hoarseness.
- Aronson in 1968 helped establish SD as an organic and not a psychiatric condition and also in later studies described the two types of SD, i.e., adductor and abductor SD.
- Dr. Herbert Dedo in 1976 introduced recurrent laryngeal nerve (RLN) sectioning as a treatment for ADSD.
- Dr. Andrew Blitzer performed the first laryngeal injection of botulinum toxin (BTX) for SD in 1984.
- Isshiki, in 1998, reported treating a case of ADSD with type 2 thyroplasty.
- In 1999, Dr. Berke described the denervation–reinnervation surgery.

Etiology

The basal ganglion plays an integral role in movement. Inputs from the cerebral cortex, especially the primary motor strip and primary somatosensory cortex, are received in the basal ganglia and the substantia nigra. The exact etiology of SD is as yet unknown. However, research by Simonyan and Ludlow[11] has shown that the primary somatosensory cortex shows consistent abnormalities in activation extent, intensity, correlation with other brain regions, and symptom severity in SD patients and, therefore, may be involved in the pathophysiology of SD. When the brains of dystonic patients were studied pathologically, although no consistent lesions were found, most frequently mentioned lesions were in the basal ganglia.[12]

In ADSD, the lack of symptoms during whispering, when the vocal folds are not vibrating, suggests that changes in laryngeal sensory feedback either from the vocal fold mucosa or from subglottal pressures in the trachea may play a role in the pathophysiology of the disorder. Further research on the role of laryngeal sensory feedback in the manipulation of symptoms needs to be performed.[8]

A genetic component does seem to be involved in some patients as 12.1% of Blitzer and Brin's 1991 series of laryngeal dystonia patients had a family history of dystonia.[10] The *DTY1* gene was first identified in one large non-Jewish family with multiple family members presenting with dystonia and has been responsible for childhood-onset dystonia in the Jewish population.[13]

A few cases with single mutations in *THAP1*, a gene involved in transcription regulation, suggest that a weak genetic predisposition may contribute to mechanisms causing a nonprogressive abnormality in laryngeal motor neuron control for speech but not for vocal emotional expression.[8]

Demographics

Though SD may be present in both males and females, it is more prevalent among the female population, with some estimates indicating the prevalence to be as high as 80%.[14] It is uncommon to find SD in children, and 45 years is the most commonage of presentation of SD. There seems to be a progression of symptoms for 2 years following which there is usually a plateau of symptoms, though the patient may complaint of a progressive increase in effort required to phonate.

SD is a relatively rare disorder; however, accurate worldwide audited numbers are not available. Some estimates are as low as 1 per 100,000 cases,[15] although accurate diagnosis is a significant roadblock to research. With the increasing awareness regarding SD being created, more cases are being accurately diagnosed and managed.

Diagnosis

Clinical

The provisional diagnosis of SD is made more often than not within a couple of minutes of talking to the patient as the diagnosis is based primarily on auditory-perceptual features.

This is possible as ADSD patients have a typical choking voice and the spasms are seen on vowels. This type affects at least 80% of persons with SD and disrupts sentences such as "we eat eggs every day."[16] This is because any sentence that has a lot of vowels dramatically worsens the voice. On asking the patient to whisper or sing, the spasms markedly decrease. In the case of ABSD patients, a typical breathy spasm is observed and is almost always accompanied by a flaring of the alae nasi. These breathy bursts take place due to prolonged voiceless consonants and while attempting to start voice after voiceless consonants such as /s/, /f/, /h/, /p/, /t/, and /k/.[17] Disruption of sentences such as "**h**e **h**ad **h**alf a **h**ead of **h**air"[18] is observed.

Flexible laryngoscopy allows an evaluation of the vocal fold movements in normal physiological phonation. The patient is asked to talk, sing, and whisper, and any change in the severity of spasms is observed. In ADSD patients, the spasms may be of only the true vocal folds or of true and false vocal folds. In severe ADSD, a complete anteroposterior and lateral compression of the supraglottis is observed. Stroboscopy may be performed using the flexible laryngoscope. In ABSD

patients, a sudden abduction is observed corresponding with the breathy spasm on phonation.

Stroboscopy confirms the spasms seen on flexible laryngoscopy, and the amplitude of the mucosal wave is seen to be decreased or occasionally absent. However, when stroboscopy is done using a Hopkins telescope through the mouth, the signs of SD may occasionally get masked as this test does not allow for normal physiological phonation.

A *team approach* in the diagnosis of SD is vital. Besides the laryngologist, a speech therapist and a neurologist form the core team in the diagnosis of SD. Occasionally, the opinion of a gastroenterologist or a psychiatrist may be sought.

> **Clinical Insights**
>
> - In ADSD, voice improves with whispering, singing, or shouting and after consuming an alcoholic beverage and worsens on the phone or in the presence of strangers.
> - Vocal tremors may accompany spasms in almost 30% of ADSD patients.
> - In ABSD, flaring of the alae nasi is seen to accompany the abductor spasms.

Differential Diagnosis

The differential diagnosis of SD includes muscle tension dysphonia (MTD), vocal tremor, Parkinson disease, Wilson disease, myasthenia gravis, motor neuron disease (MND), pseudobulbar palsy, cerebellar disorders, laryngopharyngeal reflux, laryngeal cancer, and functional voice disorders.

Muscle Tension Dysphonia

MTD may be occasionally mistaken as SD. The cardinal differences between the two are that SD is task-specific unlike MTD and in SD the strain in the voice is spasmodic unlike MTD where the strain is continuous. MTD is often associated with tenderness over the greater cornu of the hyoid and in the thyrohyoid membrane. Obliteration and tenderness in the cricothyroid membrane may also be observed. A lidocaine block of the RLN improves the voice of both ADSD and MTD patients. However, the primary treatment of MTD is laryngeal massage and speech therapy.

Vocal Tremor

Vocal tremor is an involuntary, rhythmic, oscillating movement of the vocal folds. Vocal tremors are not task-specific and are present on talking, singing, and on a sustained /eee/. This vocal tremor may be part of an essential tremor known as "benign heredofamilial tremor." This may involve only the voice or other body parts such as the head and neck also. Vocal tremor occurs in 10 to 20% of patients with essential tremor. It is essential to rule out cerebellar disease, parkinsonism, thyrotoxicosis, and drug-induced and psychogenic causes of the tremor. In 30% of SD patients, an associated vocal tremor is present.

Treatment Options

Speech therapy as a modality of treatment in ADSD patients does not meet with much success. However, it may be a viable option in patients with very early ADSD. Speech therapy is also of value in those patients who have developed wrong compensatory techniques of a breathy voice in ADSD or compensatory abductor dysphonia in ADSD.

In ABSD patients, speech therapy especially with a biofeedback mechanism has shown promising results. This has a very positive bearing in the treatment of ABSD patients who typically respond to BTX poorer than their ADSD counterparts. One of the key biofeedback techniques used for the ABSD group is to ask the patient to stand in front of the mirror and talk while making a concentrated effort in controlling the flaring of the alae nasi that accompanies each abductor spasm.

Medical treatment may benefit patients of essential tremor or those who besides having SD have a generalized dystonia. Patients of SD occasionally are also anxious or depressed and may need psychiatric treatment for the same.

Role of Botulinum Toxin in the Management of Spasmodic Dysphonia

Pharmacology of Botulinum Toxin

Clostridium botulinum is the bacteria that produce seven serologically distinct botulinum neurotoxins that are designated from A to G. These seven neurotoxins are antigenically distinct but do have similar molecular weight and a common subunit structure. These neurotoxins are synthesized as single-chain polypeptides. However, this single chain gets cleaved by trypsin or bacterial enzymes to form a bichained (one heavy chain and one light chain) molecule in which both the chains are linked by a disulfide bond. It is in this form that the molecule becomes potent.

Clinical studies have shown that BTX does not affect the synthesis or storage of acetylcholine. The toxin probably modifies the release of synaptosomes from the microtubular subsystem. Though the clinical effects of BTX are probably due to its peripheral effects, the action of BTX on the laryngeal muscle contractions cannot be assumed to have altered only muscle spasms. There may be retrograde transport affecting input to the laryngeal motor neurons.[19] In addition, as the muscle spasms are reduced not only in the laryngeal muscle injected but also in other laryngeal muscles on the opposite side of the larynx,[20] the sensory feedback from the larynx is altered by less mucosal compression and lower subglottal pressures in the trachea due to reduced hyperadduction during speech. The clinical effects are seen 24 to 72 hours following the BTX injection.

Preparation of Botulinum Toxin

BTX is commercially available as a powder in vacuum-sealed vials. The quantity of active toxin is mentioned in mouse units (mu/U) and it is essential that BTX be manufactured in a standard fashion such that each subsequent vial is of an equal potency to maintain both safety and efficacy. BTX(A) is available as Botox manufactured by Allergan (Irvine, California, United States) and also as Dysport manufactured by Ipsen, Slough, United Kingdom. In India, BTX is available in 50- and 100-mu vials, where 1mu is the median lethal dose in mice. The exact lethal dose in humans is not known but is postulated to lie near approximately 2700 U.

A 50-U vial of BTX when reconstituted with 2cc of preservative-free saline gives a concentration of 2.5 U BTX per 0.1mL of reconstituted solution. It has been recommended to use this reconstituted BTX within 4 hours of preparation.

BTX use is currently not recommended in pregnant or lactating women. Patients with myasthenia gravis, Eaton-Lambert syndrome, and MND should be treated cautiously with BTX as the neuromuscular junction is affected. Aminoglycosides may potentiate the effect of BTX as they effect neuromuscular transmission and thus are also a contraindication to BTX use.

Prolonged use of BTX may lead to antibody formation, which is seen more in the group of patients being treated by BTX for torticollis as larger doses are being used. Dezfulian et al[21] have developed an enzyme-linked immunosorbent assay that appears to be sensitive and specific in the detection of antibody.

Procedure of Botulinum Toxin Injection in Spasmodic Dysphonia Patients

Dr. Andrew Blitzer performed the first laryngeal injection of BTX for SD in 1984.[22]

The key to a successful BTX injection for SD lies in correct dose titration of BTX for every individual patient and an accurate placement of the BTX. To accurately inject the BTX in the affected muscle, most laryngologists use the laryngeal electromyography (LEMG)system while injecting. Some laryngologists, however, inject with the help of flexible laryngoscopic guidance, occasionally in association with LEMG. Dose titration is perfected once the response to standard doses of BTX on the patient has been audited. LEMG-controlled BTX injection in the management of SD is considered the gold standard.

Laryngeal Electromyography in Spasmodic Dysphonia

Electromyography (EMG) is a test measuring the micropotential reaching the muscle fibers utilizing a needle electrode placed in the muscle. When the needle is placed in the laryngeal muscle, the test is referred to as LEMG. The primary role of LEMG is in the injection of BTX in SD.

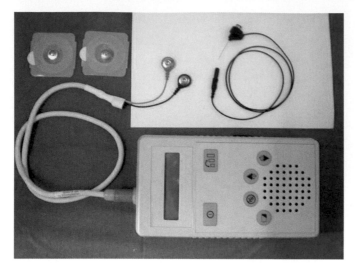

Figure 21.1 AccuGuide laryngeal electromyography system with AccuGuide cable, surface electrodes, and 27-gauge Teflon-coated monopolar needle.

However, the other therapeutic uses are in the injection of BTX in patients with cricopharyngeal spasm and contact granuloma. The diagnostic role of LEMG lies in differentiating between vocal fold paralysis and cricoarytenoid joint fixation and also in the diagnosis of various neurogenic voice disorders. It is essential that the diagnostic applications of LEMG be performed using a sophisticated, multichannel EMG system by the EMG technician in concert with the neurophysician and not by the laryngologist alone.

A conventional EMG machine or the AccuGuide system marketed by Medtronic Xomed (Jacksonville, Florida, United States) (**Fig. 21.1**),which is a portable, cost-effective, single-channel EMG device, may be used for the injection of BTX in SD patients. Various needles are available commercially for use in LEMG. A monopolar Teflon-coated 27-gauge needle is one of the most standard needle electrodes to be used. In any EMG test, the parameters studied are insertional activity, spontaneous activity at rest, response to minimal voluntary contraction, and response to maximum voluntary contraction. Rarely are laryngeal muscles at complete physiological rest. With minimal voluntary contraction, 1 or 2 motor unit potentials can be recorded, which increase with increasing strength of the contraction. Full interference pattern is the normal response of the muscle to maximal voluntary contraction where the entire screen gets filled up with waves of large action potentials such that single motor unit potentials cannot be distinguished from each other. In the case of SD, there is a normal insertional activity. However, there is a sudden increase seen in the muscle activity on asking the patient to phonate. This sudden burst of action potentials just precedes the voice spasms that are heard. If the EMG signal is put on the same time as a voice spectrogram, a greater-than-normal delay in the onset of voice production is observed, particularly in patients with ADSD.[23] In a study by Eric Nash and Christy Ludlow on laryngeal muscle activity during speech breaks in ADSD, the mean muscle activity

level was significantly greater on break than nonbreak words in ADSD patients only for the thyroarytenoid muscle ($p < 0.001$). No significant differences were found between the ADSD and control subjects during nonbreak words for any of the other laryngeal muscles studied. The results demonstrated that only the thyroarytenoid, of the muscles tested, was affected in ADSD.[24]

Botulinum Toxin in Adductor Spasmodic Dysphonia

In the ADSD group of patients, BTX is injected into the thyroarytenoid muscle bilaterally. The standard dose for the first injection is 2.5 mu bilaterally. When a 50-mu BTX vial is diluted with 2 mL of preservative-free saline, 0.1 mL of BTX will contain 2.5 mu of BTX. The position of the patient during this procedure may be supine with neck extension or sitting with neck extension. The neck of the patient and the skin over the mandible is cleaned with spirit. The EMG surface electrodes are placed on the skin overlying the mandible on the side being injected (**Fig. 21.2**). As electrical activity interferes with the EMG signal, all mobile phones, cautery, and suction machines should be switched off in the room. Initially, marking of the lower border of the thyroid and upper border of the cricoid cartilage is helpful, but this is not necessary as experience in the procedure is gained. A 27 number Teflon-coated monopolar needle is used by the author. The tip of this needle is not coated with Teflon. This needle is curved at an angulation of 30 degrees while injecting male patients (**Fig. 21.3**). While injecting female patients, the needle need not be angulated or may be angulated by 10 to 15degrees. While injecting the right vocal fold, the needle is inserted 1 to 2 mm from the midline on the right side with the tip directed 30 degrees laterally. The patient is instructed to say "eeee" as phonation stimulates

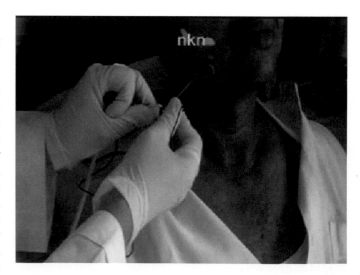

Figure 21.2 Surface electrodes applied on the skin over the surface of the mandible for right-sided injection in an adductor spasmodic dysphonia patient.

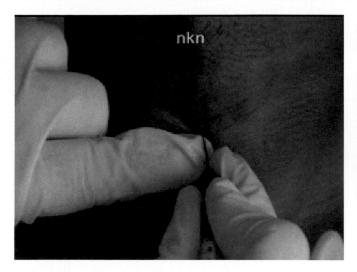

Figure 21.3 Insertion of the 27-gauge monopolar injection needle which has been bent by 30 degrees (for a male adductor spasmodic dysphonia patient), via the cricothyroid membrane, 1 mm to the right of the midline, angulated 30 degrees to the right for the right thyroarytenoid muscle injection.

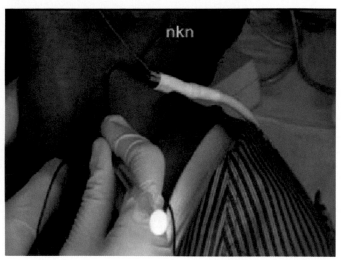

Figure 21.4 Larynx rotated toward side being injected in abductor spasmodic dysphonia.

the adductor group of muscles and a burst of activity is seen on the monitor. Aspiration before injection is advisable and the patient is instructed not to move or swallow during the procedure. A tuberculin syringe is preloaded with the amount of BTX to be injected. While using the AccuGuide system, a burst of sound is heard from the EMG system and an increasing number of bars get lit up on the liquid crystal display. This AccuGuide system has the option of being connected to the computer with a serial port interface connector so that a graphical representation of the signal may be studied on the monitor.

Botulinum Toxin in Abductor Spasmodic Dysphonia

In the case of ABSD, BTX is injected into the posterior cricoarytenoid (PCA)muscle, which is the only abductor of the larynx. If a person is very sensitive to BTX, a bilateral injection may result in stridor. Most laryngologists prefer therefore to inject ABSD patients unilaterally. There are two routes of approaching the PCA. One is through the cricothyroid membrane, passing the needle through the airway till the cricoid is hit, followed by gentle withdrawal of the needle. The primary problem with this approach is blocking of the luminal patency of the needle by pieces of cartilage. The second approach, which is commonly followed, is entering the PCA from the lateral side. If a line is made marking the posterior edge of the thyroid cartilage and another is made at the superior border of the cricoid cartilage, a transection of the two lines takes place. The upper outer quadrant of this transection is the surface marking for the insertion of the needle. While injecting the PCA, the larynx is rotated toward the side being injected (**Fig. 21.4**). When

the needle is inserted into the PCA, a signal is observed with every inspiration. The patient is asked to sniff deeply and the response to maximum stimulation is observed. Usually 3.75 mu (0.15 mL) of BTX is injected unilaterally for the first injection of BTX.

Response to Injection of Botulinum Toxin in Spasmodic Dysphonia

Following BTX injection, there is no noticeable change observed in the patient's voice for 24 to 48 hours.

In ADSD patients, this is followed by a breathy voice for a variable period of approximately 1 to 6 weeks. Though the voice is breathy, it is spasm-free. If the voice becomes very breathy, it is possible that the patient has an occasional aspiration while swallowing water or clear liquids. This is due to a large phonatory gap that has temporarily developed following BTX injection. Drinking water with a straw or spoon usually allows the patient to overcome this swallowing difficulty that may be seen in 30% of the patients. The special swallow technique is also taught to these patients. In the special swallow, the patient is asked to take a deep breath and hold it while swallowing twice before exhalation.

Following the breathy phase, the patient's voice becomes stronger and remains spasm-free. This golden period may last from 6 to 24 weeks. Finally, a return of spasms is noticed by the patient and this indicates that it is time for reinjection of BTX. Patients of ADSD show a 90 to 95% improvement following BTX injection.

In ABSD patients, a 30 to 70% improvement is observed. This is possibly due to the fact that accurate insertion of the needle into the PCA muscle is difficult coupled with the fact that most of these patients receive unilateral injections.

Though a tremulous voice may also improve with BTX injection, the results are better when the patient has both ADSD and vocal tremor.

Surgical Options for Spasmodic Dysphonia Patients

Dr. Herbert Dedo introduced *RLN sectioning* as a treatment for ADSD in 1976.[25] The phonatory gap thus created is the basis of loss of adductor spasms and a breathy but spasm-free voice. However, various studies have shown a regeneration of the cut end of the RLN with a return of spasms within 3 years in 40 to 60% of the patients.

RLN avulsion was introduced by Weed et al where the RLN was resected in the upper mediastinum and also avulsed from its insertion into the muscle in an attempt to prevent the return of spasms due to RLN regeneration seen with just sectioning. Though 78% of the patients had no return of spasm at 3 to 7 years,[26] the voice in most was too breathy, warranting a medialization procedure. However, following medialization, most patients developed a return in spasms.

Selective denervation with reinnervation was described by Berke et al in 1999. Here, the adductor branch to the thyroarytenoid muscle is bilaterally denervated and the distal stump is reinnervated to the ansa in an attempt to retain muscle tone and prevent nerve regeneration.[27]

Thyroarytenoid-Myoneurectomy

In this surgery, a variable amount of thyroarytenoid muscle fibers are destroyed in a bid to cause weakness of the adductory action of the vocal fold. An attempt is made to find and avulsion-cut the thyroarytenoid branch of the RLN. This surgery may be performed unilaterally or bilaterally using either the external or the endoscopic approach. When the external approach is used, the surgery is performed under local anesthesia. A window is made in the thyroid ala cartilage, similar to that used for a type 1 thyroplasty. The inner perichondrium of the thyroid cartilage window is then incised and removed. A bipolar cautery is then used to cauterize the thyroarytenoid muscle fibers (**Fig. 21.5**)

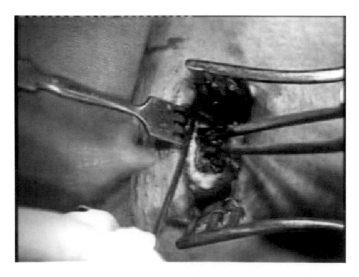

Figure 21.5 Thyroarytenoid muscle fibers being coagulated in thyroarytenoid myoneurectomy surgery.

till the patient's voice loses all its spasms and becomes slightly breathy. The advantage of doing the procedure under local anesthesia is that the voice can be tested and a decision regarding necessity of performing the procedure bilaterally can be made. An attempt is always made to find the thyroarytenoid branch of the RLN at the posteroinferior corner of the thyroplasty window. This branch is better seen using the ocular loop or microscope and is avulsed and cut. This neurectomy is believed to give a more long-lasting result postoperatively. Some surgeons like to place fat or connective tissue in the window before closure in an attempt to decrease the postoperative phonatory gap that is created.

Laser-Assisted Thyroarytenoid Myoneurectomy

The thyroarytenoid muscle fibers may also be destroyed endoscopically with the help of a CO_2 laser. Under general anesthesia, a microlaryngeal surgery is performed where the CO_2 laser is used to destroy the superolateral thyroarytenoid muscle fibers along the length of the vocal fold. Following this myectomy, the thyroarytenoid branch of the RLN is looked for, lateral to the vocal process of the arytenoid. This process is referred to as "fishing for the nerve" and is best accomplished by taking a 24-cm long hook which is used to hookup the nerve from posterior to anterior.

Thyroarytenoid myoneurectomy (TAMN) gives dramatic results on the operation table, but the long-term results are unpredictable. Spasms have been seen to return as early as 1 year after surgery. In the authors' series of six TAMNs performed (all externally), a return of spasms was seen in three patients within 1 to 2 years postoperatively. One of these patients has restarted BTX injections with good response.

Laryngeal Framework Surgery

Isshiki, in 1998,[28] performed what is now termed as a lateralization laryngoplasty for ADSD. This type 2 thyroplasty involves vertically incising the thyroid cartilage at the junction of the two alae, taking care not to enter the larynx. The vocal folds are held apart at the anterior commissure by 4-mm silicon shims (**Fig. 21.6**). The voice remains variably breathy and a return of adductor spasms may take place at an unpredictable time interval.

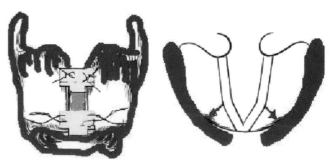

Figure 21.6 Diagrammatic representation of type 2 thyroplasty.

Research is needed to address the basic cellular and proteomic mechanisms that produce this disorder to provide intervention that could target the pathogenesis of the disorder rather than only providing temporary symptom relief.[4]

Pearls and Pitfalls

- Botulinum toxin with laryngeal electromyography control is till today considered the gold standard in the management of spasmodic dysphonia (SD).
- Muscle tension dysphonia is one of the commonest differential diagnoses of SD.
- A team of laryngologist, speech therapist, and neurologist is the key in the accurate diagnosis of SD.

References

1. Cannito MP, Johnson JP. Spastic dysphonia: a continuum disorder. J Commun Disord 1981;14(3):215–233
2. Schweinfurth JM, Billante M, Courey MS. Risk factors and demographics in patients with spasmodic dysphonia. Laryngoscope 2002;112(2):220–223
3. Traube L. Gesammelte Beitrage zur Pathologie und Physiologie.2nd ed. Berlin: Verlag Von August Hisschwald;1871:674–678
4. Schnitzler J, Hajek M, Schnitzler A. Klinischer Atlas der Laryngologie. Nebst Anleitung zur Diagnose und Therapie der Krankheiten des Kehlkopfes und der Luftrohre. Wein und Leipzig: Wilhelm Braumuller;1895
5. Gerhardt P. Bewegunggsstoerungen der stimmbaender. Nothnagels Spezielle Pathologie und Therapie.1896;13:307
6. Aronson AE. Clinical Voice Disorders. New York, NY: Thieme Medical Publishers;1985
7. Kuypers HG. Corticobular connexions to the pons and lower brainstem in man: an anatomical study. Brain 1958;81(3):364–388
8. Ludlow CL. Spasmodic dysphonia: a laryngeal control disorder specific to speech. J Neurosci 2011;31(3):793–797
9. Blitzer A, Brin MF, Fahn S, Lovelace RE. Clinical and laboratory characteristics of focal laryngeal dystonia: study of 110 cases. Laryngoscope 1988;98(6 Pt 1):636–640
10. Blitzer A, Brin MF. Laryngeal dystonia: a series with botulinum toxin therapy. Ann Otol Rhinol Laryngol 1991;100(2):85–89
11. Simonyan K, Ludlow CL. Abnormal activation of the primary somatosensory cortex in spasmodic dysphonia: an fMRI study. Cereb Cortex 2010;20(11):2749–2759
12. Marsden CD, Obeso JA, Zarranz JJ, Lang AE. The anatomical basis of symptomatic hemidystonia. Brain 1985;108(Pt 2):463–483
13. Ozelius LJ, Kramer PL, de Leon D, et al. Strong allelic association between the torsion dystonia gene (DYT1) andloci on chromosome 9q34 in Ashkenazi Jews. Am J Hum Genet 1992;50(3):619–628
14. Adler CH, Edwards BW, Bansberg SF. Female predominance in spasmodic dysphonia. J Neurol Neurosurg Psychiatry 1997;63(5):688
15. Nutt JG, Muenter MD, Aronson A, Kurland LT, Melton LJIII III. Epidemiology of focal and generalized dystonia in Rochester, Minnesota. Mov Disord 1988;3(3):188–194
16. Erickson ML. Effects of voicing and syntactic complexity on sign expression in adductor spasmodic dysphonia. Am J Speech Lang Pathol 2003;12(4):416–424
17. Rodriquez AA, Ford CN, Bless DM, Harmon RL. Electromyographic assessment of spasmodic dysphonia patients prior to botulinum toxin injection. Electromyogr Clin Neurophysiol 1994;34(7):403–407
18. Rontal M, Rontal E, Rolnick M, Merson R, Silverman B, Truong DD. A method for the treatment of abductor spasmodic dysphonia with botulinum toxin injections: a preliminary report. Laryngoscope 1991;101(8):911–914
19. Moreno-López B, Pastor AM, de la Cruz RR, Delgado-García JM. Dose-dependent, central effects of botulinum neurotoxin type A: a pilot study in the alert behaving cat. Neurology 1997;48(2):456–464
20. Bielamowicz S, Ludlow CL. Effects of botulinum toxin on pathophysiology in spasmodic dysphonia. Ann Otol Rhinol Laryngol 2000;109(2):194–203
21. Dezfulian M, Hatheway CL, Yolken RH, Bartlett JG. Enzyme-linked immunosorbent assay for detection of Clostridium botulinum type A and type B toxins in stool samples of infants with botulism. J Clin Microbiol 1984;20(3):379–383
22. Blitzer A, Brin MF, Stewart CF. Botulinum toxin management of spasmodic dysphonia (laryngeal dystonia): a 12-year experience in more than 900 patients. Laryngoscope 1998;108(10):1435–1441
23. Schaefer SD. Neuropathology of spasmodic dysphonia. Laryngoscope 1983;93(9):1183–1204
24. Nash EA, Ludlow CL. Laryngeal muscle activity during speech breaks in adductor spasmodic dysphonia. Laryngoscope 1996;106(4):484–489
25. Dedo HH. Recurrent laryngeal nerve section for spastic dysphonia. Ann Otol Rhinol Laryngol 1976;85(4 Pt 1):451–459
26. Weed DT, Jewett BS, Rainey C, et al. Long-term follow-up of recurrent laryngeal nerve avulsion for the treatment of spastic dysphonia. Ann Otol Rhinol Laryngol 1996;105(8):592–601
27. Berke GS, Blackwell KE, Gerratt BR, Verneil A, Jackson KS, Sercarz JA. Selective laryngeal adductor denervation-reinnervation: a new surgical treatment for adductor spasmodic dysphonia. Ann Otol Rhinol Laryngol 1999;108(3):227–231
28. Isshiki N, Tsuji DH, Yamamoto Y, Iizuka Y. Midline lateralization thyroplasty for adductor spasmodic dysphonia. Ann Otol Rhinol Laryngol 2000;109(2):187–193

22 Acute Inflammatory and Infective Disorders of the Larynx

Chee-Yean Eng and Muhammad Shahed Quraishi

The larynx is the narrowest part of the upper airway and is situated just anterior to the opening into the esophagus. This anatomical position means that the larynx is constantly exposed to the external environment, predisposing it to infection, environmental irritants, and potential gastric contents from gastroesophageal reflux. Edema or swelling of the larynx from inflammation can also potentially result in life-threatening upper airway obstruction.

The causes of laryngeal inflammation can broadly be divided into noninfective and infective. This can be further classified as shown in **Fig. 22.1**. The majority of noninfective inflammatory conditions of the larynx are chronic and some are described here as they form part of the differential diagnosis when patients present acutely with a short history.

Clinical Assessment

Patients of all ages can present with symptoms and signs suggestive of laryngeal inflammation. History should specifically cover throat symptoms, past medical illnesses, medication history, smoking and alcohol history, and occupation.

Laryngeal or throat symptoms include sore throat, dysphonia, dysphagia, odynophagia, globus sensation, repeated throat clearing, history of heartburn, cough, hemoptysis, and difficulty breathing or stridor. The patient may volunteer experience of laryngospasm during daytime or woken up from sleep at night. Any history of heartburn or gastroesophageal reflux disease and treatment regimen should be thoroughly explored. History of any weight loss is indicative of true dysphagia and may require radiological investigation such as contrast swallow. Dietary history is important and may be perpetuating laryngopharyngeal reflux (LPR).

The oral cavity and oropharynx examination should be performed. Flexible nasolaryngoscopy examination of the tongue base, larynx, and hypopharynx is mandatory for diagnosis and for excluding malignancy. Photographic

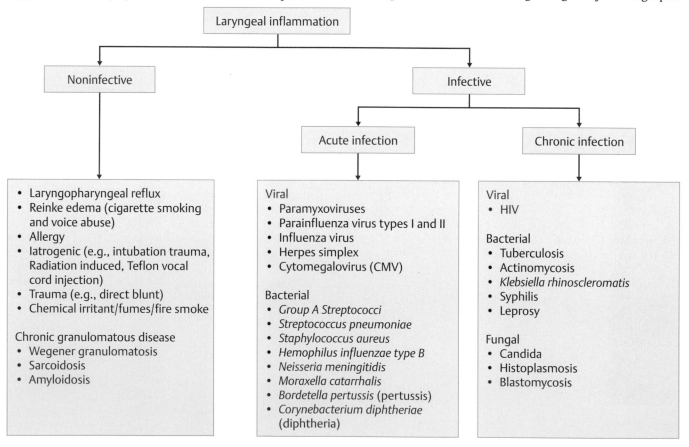

Figure 22.1 Classification of laryngeal inflammation.

documentation is recommended for record and future comparison. Bilateral neck examination to exclude cervical lymphadenopathy and malignancy should also be performed.

Noninfective Laryngitis

Laryngopharyngeal Reflux

LPR[1] is the backflow of gastric acidic refluxate, containing hydrochloric acid, pepsin, bile acids, bacteria, and pancreatic proteolytic enzymes, into the upper aerodigestive tract, resulting in damage to the thin laryngeal mucosa. The refluxate could take the form of either liquid or gas aerosol. Refluxate pepsinogen/pepsin attached to laryngeal mucosa has been shown to be the main culprit causing proteolytic tissue damage. Pepsinogen is converted to pepsin (active form) when pH drops below 4 and deactivated only when pH rises above 8.

The resulting laryngeal mucosa damage may give rise to symptoms such as globus sensation, pseudodysphagia, need for repeated throat clearing, cough, postnasal drip or "catarrh," sore throat, and dysphonia. Flexible nasolaryngoscopy examination reveals erythema and edema of both arytenoids, postcricoid region, and posterior commissure (**Fig. 22.2**). Vocal cord edema and pseudosulcus may also be visible.

Diagnosis is usually by history and examination. Contrast swallow could be used if there was suspicion of pharyngeal pouch, obstructive lesions, or esophageal malignancy. The reflux symptom index (RSI) is a patient self-assessment tool with regard to the severity of LPR. The RSI score is useful in both diagnosis and monitoring response to treatment over time.

All patients should be advised on lifestyle modifications, which have been shown to help. This includes avoiding food late at night, fatty food, and low pH drinks such as fizzy drinks and fruit juices. Depending on the severity of the disease, they could be prescribed liquid alginate preparation alone (to be taken after meal and before bedtime) or in combination with a low- or high-dose proton pump inhibitor (PPI; to be taken half an hour before meal and twice a day to ensure 24-hour cover). It may take up to 2 to 3 months before any benefit is realized and treatment may need to continue for up to 6 months. The dose of the PPI can be tailed off subsequently.

For patients who fail to respond to antireflux medical treatment, it may be useful to consider 24-hour dual-channel pH monitoring or multichannel intraluminal impedance measurement to establish objective evidence of reflux before embarking on surgical management such as fundoplication.

Clinical Pearl

- A high degree of suspicion for neoplasm should be maintained in high-risk patients who may present with symptoms of LPR.

Reinke Edema from Cigarette Smoking and Voice Abuse

Reinke edema from cigarette smoking and voice abuse[2] is a form of chronic inflammation affecting the membranous portion of the vocal cords as a result of smoking and voice abuse. The inflammatory process results in fluid accumulation within Reinke space, hence Reinke edema. Reinke space is the potential space between the basement membrane of the nonkeratinizing stratified squamous epithelium and the superficial lamina propria.

Patients are typically smokers and present with dysphonia with reduced pitch. Female patients may complain that they are regularly mistaken for a man when having telephone conversation. Flexible nasolaryngoscopy would reveal diffuse edematous vocal cords with redundant floppy vocal fold mucosa.

Significant swelling from Reinke edema may also result in stridor and acute airway obstruction requiring intubation/tracheostomy and urgent surgery (microlaryngoscopy with cold-steel technique or laser) to drain fluid from Reinke space and reduce any excess mucosa, without damaging the superficial lamina propria and vocal ligaments.

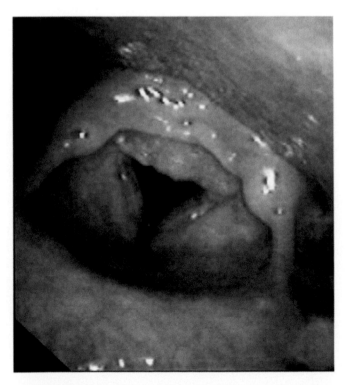

Figure 22.2 Laryngopharyngeal reflux showing postcricoid edema and significant posterior commissure hypertrophy. (*Image courtesy* of Mr. Mark Watson.)

Clinical Pearl

- Unilateral Reinke edema would warrant exclusion of neoplasm.

Allergy

Generalized allergic reaction or exposure to inhalants could trigger a type I hypersensitivity reaction leading to acute edema of the glottis or supraglottis, resulting in stridor and acute airway obstruction. Careful and close monitoring of respiratory function and pulse oximetry will be required. Immediate withdrawal and avoidance of the known allergen is indicated. Acute airway management with systemic steroids, intramuscular adrenaline, nebulized adrenaline, heliox, and antihistamine should be considered. Intubation (anesthetic involvement), cricothyroidotomy, and emergency tracheostomy may be required to secure airway.

Environmental Irritants

Toxic fumes and fire smoke can result in acute edema of the larynx. Black soot can be seen in the oral cavity and oropharynx following fire smoke inhalation. It is crucial that these patients' airway is monitored closely since laryngeal edema can develop very quickly resulting in impaired visualization of the laryngeal inlet. At-risk patients should be intubated early in Accident and Emergency to secure their airway and to reduce the risk of intubation trauma while the laryngeal inlet is still visible.

Direct Trauma

Blunt trauma of the larynx can result in hematoma and trigger an inflammatory response resulting in laryngeal soft-tissue swelling. Airway obstruction is a danger and acute airway management as per allergy is indicated. Unstable fractured laryngeal framework should be surgically repaired after airway is secured.

Iatrogenic

Inhaled Corticosteroids

The use of inhaled corticosteroids (ICSs)[3] in the treatment of asthma and chronic obstructive airways disease (COAD) is widespread. Increased dose of ICS has a positive correlation with local and systemic side effects. Systemic side effects occur because 80% of the dose delivered by conventional metered-dose inhaler is swallowed.[3]

Symptomatic local side effects occur in up to 5 to 10% of patients treated with ICS.[3] These include oropharyngeal and laryngeal candidiasis (described further in section "Fungal Infection" later in the chapter) and nonspecific inflammation of the laryngopharyngeal mucosa. These local side effects are multifactorial and related to the steroid preparations, proinflammatory effect of the propellant and lubricant constituents of the ICS, mechanical irritation because of cough, and possibly the intrinsic high susceptibility for inflammatory response of the upper airway in asthmatic and COAD patients.

These patients tend to present with hoarseness, cough, and sore throat. Flexible endoscopy may reveal erythema and white patches on the larynx. Treatments include advising patients to rinse their mouth with clear water following ICS use, education on proper inhaler use technique, and using a spacer device. Improved inhaler device design with more effective delivery mechanism has been developed, such as the breath-actuated inhalers. Some patients will benefit from replacing the metered-dose inhalers with dry powder inhalers (DPIs) since DPI does not require propellants and rely on the patient's inspiratory effort for drug delivery to the lungs.

Chemoradiation-Induced Laryngitis

It is not uncommon to see laryngeal edema and erythema following chemoradiation of the laryngopharyngeal area. Flexible laryngoscopy shows pale or erythematous swelling of the supraglottic region and saliva pooling. It can sometimes be difficult to interpret between postradiation changes and possible residual or recurrent malignant disease. In addition, it could also be due to candidal infection.[4] Postoncological magnetic resonance imaging and close monitoring with regular photographic evidence of the larynx for comparison during follow-up can help in deciding the need for biopsy. Empirical treatment of possible laryngeal candidiasis could also be tried.

Severe persistent swelling following chemoradiation may be due to permanent impaired lymphatic drainage. It would be wise for the patient to stop smoking and keep adequate vocal hygiene. Antireflux medication can be considered. Short courses of high-dose steroids may help reduce laryngeal edema and temporarily improve breathing. The patient may have swallowing impairment, aspiration, and airway obstruction in severe cases requiring tracheostomy. At times, laryngectomy may be the only option for an incompetent nonfunctioning larynx.

Foreign Body Reaction

Teflon (polytetrafluoroethylene) injection in the past for vocal cord medialization has now been discontinued since the early 1990s given its high rate of complications including granuloma formation, implant migration, severe scarring, overinjection, and airway obstruction.[5] Injection of Teflon into the vocal cords will allow it to infiltrate into all layers of vocal folds and laryngeal muscles causing foreign body granulomatous local inflammatory reaction, resulting in stiff vocal folds and subsequent poor voice outcome in the medium and long term. Surgical removal of Teflon granulomas was highly unsatisfactory given its diffuse presence and scarred vocal folds. Removal tends to be incomplete and associated with recurrent formation and granulomas requiring multiple surgeries.[5]

Apart from autologous fat, safer and more widely used implant materials nowadays include silicone, hyaluronic acid, bovine collagen, hydroxyapatite, and Gore-Tex (expanded polytetrafluoroethylene).

Chronic Granulomatous Disease

This generally refers to Wegener's granulomatosis and sarcoidosis. Management of these patients should involve a rheumatologist. Laryngeal involvement by Wegener's typically affects the subglottic area. In the active phase, flexible laryngoscopy may reveal laryngeal erythema reflecting acute inflammation. Cytoplasmic antineutrophil cytoplasmic antibodies serology may be positive. Treatment is with corticosteroids or steroid-sparing immunosuppressants. Subglottic stenosis from scarring may result following resolution.

Sarcoidosis is a systemic granulomatous disease. Involvement of the larynx can give rise to a granulomatous appearance mimicking laryngeal tuberculosis, fungal laryngitis, or squamous cell carcinoma. Chest imaging, serum angiotensin-converting enzyme level, and serum calcium level may help with the diagnosis. Treatment is with corticosteroids or steroid-sparing immunosuppressants.

Infective Laryngitis

Acute Viral Infection

Laryngotracheobronchitis (Croup)
This is a viral infection of the respiratory tract that mainly affects children aged between 6 months and 6 years.[6] Common pathogens are parainfluenza virus, respiratory syncytial virus, adenovirus, and influenza A virus. Diagnosis is clinical and they present with fever, coryza, and cough. Differential diagnoses to be considered include foreign body inhalation and epiglottitis. A chest X-ray may show subglottic edema characterized by the "steeple sign." Nasopharyngeal aspirate for viral antigen detection can be considered. Most croups are mild with no airway compromise and can be treated with humidified air at home. A child with stridor and reduced saturation should be treated with care—avoid upsetting the child and keep the child in upright position, give oxygen, and administer oral corticosteroids and nebulized adrenaline.[7] Intubation and ventilation may occasionally be required.

Acute Bacterial Infection

Supraglottitis and Epiglottitis
Supraglottitis, including epiglottitis, is an acute bacterial infection of the supraglottis resulting in supraglottic inflammation, with the potential to progress rapidly to acute airway obstruction. Common pathogens include *Haemophilus influenzae* type b (Hib), *Neisseria meningitidis*, group A streptococci, *Streptococcus pneumoniae*, *Staphylococcus aureus*, and *Klebsiella pneumoniae*.[8,9]

The introduction of Hib vaccine in 1985 has resulted in marked decrease in the incidence of epiglottitis in children. The incidence of adult epiglottitis has remained relatively stable at 2.3/100,000 per year.[10]

The patient is typically systemically unwell with pyrexia and tachycardia. They present with sore throat, dysphagia, odynophagia, hoarseness, drooling, and respiratory distress. Flexible nasolaryngoscopy shows erythema, swelling, and blisters of the epiglottis and supraglottis (**Fig. 22.3**). The larynx is tender on palpation. Readers are reminded that

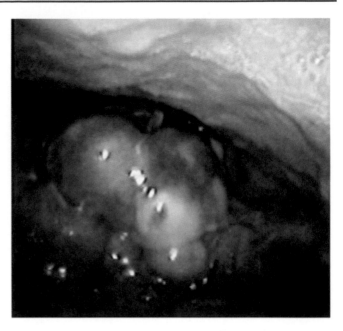

Figure 22.3   Epiglottitis. (*Image courtesy* of Mr. Mark Watson.)

it is not uncommon for patients with sore throat due to supraglottitis to be referred as "tonsillitis." The cognizant doctor would always perform a flexible nasolaryngoscopy to examine the larynx and supraglottis when the tonsils appeared normal on oral and oropharynx examination.

A pediatric patient presenting with suspected epiglottitis with drooling, respiratory distress (tachypnea, tachycardia, use of accessory muscles, recession, tracheal tug, and child prefers to sit up while stabilizing his or her chest with both hands holding onto the bed side arms), and pyrexia should be approached with care. The child should not be provoked to avoid laryngospasm. Tongue depressor examination, flexible endoscopy, and intravenous access should be postponed until the airway is secured. An experienced pediatric anesthetist should be summoned immediately ready to intubate the child to allow for further management.

Routine investigation would include a full blood count specifically looking at the white cell count, a blood culture, and a throat swab. Lateral soft-tissue neck demonstrating the "thumb sign" reflecting the swollen epiglottis is often unnecessary and only indicated if the airway has been secured and the epiglottis/supraglottis has not yet been visualized.

Admission of the patient for close airway observation is crucial. Intravenous antibiotics with second- and third-generation cephalosporin (e.g., Cefotaxime) are used. Short courses of high-dose steroids can also be used to reduce supraglottic swelling. Airway intervention including intubation, cricothyroidotomy, and tracheostomy is sometimes required to relieve acute airway obstruction and save life.

Other Bacterial Upper Respiratory Tract Infections
Pertussis and diphtheria are now uncommon since the widespread uptake of diphtheria/pertussis/tetanus (DPT) vaccination.[11] Both are notifiable diseases and involvement of an infectious disease specialist is mandatory.

Pertussis/whooping cough is caused by *Bordetella pertussis* (gram-negative bacillus). It is a pulmonary infection and presents with coryzal symptoms and paroxysmal cough that can last up to 10 to15 s each, followed by an inspiratory whoop. The diagnosis can be made by nasopharyngeal aspirate culture or polymerase chain reaction and serological testing. Treatment is to provide ventilation support as required (including intubation) and erythromycin.

Diphtheria is caused by *Corynebacterium diphtheriae* (gram-positive bacillus). This infection of the upper aerodigestive tract presents with pyrexia, sore throat, and a dirty gray membranous covering of the tonsils associated with black or green necrotic patches in the oropharynx. Infection can also spread directly into the larynx causing edema, dysphonia, and stridor. Diphtheria toxin has a significant toxic effect on the nervous system and heart. It can result in temporary paralysis of trunk and periphery muscles and permanent myocardium damage with conduction defects. Involvement of the heart increases mortality. Throat swab for microbiology and culture will help with diagnosis. Diphtheria antitoxin must be given as soon as a presumptive diagnosis has been made while waiting for microbiology confirmation. Antibiotics (penicillin or erythromycin) should also be given. Airway monitoring should be in place for early identification for the need of intubation and ventilation. Cardiac monitoring and intervention (as required) is also essential.

Chronic Bacterial Infection

Laryngeal Tuberculosis

Laryngeal tuberculosis (TB)[12] is caused by *Mycobacterium tuberculosis* (*MTB*). This is transmitted by inhaling the cough droplets, containing *MTB*, of someone with infectious TB. Respiratory TB affecting the lungs and larynx are potentially infectious. The risk of infection depends on the duration and intensity of exposure to the bacterium. The longer and more intense the exposure, the higher the risk of transmission of infection. Extrapulmonary TB affecting other organs such as bones, lymph nodes, spine, central nervous system (meninges and brain), or pericardium are rarely infectious.

When immunocompetent people are exposed to *M.Tb*, the immune system will destroy the bacteria and remove it from the body in 80% of the cases.[12] In a small proportion of people, the immune system builds a defensive barrier around the bacteria, and it is not killed but lies in a dormant state. This is known as latent TB (as opposed to the active/infectious TB). The initial bacteria can also travel in the bloodstream or lymphatic channels to other parts of the body before this defensive barrier is established to become latent TB. Latent TB is not infectious and is asymptomatic. It is estimated that one-third of the world's population (2 billion people) have latent TB. Detection of latent TB can be done by the Mantoux test (skin test) and/or blood-based immunological (interferon-gamma) test. It is estimated that up to 3% of the latent TB could become active over a 2-year period.[12]

In the immunocompromised state, such as those with HIV/AIDS and chronic poor health, malnourished, the elderly, drug abusers, and alcoholics, the risk of active TB infection is much higher.[12] These patients either failed to mount the appropriate immune response to the bacteria on initial exposure or there was breakdown of the defensive barrier in latent TB from a previous exposure. This will result in spread of the bacteria within the body causing tissue damage (e.g., cavitating lung lesions in pulmonary TB, granulomatous swelling, and ulceration in the larynx) and constitutional symptoms such as intermittent fever, night sweats, and weight loss.

Although laryngeal TB is commonly associated with active or inactive pulmonary TB, it could also occur independently without pulmonary TB (primary laryngeal TB).[13] Isolated primary laryngeal TB without pulmonary TB has been reported to occur in 15% of cases in a series of 60 laryngeal TB cases.[14] Sites commonly affected include true cords, false cords, and epiglottis.[13,15,16] The posterior commissure of the larynx has been reported to be commonly involved.[17] The modes of spread to the larynx are thought to be direct exposure to *M.Tb* (either from external cough droplets or from active pulmonary TB), hematogenous spread, or lymphatic spread.

Patients with laryngeal TB most commonly present with hoarseness, odynophagia, dysphagia, and sore throat.[15,18] In contrast, odynophagia and sore throat are not common in malignancies such as squamous cell carcinoma. Other upper aerodigestive tract symptoms in laryngeal TB also include cough, hemoptysis, and dyspnea.[17] These later symptoms are more common in patients with associated pulmonary TB. Potential upper airway obstruction with stridor can occur, albeit rarely, from swelling and granulomatous changes of the disease-infected glottis and supraglottis.

Fiberoptic examination may reveal papilloma, ulceration, generalized erythema, leukoplakia, or exophytic granulomatous lesions of the larynx and epiglottis.[14] Although unilateral vocal cord erythema (monochorditis) is a classical acute presentation of laryngeal TB (**Fig. 22.4**), the majority of patients with laryngeal TB present with granulomatous appearance (**Fig. 22.5**) and this can be very similar to squamous cell carcinoma. A firm diagnosis and confident exclusion of malignancy can only be achieved by biopsy and histological examination. Histology shows granulomas with caseating necrosis and Langhans-type giant cells. Acid-fast bacilli have been reported to be found in 88% of histological specimens containing *M.Tb* changes.[15]

Chest X-rays should be a routine investigation to look for pulmonary TB. Although microscopy and culture for acid-fast bacilli in sputum give definitive diagnosis of TB in the patient, it does not always reflect laryngeal involvement. One could also argue that the generalized erythema or ulceration could be a result of cough trauma from pulmonary TB. Therefore, a positive microscopy and culture result may merely indicate pulmonary TB since the sputum could have been coughed up from the lungs. As such, histological examination with *M.Tb* features of laryngeal tissue is vital to confirm true laryngeal

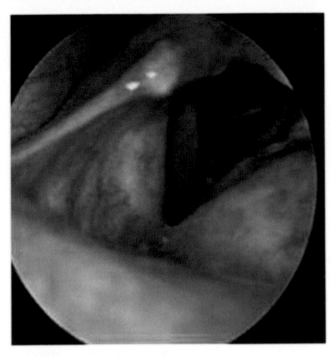

Figure 22.4 Laryngeal tuberculosis showing right monochorditis. (*Image courtesy* of Dr. Abir K. Bhattacharyya.)

involvement. Other differential diagnoses include Wegener's granulomatosis, sarcoidosis, fungal infection, and syphilis. These can also be excluded from histological examination.

The diagnosis of laryngeal TB, which is a form of respiratory TB, would mandate a referral to an infectious disease physician trained in TB management. It is likely

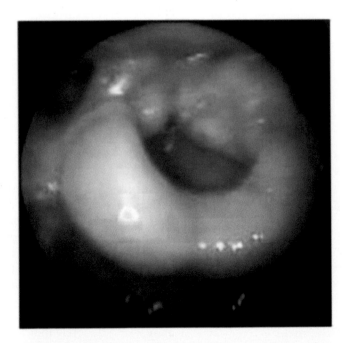

Figure 22.5 Laryngeal tuberculosis showing epiglottis edema, arytenoid edema, left arytenoid ulceration, lack of erythema, and a pale appearance. (*Image courtesy* of Prof. Alok Thakar.)

that a multidisciplinary approach will be taken by the TB team with involvement of specialized nurses and health visitors. Contact tracing will also be initiated upon confirmation of diagnosis. Treatment should be commenced as soon as possible without the need to wait for culture results. A 6-month, four-drug initial regimen (6 months of isoniazid and rifampicin supplemented in the first 2 months with pyrazinamide and ethambutol) is recommended.[12] Improvement and resolution of laryngeal abnormalities have been reported to occur within 2 to 4 weeks of treatment.[13,15,16,19] Completion of the treatment course is essential to avoid development of drug-resistant TB. Directly observed therapy is sometimes indicated to ensure compliance with treatment, given the socioeconomic status of this patient group. No routine follow-up is required following successful treatment and patients are educated and advised to self-monitor. Those with drug-resistant TB should be followed up for 12 months. Those with multidrug-resistant TB should have prolonged follow-up.

Complications from untreated infection may progress to vocal cord paralysis from cricoarytenoid joint destruction, muscular involvement, or recurrent laryngeal nerve damage.[15] Laryngeal web, posterior glottic stenosis, and subglottic stenosis may also occur as a result.[14] It is therefore important to recognize the condition and manage this early to avoid complications and spread of infection.

Fungal Infection

Mycotic infection can occur in the larynx. These included candidiasis (most common), histoplasmosis,[11] and blastomycosis.[11]

Histoplasmosis is mainly a pulmonary fungal disease caused by *Histoplasma capsulatum*. It may present with nodular granuloma in the larynx when it is involved. Dissemination of the infection can occur to cause meningitis, endocarditis, pericarditis, and arthropathies.

Blastomycosis is caused by *Blastomyces dermatitidis*. This is again primarily a pulmonary fungal infection. Extrapulmonary involvement is most likely through dissemination of disease. Laryngeal involvement could be due to direct exposure to the fungus and hematogenous or lymphatic spread from lungs. Skin involvement can also be due to direct inoculation from dog bites or accidental skin exposure to the organism in laboratory or at autopsy. Laryngeal appearance may mimic squamous cell carcinoma.

The management approach to laryngeal fungal infection would be to perform biopsies to exclude malignancy when there is any doubt. Microscopy and culture may reveal the fungal organism. Chest imaging (chest X-ray or chest computed tomography) may show multiple small calcification and mediastinal granulomas in histoplasmosis.

Treatment with itraconazole in immunocompetent patients approaches 90% success rate.[11] Alternative antifungal drug includes fluconazole (available in both oral and intravenous forms) and amphotericin B intravenous infusion. An infectious disease specialist is invariably involved in the management of these patients.

Candidiasis

Symptoms of laryngeal candidiasis include hoarseness or dysphonia, chronic cough, shortness of breath, sore throat, and globus sensation. Predisposing factors for laryngeal candidiasis include a breach in the mucosal integrity of the larynx, immunodeficiency, use of immunosuppressants, postradiotherapy in the laryngeal area,[4] use of ICSs, and long-term use of antibiotics.[20,21]

Direct visualization (e.g., flexible laryngoscopy) of the larynx may reveal white patches on a background of laryngeal erythema and edema. Common sites affected included the supraglottis, glottis, subglottis, and hypopharynx (**Fig. 22.6**). These white patches may mimic leukoplakia. They can also present with hyperplastic, exophytic, or papillomatous lesions suspicious of laryngeal carcinoma. In cases like these, it will be necessary to biopsy the larynx to exclude malignancy. Histological features of fungal infection may include epithelial hyperplasia, parakeratosis, cellular atypia, neutrophil infiltration, or focal dysplasia.[22] *Candida* stain weakly with hematoxylin and eosin (H&E) and therefore can sometimes be missed. It would be useful to perform additional stain of a confident deep laryngeal biopsy with periodic acid–Schiff (PAS) or Gomori's methenamine silver to look for candida.[22] Microscopy and culture will help determine the actual fungal species and sensitivity to antifungal medication.

Treatment of laryngeal candidiasis includes vocal hygiene with good hydration. Oral nystatin (4 to 6 mL of

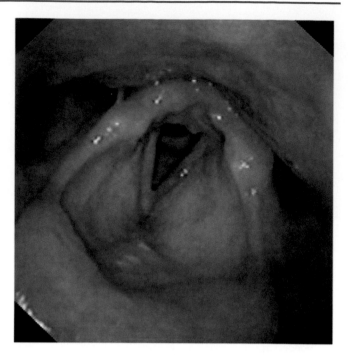

Figure 22.7 Fungal laryngitis—posttreatment. (*Image courtesy of* Mr. Mark Watson.)

100,000 units/mL qds) and/or systemic oral fluconazole (100 to 200 mg/d) for laryngeal candidiasis given for between 1 and 4 weeks is effective with up to 95% response rate after a single course of treatment (**Fig. 22.7**).[21,23] Treating or controlling any predisposing factors, if possible, would also help (e.g., ensuring good control of blood sugar in diabetic patients). It is wise to involve a infectious disease specialist in the management of these patients.

Conclusion

LPR, acute viral upper respiratory tract infection, and acute epiglottitis are common causes for laryngeal inflammation. Management of chronic laryngeal infection such as laryngeal tuberculosis or fungal laryngitis should involve the infectious disease specialist.

Acknowledgments
We would like to acknowledge and thank Mr. Mark Watson for kindly providing and allowing us to use clinical photographs in **Figs. 22.2, 22.3, 22.6,** and **22.7**.

We would like to acknowledge and thank Dr. Abir K. Bhattacharyya for kindly providing and allowing us to use the clinical photograph in **Fig. 22.4**.

We would also like to acknowledge and thank Prof. Alok Thakar for kindly providing and allowing us to use the clinical photograph in **Fig. 22.5**.

References

1. Pearson JP, Parikh S, Orlando RC, et al. Review article: reflux and its consequences—the laryngeal, pulmonary and oesophageal manifestations. Conference held in conjunction with the 9th

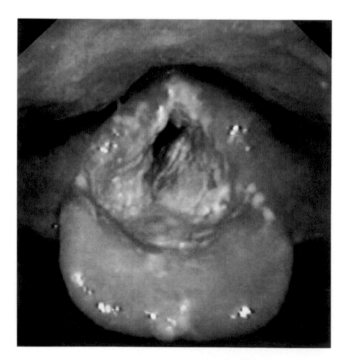

Figure 22.6 Fungal laryngitis—pretreatment. (*Image courtesy of* Mr. Mark Watson.)

International Symposium on Human Pepsin (ISHP) Kingston-upon-Hull, UK, 21-23 April 2010. Aliment Pharmacol Ther 2011;33(Suppl 1):1–71

2. MacKenzie K. Chronic laryngitis. In: Scott-Brown WG, Gleeson M, Browning GG, Hibbert J, eds. Scott-Brown's Otolaryngology, Head and Neck Surgery. Vol 2. 7th ed. London: Hodder Arnold; 2008:2264–2265

3. Roland NJ, Bhalla RK, Earis J. The local side effects of inhaled corticosteroids: current understanding and review of the literature. Chest 2004;126(1):213–219

4. Divi V, Gupta R, Sataloff RT, Pebdani P. Laryngeal candidiasis. Ear Nose Throat J 2010;89(11):526

5. Netterville JL, Coleman JR Jr, Chang S, Rainey CL, Reinisch L, Ossoff RH. Lateral laryngotomy for the removal of Teflon granuloma. Ann Otol Rhinol Laryngol 1998;107(9 Pt 1):735–744

6. Knutson D, Aring A. Viral croup. Am Fam Physician 2004;69(3):535–540

7. Brown JC. The management of croup. Br Med Bull 2002;61:189–202

8. Swift AC. Acute infections of the larynx. In: Scott-Brown WG, Gleeson M, Browning GG, Hibbert J, eds. Scott-Brown's Otolaryngology, Head and Neck Surgery. Vol 2. 7th ed. London: Hodder Arnold; 2008:2248–2257

9. Trollfors B, Nylén O, Carenfelt C, et al. Aetiology of acute epiglottitis in adults. Scand J Infect Dis 1998;30(1):49–51

10. Hugosson S, Olcén P, Ekedahl C. Acute epiglottitis—aetiology, epidemiology and outcome in a population before large-scale *Haemophilus influenzae* type b vaccination. Clin Otolaryngol Allied Sci 1994;19(5):441–445

11. Mandell GL, Bennett JE, Dolin R. Mandell, Douglas, and Bennett's Principles and Practice of Infectious Diseases. 7th ed. Philadelphia, PA: Churchill Livingstone/Elsevier; 2010

12. (NICE) NIoCE. Tuberculosis—Clinical diagnosis and management of tuberculosis, and measures for its prevention and control. In: (NICE) NIoCE, ed. Vol NiCE Clinical Guideline 117. Royal College of Physicians of London: National Institute of Clinical Excellence (NICE); 2011

13. Edizer DT, Karaman E, Mercan H, Alimoglu Y, Esen T, Cansiz H. Primary tuberculosis involving epiglottis: a rare case report. Dysphagia 2010;25(3):258–260

14. Lim JY, Kim KM, Choi EC, Kim YH, Kim HS, Choi HS. Current clinical propensity of laryngeal tuberculosis: review of 60 cases. Eur Arch Otorhinolaryngol 2006;263(9):838–842

15. Wang CC, Lin CC, Wang CP, Liu SA, Jiang RS. Laryngeal tuberculosis: a review of 26 cases. Otolaryngol Head Neck Surg 2007;137(4):582–588

16. Uslu C, Oysu C, Uklumen B. Tuberculosis of the epiglottis: a case report. Eur Arch Otorhinolaryngol 2008;265(5):599–601

17. Bhat VK, Latha P, Upadhya D, Hegde J. Clinicopathological review of tubercular laryngitis in 32 cases of pulmonary Kochs. Am J Otolaryngol 2009;30(5):327–330

18. Ling L, Zhou SH, Wang SQ. Changing trends in the clinical features of laryngeal tuberculosis: a report of 19 cases. Int J Infect Dis 2010;14(3):e230–e235

19. Huon LK, Huang SH, Wang PC, Chen LC. Clinical photograph. Laryngopharyngeal tuberculosis masquerading as chronic laryngopharyngitis. Otolaryngol Head Neck Surg 2009;141(4):537–538

20. Neuenschwander MC, Cooney A, Spiegel JR, Lyons KM, Sataloff RT. Laryngeal candidiasis. Ear Nose Throat J 2001;80(3):138–139

21. Wong KK, Pace-Asciak P, Wu B, Morrison MD. Laryngeal candidiasis in the outpatient setting. J Otolaryngol Head Neck Surg 2009;38(6):624–627

22. Pabuçcuoğlu U, Tuncer C, Sengiz S. Histopathology of candidal hyperplastic lesions of the larynx. Pathol Res Pract 2002;198(10):675–678

23. Chandran SK, Lyons KM, Divi V, Geyer M, Sataloff RT. Fungal laryngitis. Ear Nose Throat J 2009;88(8):1026–1027

23 Granulomatous Diseases of the Larynx

Nupur Kapoor Nerurkar and Gauri Kapre

Ever since Manuel Garcia devised the laryngeal mirror in 1854, physicians began to develop an interest in diagnosing and localizing lesions of the larynx. There was a realization that all patients with an altered voice pattern need not have the same pathology. Infections, neoplasms, movement disorders, to name a few, gradually began to be diagnosed by visualizing the larynx and from thereon grew the science of laryngology.

The term *granuloma* is derived from the Latin word "granulum," referring to a small particle such as a grain. Such granulomas are formed as a result of a systemic immunological response to a specific or nonspecific antigen. Chronic granulomatous conditions of the larynx form a part of such systemic diseases with specific laryngeal lesions. Often, the physical presentations of these conditions mimic laryngeal cancer and hence early diagnosis is of utmost importance to ensure correct treatment.

Among the granulomatous diseases affecting the larynx, the ones which are more clinically relevant for a laryngologist will be discussed and elaborated here. These include tuberculosis, sarcoidosis, fungal laryngitis, Wegener granulomatosis, leprosy, syphilis, and rhinoscleroma.

Laryngeal Tuberculosis

As early as in the 17th century, Morgagni described laryngeal lesions caused by tuberculosis. Louis, in the mid-19th century, established the correlation between pulmonary and laryngeal tuberculosis and explained the pathophysiology of such laryngeal lesions.

With the ever-increasing incidence of HIV and AIDS leading to an increase in the immunocompromised population, researchers have noted a resurgence in the incidence of tuberculosis in all its manifestations, especially the extrapulmonary variety.[1] Laryngeal tuberculosis is a disease commonly affecting young adults. However, studies have shown an increasing incidence in patients in the fifth and sixth decades of life.[2] Before the advent of highly efficacious antitubercular chemotherapy, the incidence of extrapulmonary tuberculosis was reported as nearly 30%,[3] which has now decreased dramatically. Although laryngeal tuberculosis is now relatively uncommon (accounting for only up to 1 to 10% of all patients having tuberculosis),[4] it is, nevertheless, the most common ENT manifestation of the disease, discounting cervical lymphadenopathy.

Clinical Features

Most chronic granulomatous diseases of the larynx present with hoarseness and vocal fatigue, occasionally associated with cough. Odynophagia and odynophonia are also commonly encountered symptoms. These symptoms

stand true also for laryngeal tuberculosis. Most patients usually have coexistent cavitatory lesions in the lungs. Such patients may present with hemoptysis, breathlessness on exertion, and productive cough. Constitutional symptoms such as anorexia, weight loss, evening rise of temperature, and general debility in patients with chronic laryngitis are pointers toward suspecting tuberculosis.

In the preantibiotic era, the most common cause of laryngeal tuberculosis was the pooling of secretions in the posterior glottis due to the patient being in the recumbent position. Perhaps for this reason, the posterior larynx was the commonest site of tubercular lesions of the larynx. In recent times, however, as morbidity associated with the disease has reduced, this theory no longer holds true. The spread of the disease to the larynx is thought to be more via the hematogenous and lymphatic route and hence we find lesions more anteriorly, especially over the vocal folds.[5] Lindell et al[6] have mentioned that the site of the disease is the true vocal folds in 47.1% of the cases, the epiglottis in 39.4%, and the false vocal folds in 29.2%. The disease may even spread to the pharynx, tonsils, or palate; however, its spread to the subglottis is uncommon.

Diffuse asymmetric involvement of the vocal folds, which may be unilateral or bilateral, is the typical clinical picture seen in tubercular laryngitis. In the early stages of the disease, there are signs of severe and extensive inflammation and congestion over the vocal folds (**Fig. 23.1**). There is exudation and round cell infiltration in the subepithelial layers of the superficial lamina propria. The edematous-looking thickened epiglottis has been traditionally referred to as "turban epiglottis."[7] Hermani and Sawitra reported that exophytic lesions are more common than the ulcerative type.[4]

These lesions, especially if unilateral, might quite often be mistaken for a malignancy. Inflammatory infiltration eventually heals with fibrotic changes.

Investigations

A video laryngoscopic examination using a flexible laryngoscope or a 70-degree Hopkins rod examination is a must. It is important to note the site of the lesion, the involvement of contiguous structures, and also the impairment of vocal fold mobility, if any. A biopsy should be taken from the representative part of the lesion. *Mycobacterium tuberculosis* bacilli are detected on acid-fast staining of the biopsied tissue. Histopathology shows granulomatous foci intramucosally with lymphocytic infiltrate, epithelioid cells, and Langhans giant cells.

Systemic evaluation for tuberculosis should be done in all patients and family members should be screened for possible infection. This includes routine investigations such

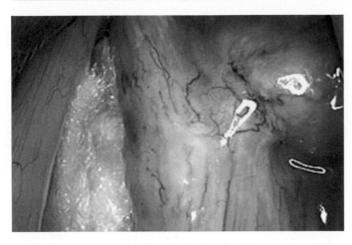

Figure 23.1 Laryngeal tuberculosis showing inflammation of the right vocal fold with a granulomatous lesion on the superior surface extending into the right ventricle.

as complete blood count (which reveals lymphocytosis and an elevated erythrocyte sedimentation rate [ESR]), tuberculin test, and sputum examination for acid-fast bacilli (AFB). Sputum-positive rates may be as high as 90 to 95%.[5]

Radiological investigations include plain radiographs of the chest and neck as well as computed tomography (CT) and MRI evaluation of the larynx. About 40 to 70% of patients had a fibrotic or fibrocavitatory lesion on chest X-ray.[6] It is important to note that the integrity of the laryngeal skeleton is always maintained in cases of laryngeal tuberculosis, unlike malignancies. In untreated or inadequately treated cases, some amount of laryngeal stenosis or cricoarytenoid joint fixation may be noted.

Due to the increasing trend of extrapulmonary tuberculosis in immunocompromised patients, all patients of laryngeal tuberculosis must be evaluated for HIV and AIDS.

Treatment

Once the diagnosis is confirmed, appropriate antitubercular chemotherapy should be immediately instituted. The standard HRZE (isoniazid, rifampicin, pyrazinamide, and ethambutol) regimen for extrapulmonary tuberculosis is started. The response to the treatment is usually quite good and, indeed, a favorable response to the therapy is a confirmation of the diagnosis. Monitoring liver enzymes during the treatment is important.

Sarcoidosis

Sarcoidosis is a multisystem disease of unknown etiology, characterized by noncaseating epithelioid granulomas. The respiratory system is affected in more than 90% of the cases with granuloma formation within the lung parenchyma as well as the hilar lymph nodes.[8] Skin, liver, eyes, and heart are less frequently involved. Sarcoidosis of the upper airway is quite rare.

Clinical Features

As the pulmonary system is most commonly affected, patients most often present with a persistent dry cough or, in some cases, dyspnea on exertion. Constitutional symptoms such as fatigue and weight loss may also be seen. Pulmonary fibrosis is the most severe complication of the disease. Airway involvement in sarcoidosis initially manifests as mucosal edema, inflammation, and erythema with granuloma formation which heals with fibrosis. Endobronchial granuloma formation may take place which heals with fibrosis, ultimately giving rise to bronchial stenosis in 14% of the cases.[8]

Among the extrapulmonary manifestations, lymph node enlargement remains the commonest (about 70% of the cases), as with tuberculosis.[9]

Nasal passages, oropharynx, and larynx are affected in about 6% of sarcoidosis patients.[10] Laryngeal lesions may be found on the epiglottis, aryepiglottic folds, false vocal folds, and subglottis (**Fig. 23.2**). The epiglottis and aryepiglottic folds are thickened with granularity and yellowish red nodule formation. Sometimes the nodular lesions in the supraglottic larynx will lead to airway obstruction and a tracheostomy may be required to relieve the stridor. The true vocal folds are less frequently involved.[11] In contrast to tuberculosis, where laryngeal lesions are virtually always associated with a pulmonary focus, laryngeal sarcoid nodules can exist without any pulmonary infiltrates.

Investigations

Confirmation of the disease is only possible by doing a histopathological examination of the tissue. Noncaseating granulomas with a surrounding epithelioid reaction with lymphocytic infiltration are characteristic.

Radiological investigations such as X-ray and high-resolution CT of the chest aid in diagnosing the systemic effects of the disease. Asymmetric pulmonary interstitial

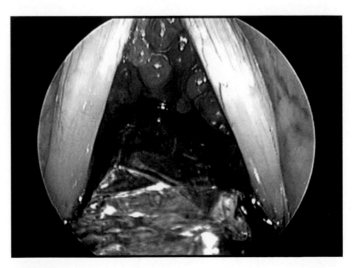

Figure 23.2 Granulomatous tissue seen in the subglottis of a patient of laryngeal sarcoidosis.

or parenchymal infiltrates, fibrotic changes with traction bronchiectasis, or luminal narrowing of the airway are noted. Hilar lymphadenopathy, compressing upon the airway causing luminal narrowing, may be seen. Bronchoalveolar lavage fluid shows lymphocytosis with a CD4+/CD8+ ratio higher than 3.5 in 50% of the cases. Serum angiotensin-converting enzyme levels are raised and are found to correlate with disease activity.[9]

Treatment

Approximately 30 to 70% of patients never require therapy as the disease process is self-limiting.[9] The symptoms will usually resolve within a 1- to 3-year period with only 10 to 20% of patients suffering permanent sequelae. In patients with significant pulmonary infiltrates or serious extrapulmonary manifestations, systemic corticosteroids are administered for a minimum duration of 12 months. Methotrexate, azathioprine, cyclophosphamide, infliximab, and eternacept have all been used with varying efficacy in sarcoidosis, especially with extrapulmonary manifestations. A period of 3 years after discontinuation of the therapy should have passed before the patient is declared as healed.

The laryngeal lesions will usually respond to a course of prolonged systemic steroids. Some studies have also advocated intralesional steroid injection. If the response is suboptimal, or if the laryngeal lesion is large enough to cause airway obstruction, surgical resection by the transoral route with or without the laser may be done. Tracheostomy may be required to tide over the crisis of acute airway obstruction. In the case of stenosed airways, serial dilatations may be required. Some studies have used external beam irradiation for the control of local laryngeal lesions, while others believe that this will lead to further fibrosis.

Fungal Laryngitis

Fungal laryngitis is more common in immunocompromised patients such as those with HIV, diabetes, and patients on long-term steroid therapy. Some studies have reported an 89% incidence of fungal laryngitis in patients on inhaled steroids.[12] Candidiasis in the larynx is more common than histoplasmosis and blastomycosis.

Candidiasis

Candida albicans is the causative fungus. Clinical features include hoarseness, dysphonia, dysphagia, and, very rarely, respiratory distress. On laryngoscopy, the laryngeal mucosa is edematous, hyperemic with whitish adherent plaques or a greyish white pseudomembrane formation (**Fig. 23.3**). Cytology (brush cytology) and culture from the lesion are less invasive procedures for diagnosis. However, sometimes it may be essential to get a tissue biopsy for diagnosis.

A large part of the treatment is supportive, directed toward treating the predisposing illness. Surgical intervention is rarely required and antifungal drugs ranging from ketoconazole to amphotericin B are effective.

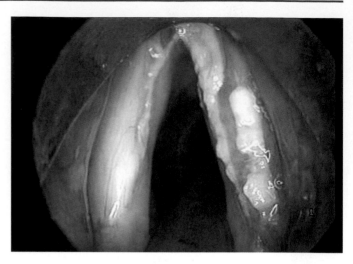

Figure 23.3 White plaques on both the vocal folds in a case of candidiasis of the larynx.

Printed with permission from Jaypee. Nerurkar N, Kapre G. Leukoplakia of the vocal folds. In: Hathiram BT, Khattar VS, eds. *Atlas of Operative Otorhinolaryngology and Head & Neck Surgery*. Vol. 2. New Delhi, India: Jaypee Brothers Medical Publishers; 2013:Chapter 113.

Histoplasmosis

This is a rare infection caused by the dimorphic fungus, *Histoplasma capsulatum*. The impact of the disease depends upon the nutritional status, age, and immunological profile of the patient. Painful swallowing and speech, dysphonia, and, rarely, respiratory obstruction are the presenting symptoms. Systemic involvement is also common, with many patients showing hepatosplenomegaly. The laryngeal lesions are more common over the epiglottis and anterior larynx and the mucosa appears edematous and inflamed. Painful necrotic ulcers with raised edges may be seen. Diagnosis can only be confirmed by identifying the organism from a smear taken from the center of the ulcer or from a tissue biopsy of the lesion. Treatment is in the form of intravenous amphotericin B, though some authors proposed a long-term oral ketoconazole therapy as an alternative.

Blastomycosis

This fungal infection is more common in Northern America and is caused by *Blastomyces dermatidis*. Pulmonary lesions are most common, although multisystem involvement is known. Laryngeal lesions are seen mostly over the vocal folds. There is a formation of erythematous granulomas that ulcerate and form microabscesses. The fungus can be isolated from these abscesses.

Wegener Granulomatosis

Wegener granulomatosis, more recently renamed as granulomatosis with polyangiitis, is a systemic disease commonly affecting the lungs, kidneys, and sinuses. It is characterized by a necrotizing and granulomatous vasculitis of the renal and airway vessels. Involvement of the upper

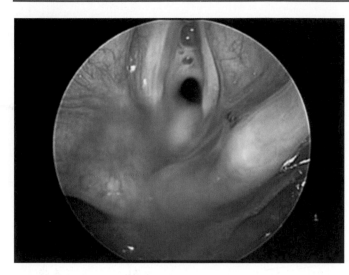

Figure 23.4 Subglottic stenosis in a patient of Wegener granulomatosis.

Printed with permission from Jaypee. Garg S, Nerurkar N. Childhood Wegener's Granulomatosis in Subglottic Stenosis. *International Journal of Laryngology and Phonosurgery* 2011;1(2):71–73.

airway is often misdiagnosed, as biopsies from this region may not display the classic vasculitis pattern.[13] Isolated involvement of the upper airway remains an unusual manifestation of the disease process.

Clinical Features

Pulmonary cavitatory infiltrates lead to dry cough, hemoptysis, and breathlessness. Renal symptoms dominate the clinical picture with hematuria and proteinuria caused by immune-mediated glomerulonephritis. Ocular, skin, cardiac, and CNS involvements may be seen. Laryngeal involvement, whenever present, is seen in the upper trachea and subglottis. Symptoms range from a slight progressive hoarseness of the voice with dyspnea on exertion to full-blown stridor needing emergency tracheostomy. The subglottic region, especially at the level of the ring-shaped cricoid cartilage, is more prone to critical airway narrowing caused by circumferential stenosis, as is seen in about 20% of patients (**Fig. 23.4**).[14] Often, the disease can be localized to the posterior subglottis. The mucosa becomes boggy, erythematous, and sometimes ulcerated. On occasion, granulomas may become large enough to produce a mass lesion. Involvement of the vocal folds or bronchi is quite uncommon.[13] Other ENT manifestations are in the form of pansinusitis, nasal septal perforation, and eustachian tube blockage, leading to serous otitis media.

Investigations

A CT scan of the chest and neck will show the area of stenosis and pulmonary lesions, if any. However, direct endoscopic visualization is a must for taking a biopsy from the site to clinch the diagnosis. Histopathologically, often, nonspecific acute and chronic inflammatory changes with granulomas

are seen, but rarely vasculitis. This makes it difficult to rule out other differentials such as tuberculosis, sarcoidosis, or even posttraumatic subglottic stenosis.

Pulmonary function tests will reveal airflow obstruction, if any, due either to the pulmonary infiltrates or airway narrowing. Antineutrophil cytoplasmic antibody levels are raised, especially in the presence of active glomerulonephritis, but cannot be considered as markers for disease activity.

Treatment

Immunosuppressive therapy using intravenous cyclophosphamide (or even azathioprine) and glucocorticoids is most effective. However, it has been noted that laryngeal lesions do not respond well even to aggressive systemic immunosuppressive therapy. Intralesional steroid injection has a certain role, especially when coupled with tracheal dilatation. Laser excision of the stenosis has not proved beneficial, with most surgeons reporting severe subsequent scarring and narrowing of the airway. Tracheostomy is needed to relieve airway obstruction. Before contemplating any major open surgery, such as tracheoplasty or cricotracheal resection with primary anastomosis, stabilization of the disease pathology is advisable.

Leprosy

Leprosy is caused by *Mycobacterium leprae*, an acid-fast and obligate intracellular bacillus. Although there have not been any reported cases of isolated laryngeal leprosy in medical literature, it is important for the modern-day laryngologist to be aware of the possibility of this condition.

Clinical Features

The disease usually presents with hypopigmented skin patches with raised or erythematous margins that are hypoesthetic. Enlargement of the peripheral nerves with resultant neuropathies, wrist and foot drop, trophic nonhealing ulcers, and even loss of digits are all hallmarks of leprosy. In the nasal cavity, symptoms mimicking atrophic rhinitis are seen with cartilage destruction, septal perforations, and a saddle nose deformity.

The presenting symptoms of laryngeal lesions are usually a husky hoarse voice, cough, and dyspnea. Hawking and a foreign body sensation are common complaints. A study by Soni et all found laryngeal leprosy in 36% of patients with positive slit-skin smear.[15] The disease process usually starts in the nasal cavity and works its way down the airway involving the supraglottic larynx, especially the epiglottis which is thickened in almost all cases. However, vocal fold involvement is rare. Nodules eventually ulcerate and cause scarring, leading to stenosis in some cases, which may present with respiratory distress.

Bretan et al suggested that the mycobacterium invades the mucosa of the larynx and infiltrates into the sensory nerve endings possibly causing impaired mobility of the vocal folds and diminished sensation of the laryngeal mucosa, which may contribute to aspiration and oropharyngeal dysphagia.[16]

Investigations

The diagnosis of leprosy is clinical. Demonstration of the acid-fast bacilli in the tissue along with typical epithelioid granuloma formation is characteristic.

Treatment

The regimen for leprosy consists of dapsone, clofazimine, and rifampicin, which are highly efficacious in curing the laryngeal lesions as well.

Syphilis

Syphilis is a chronic infectious disease caused by the spirochete *Treponema pallidum*. It is a sexually transmitted disease or may be passed on from the mother to the fetus (congenital syphilis).

Clinical Features

The incidence of syphilis has dropped reasonably over the years and yet with the upsurge of HIV infections, it is again on a rise. Syphilis has three stages in disease progression, which are primary (the syphilitic chancre), secondary (laryngeal syphilis may appear in this stage), and tertiary.

Patients suffering from laryngeal syphilis complain of a husky, raucous, or slightly hoarse voice sometimes accompanied by discomfort during swallowing. There is no pain in the throat. Syphilitic laryngitis is seen as a descending mucosal infection from the oral cavity and pharynx and hence more often than not, oral ulcers are found to be present. Not surprisingly, therefore, supraglottic lesions are more common.[17] The mucosa is hyperemic, erythematous, and edematous. Papules appear over the free border of the epiglottis and eventually erode to form ulcers, giving it a punched-out appearance. There is granuloma formation over the mucosa of the supraglottis, which, if left untreated, proceeds to perichondritis and chondritis of the thyroid and cricoid cartilage.

Investigations

Diagnosis of the local laryngeal lesion can be confirmed only by biopsy and demonstration of the spirochete in the tissue on dark field microscopy.

Although the *T. pallidum* hemagglutination test and the fluorescent treponemal antibody absorption test are more sensitive in detecting the disease, Venereal Disease Research Laboratories (VDRL) is a good screening tool and titers show a close correlation with disease activity. The patient should also be screened for other sexually transmitted diseases, especially HIV.

Treatment

Penicillin G is the drug of choice for the treatment of syphilis in all stages, with an efficacy that remains unchallenged through the past six decades of its use.

Rhinoscleroma

Rhinoscleroma is an infectious disease caused by the microorganism *Klebsiella rhinoscleromatis* (Frisch's bacillus), more commonly seen in poorer developing parts of the world.

Clinical Features

K. rhinoscleromatis has an affinity for the nasal mucosa, although it can affect the mucosa of the entire respiratory tract. Some authors have reported statistics suggesting a 95 to 100% nasal affliction in patients. The pharynx is affected in 18 to 43%, the larynx in 15 to 80%, the trachea in 12%, and the bronchi in 2 to 7% of the cases.[18] Other sites such as the paranasal sinuses or the eustachian tubes may be affected as well.

The disease is characterized by three clinical stages:

Stage 1: Catarrhal stage
Stage 2: Granulomatous stage
Stage 3: Sclerotic stage

In the catarrhal stage, there is a foul-smelling, mucopurulent nasal discharge, nasal obstruction, and occasional epistaxis.

Most patients present with the second stage, also known as the granulomatous, proliferative, or nodular stage. In this stage, there is nodule or granuloma formation over the mucosa of the respiratory tract, more commonly in the nose. The granulomas over the larynx are in the form of irregular polypoidal masses, which give rise to a productive cough, occasionally with hemoptysis, dysphonia, and even stridor.

Finally, the disease progresses into the sclerosing or cicatrizing stage. This is the stage with the most severe symptoms. The granulomas formed earlier heal with massive fibrosis and scarring, giving rise to an airway compromise which may be severe enough to warrant surgical intervention in the form of tracheostomy. Studies have suggested that subglottic or glottis stenosis is more common. Vocal fold mobility is reduced due to scarring and a severe diffuse stenosis is seen on endoscopy. Tracheal stenosis is usually seen to be limited to the first few tracheal rings and tracheobronchial stenosis is quite rare.[19]

Investigations

Histopathological examination of a biopsy taken from the affected mucosa is the way to make a definite diagnosis. The classic "Mikulicz cells," which are large, foamy, vacuolated macrophages, are seen within the granulomas and "Russell bodies," which are plasma cells with eosinophilic material, are seen within the cytoplasm. In the cicatrizing stage, there

Table 23.1 Summary of the Slient Features of All Granulomatous Diseases of the Larynx

	Supraglottis	Vocal Folds	Subglottis	Lower Airway	Special Tests
Tuberculous laryngitis	Turban epiglottis	Asymmetric involvement	Usually not involved	Cavitatory lesions, mediastinal lymphadenopathy	CBC, ESR, chest X-ray, chest CT scan, sputum AFB, bronchial lavage for AFB
Laryngeal sarcoidosis	May be involved	Usually not involved	Often involved	Hilar lymphadenopathy, traction bronchiectasis, bronchial stenosis, pulmonary infiltration may be absent	Serum ACE levels, bronchial lavage for lymphocytosis
Fungal laryngitis	Usually involved	Usually involved	Usually not involved	Usually not involved	Brush cytology
Wegener granulomatosis	Usually not involved	Usually not involved	Often involved	Pulmonary cavitatory infiltrates	Renal profile, nasal evaluation, neck and chest CT scan

CBC, complete blood count; ESR, erythrocyte sedimentation rate; CT, computed tomography; AFB, acid-fast bacilli; ACE, angiotensin-converting enzyme.

is severe fibrosis with scar tissue and an absence of Mikulicz cells and Russell bodies.

Treatment

The drug of choice is ciprofloxacin. Tetracyclines have also shown good improvement. Duration of the therapy has been proposed as 6 months or until the tissue biopsy becomes negative. For the severe acute airway stenosis, hospitalization with administration of intravenous steroids and surgical intervention in the form of tracheostomy may be required. Laser excision of the stenosis has shown good results. Tracheal and bronchial stenosis may require several sittings of dilatation and a regular follow-up is essential.

Summary

As granulomatous diseases of the larynx often mimic laryngeal malignancy, a tissue biopsy is mandatory for histopathological studies (**Table 23.1**). However, when there is a high suspicion of tuberculous laryngitis, an X-ray of the chest, ESR, and sputum AFB samples may aid the diagnosis. In immunocompromised patients or those using steroid sprays, fungal laryngitis should remain high on the differential and may be diagnosed by a brush biopsy. Keeping our antennae up for the possibility of a granulomatous disease of the larynx helps avoid delayed and wrong treatment for patients.

References

1. Barnes PF, Bloch AB, Davidson PT, Snider DE Jr. Tuberculosis in patients with human immunodeficiency virus infection. N Engl J Med 1991;324(23):1644–1650
2. Kandiloros DC, Nikolopoulos TP, Ferekidis EA, et al. Laryngeal tuberculosis at the end of the 20th century. J Laryngol Otol 1997;111(7):619–621
3. Moon WK, Han MH, Chang KH, et al. Laryngeal tuberculosis: CT findings. AJR Am J Roentgenol 1996;166(2):445–449
4. Hermani B, Sawitra D. Laryngeal tuberculosis: an important issue. Acta Med Indones 2006;38(1):29–32
5. Soda A, Rubio H, Salazar M, Ganem J, Berlanga D, Sanchez A. Tuberculosis of the larynx: clinical aspects in 19 patients. Laryngoscope 1989;99(11):1147–1150
6. Lindell MM Jr, Jing BS, Wallace S. Laryngeal tuberculosis. AJR Am J Roentgenol 1977;129(4):677–680
7. Beg MHA, Marfani S. The larynx in pulmonary tuberculosis. J Laryngol Otol 1985;99(2):201–203
8. Polychronopoulos VS, Prakash UBS. Airway involvement in sarcoidosis. Chest 2009;136(5):1371–1380
9. Nunes H, Bouvry D, Soler P, Valeyre D. Sarcoidosis. Orphanet J Rare Dis 2007;2:46
10. Hunninghake GW, Costabel U, Ando M, et al. ATS/ERS/WASOG statement on sarcoidosis. American Thoracic Society/European Respiratory Society/World Association of Sarcoidosis and other Granulomatous Disorders. Sarcoidosis Vasc Diffuse Lung Dis 1999;16(2):149–173
11. Devine KD. Sarcoidosis and Sarcoidosis of larynx. Laryngoscope 1965;75:533–569
12. Nair AB, Chaturvedi J, Venkatasubbareddy MB, Correa M, Rajan N, Sawkar A. A case of isolated laryngeal candidiasis mimicking laryngeal carcinoma in an immunocompetent individual. Malays J Med Sci 2011;18(3):75–78
13. Hellmann D, Laing T, Petri M, Jacobs D, Crumley R, Stulbarg M. Wegener's granulomatosis: isolated involvement of the trachea and larynx. Ann Rheum Dis 1987;46(8):628–631
14. Blaivas AJ, Strauss W, Yudd M. Subglottic stenosis as a complication of Wegener's granulomatosis. Prim Care Respir J 2008;17(2):114–116
15. Soni NK. Leprosy of the larynx. J Laryngol Otol 1992;106(6):518–520
16. Bretan O, De Souza LB, Lastória JC. Laryngeal lesion in leprosy and the risk of aspiration. Lepr Rev 2007;78(1):80–81
17. Caldarelli DD, Friedberg SA, Harris AA. Medical and surgical aspects of the granulomatous diseases of the larynx. Otolaryngol Clin North Am 1979;12(4):767–781
18. Maguina C, Cortez-Escalante J, Osores-Plenge F, et al. Rhinoscleroma: eight Peruvian cases. Rev Inst Med Trop Sao Paulo 2006;48(5):295–299
19. Yigla M, Ben-Izhak O, Oren I, Hashman N, Lejbkowicz F. Laryngotracheobronchial involvement in a patient with nonendemic rhinoscleroma. Chest 2000;117(6):1795–1798

24 Infections of the Fascial Spaces of the Head and Neck

Mriganka De and Anita Sonsale

Neck spaces are potential fascial planes extending from the skull base to the mediastinum. These potential spaces lie between the layers of the superficial fascia and deep layers of the cervical fascia surrounding the structures of the neck. The fascial layers limit and also direct the spread of infection. These spaces include submandibular, parapharyngeal, retropharyngeal, and prevertebral spaces. Infection of these spaces may vary from lymphadenitis, neck abscess, lethal necrotizing fasciitis, jugular venous thrombosis to descending mediastinitis.[1-3] The knowledge of the neck spaces is invaluable to understand the spread of infection and to prevent potential life-threatening conditions. Neck infections were more common in the preantibiotic era. Even today, it still presents as a challenging condition.[1-5] Once the infection or an abscess is formed in one fascial plane, it can potentially spread to other areas with a potentially lethal, especially airway, compromise.[6] It can affect the pediatric as well as adult population; however, the cause may vary. In the pediatric population, the most common cause of infection is cervical lymphadenitis, and in adults, the infection is of odontogenic and peritonsillar origin. Submandibular space infections are common.[4] Recurrent neck space infections may have underlying congenital cysts that usually need further investigation and treatment.

Anatomy of the Neck Spaces

The anatomy of the neck spaces is helpful in understanding the source, direction, and spread of infection (**Table 24.1**).

Submandibular Space

It is the space of the floor of the mouth. It is bounded superiorly by the mucosa of the floor of the mouth, anteriorly by the mylohyoid and the anterior belly of the digastric

Table 24.1 Anatomy of the Fascial Neck Spaces

Neck spaces	Boundaries	Contents
Submandibular space	Superior: oral mucosa Inferior: anteriorly by mylohyoid and anterior belly of the digastric muscle Posteriorly: posterior belly of the digastric muscle and stylomandibular ligament Medial: hyoglossus and mylohyoid Lateral: skin, platysma, and mandible	Superior sublingual space: sublingual gland Inferior inframylohyoid space: submandibular gland
Parapharyngeal space	Superior: skull base Anterior: pterygomandibular raphe Posterior: prevertebral fascia Medial: superior constrictor, pharyngobasilar fascia Lateral: deep lobe of the parotid gland, mandible	Prestyloid compartment: fat, lymph nodes Internal maxillary artery: pterygoid muscles Poststyloid compartment: carotid artery Internal jugular vein: cranial nerves IX, X, XI, XII Sympathetic chain
Retropharyngeal space	Superior: skull base Inferior: superior mediastinum, tracheal bifurcation Anterior: pharynx, esophagus Posterior: alar fascia Lateral: carotid fascia	Lymph nodes
Prevertebral space	Superior: skull base Inferior: coccyx Anterior: prevertebral fascia Posterior: vertebral bodies	Alveolar tissue
Carotid space	Anterior: sternocleidomastoid Posterior: prevertebral space Medial: visceral space Lateral: sternocleidomastoid	Carotid artery, internal jugular vein, nerve X, ansa cervicalis

Adapted from Lee KJ, Lee MS. *Essential Otolaryngology: Head and Neck Surgery.* New York, NY: McGraw-Hill; 2003.

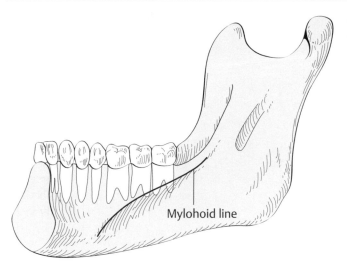

Figure 24.1 Relationship of the mylohyoid line to the molars.

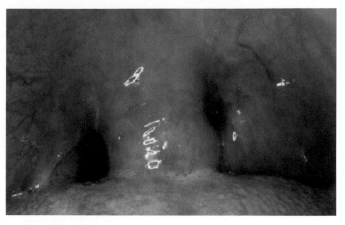

Figure 24.2 Left peritonsillitis. The patient presented with odynophagia, fever, and a degree of trismus. It is the most common cause of deep neck space infections in adults.

muscle, posteriorly by the posterior belly of the digastric muscle and the stylomandibular ligament, medially by the hyoglossus and mylohyoid. It is in continuity with the floor of the mouth along the posterior edge of the mylohyoid. The relationship of the apices of the teeth to the mylohyoid line determines the source of infection from dental origin. The apices of the teeth anterior to the second molar lies superior to the mylohyoid line and the apices of the second and third molars extend below the mylohyoid line as shown in **Fig. 24.1**. Hence infection at the apices of the teeth anterior to the second molar would present with infection in the floor of the mouth, and infection posterior to the second molar would present with infection in the submandibular triangle of the neck.[7]

Clinical Insights

Ludwig angina can lead to a potential airway compromise. The infection presents with a sudden onset of the inability to swallow and dribbling. This is because the infection in the sublingual space pushes the tongue to the roof of the mouth and posteriorly causes an airway compromise. It is one of the otolaryngological emergencies. The need of the hour is an experienced anesthetist and ENT surgeon ready for fiberoptic intubation and, if unsuccessful, for tracheostomy to secure the airway, followed by incision and drainage of the abscess.

Parapharyngeal Space

It is an inverted pyramidal space with its base at the petrous temporal bone of the skull base and its apex at the hyoid bone. It is bounded anteriorly by the pterygomandibular raphe, posteriorly by the prevertebral fascia, and laterally by the deep lobe of the parotid gland.[7] Infection in this space is usually secondary to tonsillar/peritonsillar infections,[4,5] as shown in **Fig. 24.2**.

Retropharyngeal Space

This space is situated behind the pharynx and the esophagus and in front of the prevertebral fascia. It is bounded superiorly by the base of the skull, inferiorly by the superior mediastinum, tracheal bifurcation, anteriorly by the pharynx and the esophagus, posteriorly by the alar fascia (deep layer of the deep cervical fascia), and laterally by the carotid sheath as shown in **Fig. 24.3**. Its contents are fat and lymph nodes in the suprahyoid portion.[7] The greatest number of lymph nodes is found in children under the age of 4 years.

The danger space is between the alar fascia and the true prevertebral fascia. It extends from the skull base to the posterior diaphragm where the alar fascia and the prevertebral fascia fuse together. The prevertebral space is bounded anteriorly by the prevertebral fascia and posteriorly

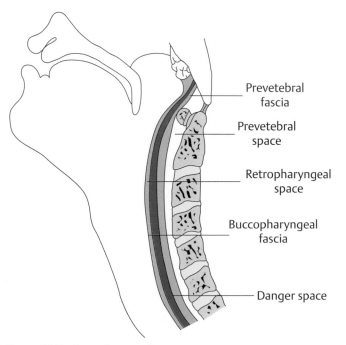

Figure 24.3 Retropharyngeal space.

by vertebral bodies and prevertebral muscles and transverse process, and extends through the entire vertebral column and fuses with the anterior longitudinal ligament at T3.[7]

Deep Neck Space Infection

The involvement of a specific neck space can be usually helpful to identify the source of infection. The fascial layers of the neck (**Fig. 24.4**) act as a barrier to infection, but once the infection is formed, the fascial layers facilitate its spread. Hence anatomical understanding of the neck space and its contents is crucial to the management of infection.

The presentation and etiology of neck space infections defer between pediatric and adult patients. The most common cause of infection in adults is idiopathic followed by odontogenic,[1-5] as shown in **Fig. 24.5**.

Neck Space Infections in Children

The most common cause of infection is cervical lymphadenitis. The typical history is a rapid onset of neck mass, fever, and raised inflammatory markers followed by upper respiratory tract infection. Infection in the parapharyngeal space is usually secondary to odontogenic or tonsillar infection. It is characterized by pyrexia, dehydration, and torticollis with or without external neck swelling. If the index of suspicion for an abscess is high, a computed tomography (CT) scan with contrast is helpful to diagnose a deep-seated abscess.[8-10] External neck incision and drainage with a broad-spectrum antibiotic coverage is the treatment of choice.

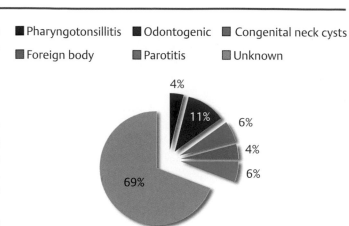

Figure 24.5   Etiology of deep neck infections.
Adapted from Lee KJ, Kim DH, Lim CS. Predisposing factors of complicated deep neck infection. An analysis of 158 cases. *Yonsei Med J.* 2007;48(1):55–62.

In children with a peritonsillar abscess, examination can be challenging because of the trismus. If quinsy is suspected, an experienced pediatric anesthesiologist would be needed to anesthetize the child, as there is a high risk of airway compromise and aspiration.[9] In this population, drainage of the peritonsillar abscess and "hot" tonsillectomy is the preferred course of action.

Special mention is needed for children under the age of 2 years. Retropharyngeal abscess, an uncommon but lethal deep space infection, can occur (95%) in this age group.[2,11] It is due to suppuration of the lymph nodes between the pharynx

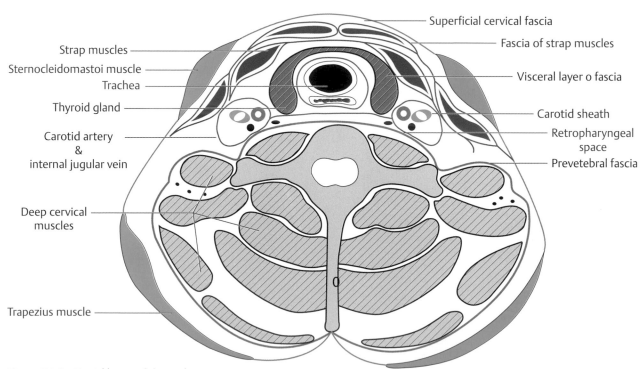

Figure 24.4   Fascial layers of the neck.
Adapted from Lee KJ, Lee MS. *Essential Otolaryngology: Head and Neck Surgery.* New York, NY: McGraw-Hill; 2003.

and the prevertebral fascia. A high index of suspicion is needed in children presenting with high fever, drooling, characteristic neck posture, and raised inflammatory markers. A lateral neck X-ray may fail to reveal the retropharyngeal abscess and hence a CT scan is helpful in the diagnosis of the retropharyngeal abscess. The CT scan should be performed under general anesthesia by a skilled pediatric anesthetist, preferably in the presence of pediatric otolaryngologist.[9–11] The child would require admission for intravenous antibiotics and rehydration and a careful observation, as well as for incision and drainage of the abscess.

Atypical mycobacterial infection is surprisingly common in children. The causative organisms are *Mycobacterium bovis* and *Mycobacterium avium intracellulare*, which are widely present in soil and limescale deposits in the shower head.[11] The organisms enter via oral ingestion and pass to the regional lymph nodes. Atypical mycobacterial infection typically presents in children with a neck lump with a violet-red skin discoloration and skin breakdown. The diagnosis is based on clinical suspicion based on the clinical features with minimal systemic symptoms and long history. Incision and drainage or aspiration should be avoided due to the possibility of sinus formation and compromised cosmetic result. A prolonged antibiotic treatment (3 to 9 months) with a single agent (clarithromycin, ciprofloxacin) or a multiagent (clarithromycin plus ethambutol, isoniazid plus rifabutin) is recommended. These children require a close follow-up.[11]

Young children under the age of 16 months with or without lateral neck abscesses are at risk of having *Staphylococcus aureus* or even methicillin-resistant *S. aureus* infection.[12]

Neck Space Infections in Adults

The most common deep neck space to be involved in adults is the parapharyngeal space, followed by the submandibular space.[1–6] Odontogenic and pharyngotonsillar infections are the leading cause of deep neck space infections. Patients with diabetes mellitus and immunocompromised status are more likely to develop multispace infections and hence a prolonged hospital stay.[4]

Understanding the salient features of deep neck space anatomy is a useful guide to the source of infection.

Infection of the teeth anterior to the second molar involves the sublingual space and may lead to Ludwig's angina. Infection of the second or the third molar tends to involve the submandibular or parapharyngeal space.[8]

Presenting features include a history of upper respiratory tract infection, dental infection, or trauma (including surgery). Examination of these patients is aimed at identifying the source of infection, the extent of infection, and impending airway obstruction. The presence of the trismus can compromise an oral examination. Any suggestion of "hot potato" speech warrants flexible nasolaryngoscopy to rule out any impending airway obstruction. The mainstay of the treatment is broad-spectrum intravenous antibiotics, hydration, protection of the airway, and incision and drainage of the abscess.[1–6]

Investigations

The history, presenting features, and high index of suspicion of deep neck space infections necessitate admission and further investigation. The presence of external swelling may indicate the presence of the abscess, and therefore it may be useful to perform an ultrasound of the neck (**Fig 24.6**). However, if the external swelling is absent, or in the presence of extensive swelling (multispace involvement), a CT scan is the investigation of choice. The CT scan with contrast gives good anatomical understanding of the space and the presence of complications such as jugular venous thrombosis and mediastinitis (see **Figs. 24.7** and **24.8**).

Retropharyngeal space infection is seen posteromedially to the parapharyngeal space and causes the displacement of prevertebral muscles posteriorly. Prevertebral space infection causes the displacement of prevertebral muscles anteriorly and involves the muscles with or without the vertebral body. The common organisms isolated are *Klebsiella*

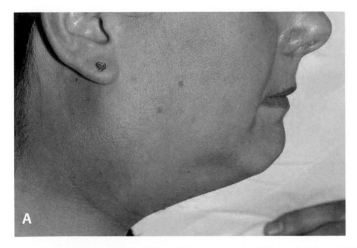
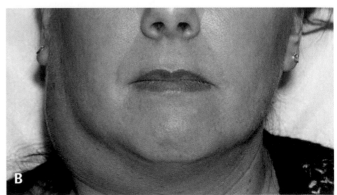

Figure 24.6 Inflamed swelling of the right neck: (A) lateral view and (B) front view.

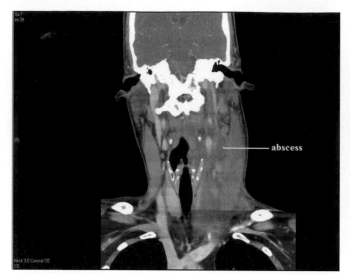

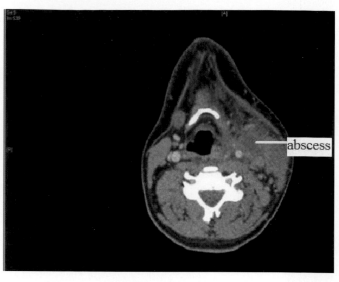

Figure 24.7 Coronal section of a computed tomography scan image with a left neck abscess in the submandibular space. The arrow indicates the abscess cavity. The section reveals the hypodense area lateral to the carotid artery and under the cover of the sternocleidomastoid muscle. The patient required incision and drainage and intravenous antibiotics.

Figure 24.8 Axial computed tomography (CT) scan section with a left neck abscess. The arrow indicates the abscess cavity. The axial CT image is from the same patient as in **Figure 24.7**. The abscess cavity is lateral to the carotid artery and deep to the sternocleidomastoid muscle.

pneumoniae, Streptococcus milleri group bacteria, and anaerobic bacteria.[1–5,7] *Streptococcus aureus* has been found in children with complications.[12] In an immunocompromised or recurrent abscess, the pus from the site is helpful for the purpose of antibody sensitivity.[7]

Clinical Insight

Patients with immunocompromised status, systemic disease (HIV), and uncontrolled diabetes mellitus are more likely to have multispace infection, complications, and a prolonged hospital stay. The threshold for a CT scan, especially in these cases, should be low.

Clinical Pearls

- Anatomy of fascial neck spaces is a key to better understanding of the fascial space infection and its management.
- Computed tomography scan is the preferred investigation in patients with potential multispace infections and complications.
- Maintenance and protecting the airway is crucial to the management of deep fascial space infections.
- Intravenous antibiotics are the mainstay of the treatment along with incision and drainage of the abscess.
- Length of the treatment depends on the causative organism and immunological status of the patient.

Conclusion

Despite improvement in dental care and the presence of antibiotics, deep neck space infections still persist and can cause significant morbidity.[1–6] Deep neck space infections can affect all age groups and can cause potentially life-threatening complications and airway compromise. It is important to understand the anatomy of the deep neck space to enable us to know the depth and extend of infections so as to manage them effectively to avoid morbidity. CT scan is the preferred investigation in cases with potential complications and multispace involvement and a high index of possible retropharyngeal infections. Airway obstruction should be anticipated in infection involving the floor of the mouth and in multispace deep neck infections.[6] The mainstay of the treatment is broad-spectrum intravenous antibiotics, secured airway, and surgical drainage of the abscess.[1–5]

References

1. Bakir S, Tanriverdi MH, Gün R, et al. Deep neck space infections: a retrospective review of 173 cases. Am J Otolaryngol 2012;33(1): 56–63
2. Eftekharian A, Roozbahany NA, Vaezeafshar R, Narimani N. Deep neck infections: a retrospective review of 112 cases. Eur Arch Otorhinolaryngol 2009;266(2):273–277
3. Lee JK, Kim HD, Lim SC. Predisposing factors of complicated deep neck infection: an analysis of 158 cases. Yonsei Med J 2007;48(1):55–62
4. Lee YQ, Kanagalingam J. Deep neck abscesses: the Singapore experience. Eur Arch Otorhinolaryngol 2011;268(4):609–614
5. Srivanitchapoom C, Sittitrai P, Pattarasakulchai T, Tananuvat R. Deep neck infection in Northern Thailand. Eur Arch Otorhinolaryngol 2012;269(1):241–246

6. Karkos PD, Leong SC, Beer H, Apostolidou MT, Panarese A. Challenging airways in deep neck space infections. Am J Otolaryngol 2007;28(6):415–418

7. Yang SW, Lee MH, See LC, Huang SH, Chen TM, Chen TA. Deep neck abscess: an analysis of microbial etiology and the effectiveness of antibiotics. Infect Drug Resist 2008;1:1–8

8. Lee KJ. Essential Otolaryngology: Head and Neck Surgery. 9th ed. New York, NY: McGraw-Hill; 2008

9. Baldassari CM, Howell R, Amorn M, Budacki R, Choi S, Pena M. Complications in pediatric deep neck space abscesses. Otolaryngol Head Neck Surg 2011;144(4):592–595

10. Uzomefuna V, Glynn F, Mackle T, Russell J. Atypical locations of retropharyngeal abscess: beware of the normal lateral soft tissue neck X-ray. Int J Pediatr Otorhinolaryngol 2010;74(12):1445–1448

11. Melia L, Kubba H. Neck abscess in children. ENT & Audiology News. 3 August 2011;20(3):46–47

12. Duggal P, Naseri I, Sobol SE. The increased risk of community-acquired methicillin-resistant Staphylococcus aureus neck abscesses in young children. Laryngoscope 2011;121(1):51–55

25 Benign Lesions of the Larynx

Natasha Choudhury and Khalid Ghufoor

Assessment

Most patients with benign laryngeal disorders present with dysphonia. All patients should undergo a complete assessment, including a head and neck examination to exclude an underlying malignant neoplastic process. Following this, patients should ideally be managed within a voice clinic, with a suitably qualified voice therapist.

A thorough history of all patients presenting with a voice problem is essential. The quality, timing, and frequency of exacerbating and relieving factors must be explored. Contributing factors including smoking, caffeine intake, gastroesophageal reflux disease (GERD), thyroid disease, and regular medications must be documented. Vocal history with particular attention to patterns of vocal behavior should be recorded, as well as attention to vocal hygiene. Vocal abuse behaviors result in damage to the laryngeal mucosa, and this is associated with excessive talking, prolonged or excessive loudness, use of inappropriate pitch, excessive cough, and frequent throat clearing.

A detailed examination of the patient's vocal folds with videolaryngoscopy and stroboscopy should be conducted as routine. In select cases, laryngeal electromyography and quantitative voice measurements may be indicated. Videodocumentation of preoperative findings and a high-quality voice recording are essential. Visualization of the larynx by the patient also enables them to appreciate and understand their pathology and can subsequently improve compliance with voice therapy.

Almost all patients with benign laryngeal pathology should be considered for a trial of voice therapy, before surgery is considered. Education regarding vocal hygiene, hydration, and avoidance of vocal abuse is a necessary baseline. Patients must understand how certain behaviors may have contributed to their vocal fold pathology. Voice therapy to address how these factors may have contributed and correction of these may be all that is required for many patients.

If this is not sufficient to resolve symptoms, and surgery is indicated, patients should also be considered for postoperative voice therapy, to address contributing factors and prevent recurrence of their pathology.

Anatomy

We now have a more comprehensive understanding of the laryngeal anatomy, specifically the microarchitecture of the vocal folds. This knowledge of anatomy has evolved over the past several decades, since Hirano's description of the complex layered microanatomy of the human vocal fold,[1] which is of paramount importance in phonation.

The true vocal fold is composed of five separately identifiable layers. The deepest layer consists of the thyroarytenoid muscle, also functionally known as the "body." Contraction of this muscle stiffens and thickens the vibratory margin of the cord. Overlying this muscle is the lamina propria, which is subdivided into three layers (superficial, middle, and deep), based on the molecular composition of each. The deep layer is largely composed of dense collagen fibers. The middle layer also contains some collagen fibers but is distinguishable by its high elastin content. Together, the deep and middle layers form the vocal ligament or "transition," a recognized and important landmark in vocal fold surgery, and also a transition between the deepest muscle layer and the "cover" (epithelium and superficial lamina propria). The superficial lamina propria is composed mainly of amorphous glands and a few fibrils. The most superficial of all the layers is the overlying stratified nonkeratinizing squamous epithelium that overlies the superficial lamina propria, and together these form the "cover." The layered structure of the vocal fold allows the superficial layer to oscillate independently during phonation.

Principles of Phonosurgery

Understanding the layered microarchitecture of the true vocal fold and its role in normal voice production has led to much emphasis on refined surgical techniques for maximal preservation of normal tissue. The principles of phonosurgery aim to preserve the uninvolved epithelial covering, while removing an underlying lesion. Using this conservative approach, little or no trauma to the normal mucosa and superficial layer of the lamina propria should occur. For almost all benign laryngeal lesions, one should remain superficial to the vocal ligament, which will avoid scar formation, without stimulating fibroblasts in the intermediate layer of the lamina propria, or deeper. There is currently no role for stripping of mucosa of the vocal fold, for benign disease.

Anesthesia

Local anesthesia with sedation can be used to perform direct laryngoscopy for endoscopic microlaryngeal surgery, but this is not widely favored or practiced within the United Kingdom. Most endoscopic procedures for benign laryngeal pathology are performed under general anesthesia as a day case procedure. This requires a close working relationship and cooperation of both the otolaryngologist and the anesthetist for the shared airway.

There are several approaches that can be employed and this is determined by the individuals' experience and preference. Endotracheal intubation provides the safest, most stable ventilation under general anesthesia. A microlaryngoscopy tube, of 5.0 mm internal diameter, can be placed in the posterior glottis and usually provides an adequate view for most pathologies. If transoral laser surgery is planned, specifically designed laser-resistant endotracheal tubes can be used. An alternative approach is general anesthesia without intubation, using the Venturi jet ventilation technique, which allows for a clear view of the larynx. This can be delivered in one of two ways: supraglottic jet ventilation can be employed using a sanders jetting needle secured through a side-arm channel of the laryngoscope, positioned above the level of the vocal folds. This allows for a completely unobstructed laryngeal view for the surgeon. Alternatively, a disposable jet catheter can be placed through the vocal folds to deliver transglottic jet ventilation. The advantage of this is that jet ventilation is initiated below the level of the vocal folds, and therefore there is less mechanical interference at the vibratory margin, when performing surgery.

Clinical Insights

The author (K.G.) prefers supraglottic jet ventilation for laser-assisted surgery as this helps in the dispersal of plume from the surgical field. Delicate microlaryngeal surgery, however, is best achieved with subglottic tracheal jet ventilation.

Laryngeal Instrumentation for Dissection

Technical advances and improved outcome assessments have resulted in great advances in phonosurgery. Suspension laryngoscopy, appropriate anesthetic techniques, microscopic vision, and our improved knowledge of laryngeal microanatomy have led to surgical refinements in endoscopic techniques, with a variety of alternative tools being used. The most widely practiced techniques include cold steel dissection and the carbon dioxide (CO_2) laser.

Cold steel dissection instruments have long been available. In recent times, these instruments have become more refined for the delicate microsurgery that is now practiced, and these should include a selection of sharp, precise microsurgery instruments. However, with the advent of high-magnification microscopes and high-precision microlaryngeal instrumentation, the carbon dioxide laser has become an alternative surgical tool, which should be used as a high-precision surgical knife, in experienced hands. However, the operating surgeon must have a good understanding of the effects of wattage, spot size, and mode (continuous or pulsed) and indeed the indications and limitations of this surgical tool. One important consideration is that the CO_2 laser does introduce a potential risk of peripheral tissue damage, from dissipated thermal injury, and for this reason some laryngologists have traditionally not favored its use in benign laryngeal pathology. However,

others argue that now with the advent of the microspot laser with a spot size of less than 250 µm, the potential heat distribution to the deepest layers of the lamina propria is significantly reduced, making this a safe and effective tool in patients with superficial benign vocal fold lesions. Furthermore, the newer microspot and scanning devices provide a range of spot sizes and laser beam shapes, which can enhance the delivery of laser energy while minimizing carbonization, charring, or thermal collateral effects.

There is still much debate regarding the relative merits of these two mainstream techniques. Only a limited number of studies have directly compared the efficacy of microdissection with microspot CO_2 laser surgery in the larynx, and these have consistently shown comparable results, with no significant differences in clinical outcomes between the two surgical tools.[2,3] There are only two prospective randomized trials comparing CO_2 laser surgery with conventional microdissection techniques. The first of these was reported in 1999 by Hörmann et al, who evaluated pre- and postoperative vocal function using direct videolaryngoscopy, maximal phonation, and speech and singing voice fields.[4] The results from this study showed an improvement in postoperative vocal function with both techniques, but this was only statistically significant in their cold surgery group. A similar prospective randomized study was reported in 2000 by Benninger who compared aerodynamic, perceptual, and videostroboscopic outcome measures between microspot CO_2 laser excision and cold steel microdissection for a variety of superficial benign vocal fold lesions.[5] Interestingly, his data showed no demonstrable difference in clinical outcomes or indeed in the recovery time comparing the two surgical techniques. On balance, the literature largely supports the use of laser in the treatment of superficial benign laryngeal pathologies, and its use is now far more acceptable to most phonosurgeons.

More recently, some surgeons now also advocate the use of powered instruments, such as the laryngeal microdebrider. This can be used for a variety of laryngeal pathologies, including malignancy. However, for benign lesions of the larynx, it is most widely used in the treatment of laryngeal papillomas. However, the safe and efficient use of this powered instrument requires a clear understanding of the instrumentation, including the different blade options and instrument settings. In recent years, the use of the microdebrider for laryngeal papillomas is becoming increasingly favored compared with the laser, as it avoids the risks of laser-associated thermal injury. A few retrospective studies have compared microdebrider with laser treatment for respiratory papillomas. These have shown that microdebrider resection was associated with significantly reduced operative times and potentially reduced cost implications,[6] as well as a reduced incidence of soft-tissue complications.[7] A more recent prospective study also supported the use of the microdebrider, as this was associated with significantly better objective voice outcomes postoperatively.[8] The only randomized, prospective study comparing microdebrider with CO_2 laser removal of recurrent respiratory papillomas also demonstrated greater improvement in voice quality and shorter procedure times,[9] thus supporting the use of the microdebrider as a safe and potentially more cost-effective tool. Cautious use of this device is needed to avoid resection of normal epithelium.

All techniques require extreme care and a skilled surgeon. Individually, they are all excellent tools if used in the correct way, with due consideration to the microanatomy of the vocal folds and the principles of phonosurgery. The use of all types of instrumentation should be within the armamentarium of every phonosurgeon, and the use of each tool should be modified according to the pathology that is being treated.

Clinical Insights

The author (K.G.) prefers the use of the CO_2 laser particularly for extensive pathology or premalignant conditions of the larynx. Any surgical intervention on the free edge of the musculomembranous vocal fold requires great care, with laser settings adjusted to minimize collateral trauma. Use of lowest power settings to effect change to the lesion (~2.5 W) and in either single pulse or superpulse (0.4/0.1 seconds) minimize collateral trauma. Most recently, scanned beams of linear 1 or 2 mm length or curvilinear 1 to 3 mm length have provided an excellent tool for bloodless excision of benign lesions with hardly any trauma or disturbance of the adjacent vocal fold epithelium.

Vocal Fold Nodules

Vocal fold nodules (singer's nodules) are benign, localized, and superficial "growths" on the medial surface of the true vocal folds that are believed to result from phonotrauma. Nodules are typically bilateral and usually small and gray-white in color (**Fig. 25.1**), with hyperplastic epithelium and underlying chronic inflammatory infiltrate. They are classically located at the junction of the anterior and middle thirds of the vocal

fold, i.e., midpoint of the membranous vocal fold, and are confined to the superficial squamous epithelium. Nodules are most commonly observed in middle-aged women and children (boys more frequently than girls), who are prone to vocal abuse.

Patients with vocal fold nodules commonly present with dysphonia. This results from their effect on interrupting the vibratory pattern of the vocal fold from both their mass effect and impeding full glottic closure during phonation. Their occurrence is typically related to vocal abuse and misuse. Therefore, attention to underlying causative factors, through voice therapy and education, plays an integral role in the treatment plan. If diagnosed correctly, more than 90% will resolve or become asymptomatic with voice therapy alone. If, however, there is unacceptable vocal impairment despite compliance with medical treatment and voice therapy, surgery may be considered. The nodules can be removed using microsurgical techniques, with minimal normal tissue disruption, usually with cold steel microdissection, although the CO_2 laser can also be used. The center of the nodule should be held with grasping microforceps and pulled medially toward the opposite cord. Microscissors can be used to cut the mucosa close to its base, thus preserving the normal mucosa. The opposite side nodule can also be removed at the same time. Postoperative voice rest is recommended for 48 hours and correction of voice production techniques with voice therapy is essential, to prevent recurrence.

Vocal Fold Polyps

Vocal fold polyps are generally unilateral and represent localized areas of edematous polypoidal changes, superficial to the vocal ligament, usually resulting from phonotrauma. They typically involve the free edge of the vocal fold mucosa (**Fig. 25.2**), although they may also occur on the superior or inferior aspect of the vocal fold. They are more common in men, in smokers, and in the young and middle-aged groups. Careful examination may also reveal a contact response resulting in a "contrecoup" lesion on the contralateral vocal fold (**Fig. 25.3**).

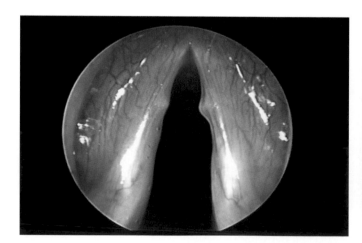

Figure 25.1   Bilateral vocal fold nodules.

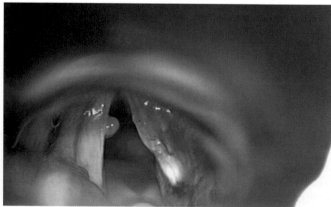

Figure 25.2   Left vocal fold polyp, arising from the free edge of the vocal fold mucosa.

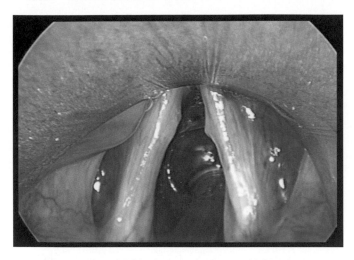

Figure 25.3 Left mid-fold edema and right vocal fold polyp.

Patients with vocal fold polyps commonly present with dysphonia, both from their mass effect and also from impeding full glottic closure during phonation. They can also rarely cause symptoms of airway obstruction, if very large. For most patients, initial voice therapy should be considered, with the exception of lesions affecting airway patency or those where underlying malignancy may be suspected. If surgical excision is indicated, this can be undertaken using cold instrument techniques or with the laser. The polyp can be grasped using microforceps and gentle traction applied to medialize the lesion toward the opposite cord. The base of the polyp can be dissected and removed from the mucosa overlying the vocal ligament, with microscissors or laser, with the aim of preservation of normal mucosal integrity. Sometimes, vocal fold polyps may be accompanied by an obvious central feeding blood vessel. Prominent feeding vessels should be vaporized with the laser (1 W, defocused), to prevent recurrent hemorrhage and polyp reformation. If the vessel is found near the free edge of the vocal fold, medially, it may be prudent to dissect the vessel through a laterally placed incision and microflap. Cautery or removal of the vessel through this approach minimizes the risk of disrupting the mucosal wave. Once the vocal polyp has been excised, voice rest for at least 48 hours should be recommended, with postoperative voice therapy to address and correct any habits of vocal misuse.

Reinke Edema

This is a diffuse edematous change of the vocal fold, which is usually bilateral. It results from accumulation of fluid within Reinke space, the potential space between the vocal ligament and the overlying mucosa (**Fig. 25.3**). This chronic inflammatory response occurs as a result of the poor lymphatic drainage of the vocal folds. The underlying etiology for Reinke edema is unknown, but there is a strong association with cigarette smoking and heavy voice use, with a clear predilection among middle-aged women. Patients typically present with dysphonia from disruption of the mucosal wave, or a mass effect in extreme cases.

A combination of treatment modalities is required for this condition. Smoking cessation is key and in mild cases, this combined with speech therapy can be sufficient. However, in severe cases, surgery may be indicated. Some laryngologists advocate surgery on only a single vocal fold at a time, as surgical treatment for this condition can result in vocal fold stiffening. Therefore, staged surgery allows for healing and voice recovery, before planning surgery to the opposite side. However, this approach is still widely debated and others deny any contraindication to operating on both folds at the same time, as long as care is taken to avoid injury to the underlying vocal ligament and the anterior commissure.

Surgery can be undertaken using cold techniques or the CO_2 laser. The aim of surgery is to remove the fluid and reduce the excess mucosa, with minimal damage to the underlying laryngeal architecture. This technique was originally described by Hirano.[10] It involves a lateral cordotomy, where a linear incision is made along the lateral aspect of the superior surface of the vocal fold, with a sharp, sickle knife. The superficial mucosa can then be elevated with a blunt dissector and Reinke space entered (the lateral microflap). The submucosal fluid contents can be aspirated with fine suction or using cupped forceps. The mucosal edges can then be replaced. If there is excess, redundant mucosa, this can be trimmed with microscissors and the mucosal edges reapproximated. Following surgery, voice rehabilitation should be undertaken.

Laryngeal Cysts

Two types of intracordal cysts can form within Reinke space, mucus retention cysts or epidermoid cysts, depending on their origin. Mucus retention cysts are often translucent and lined by cuboidal or columnar epithelium. Epidermoid cysts contain epithelium or accumulated keratin in the subepithelial layer. The term intracordal cyst refers to their location just below the cover of the vocal fold within Reinke space and superficial to the vocalis muscle.

The formation of epidermoid cysts is associated with repeated trauma from vocal abuse or misuse (**Fig. 25.4**). Mucus

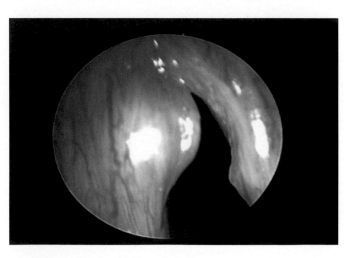

Figure 25.4 Left vocal fold epidermal cyst.

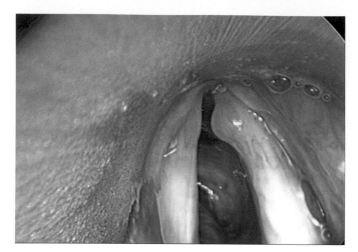

Figure 25.5 Right vocal fold mucosal cyst.

retention cysts may occur spontaneously or be related to poor vocal hygiene (**Fig. 25.5**). They are presumed to arise from an obstructed mucus secreting gland. A focal thickening may occur as a reaction to trauma from the cyst on the contralateral cord. Patients with intracordal cysts may present with dysphonia. However, in many cases, there may be no significant effect on the voice, in which case there is no indication for treatment.

Cysts may appear as a translucent swelling or fullness of the vocal fold on direct laryngoscopy. However, intracordal cysts may be difficult to visualize and videostroboscopy is essential in making the diagnosis, where the mucosal wave overlying the cysts is decreased or absent.

Medical therapy includes reversing or eliminating precipitants, including allergy, reflux, and maintaining good vocal hygiene. Speech therapy is necessary to reduce abusive behaviors, improving vocal efficiency, and modifying vocal habits. Surgery should be reserved for patients who complain of persistent significant symptoms despite aggressive medical and voice therapy. The aim of surgical excision is preservation of the mucosal cover with minimal disruption of the underlying tissue. A mucus retention cyst can be removed either with cold microinstruments or with laser, remaining superficial to the ligament. An epidermoid submucosal cyst can be approached via a lateral microflap where an incision is made on the superior surface of the vocal fold away from its medial edge. The flap is elevated and the lesion excised, before replacing the flap. Some laryngologists, however, have debated that elevating a microflap in this way may disrupt the attachment of the underlying basement membrane to the superficial lamina propria through interlinked collagen loops. To address this, Sataloff et al devised and described the mini-microflap technique to minimize tissue manipulation and prevent possible basement membrane injury with good results reported using this method.[11] This involves elevating a small section of the epithelium directly over the lesion, via a medially based incision. The plane of the mini-microflap is in the superficial lamina propria layer, deep to the basement membrane, so in theory leaving these attachments untouched.

Laryngoceles

A laryngocele is an abnormal air-filled dilatation or herniation of the appendix of the ventricle of Morgagni. They communicate with the laryngeal lumen when they become air filled. Less commonly, if the neck of the sac is blocked, the sac can fill with fluid (mucocele) or become infected and pus filled, forming a laryngopyocele. Laryngoceles can manifest internally and are totally contained within the thyroid cartilage framework. An external laryngocele extends through the thyrohyoid membrane and may present as a neck mass, extending as high as the submandibular triangle. They may also be mixed, with an external and internal component.

There are several proposed mechanisms for laryngocele formation. In neonates, they are thought to be remnants of lateral air sacs, seen in other primates. In adults, they are more commonly acquired lesions associated with increased intraluminal pressure and are therefore widely recognized to be more prevalent among brass and woodwind instrument players. There is also an association of laryngoceles with laryngeal carcinoma and this must be excluded in patients presenting with laryngoceles; they are thought to occur secondary to malignancy within the laryngeal ventricle.[12]

Presentation of laryngoceles can occur at any age, but the peak incidence is in the sixth decade, most commonly in men. An external or combined laryngocele can present as an intermittent neck swelling, which can be inflated by the patient, by performing the Valsalva maneuver, and emptied into the larynx by external compression. Distension of an internal laryngocele can result in symptoms of airway obstruction, hoarseness, and dysphagia or a lump sensation in the throat.

Surgery is the only definitive treatment for laryngoceles and is recommended in patients who have experienced infections, resulting in laryngopyoceles. A magnetic resonance imaging or computed tomography scan should be obtained to delineate the extent of the lesion before surgery. In acute cases, if the infection has progressed resulting in abscess formation, aspiration or drainage via an external approach may be necessary, with tracheostomy if there is airway obstruction. Once the acute infective episode has resolved, the laryngocele can be excised. Traditionally, this has been by an external approach; if the airway is at risk, a temporary tracheostomy may be needed. More recently, complete endoscopic excision using the CO_2 laser has been described for the management of both internal and external laryngoceles.[13]

Clinical Insights

The author (K.G.) prefers the laser to deal with all varieties of laryngocele. The large external laryngocele can be effectively dealt with by transoral laser resection techniques. Importance must be paid to the neurovascular bundle which is in close proximity to the site of exit of external laryngoceles through the thyrohyoid membrane. Ligaclip application to prominent vessels and suction monopolar diathermy of >1 mm vessels may be necessary as they are less likely to be effectively controlled by the CO_2 laser. All laser dissection should be applied closely to the laryngocele wall.

Granuloma

Contact granulomas are benign lesions located on the posterior third of the vocal fold, which corresponds to the vocal process of the arytenoid cartilage. They are usually unilateral lesions that appear pale or sometimes as a red pedunculated mass visible in this typical location (**Fig. 25.6**). Common etiologies include gastroesophageal reflux, traumatic or prolonged intubation, previous laryngeal surgery, and voice misuse. Contact ulceration often precedes granuloma formation and is associated with vocal abuse. This occurs when the thin mucosa overlying the firm cartilage is traumatized, resulting in mucosal breakdown. Consequently, an ulcer can form accompanied with granulation formation. Granulomas may be unilateral or bilateral, particularly if intubation trauma is the underlying cause.

Hoarseness is not a common symptom as the granuloma is usually located on the cartilaginous part of the glottis and therefore does not affect vibration. Intervention is indicated even in relatively asymptomatic disease, to prevent further complications arising, including airway obstruction, bleeding, or posterior laryngeal stenosis. However, before surgical excision, causative and contributing factors should be addressed. Reflux should be treated and voice therapy instituted. If the lesions fail to resolve, they should be surgically excised. Surgical resection of these lesions is amenable to the CO_2 laser, particularly as these lesions do not generally occur on the vibratory margin, and therefore, scarring is less of an issue. Furthermore, these lesions are often friable and therefore the laser can be convenient in minimizing bleeding. However, conversely, it must be remembered that these occur in a nonhealing area and therefore caution should be applied to avoid potential thermal injury effects at the base of the lesions, to the underlying perichondrium.

Nonetheless, following surgical resection, granulomas frequently recur, and therefore a combination of surgery together with antireflux treatment, injection of steroids into the base, speech therapy, and even botulinum toxin injections into the lateral cricoarytenoid muscle to decrease the force of adduction may all be considered.

Recurrent Respiratory Papillomatosis

Laryngeal papillomatosis is a benign epithelial tumor, presenting with a warty or condylomatous mass (**Fig. 25.7**). Papillomas are exophytic lesions, which can occur at areas of constriction in the aerodigestive tract, associated with increased airway turbulence, drying and cooling of mucosa, and at the change of the ciliary to squamous epithelium.[14] Their primary site of involvement is the larynx, but aggressive papillomata can involve the trachea, distal bronchi, pharynx, or tonsils. Laryngeal papillomas classically result in symptoms of progressive hoarseness, stridor, and respiratory distress.

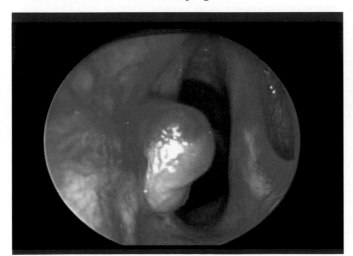

Figure 25.6   Left vocal fold granuloma, located in the posterior third of the glottis.

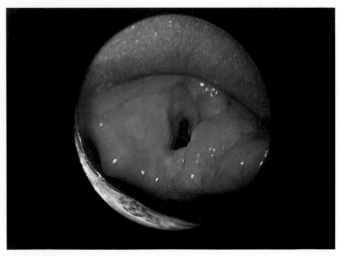

Figure 25.7   Laryngeal papillomatosis.

Recurrent respiratory papillomatosis (RRP) is a disease of viral etiology caused by human papillomavirus (HPV) subtypes 6 and 11. HPV type 11 is known to be associated with a worse prognosis, in terms of both distal airway spread and malignant transformation potential. Other subtypes of HPV implicated in RRP are HPV 16 and 18, which also have a recognized malignant potential. The precise mode of HPV transmission still remains unclear, but it is thought that the most likely method of fetal–maternal transmission is by direct contact via the birth canal. However, it is now clear that there are additional factors that must also be important in the development of RRP including patient immunity, timing, length and volume of viral exposure, and local trauma. Interestingly, the condition tends to more commonly affect the firstborn child in the family and the use of cesarean section does not reduce the incidence of transmission.

RRP can occur at any age, but it typically demonstrates a bimodal distribution in presentation. The two distinct, recognized forms include juvenile-onset RRP and adult-onset RRP. Adult-onset RRP could reflect activation of the virus present at birth or infection acquired in adolescence or adulthood.

RRP is the commonest benign laryngeal neoplasm in children and most commonly presents between the ages of 2 to 4 years, with an equal male to female ratio. Adult RRP peaks between ages 20 and 40 years with a male preponderance (4:1). Although histologically lesions appear similar in children and adults, their clinical course is different. In children, the disease is more common and usually much more aggressive, with patients often requiring multiple surgeries, with the disease usually becoming quiescent in adolescence. In contrast, adult-onset RRP behaves more indolently.

Malignant transformation of laryngeal or pulmonary RRP is rare, affecting 1 to 7% of patients with RRP.[15] Typically, malignant transformation occurs in patients with advanced disease, usually with pulmonary extension, who may later be diagnosed with lung carcinoma. The lung carcinoma will have the same viral etiology found within it, most commonly HPV 11, rather than HPV type 6.

Surgery is the standard treatment for laryngeal papillomatosis and is indicated when they interfere with voice quality or airway patency. Several surgical approaches can be used including the powered microdebrider, CO_2 laser, and also microsurgical instruments for smaller, single lesions. The aim should be to remove any papillomata that debilitate, sparing mucosa wherever possible. If the laser is used, all cases should be performed using an endoscope with a smoke evacuation channel, along with protective laser masks. Laser resection should use settings of 4 W on superpulsed laser. Individual papillomas can be gently grasped and the laser used to excise the lesions at their base. Alternatively, some surgeons directly vaporize all the areas of papillomatous involvement on the vocal folds, taking care to avoid the anterior commissure, to minimize the risk of webbing. Furthermore, one must be cautious to avoid injury to deeper underlying structures (vocal ligament and muscle) to prevent permanent dysphonia or deeper

recurrence. In cases of frequently recurring papilloma where regular debulking is required, some may favor the use of the microdebrider. This can be achieved using a 3.5- or 4.0-mm angle tip laryngeal blade at 5000 rpm.

Several adjuvant treatments have also been considered for use in select cases, but most of these are still experimental. Cidofovir is a cytosine analogue active against several DNA viruses. This antiviral agent can be injected directly into the base of the papillomatous lesions, with some promising results. There are some prospective studies, which have shown intralesional cidofovir to promote regression of papillomas and reduce frequency of surgical debulking.[16,17] However, the use of cidofovir for laryngeal injections is an off-label use. The medication is reported to have some serious side effects, although they are unlikely to occur in the minimal doses commonly used for laryngeal surgery. Nonetheless, parents and patients need to be fully informed. The recommended doses for laryngeal use are 2.5 to 5.0 mg/mL. Other alternative therapies include the use of interferon, which has antiviral, antiproliferative, and immunomodulatory effects. However, to date, the evidence is still lacking for a clear beneficial effect. Healy et al did not show any curative effect when interferon was used alone or as an adjuvant treatment.[18] Effective control of GERD is also considered an adjuvant treatment for laryngeal papillomatosis. Acid reflux is thought to exacerbate laryngeal RRP, and therefore control has also been explored as a treatment option. One prospective study showed improved control and sometimes remission when GERD is controlled.[19]

Some individual patients may have gained some benefit from these adjuvant therapies. However, clear evidence for their benefit is still in the experimental stages.

Vascular Lesions

Microvascular lesions of the true vocal folds include a variety of pathologies, including varices, ectasias, and spider telangiectasias. Most vascular lesions are located in the middle of the musculomembranous vocal fold, usually on the superior and lateral surface. This middle segment of the musculomembranous portion of the vocal fold is referred to as the "striking zone,"[20] as it is thought to be the area where maximal shearing forces are generated in the superficial layer of the lamina propria, during the mucosal wave. It is therefore thought that most vascular lesions of the vocal folds are related to mechanical trauma to the microvasculature, hence their prevalence among professional vocalists. The anatomic variations between the various microvascular lesions of the vocal folds are very subtle, and their presentation and management for all are broadly the same.

Microvascular lesions of the true vocal folds have a variable clinical presentation. They can be entirely asymptomatic or cause problems from hemorrhage or their mass effect. This can result in dysphonia through disruption of the vibratory pattern and closure of the true vocal folds. Repeated trauma leads to new blood vessel formation and weakening of the blood vessel walls. In symptomatic patients, surgical intervention is indicated. Recurrent hemorrhage from these vessels can be managed by laser extirpation of the abnormal blood vessels with CO_2 laser, using defocused 1-W laser bursts. Care should be taken to avoid heat transfer to the intermediate and deep layers of the lamina propria, and protection can be accomplished with submucosal infiltration.

Vocal Sulcus

This is a groove that occurs along the vocal fold mucosa. Although this can be a subtle lesion, it can result in restriction of the mucosal wave and voice dysfunction. Its etiology is unclear, but it can be classified into three types. The first is physiological or pseudosulcus. This nonpathological entity is often associated with reflux. The second is a sulcus vergeture, which is a deficient area down to the superficial layer of the lamina propria. The third is a sulcus vocalis, which is an epithelial-lined pocket extending down to the deeper layers of the vocal ligament, and it is thought that this type may be related to a ruptured congenital cyst.

The management approach for patients with vocal sulcus has evolved with time. Previously, surgical intervention was not recommended, but now it is generally agreed that patients with significant symptoms should be offered surgical options. However, sulci are difficult to treat, with an unreliable outcome.

The management of patients with symptomatic vocal sulcus should address compensatory hyperfunction through voice therapy, failure of glottic closure through medialization techniques, and recreation of a mucosal wave through surgery on the vibratory margin. Numerous phonosurgery techniques have been described and none are considered a single definitive treatment. The simplest approach is to dissect and elevate the mucosa off the deeper layer to which it is adherent; however, this technique is frequently unsuccessful. Alternatively, the area of the sulcus can be resected and the mucosa on either side reapproximated. This technique works better than simple elevation, but also does not produce consistent results. Others favor collagen or fat injections to boost the underlying deeper layers, but this also produces variable results. Pontes and Behlau advocate a technique that involves multiple parallel cross incisions, throughout the length of the sulcus, running perpendicular to the plane of the vocal fold.[21] The multiple relaxing incisions break up the linear scar of the vocal fold and can result in voice improvement. The surgical recommendations for this condition continue to evolve and patients should be informed of this, as part of their decision making in proceeding with intervention.

Rare Benign Laryngeal Lesions

Amyloidosis

Laryngeal amyloidosis is usually primary and localized, but can occur as part of a more systemic process. The larynx is the most common site in the respiratory tract for amyloid deposition. Amyloid deposits can occur at any of the various subsites of the larynx and result in dysphonia from their mass effect. In advanced cases, there may also be an effect on the airway.

The amyloid deposits are highly proteinaceous aggregates with a high fluid content. They can result in a diffuse submucosal process or discrete submucosal masses. The treatment is microlaryngeal surgery to remove the deposits, with either cold techniques or laser. The laser has the advantage of vaporizing the high fluid content within the deposits. The diagnosis must be confirmed histologically with Congo Red dye, which demonstrates "apple green birefringence" seen with a polarizing microscope. All cases of laryngeal amyloidosis should also have a thorough systemic evaluation.

Chronic Granulomatous Disease

These are a group of systemic conditions, which rarely affect the larynx. They should be considered particularly in immunocompromised patients.

Tuberculosis

Patients with pulmonary tuberculosis (TB) can rarely also have laryngeal involvement, resulting in dysphonia, odynophagia, and otalgia. On examination, there may be a diffusely red and edematous larynx, usually affecting the posterior third of the glottis. There may also be evidence of ulceration and necrosis, and therefore malignancy must be excluded. The diagnosis must be confirmed histologically, and a safe airway should be secured. Histologically, the presence of granulomas with areas of caseating necrosis, Langhans-type giant cells, and acid-fast bacilli will confirm the diagnosis. Treatment is medical, with antituberculous medical therapy.

Sarcoidosis

Sarcoidosis is a slow, progressive systemic condition, in which the larynx is involved in less than 5% of cases. The laryngeal appearances are similar to those of TB, with the supraglottic structures being most commonly involved, in particular, the epiglottis. The diagnosis should be made histologically, with evidence of noncaseating granulomas. Treatment should be guided by symptoms, ensuring there is a safe airway, with endoscopic resection or tracheostomy, and corticosteroids if required.

Wegener Granulomatosis

Wegener granulomatosis is a multisystem autoimmune disease that can affect the upper and lower respiratory tracts and kidneys. The larynx is involved in up to 25% of cases, particularly in the subglottic region. Patients may complain of dysphonia, although more commonly there are symptoms of airway obstruction. The diagnosis can be made from biopsies, showing necrotizing granuloma and vasculitis. The cytoplasmic antineutrophil cytoplasmic antibody is also specific for Wegener granulomatosis and should therefore be confirmed, along with a systemic evaluation. Treatment for localized laryngeal disease is endoscopic resection with intralesional corticosteroid injections and securing a safe airway.

Conclusion

Careful evaluation of patients with benign laryngeal pathology in a combined voice clinic is mandatory to providing comprehensive management for the dysphonic condition. Most patients will benefit from voice therapy and treatment of cofactors that contribute to or exacerbate the primary pathology. Surgical intervention appropriate to the condition should utilize the array of techniques available from laser, cold steel, and powered instrumentation. The phonosurgeon should be familiar with all surgical options available and use the most appropriate technique, ensuring minimal damage to healthy vocal fold tissue.

References

1. Hirano M. Morphological structure of the vocal cord as a vibrator and its variations. Folia Phoniatr (Basel) 1974;26(2):89–94

2. Robinson PM, Weir AM. Excision of benign laryngeal lesions: comparison of carbon dioxide laser with conventional surgery. J Laryngol Otol 1987;101(12):1254–1257

3. Keilmann A, Biermann G, Hörmann K. [CO_2 laser versus conventional microlaryngoscopy in benign changes of the vocal cords]. Laryngorhinootologie 1997;76(8):484–489

4. Hörmann K, Baker-Schreyer A, Keilmann A, Biermann G. Functional results after CO_2 laser surgery compared with conventional phonosurgery. J Laryngol Otol 1999;113(2):140–144

5. Benninger MS. Microdissection or microspot CO_2 laser for limited vocal fold benign lesions: a prospective randomized trial. Laryngoscope 2000;110(2 Pt 2, Suppl 92):1–17

6. Patel N, Rowe M, Tunkel D. Treatment of recurrent respiratory papillomatosis in children with the microdebrider. Ann Otol Rhinol Laryngol 2003;112(1):7–10

7. El-Bitar MA, Zalzal GH. Powered instrumentation in the treatment of recurrent respiratory papillomatosis: an alternative to the carbon dioxide laser. Arch Otolaryngol Head Neck Surg 2002;128(4):425–428

8. Holler T, Allegro J, Chadha NK, et al. Voice outcomes following repeated surgical resection of laryngeal papillomata in children. Otolaryngol Head Neck Surg 2009;141(4):522–526

9. Pasquale K, Wiatrak B, Woolley A, Lewis L. Microdebrider versus CO_2 laser removal of recurrent respiratory papillomas: a prospective analysis. Laryngoscope 2003;113(1):139–143

10. Hirano M. Microsurgery of the Larynx. Videotape, New York, NY: The Voice Foundation; 1982

11. Sataloff RT, Spiegel JR, Heuer RJ, et al. Laryngeal mini-microflap: a new technique and reassessment of the microflap saga. J Voice 1995;9(2):198–204

12. Celin SE, Johnson J, Curtin H, Barnes L. The association of laryngoceles with squamous cell carcinoma of the larynx. Laryngoscope 1991;101(5):529–536

13. Martinez Devesa P, Ghufoor K, Lloyd S, Howard D. Endoscopic CO_2 laser management of laryngocele. Laryngoscope 2002;112(8 Pt 1):1426–1430

14. Kashima H, Mounts P, Leventhal B, Hruban RH. Sites of predilection in recurrent respiratory papillomatosis. Ann Otol Rhinol Laryngol 1993;102(8 Pt 1):580–583

15. Gerein V, Rastorguev E, Gerein J, Draf W, Schirren J. Incidence, age at onset, and potential reasons of malignant transformation in recurrent respiratory papillomatosis patients: 20 years experience. Otolaryngol Head Neck Surg 2005;132(3):392–394

16. Tasca RA, Clarke RW. Recurrent respiratory papillomatosis. Arch Dis Child 2006;91(8):689–691

17. Soma MA, Albert DM. Cidofovir: to use or not to use? Curr Opin Otolaryngol Head Neck Surg 2008;16(1):86–90

18. Healy GB, Gelber RD, Trowbridge AL, Grundfast KM, Ruben RJ, Price KN. Treatment of recurrent respiratory papillomatosis with human leukocyte interferon. Results of a multicenter randomized clinical trial. N Engl J Med 1988;319(7):401–407

19. McKenna M, Brodsky L. Extraesophageal acid reflux and recurrent respiratory papilloma in children. Int J Pediatr Otorhinolaryngol 2005;69(5):597–605

20. Hochman I, Sataloff RT, Hillman RE, Zeitels SM. Ectasias and varices of the vocal fold: clearing the striking zone. Ann Otol Rhinol Laryngol 1999;108(1):10–16

21. Pontes P, Behlau M. Treatment of sulcus vocalis: auditory perceptual and acoustical analysis of the slicing mucosa surgical technique. J Voice 1993;7(4):365–376

26 Premalignant Lesions of the Larynx

Jahangir Ahmed and Khalid Ghufoor

Exactly 43 years after Durant described the first documented case of laryngeal leukoplakia as "white cicatrices" adjacent to a malignant laryngeal lesion,[1] Jackson in 1923 conceptualized premalignancy of the larynx as akin to "a large number of citizens leaving their regular daily routine and mobilizing preparatory to invasion."[2] In 2008, cancer of the larynx accounted for 1.2% of all new malignancies diagnosed worldwide and was responsible for 82,000 deaths.[3] The best chance of curing any cancer is via its early detection and eradication as morbidity and mortality are proportionately related to stage.[4] The former is pertinent to the larynx, as laryngectomy is a devastating consequence for many patients in the curative treatment of advanced laryngeal cancer. Thus, appropriate management of precancerous laryngeal lesions in those patients fortunate enough to present at this stage is obviously vital.

A cancerous lesion is a culmination of multiple genetic changes leading to the selection of a clonal population of cells that have broken free from local host-specific growth control mechanisms.[5] Classifying the morphological correlates of this sequence of events has generated much debate among pathologists and the wider scientific community. Classification schemes are only useful if they provide prognostic information and can thus impact on subsequent management. In 1952, Kleinsasser devised a systematic classification for precancerous lesions of the laryngeal squamous epithelium. There were three tiers that sequentially progressed as follows: simple squamous cell hyperplasia, hyperplasia with atypia, and finally carcinoma in situ (CIS).[6] Numerous classification schemes have evolved from this fundamental premise, but to date none have found universal acceptance. Currently, two are prominently used throughout the world (discussed later). Much focus in recent years has been placed on the molecular events characterizing laryngeal precancerous lesions, aiming to enhance the predictability of the fairly subjective morphological criteria that govern these existing schemes.[7]

The larynx serves to protect the airway and to commence vocalization and provides the ability to generate raised intrathoracic pressure as in a Valsalva maneuver. These vital functions may all be compromised by overaggressive treatment of preneoplastic lesions, some of which may ultimately even regress.[8] This chapter discusses the presentation, aspects of diagnosis including the aforementioned histological difficulties, and principles for managing preneoplastic laryngeal lesions.

Anatomy

While the detailed functional anatomy and physiology of the larynx are discussed elsewhere, an appreciation of macro and microanatomy is necessary for understanding surgical management.

The larynx may be grossly divided into the supraglottis, the glottis, and the subglottis, separated respectively and arbitrarily by two horizontal lines: one passing through the level of the apices of the laryngeal ventricles and another at 1 cm below the free edge of the vocal folds. Within the glottis lie the true vocal folds that extend anteriorly from the vocal processes of the arytenoid cartilages to form a confluent attachment at the inner surface of the junction between the laminae of the thyroid cartilages (the anterior commissure). The posterior commissure lies between the arytenoid cartilages and is limited posteriorly by the mucous membrane bridging them. The rima glottidis is the triangular airspace between the vocal folds anteriorly and the vocal processes and the base of the arytenoid cartilages posteriorly. Being the narrowest section of the upper airway, it affords most resistance to airflow and thus airborne carcinogens. This is perhaps one of the reasons why the glottis and in particular the vocal folds are the commonest sites of laryngeal carcinoma and indeed preneoplastic lesions. Although the vocal folds constitute two-thirds of the length of the rima glottidis, the wider posteriorly located interarytenoid space has a much larger area through which most of the volume of air passes during respiration. The vocal folds and their intervening space are responsible for creating the necessary vibratory cycles for phonation.

The anterior commissure is an important surgical landmark. It may be difficult to access and incomplete visualization often leads to uncertainty in the complete surgical clearance of any disease sited here. It is also a source of significant postoperative morbidity if inappropriately managed. The anterior commissure comprises the convergence of the vocal ligaments with the thyroepiglottic ligaments from either side. These ligaments ultimately unify to form the anterior commissure tendon (Broyles ligament), which is a thick gland-free region that resists tumor spread. However, superior and inferior to the Broyles ligament, the glottic mucosa reflects onto bare thyroid cartilage which at this point is devoid of inner perichondrium. It is here that the tumor may easily invade the thyroid cartilage to significantly upstage disease.

The mucosa covering the larynx consists of two types. Stratified nonkeratinizing squamous epithelium lines the vocal folds and much of the epiglottic surface, signifying their position in areas that are subjected to repetitive abrasive forces, that is, contact of the vocal folds upon closure of the rima glottidis in the former case. The remainder of the laryngeal surface is covered by ciliated columnar respiratory epithelium. Squamous carcinoma of the larynx commonly occurs at the transition between the squamous and respiratory epithelium on the ventricular surface of the true vocal folds (the inferior arcuate line). Mucinous glands are found in the saccule of the ventricles (which are guarded by the false vocal folds), the laryngeal surface of the epiglottis, and the infraglottic surface of the vocal folds. The free edge is void of glands needing to remain smooth to optimize its ability to oscillate during the phonatory cycle. The vocal folds are also largely devoid of lymphatics and thus cervical lymphadenopathy for early-stage glottic carcinoma is relatively rare. The level of the rima glottidis is a watershed that marks the junction of the different embryological origins of the superior and inferior larynx.

The vast majority of surgical procedures on preneoplastic laryngeal lesions will involve the vocal folds. It is thus important to understand their layered histological structure to minimize functional damage. Nonkeratinizing squamous epithelium lines the surface. The lamina propria lies deep to this and is divided into the superficial (Reinke space, which consists of fluid amorphous material), intermediate (elastic fibers), and deep (firm collagenous fibers) layers. The intermediate and deep layers form the vocal ligament. Deeper still lies the vocalis muscle. Functionally, the vocal fold acts as three layers: the cover (squamous epithelium and superficial layer of the lamina propria) slides and vibrates on the transition zone (intermediate and deep layers of the lamina propria) and the body (the vocalis muscle).

Definitions and Histology

A variety of malignant neoplasms may arise in the larynx (**Table 26.1**), reflecting the different tissues from which they originate. The vast majority, however, are squamous carcinomas (up to 95%) and predominantly arise on the true vocal folds. All other histological subtypes will necessarily develop via a premalignant phase, but due to the paucity of such cases in the literature they have not been studied and characterized to the same extent as premalignant squamous

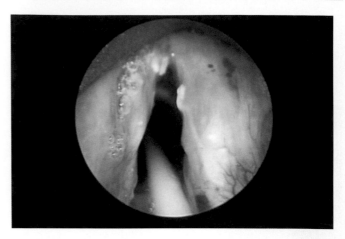

Figure 26.1 Leukoplakic vocal folds associated with widespread mild underlying dysplasia.

carcinomatous lesions. The remainder of this chapter will therefore focus on the latter.

Histologically, neoplasms that do not fulfill the criteria for frank malignancy are referred to as dysplastic. Lesions are dysplastic when there is evident cytological and tissue architectural atypia without invasion. CIS lies at the extreme end of the dysplastic spectrum, where morphological features of malignancy are displayed by an epithelial lesion that has not yet breached the underlying basement membrane.[9]

Laryngeal dysplastic epithelium manifests clinically in three main forms: leukoplakia (white patches), erythroplakia (red), and mixed leukoerythroplakia (speckled).[9] Leukoplakia (**Fig. 26.1**) represents keratin production (which is not normally produced by laryngeal squamous epithelium), whereas erythroplakia (**Fig. 26.2**) indicates enhanced vascularity. Although keratinization is the histological counterpart of leukoplakia, its extent does not correlate with the underlying degree of dysplasia. Indeed the rare purely erythroplakic area, although clinically less impressive than a thickened, raised patch of leukoplakia, has a much higher

Table 26.1 Histological Subtypes of Laryngeal Malignancies

- Squamous carcinoma
  - Histological variants: verrucous, spindle, and basaloid
- Mucoepidermoid
- Adenoid cystic
- Sarcomas
  - Rhabdomyosarcoma
  - Chondrosarcoma
- Lymphoma
- Neuroendocrine
  - Carcinoid
  - Small cell

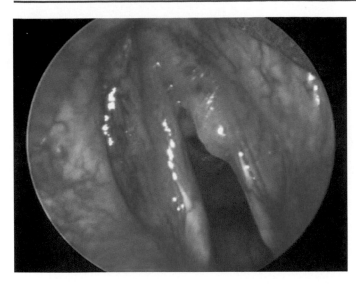

Figure 26.2 Erythroplakia associated with severe underlying dysplasia.

chance of representing severe dysplasia/CIS.[10] Some clinical features are indicative of high-risk epithelium: erythroplakia, surface granularity, large surface area; but in general clinical correlation (**Figs. 26.1** to **26.3**) with the underlying state of the epithelium is relatively poor.[7,11] For this reason a biopsy is mandatory in all suspected cases. Most dysplastic squamous epithelial lesions arise on the true vocal folds, but they may occasionally be found in other laryngeal subsites normally covered with squamous epithelium (e.g., the epiglottis) or in areas of squamous metaplasia that usually occur as a consequence of repeated physical insult.

Dysplastic epithelium represents an increased risk of malignant transformation compared with nondysplastic epithelium.[8] However, the term dysplasia covers a broad range of morphological atypia that do not always lie neatly on a spectrum from normal epithelium to CIS. There have been numerous attempts at grading such changes ever since Kleinsasser's landmark work.[12] The ideal grading system should have prognostic value regarding the risk of malignant transformation and demonstrate good interobserver and intraobserver reproducibility. Unfortunately, nearly 60 years and over 24 attempts later, such a morphological grading system does not exist. Thus, laryngeal dysplasia remains one of the most hotly debated subjects within head and neck pathology. The two major grading systems for laryngeal dysplasia in use in the United Kingdom are the World Health Organization and the Ljubljana classifications.[13]

The WHO classification has three dysplastic categories: mild, moderate, and severe, straddled on either side by hyperplasia and CIS. Squamous hyperplasia here simply represents an increased number of cells that may occur in the spinous layer (acanthosis) or in the parabasal/basal layers (basal cell hyperplasia). There is no cellular atypia or architectural disturbance, although there is often a degree of superficial keratin formation. Histological features found in dysplasia, which suggest malignant potential, include abnormal mitotic figures, in terms of both morphology and numbers, nuclear pleomorphism, and stromal inflammation.

Mild, moderate, and severe dysplasia represent a spatial increase in dysplastic epithelium, with cytological and architectural disturbance limited to the lower one-third (basal/parabasal), the lower two-thirds, and extending throughout the epithelium, respectively. The degree of cytological atypia also increases with increasing grade. By these definitions, the distinction between severe dysplasia and CIS is somewhat blurred and indeed many pathologists and clinicians manage these entities similarly.[14] The WHO classification evolved from the classification for lesions of the cervix, that is, cervical intraepithelial neoplasia (CIN), with the laryngeal adaptation for CIN 1, 2, 3 replaced by squamous intraepithelial neoplasia (SIN) 1, 2, 3.[15] Kambic and Lenart in 1971[16] felt that this categorization did not divide patients with laryngeal dysplasia into distinct prognostic groups, and their own adaptation was further modified by a working group on head and neck pathology from the European Society of Pathology in 1997[17] to form the Ljubljana classification, which in essence is a two-tier classification of laryngeal dysplasia. Abnormal laryngeal epithelium is subcategorized as follows: (1) basal/parabasal hyperplasia (minimal risk of malignant transformation) or (2) atypical hyperplasia or "risky" epithelium, featuring cellular atypia which does not span the entire width. Simple squamous hyperplasia in the Ljubljana classification is confined to the spinous layer, whereas CIS is defined as "full-thickness" atypia without invasion, thus overlapping with the WHO's "severe dysplasia" and is prognostically significantly different from the other categories. **Table 26.2** summarizes the two classification schemes.

There is no easy overlap between these and other classification systems, but dichotomous systems such as the Ljubljana classification or indeed dichotomizing the WHO classification system (e.g., severe/CIS versus mild/moderate)

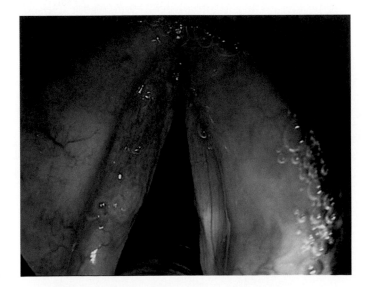

Figure 26.3 Early invasive (T1) carcinoma of the left vocal fold.

Table 26.2   Comparison of Two Popular Classification Systems Used for Premalignant Laryngeal Epithelium

The WHO Classification (2005)	The Ljubljana Classification
• Squamous cell hyperplasia	• Squamous cell (simple) hyperplasia

• Dysplasia
  ◦ Mild dysplasia
  ◦ Moderate dysplasia
  ◦ Severe dysplasia
	• Abnormal epithelium
	  ◦ Basal/parabasal cell hyperplasia
	  ◦ Atypical hyperplasia ("risky" epithelium)

• Carcinoma in situ	• Carcinoma in situ

appears to be far better in reliability studies.[18] This indicates the relative uncertainty of categorizing middle-grade or "moderate" dysplasia. As expected, agreement reliability for any particular grading system improves following group training sessions.[17] The importance of accurate histological grading cannot be stressed enough, as it is the single most important determinant of subsequent patient management.

Clinical Insight

The senior author (K.G.) maintains a close collaboration with dedicated head and neck pathologists to ensure consistency of pathology reporting. These patients can be challenging and multidisciplinary meetings allow concerns regarding the nature of laryngeal dysplasias to be voiced in the context of a patient's clinical condition, comorbidities, and risk factors, all of which influence future management.

Epidemiology

There is a paucity of epidemiological data on preneoplastic laryngeal lesions. However, the incidence of frank laryngeal malignancy varies throughout the world, presumably as a consequence of exposure to differential quantities and types of carcinogenic agents. The nature of the carcinogenic insult will also determine the site of the lesion within the larynx. Thus inhaled smoke, to which most resistance occurs at the glottis, is most likely to cause vocal cord lesions, whereas supraglottic lesions are more likely to result from ingested carcinogens such as alcohol.[19] In the United Kingdom, the age-standardized incidence of laryngeal carcinoma for men was 5.3/100,000 and for women 1/100,000 in 2005.[19] The male to female ratio is likely to decline, however, due to the relative increase in female smokers of late. As with most other carcinomas, the incidence increases with age. In one of the largest single-center series of leukoplakic lesions of the larynx, comprising a total of 1268 patients, the male to female ratio was 4.6, but women developed pathology at an earlier age (mean 44.8 vs 51.5 years). Here, the overall incidence, based on the catchment area of the host institute, was 2.61/100,000 for simple hyperplasias and 0.86/100,000 for atypical hyperplasias.[7]

Etiology

The risk factors for laryngeal dysplasia will necessarily be the same as that of laryngeal carcinoma. Laryngeal neoplasia is a preventable disease in the vast majority of cases, implicating environmental factors in causation. The strongest association is with tobacco smoking. Burning cigarettes releases tar that contains carcinogenic polycyclic aromatic hydrocarbon compounds. These are degraded into intracellular chemicals that bind to and damage DNA and RNA molecules. Several observational studies report a dose-dependent increase in the risk of laryngeal cancer with tobacco smoking.[20] Alcohol and smoking appear to act synergistically to enhance the risk of laryngeal cancer,[21,22] although as mentioned above, patients whose predominant risk factor is alcohol are more likely to develop supraglottic carcinoma.[23] Although alcohol, like cigarette smoke, directly instigates carcinogenic pathways, concurrent malnutrition, including defective vitamin status, is also likely to play a significant role.[24]

There is a growing and convincing body of evidence implicating human papillomavirus (HPV) in oropharyngeal carcinomas.[25] HPV-positive and HPV-negative cancers in this site appear to be different clinical entities, with distinct prognoses.[26] As with squamous carcinoma of the cervix, serotypes 16 and 18 appear to be the most carcinogenic. This HPV-positive versus HPV-negative carcinoma dichotomy is not as clear-cut in the larynx. The prevalence of HPV in laryngeal carcinoma specimens varies from 0 to 58%, depending on the population and method of detection utilized, with an overall reported prevalence of around 25%.[7] A recent systematic review revealed only a weak correlation between HPV and laryngeal carcinoma.[25] Serotype 16 is the most commonly isolated subtype. In contrast, the serotypes most prevalent in recurrent respiratory papillomatosis are 6 and 11. Recurrent respiratory papillomatosis (**Fig. 26.4**) may rarely transform into squamous carcinoma, particularly if patients have been irradiated, but these two disease entities are thought to have different mechanistic origins.[27] It should be noted that HPV has been detected in up to 25% of individuals with clinically and histologically normal laryngeal epithelium.[28]

That chronic laryngopharyngeal reflux may play a role in laryngeal carcinoma was first highlighted by Olson in 1983.[29] Several uncontrolled case series report high prevalences of gastroesophageal reflux disease (GERD) in patients with

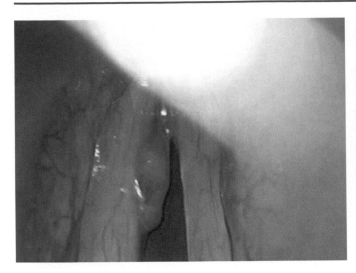

Figure 26.4   Laryngeal papillomatosis.

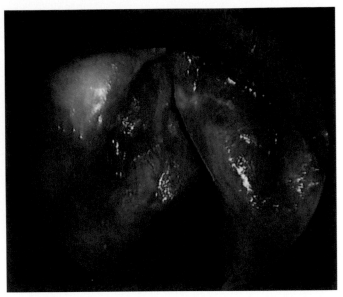

Figure 26.5   Moderate dysplasia with localized edema of the left vocal fold.

laryngeal carcinoma.[30] However, given the relatively high prevalence of GERD in the general population, it is difficult to attribute a direct etiological role. Larger sample sizes, with well-matched controls, are necessary for further clarity.

Other environmental risk factors implicated in the development of laryngeal neoplasia include air pollution, malnutrition, occupational carcinogenic agents such as asbestos, and lower socioeconomic class.[19] Ionizing radiotherapy to neighboring anatomical regions, for example, for thyroid carcinoma, also increases the risk of laryngeal neoplasia, particularly for sarcomas.[31] Although environmental influences predominate in etiology, some patients have heritable genetic characteristics that confer susceptibility, for example, enzymatic polymorphisms in the detoxification of alcohol- and smoke-derived carcinogens.[32]

Presentation and Investigations

Patients will often present by referral from their primary care physicians with a prolonged history of fluctuating dysphonia. They may have received antibiotic treatment for presumed acute laryngitis as soreness is often an accompanying feature. Other symptoms include a sensation of a laryngeal foreign body and chronic cough. These symptoms usually occur in the context of tobacco smoking and/or significant alcohol consumption.

At present, the gold standard for diagnosis is direct laryngoscopy and biopsy, usually performed under general anesthesia. Alternatively, it may also be performed under local anesthesia with a transnasal endoscope containing an aperture for the passage of a biopsy forceps. Most lesions occur on the superior surface of the true membranous vocal folds and may be clinically single or multiple and red, white, or speckled, with varying degrees of surface texture (**Figs. 26.1** to **26.3**). Although the uncommon purely erythroplakic lesion most likely represents severe dysplasia/CIS or even early-stage carcinoma, clinical appearances in general do not correlate very well with the underlying histology, as illustrated by **Figs. 26.5** to **26.7**. Therefore, a biopsy is mandatory. The availability of angled rigid fiberoptic endoscopes, in conjunction with specialist anesthetic maneuvers, should enable the surgeon to obtain supraglottic and infraglottic views. Ideally, laryngoscopy should be combined with pharyngoscopy and upper esophagoscopy to exclude synchronous lesions. Photodocumentation should include pictures taken before and after any biopsies.

In many cases, the initial microlaryngoscopy and biopsy serve as both diagnostic and definitive treatment. To maintain that paradigm, the surgeon will need to obtain a large enough excision biopsy and not miss any areas of preneoplastic change that are not macroscopically obvious.

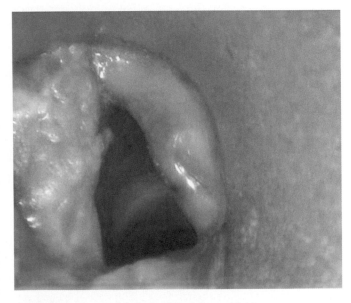

Figure 26.6   Severe dysplasia of the left vocal fold.

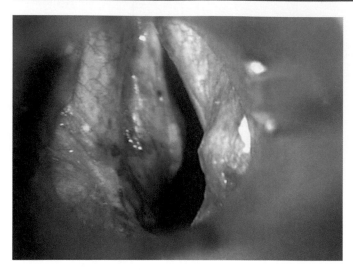

Figure 26.7   T1-laryngeal carcinoma of the left vocal fold.

It is important to therefore take multiple biopsies in a systematic fashion from different subsites. Normal-looking adjacent epithelium may indeed be dysplastic, reflecting a wide "field" change.[33] However, overzealous excisions will need to be balanced against vocal fold mucosal preservation to maintain vocal function, particularly in patients with high vocal demands. To achieve this balance, adjunctive techniques to microlaryngeal surgery have and are continuing to be developed. One technique takes advantage of the ability of certain compounds (fluorophores) in cells to emit long-wave scattered light, when exposed to shorter wave blue light.[34] This phenomenon is known as "autofluorescence." The predominant color of the light emitted depends on the concentrations of fluorophores, which differ between normal and neoplastic cells (including moderate and higher grades of dysplasia). Thus, upon exposure to blue light, normal mucosa fluoresces green, whereas neoplastic mucosa appears violet. In a similar vein, upon application of aminolevulinic acid, neoplastic cells fluoresce orange red (due to the selective accumulation of protoporphyrin), in comparison to the green fluorescence from normal epithelium. These techniques appear to be highly sensitive, with reports quoting figures as high as 97%.[34] However, high false-positive rates consequent to enhanced vascularity and inflammation may preclude their universal use.[35]

Techniques that aim to provide in situ, real-time examination of the cytological and histological architecture of the superficial layers of the epithelium may also prove useful. Contact endoscopy uses highly magnified images (up to 150×) from a rigid endoscope placed in direct contact with the vocal fold epithelium following staining with 1% methylene blue dye. High sensitivities (80 to 100%) and specificities (81 to 100%) have been cited in the recent literature.[36] Notable disadvantages include its relative inability to detect mild atypia, which usually commences in the deeper basal epithelial layers. The lack of basal layer assessment means that it cannot distinguish between severe dysplasia, CIS, and invasive carcinoma, all of which require histological depth assessment.[37] There is obviously a learning curve involved, and many otolaryngologists may not feel comfortable at making histological assessments in the absence of a pathologist.

Although not in mainstream use, such techniques will continue to be developed in a bid to minimize the extent and quantity of laryngeal biopsies taken for initial diagnosis, management, and subsequent follow-up of patients with preneoplastic and neoplastic lesions of the larynx.

Molecular Biomarkers

It is estimated that at least 6 to 10 independent genetic mutations are required in a single cell for squamous cell carcinoma development in the upper aerodigestive tract.[38] They will eventually manifest themselves as different morphological grades of dysplasia before malignant transformation, which may take as long as 25 years.[5] As with malignancy in general, these genetic events culminate in the activation of oncogenes and/or inactivation of tumor suppressor genes to effect carcinomatous change. As these molecular events precede frank morphological change, their identification (or of surrogate markers) in preneoplastic lesions may provide useful prognostic information about a particular lesion and thus influence further management. Biological markers that simply mirror microscopic change offer limited prognostic information; in other words, only those whose presence predicts progression offer useful clinical information. A detailed discussion is beyond the scope of this chapter, but cited below is a brief synopsis of some of the key genetic and molecular events that may guide the development of useful prognostic biomarkers of malignant progression.

An enhanced accumulation of chromosomal abnormalities has been correlated with higher grades of laryngeal dysplasia.[5,33] Aneuploidy, for example, preceded malignant transformation and progressively increased with the severity of dysplasia in one study.[39] Alterations in chromosomal regions frequently include those encoding tumor suppressor genes. The most common in head and neck cancer occurs in the 9p21 locus, resulting in the loss of the *p16* gene,[5,33] which limits cell cycle progression. 9p21 loss appears early and may even be found in hyperplastic mucosa before atypia.[40] Other loci altered early include 3p (containing at least three tumor suppressor genes) and 17p13, where the gene encoding p53, "the guardian of the cell," is located.[40] p53 controls the cell's ability to repair and undergo apoptosis as a consequence of DNA damage and its dysfunction leads to genetic instability. About 50 to 80% of head and neck carcinomas contain mutations of p53 and their presence may signify transition from preinvasive to invasive lesions.[41]

In contrast to allelic loss, amplification of loci encoding proto-oncogenes (which drive cellular growth and proliferation) may contribute to preneoplastic and neoplastic epithelial change. Thus, amplification of 11q13 containing the cyclin D1 gene (a cell cycle regulator) is found in 30 to 50% of cases.[42] Similarly, overexpression of the epidermal growth factor receptor appears to correlate with severity of epithelial dysplasia.[43]

Enhanced cell proliferation is one of the hallmarks of dysplasia. Traditionally, this was assessed by counting mitotic figures; however, the discovery of the nuclear antigen Ki-67, expressed exclusively by proliferating cells, now enables objective quantification. Ki-67 expression is found throughout the mucosa (superficial and deep) in dysplasia, whereas its expression is limited to the basal layer in simple epithelial hyperplasia.[44] Thus, positive histochemistry of superficial suspect epithelium may be a useful indicator of progression.

Numerous other putative molecular markers of laryngeal dysplasia have been studied with regard to prognostic information.[7] However, in a recent systematic review, only p53, cyclin D1, and cortacin (a protein that plays a role in cell motility) demonstrated any statistically significant results with regard to prognostication, and even these studies were of limited quality.[45] Thus at present there is currently no single molecular biomarker that can reliably predict the future of laryngeal dysplastic lesions. Larger, prospective studies with consistent outcome reporting will be necessary to provide clarity in this area.

Clinical Insight

The senior author (K.G.) prefers direct endoscopic techniques with histological confirmation of diagnosis before proceeding to more radical or definitive treatments. This enables a discussion with patients at a later date, about future treatment, and the effect on function. Where a diagnosis has already been made before definitive endoscopy, frozen section histopathology is very useful in determining the extent of surgery, particularly for malignant neoplasms.

Management

As recently as a few decades ago, the management of laryngeal dysplasia, most of which occurs on the vocal folds, consisted of denuding the epithelium by "vocal cord stripping." This reflected the concern that if left alone, lesions would inevitably progress to invasive carcinoma and moreover that adjacent epithelium was also at high risk for transformation. However, histopathological and prognostication studies reveal a more complex picture.[7] Many lesions are at minimal risk, if at all, of progression. Contemporary surgical practice reflects knowledge of the ultrastructure of the vocal fold and mechanisms of phonation and thereby aims to preserve as much laryngeal epithelium (and consequently vocal function) as possible.

There are several controversial issues in the management of laryngeal dysplasia, not least exacerbated by the difficulty in histological classification mentioned earlier. Meaningful comparisons of prospective studies and thus systematic analysis have been challenging due to the heterogeneity of the methodology used, that is, the use of different histological grading criteria, differing initial treatment modalities, and variable duration of follow-up. This is highlighted by a recent survey of otolaryngologists, which revealed a wide variation in practice across the United Kingdom.[46] Laryngeal dysplasia was managed by dedicated head and neck surgeons or laryngologists in only 61% of ENT units and 53.6% of respondents managed less than 10 cases per year. Most surgeons used either sharp ("cold") dissection or the CO_2 laser to effect primary surgical excision. However, for persistent or widespread high-grade lesions, management varied from periodic sampling to irradiation. Only a fifth of the respondents used measures of functional outcome postintervention, and follow-up was also nonstandardized. The vast majority of respondents (98.2%) worked at centers that used the WHO classification, which is also the case at our institute.

In a bid to standardize practice, a consensus meeting of UK otolaryngologists and pathologists involved in the care of head and neck cancer was recently held and guidance issued.[14] This mirrors our own clinical practice.

Otolaryngologists involved in the care of laryngeal dysplasia should ideally be a member of the head and neck oncology multidisciplinary team (MDT). At initial presentation, single or indeed multiple foci should be completely excised if possible, whereas in the case of widely confluent or widespread disease, multiple biopsies should be taken both from the center and from the margins of the lesion (straddling normal mucosa). Definitive surgical resection should be performed after histological confirmation of the nature of large lesions. Histological specimens should be clearly labeled and anatomically orientated on a board with a diagram of the aerodigestive tract biopsy sites. The use of either sharp instrument dissection or CO_2 laser is acceptable, as long as viable histological specimens are obtained. Vocal cord stripping and indiscriminate laser ablation of the cords are not recommended as they are likely to cause collateral damage and eventual voice dysfunction. Radiotherapy is generally not recommended for primary treatment, but it may be considered in exceptional circumstances, for example, if comorbidities prevent further surgical extirpation, where surgical access to a clinically suspicious lesion is impossible, or in the management of widespread high-grade lesions, especially if the patient refuses to give up smoking. Although primary radiotherapy offers excellent cure rates and preserves anatomy for these noninvasive lesions, there may be adverse functional outcomes[47] in addition to other side effects. Postradiotherapy effects on tissue and epithelium, such as edema, inflammation, telangiectasia, and scarring, may confound posttreatment monitoring, and radiotherapy itself may promote neoplastic change.[48] Furthermore, this modality cannot be used again should the patient subsequently develop invasive carcinoma. Hence, the decision to treat with radiotherapy should be made after careful discussion in an MDT meeting.

In all cases, patients should be counseled regarding the risk/benefits of the proposed management whether observation, radiotherapy, or surgery. This includes the potential for worsening dysphonia, recurrence, and malignant transformation and the need for further interventions. Contributory risk factors should be actively sought and managed, for example, smoking cessation and GERD.

Recurrent focal low-grade dysplasia could be excised if possible, whereas more widespread disease could be regularly followed up, with further excision reserved for changes in endoscopic appearance or in clinical symptoms. "Low grade" in our practice corresponds to the WHO classifications of mild/moderate dysplasia. Recurrent focal severe dysplasia/CIS should be treated as a T1a carcinoma and excised with clear margins. A serious discussion with the patient about radiotherapy should be made in recurrent widespread severe dysplasia, especially if they continue to smoke. It is important to eradicate severe dysplastic epithelium or CIS as some case series reveal an eventual laryngectomy rate as high as 82% for patients in whom the disease has progressed.[19]

Endoscopic Technique

The treatment approach will be determined by the level of expertise, available facilities, the site and multiplicity of dysplasia, and access to these lesions. For preneoplastic lesions and early laryngeal cancer, the success of surgery should be judged by the final vocal outcome, as all treatment modalities (transoral excision and radiotherapy) offer similar control rates,[49,50] although it should be noted that there are currently no methodologically sound randomized controlled trials. Sadri et al[51] reviewed the literature on treatment of laryngeal dysplasia/CIS and found radiotherapy to have a higher local control rate (93.52%) than transoral laser (80.88%). However, it is again difficult to draw firm conclusions from mainly retrospective case series, compounded by heterogeneity of diagnostic and treatment modalities.

A small amount of extra tissue excised at the deep margin may have a profound effect on voice while not necessarily improving cure rate. Preservation of the layered microstructure of vocal fold epithelium is therefore important, especially for isolated lesions. A useful adjunctive technique is injection of Reinke space with saline/adrenaline, which hydrodissects the epithelium containing the noninvasive epithelial lesion off the lamina propria. The fluid may enhance visualization of the margins of the lesion (due to the epithelium placed under tension) and acts as a heat sink in laser procedures. Hydrodissection is useful when performing microflap techniques that allow inspection of the subepithelial layers to exclude deeper infiltration. The lesion should be excised using precise tangential cuts in toto, but the medial contact surface of the vocal folds should not be violated (unless the lesion is located on this free edge). Sharp (cold) excision uses readily available, relatively inexpensive instruments that enable accurate removal of lesions by the skilled dextrous operator, with minimal collateral effects to normal tissue. Dissection may be facilitated by the CO_2 laser in superpulse mode. A variety of micromanipulating/scanning devices that generate shaped-incision beams may be used to precisely cut lesions without causing hemorrhage, carbonization, or charring, thus minimizing thermal collateral damage. These latter techniques are particularly useful in revision procedures, in postradiotherapy tissue, and where deeper dissection is required. All of these techniques are potentially repeatable and still leave the option of further treatment with radiotherapy.

Anterior commissure disease poses special problems. Here, recurrence and thus progression to cancer is reported to be more likely.[52] This may, however, be due to inadequate initial clearance and indeed understaging of frankly malignant disease. Furthermore, although Broyles ligament is a tough barrier to tumor extension, superior and inferior to it are areas of relative weakness where malignancy may rapidly upstage if left behind. On the other hand, overaggressive treatment may cause scarring and webbing, resulting in a poor voice outcome. The anterior commissure is notoriously difficult to visualize and the patient's anatomy often impairs access of surgical instruments. Specially designed anterior commissure scopes may facilitate access. Furthermore, prominent false vocal cords may impair visualization due to their overhang. We advocate removing the anterior vestibular folds with the CO_2 laser.[53] Suitable excision biopsies may then be confidently taken, or staged resection planned if disease affects both vocal cords. In the latter scenario, if preservation of voice is paramount (e.g., due to professional demands), then radiotherapy could be considered a primary treatment modality after carefully counseling the patient.

Clinical Insight

The senior author (K.G.) uses a variety of endoscopes with supraglottic jet ventilation for unparalleled views of all areas of the larynx. Where disease is noninvasive, local anesthetic and adrenaline solution infiltration in the subepithelial plane improves resection of isolated lesions and minimizes removal of normal epithelium. The infiltration also helps disperse heat, preventing collateral thermal damage when a laser is deployed. The carbon dioxide laser, at low power settings, in superpulse mode, helps minimize damage to vocal fold epithelium and ligament, especially when voice preservation is a significant issue for the patient. Newer lasers produce less charring or carbonization of tissue, aiding precision excision with minimal collateral damage. Scanning devices with shaped laser beams enhance the delivery of laser energy and help accurate removal of lesions close to their margins.

Other Treatment Modalities

Photodynamic therapy (PDT) is a minimally invasive therapy, which in simple terms uses an external beam of light of a certain wavelength to activate light-sensitive drugs pervading tissue to effect the destruction of malignant or other diseased cells. These compounds are designed to be selectively taken up by rapidly dividing, metabolically active cells and when activated produce reactive oxygen radicals. Normal tissue should thus be relatively spared. Several phase two clinical trials of head and neck cancers have demonstrated efficacy in the treatment of early oropharyngeal cancers.[54] Of early (CIS, T1, or T2) laryngeal cancers treated with PDT (171 patients), 89% had a complete sustained response.[54] Phase three randomized controlled trials are now required, but this modality holds promise.

Fiber-based pulsed dye lasers in conjunction with distal chip endoscopy have been used to treat laryngeal dysplasia in the office setting under local anesthesia. They probably cause angiolysis of the microvasculature supplying the lesion.[55] This treatment modality is suitable for patients requiring multiple repeat laryngeal procedures and also appears to minimize the risk of web formation in anterior commissure disease.[56] It is therefore particularly useful in the management of recurrent respiratory papillomatosis,[56] but has also demonstrated efficacy in laryngeal dysplasia[57,58] and early glottic cancer.[55]

Voice Outcomes

When sharp dissection is confined to the superficial lamina propria, perceptual voice assessment is usually normal, although there may be mild stroboscopic impairment of the mucosal wave in both amplitude and magnitude. These and other vocal parameters are expected to worsen with more extensive surgery. The use of the CO_2 laser by experienced surgeons when limited to the superficial mucosal layer should not adversely affect vocal function,[59] although many patients with preneoplastic vocal cord lesions already have phonatory dysfunction at presentation. Many of the studies assessing voice in this context are case series of patients with invasive laryngeal carcinomas treated by relatively aggressive interventions, and their outcomes may therefore not be directly applicable to preneoplastic lesions. Xu et al[60] performed CO_2-mediated epithelial ablation in 50 patients with dysplastic laryngeal lesions following intraoperative frozen section. Perceptual vocal quality improved after 1 month in all, when acoustic analysis was nearly normal compared with healthy control subjects. Contrary to current perceptions, a recent meta-analysis of comparative studies did not reveal any significant differences in voice perception and acoustic analysis between transoral laser surgery and radiotherapy for T1a glottic cancer.[49]

All patients, regardless of treatment modality, should have preoperative and postoperative voice assessments consisting of at least a voice function inventory but ideally also acoustic and videostroboscopic analyses. Peritreatment speech and language therapy support is vital for the long-term rehabilitation of these patients.

Follow-Up

A total of 35 to 54% of all suspect biopsies will display some degree of dysplasia.[19] Dysplastic lesions do not all undergo a simple linear progression in severity from simple hyperplasia to CIS and ultimately invasive malignancy. Thus, a "one treatment fits all" approach cannot be adopted. Prognostic information of specific lesions is compounded by the variable inter- and intrarater reliability of current grading schemes.[61] Furthermore, the literature reveals significant variability in initial treatment modalities and length of follow-up. These factors probably account for the reported malignant transformation rate in the literature of between 2 and 74%.[62]

In the largest single-unit series of vocal cord dysplasias (1268 patients) who were followed up to 25 years, the malignant transformation rate was reported as 1.1% for simple/parabasal hyperplasia and 9.5% for atypical hyperplasia (the mean follow-up was 6.2 years).[7] In this series, the atypical hyperplasic group was predominantly treated by vocal cord stripping. Two-thirds of CISs treated expectantly will transform into invasive cancer.[63] A recent systematic review reported a mean overall transformation rate of dysplasia to invasive carcinoma of 14%: 10.6% for low-grade lesions (WHO: mild/moderate) and 30.4% for high-grade lesions (WHO: severe and CIS).[62] The overall mean time to transformation was 5.8 years, ranging from 1.8 to 14.4 years, with no significant differences when subcategorized by grade. The authors acknowledge, however, that the quality of the analyzed data was relatively poor.

Due to the difficulties in reliably grading dysplasia into multiple categories, for the purposes of management, our unit dichotomizes the WHO system into a two-tier grading system: low grade (WHO mild/moderate) versus high grade (severe/CIS). As previously mentioned, we advocate that severe dysplasia/CIS should be treated as a T1 carcinoma, as many cases retrospectively demonstrate histological foci of invasion. Thus in our center, patients with laryngeal dysplasia are placed into low or high histological risk groups. In the absence of associated risk factors such as smoking or heavy alcohol consumption, low-risk patients (with low-grade lesions as defined above) may be discharged after 6 months of follow-up, with instructions to return should there be a change in symptoms. Longer follow-up will be required if these patients continue to smoke or if a lesion(s) is visible on endoscopy. For the higher histological risk group, their follow-up should mirror that for T1 carcinoma which in our institute consists of monthly/bimonthly attendance in the first 2 years (during which time recurrence is most likely to occur) and prolonged intervals thereafter until discharge at the end of 5 years. In our experience, many of these patients often end up being followed up for longer periods as a consequence of recurrence or new lesions. At each visit, the upper aerodigestive tract should be visualized using endoscopy, the neck palpated, and the larynx photodocumented or at the very least, a pictorial representation of the current state of the larynx made in the medical records. Perceptual and physiological (if available) assessments of voice should also be made at least biannually. High-risk patients should be followed up in dedicated head and neck oncology clinics.

Conclusion

Regardless of the heterogeneity in study methodology, the literature reveals that dysplastic laryngeal lesions are at significant risk of transforming into frank malignancies. This risk generally increases with the grade of dysplasia and the continual presence of concomitant risk factors. It is no longer acceptable to indiscriminately and widely ablate laryngeal lesions as this will inevitably lead to functional demise. The outcome of any treatment for what is essentially a nonmalignant lesion has to be measured by functional preservation. For this reason it is important to attain accurate histological categorization to dictate aggressiveness of subsequent management. At present there is no worldwide consensus in grading of precancerous laryngeal lesions based on morphological assessment. This will partially account for similar heterogeneity in treatment modalities. The use of molecular biomarkers that reflect our increasing understanding of cell and molecular biology of head and neck cancer may in future offer better prognostic criteria and lead to a universal classification of laryngeal precancerous lesions. In the absence of such defined biomarkers, close collaboration with a dedicated head and neck pathologist is mandatory for the laryngologist.

The old adage that "prevention is better than cure" is highly appropriate for laryngeal malignancies, where accurate diagnosis, management, and follow-up of preneoplastic laryngeal lesions by a multidisciplinary head and neck team have a very real chance of obviating the significant morbidity and mortality associated with malignant progression.

References

1. Durant G. Case of cancer of the larynx. Arch Otolaryngol 1880;1: 61–62
2. Jackson C. Cancer of the larynx: is it preceded by a recognizable precancerous condition? Ann Surg 1923;77(1):1–14
3. Ferlay J, Shin HR, Bray F, Forman D, Mathers C, Parkin DM. Estimates of worldwide burden of cancer in 2008: GLOBOCAN 2008. Int J Cancer 2010;127(12):2893–2917
4. Ferlito A, Doglioni C, Rinaldo A, Devaney KO. What is the earliest non-invasive malignant lesion of the larynx? ORL J Otorhinolaryngol Relat Spec 2000;62(2):57–59
5. Ha PK, Califano JA III. The molecular biology of laryngeal cancer. Otolaryngol Clin North Am 2002;35(5):993–1012
6. Kleinsasser O. [The classification and differential diagnosis of epithelial hyperplasia of the laryngeal mucosa on the basis of histomorphological features. II]. Z Laryngol Rhinol Otol 1963;42:339–362
7. Gale N, Michaels L, Luzar B, et al. Current review on squamous intraepithelial lesions of the larynx. Histopathology 2009;54(6):639–656
8. Kambic V, Gale N. Significance of keratosis and dyskeratosis for classifying hyperplastic aberrations of laryngeal mucosa. Am J Otolaryngol 1986;7(5):323–333
9. Eversole LR. Dysplasia of the upper aerodigestive tract squamous epithelium. Head Neck Pathol 2009;3(1):63–68
10. Wenig BM. Squamous cell carcinoma of the upper aerodigestive tract: precursors and problematic variants. Mod Pathol 2002;15(3):229–254
11. Cupić H, Kruslin B, Belicza M. Epithelial hyperplastic lesions of the larynx in biopsy specimens. Acta Otolaryngol Suppl 1997;527: 103–104
12. Bosman FT. Dysplasia classification: pathology in disgrace? J Pathol 2001;194(2):143–144
13. Gale N, Pilch BZ, Sidransky D, Westra WH, Califano J. Epithelial precursor lesions. In: Barnes L, Eveson JW, Reichart P, Sidransky D, eds. World Health Organization Classification of Tumour, Pathology and Genetics of Head and Neck. Lyon: IARC; 2005:140–143
14. Mehanna H, Paleri V, Robson A, Wight R, Helliwell T. Consensus statement by otorhinolaryngologists and pathologists on the diagnosis and management of laryngeal dysplasia. Clin Otolaryngol 2010;35(3):170–176
15. Crissman JD, Visscher DW, Sakr W. Premalignant lesions of the upper aerodigestive tract: pathologic classification. J Cell Biochem Suppl 1993;17F:49–56
16. Kambic V, Lenart I. [Our classification of hyperplasia of the laryngeal epithelium from the prognostic point of view]. J Fr Otorhinolaryngol Audiophonol Chir Maxillofac 1971;20(10): 1145–1150
17. Hellquist H, Cardesa A, Gale N, Kambic V, Michaels L. Criteria for grading in the Ljubljana classification of epithelial hyperplastic laryngeal lesions. A study by members of the Working Group on Epithelial Hyperplastic Laryngeal Lesions of the European Society of Pathology. Histopathology 1999;34(3):226–233
18. McLaren KM, Burnett RA, Goodlad JR, et al; Scottish Pathology Consistency Group. Consistency of histopathological reporting of laryngeal dysplasia. Histopathology 2000;37(5):460–463
19. Sheahan P, Ganly I, Rhy Evans PH, Patel SG. Tumours of the larynx. In Montgomery PQ, Rhys Evans PH, Gullane PJ (eds). Principles and Practice of Head and Neck Surgery and Oncology. 2nd ed. London, UK: Informa Health Care; 2009:257–290
20. Polesel J, Talamini R, La Vecchia C, et al. Tobacco smoking and the risk of upper aero-digestive tract cancers: a reanalysis of case-control studies using spline models. Int J Cancer 2008;122(10):2398–2402
21. Maier H, Tisch M. Epidemiology of laryngeal cancer: results of the Heidelberg case-control study. Acta Otolaryngol Suppl 1997;527:160–164
22. Talamini R, Bosetti C, La Vecchia C, et al. Combined effect of tobacco and alcohol on laryngeal cancer risk: a case-control study. Cancer Causes Control 2002;13(10):957–964
23. La Vecchia C, Zhang ZF, Altieri A. Alcohol and laryngeal cancer: an update. Eur J Cancer Prev 2008;17(2):116–124
24. Brugere J, Guenel P, Leclerc A, Rodriguez J. Differential effects of tobacco and alcohol in cancer of the larynx, pharynx, and mouth. Cancer 1986;57(2):391–395
25. Hobbs CG, Sterne JA, Bailey M, Heyderman RS, Birchall MA, Thomas SJ. Human papillomavirus and head and neck cancer: a systematic review and meta-analysis. Clin Otolaryngol 2006;31(4):259–266
26. Mannarini L, Kratochvil V, Calabrese L, et al. Human Papilloma Virus (HPV) in head and neck region: review of literature. Acta Otorhinolaryngol Ital 2009;29(3):119–126

27. Syrjänen S. Human papillomavirus (HPV) in head and neck cancer. J Clin Virol 2005;32(Suppl 1):S59–S66

28. Nunez DA, Astley SM, Lewis FA, Wells M. Human papilloma viruses: a study of their prevalence in the normal larynx. J Laryngol Otol 1994;108(4):319–320

29. Olson NR. Effects of stomach acid on the larynx. Proc Am Laryngol Assoc 1983;104:108–112

30. Qadeer MA, Colabianchi N, Vaezi MF. Is GERD a risk factor for laryngeal cancer? Laryngoscope 2005;115(3):486–491

31. Baker DC Jr, Weissman B. Postirradiation carcinoma of the larynx. Ann Otol Rhinol Laryngol 1971;80(5):634–637

32. Geisler SA, Olshan AF, Cai J, Weissler M, Smith J, Bell D. Glutathione S-transferase polymorphisms and survival from head and neck cancer. Head Neck 2005;27(3):232–242

33. Califano J, van der Riet P, Westra W, et al. Genetic progression model for head and neck cancer: implications for field cancerization. Cancer Res 1996;56(11):2488–2492

34. Malzahn K, Dreyer T, Glanz H, Arens C. Autofluorescence endoscopy in the diagnosis of early laryngeal cancer and its precursor lesions. Laryngoscope 2002;112(3):488–493

35. Delank W, Khanavkar B, Nakhosteen JA, Stoll W. A pilot study of autofluorescent endoscopy for the in vivo detection of laryngeal cancer. Laryngoscope 2000;110(3 Pt 1):368–373

36. Szeto C, Wehrli B, Whelan F, et al. Contact endoscopy as a novel technique in the detection and diagnosis of mucosal lesions in the head and neck: a brief review. J Oncol 2011;2011:196302

37. Hughes OR, Stone N, Kraft M, Arens C, Birchall MA. Optical and molecular techniques to identify tumor margins within the larynx. Head Neck 2010;32(11):1544–1553

38. Renan MJ. How many mutations are required for tumorigenesis? Implications from human cancer data. Mol Carcinog 1993;7(3):139–146

39. Crissman JD, Zarbo RJ. Quantitation of DNA ploidy in squamous intraepithelial neoplasia of the laryngeal glottis. Arch Otolaryngol Head Neck Surg 1991;117(2):182–188

40. Yoo WJ, Cho SH, Lee YS, et al. Loss of heterozygosity on chromosomes 3p,8p,9p and 17p in the progression of squamous cell carcinoma of the larynx. J Korean Med Sci 2004;19(3):345–351

41. Boyle JO, Hakim J, Koch W, et al. The incidence of p53 mutations increases with progression of head and neck cancer. Cancer Res 1993;53(19):4477–4480

42. Bartkova J, Lukas J, Müller H, Strauss M, Gusterson B, Bartek J. Abnormal patterns of D-type cyclin expression and G1 regulation in human head and neck cancer. Cancer Res 1995;55(4):949–956

43. Gallo O, Franchi A, Chiarelli I, et al. Potential biomarkers in predicting progression of epithelial hyperplastic lesions of the larynx. Acta Otolaryngol Suppl 1997;527:30–38

44. Zidar N, Gale N, Cör A, Kambic V. Expression of Ki-67 antigen and proliferative cell nuclear antigen in benign and malignant epithelial lesions of the larynx. J Laryngol Otol 1996;110(5):440–445

45. Nankivell P, Weller M, McConkey C, Paleri V, Mehanna H. Biomarkers in laryngeal dysplasia: a systematic review. Head Neck 2011;33(8):1170–1176

46. Paleri V, Mackenzie K, Wight RG, Mehanna H, Pracy P, Bradley PJ; ENT-UK Head and Neck Group. Management of laryngeal dysplasia in the United Kingdom: a web-based questionnaire survey of current practice. Clin Otolaryngol 2009;34(4):385–389

47. Lehman JJ, Bless DM, Brandenburg JH. An objective assessment of voice production after radiation therapy for stage I squamous cell carcinoma of the glottis. Otolaryngol Head Neck Surg 1988;98(2):121–129

48. Hellquist H, Lundgren J, Olofsson J. Hyperplasia, keratosis, dysplasia and carcinoma in situ of the vocal cords—a follow-up study. Clin Otolaryngol Allied Sci 1982;7(1):11–27

49. Abdurehim Y, Hua Z, Yasin Y, Xukurhan A, Imam I, Yuqin F. Transoral laser surgery versus radiotherapy: systematic review and meta-analysis for treatment options of T1a glottic cancer. Head Neck 2012;34(1):23–33

50. Dey P, Arnold D, Wight R, MacKenzie K, Kelly C, Wilson J. Radiotherapy versus open surgery versus endolaryngeal surgery (with or without laser) for early laryngeal squamous cell cancer. Cochrane Database Syst Rev 2002;(2):CD002027

51. Sadri M, McMahon J, Parker A. Management of laryngeal dysplasia: a review. Eur Arch Otorhinolaryngol 2006;263(9):843–852

52. Myssiorek D, Vambutas A, Abramson AL. Carcinoma in situ of the glottic larynx. Laryngoscope 1994;104(4):463–467

53. Zeitels SM. Infrapetiole exploration of the supraglottis for exposure of the anterior glottal commissure. J Voice 1998;12(1):117–122

54. Biel MA. Photodynamic therapy of head and neck cancers. Methods Mol Biol 2010;635:281–293

55. Zeitels SM, Burns JA, Lopez-Guerra G, Anderson RR, Hillman RE. Photoangiolytic laser treatment of early glottic cancer: a new management strategy. Ann Otol Rhinol Laryngol Suppl 2008;199:3–24

56. Hartnick CJ, Boseley ME, Franco RA Jr, Cunningham MJ, Pransky S. Efficacy of treating children with anterior commissure and true vocal fold respiratory papilloma with the 585-nm pulsed-dye laser. Arch Otolaryngol Head Neck Surg 2007;133(2):127–130

57. Zeitels SM, Akst LM, Burns JA, Hillman RE, Broadhurst MS, Anderson RR. Office-based 532-nm pulsed KTP laser treatment of glottal papillomatosis and dysplasia. Ann Otol Rhinol Laryngol 2006;115(9):679–685

58. Koufman JA, Rees CJ, Frazier WD, et al. Office-based laryngeal laser surgery: a review of 443 cases using three wavelengths. Otolaryngol Head Neck Surg 2007;137(1):146–151

59. Damm M, Sittel C, Streppel M, Eckel HE. Transoral CO_2 laser for surgical management of glottic carcinoma in situ. Laryngoscope 2000;110(7):1215–1221

60. Xu W, Han D, Hou L, Zhang L, Yu Z, Huang Z. Voice function following CO_2 laser microsurgery for precancerous and early-stage glottic carcinoma. Acta Otolaryngol 2007;127(6):637–641

61. Kujan O, Oliver RJ, Khattab A, Roberts SA, Thakker N, Sloan P. Evaluation of a new binary system of grading oral epithelial dysplasia for prediction of malignant transformation. Oral Oncol 2006;42(10):987–993

62. Weller MD, Nankivell PC, McConkey C, Paleri V, Mehanna HM. The risk and interval to malignancy of patients with laryngeal dysplasia; a systematic review of case series and meta-analysis. Clin Otolaryngol 2010;35(5):364–372

63. Hintz BL, Kagan AR, Nussbaum H, Rao AR, Chan PY, Miles JA. A "watchful waiting" policy for in situ carcinoma of the vocal cords. Arch Otolaryngol 1981;107(12):746–751

27 Laryngeal Trauma

Guri S. Sandhu and S. A. Reza Nouraei

The larynx protects the airway from aspiration, acts as the respiratory gateway to the lungs, and is the primary organ of phonation.[1] Laryngeal trauma can disrupt one or all of these function and, in the context of airway compromise, is acutely life-threatening.[2-4] If not promptly recognized and adequately treated, it can also cause significant long-term morbidity.[4-6] Laryngeal trauma often co-occurs with cervical and intracranial injuries and frequently forms part of polytrauma.[4] It is therefore important that all patients with suspected laryngeal injury be managed by a multidisciplinary trauma team according to Advanced Trauma Life Support (ATLS) guidelines.

Mechanisms of Injury

Laryngeal trauma can be broadly divided into external trauma, which can be blunt or penetrating, and internal trauma, which can be caused by iatrogenic, thermal, caustic, or foreign body injuries.

External Laryngeal Trauma

External laryngeal trauma has a population incidence of 1 in 137,000 in adults[4] and accounts for 0.5% of trauma admissions in children.[7] The larynx—which is superiorly, inferiorly, posteriorly, and laterally well protected by the mandible, sternum, the cervical spine, and strap muscles of the neck—is susceptible to crushing anterior cervical trauma. Rapid motor vehicle deceleration can thrust the neck against the steering wheel or dashboard if driving without a seat belt. Another important mechanism of injury is the clothesline injury, in which a rider encounters a fixed horizontal object at neck level. Suicidal or homicidal strangulations can also cause laryngeal trauma. Clothesline injuries are often associated with major neck trauma, which may not be initially apparent.[8,9] Homicidal strangulation is more likely to cause laryngotracheal separation and neurovascular trauma when compared with suicidal strangulation.[10] All strangulation injuries can cause loss of airway due to laryngeal edema some time after the event, despite minimal initial findings.[11-13] Laryngeal injury can be confounded by the process of laryngeal calcification, which begins during the third decade of life and can lead to creation of stress risers leading to laryngeal comminution.[14]

Over the past decades, however, with improvements in public education, reductions in speed limits, and mandatory use of seat belts, the number of blunt laryngeal trauma cases has declined, and penetrating laryngeal trauma, which is due predominantly to interpersonal violence or war, has become the predominant form of laryngeal trauma.[2,3,6,15-23] Penetrating trauma is more likely to damage additional cervical structures, with the extent of injury being proportional to both the weight and velocity of the penetrating projectile ($E = \frac{1}{2} mv^2$).

Diagnosis

Clinical presentation of laryngeal trauma ranges from cardiopulmonary arrest due to airway obstruction to subtle changes in voice quality. The most common presenting feature of laryngeal trauma is hoarseness (85%), followed by dysphagia (52%), anterior cervical pain (42%), breathlessness (21%), and hemoptysis (18%).[5]

Management

Examination and initial management of laryngeal trauma should follow ATLS guidelines to ensure that concomitant injuries are not missed (**Table 27.1**).[4] The overriding priority is to establish a safe airway with cervical spine protection and this may, and often does, necessitate performing an emergent tracheotomy under local anesthesia. Endotracheal intubation is not favored in this situation, as it can exacerbate a laryngeal injury[24] and precipitate total airway obstruction. If endotracheal intubation has been performed, it is converted at the earliest opportunity to a tracheotomy to prevent long-term laryngeal injury. No manipulation of the neck is permissible until the cervical spine has been cleared.

Table 27.1 Concomitant Primary Diagnoses Recorded along with Laryngeal Trauma[4]

Injury	(%)
Open neck injury	18
Maxillofacial fractures	18
Intracranial injuries	17
Cervical spine fracture	13
Chest injury	13
Other facial injury	10
Skull fracture	7
Open pharyngeal injury	4

The neck is inspected for evidence of injury such as skin abrasions, bruising, and entry and exit wounds in penetrating trauma, and is palpated for crepitations, laryngeal tenderness, and any obvious changes in laryngeal anatomy such as loss of the prominence. Open wounds should not be explored at this stage, as instrumentation may restart hemorrhage. Flexible nasoendoscopy is then performed, and the oropharynx and hypopharynx are examined for injuries. The laryngeal mucosa is examined for lacerations and hematomas, and particular care is taken to assess the vibratory edge of the vocal cords and the anterior commissure. Arytenoid adduction is examined during phonation, and abduction is assessed by asking the patient to sniff. Impairment of arytenoid mobility may be secondary to structural damage or due to recurrent laryngeal nerve injury. Note is taken of any exposed or protruded cartilage or submucosal distortion of the framework. A sign of cartilaginous injury is the failure of the vocal cords to meet in the same horizontal plane.

In our practice, multislice computed tomography (CT) (**Fig. 27.1**) is performed in all patients presenting with "impending airway obstruction" once the airway has been secured, and in those patients with a "stable airway" who are found, on flexible nasoendoscopy, to have endolaryngeal abnormalities, since imaging may reveal further laryngeal injuries and most importantly clear the cervical spine. This is particularly pertinent consideration, as up to 13% of patients with laryngeal trauma can have an associated cervical spine injury and that the spinal injury may be masked by the presence of a distracting laryngeal injury.[4,25] CT scanning can be deferred only in those patients with unalarming history and minor physical findings. Laryngeal trauma can be classified according the Schaefer-Fuhrman[24,26] (**Table 27.2**) or the Lee-Eliashar systems.[27]

Managing Laryngeal Trauma

The first priority in managing laryngeal trauma is to assess and secure the airway while protecting the cervical spine. We take a stepwise approach to securing the airway based

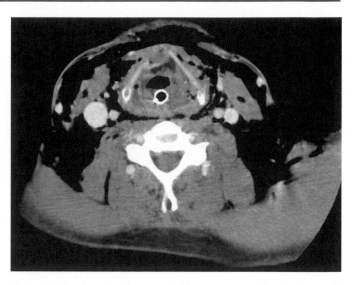

Figure 27.1 Computed tomographic appearance of a patient with acute external laryngeal trauma.

on information available at the different stages of clinical assessment (**Fig. 27.2**). A stridulous patient with respiratory distress at presentation should immediately proceed to have a tracheotomy under local anesthesia. If the airway is judged to be stable following initial history and examination, the patient has a flexible nasoendoscopy. In a small number of cases, unexpected airway-encroaching injuries are identified at this stage and the patient proceeds to have a tracheotomy. More subtle endolaryngeal injuries are further assessed with CT and again, if airway-encroaching injuries are identified, the patient proceeds to have a tracheotomy.

The decision on the most appropriate therapy for laryngeal trauma rests on assessing the stability of, and the extent of injury to, the *laryngeal framework*, the extent of *mucosal injuries*, the presence or otherwise of injury to the *vibratory apparatus*, and the integrity of the *laryngotracheal junction*. Jewett et al showed that 37% of patients with laryngeal trauma could be managed with no airway intervention and a further one-sixth of patients required only a tracheotomy.[4]

Table 27.2 Schaefer-Fuhrman Classification of Laryngeal Trauma

Group 1	Minor endolaryngeal hematomas or lacerations No detectable fracture
Group 2	Edema, hematoma, minor mucosal disruption without exposed cartilage Nondisplaced fracture Varying degrees of airway compromise
Group 3	Massive edema, large mucosal lacerations, exposed cartilage Displaced fracture(s) Vocal cord immobility

Group 4	Same as Group 3 but more severe with:
	    Severe mucosal disruption
	    Disruption of the anterior commissure
	    Unstable fracture, two or more fracture lines

Group 5	Complete laryngotracheal separation

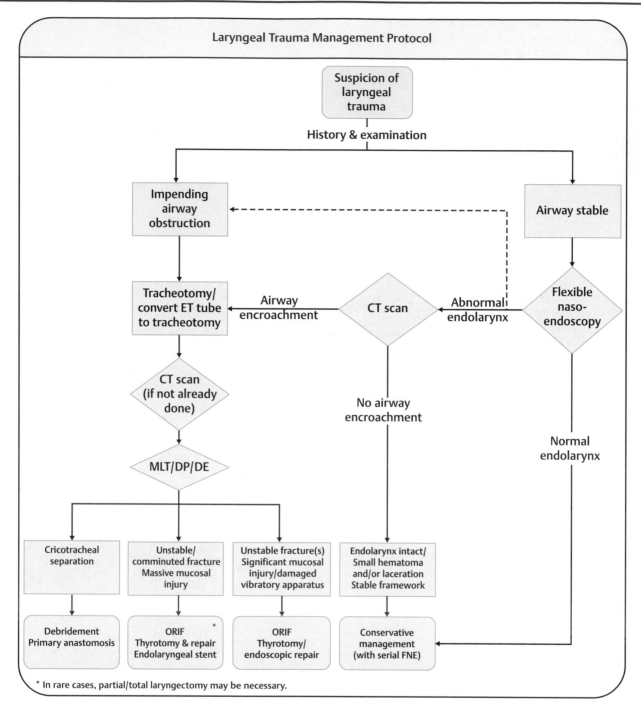

Figure 27.2 A protocol for managing laryngeal trauma. CT, computed tomography; DE, direct esophagoscopy; OP, direct pharyngoscopy; ET, endotracheal; FNE, flexible naso-endoscopy; MLT, microlaryngoscopy and tracheoscopy; ORIF, open reduction and internal fixation.

Patients with a normal endolarynx on nasoendoscopy and patients with minimal endolaryngeal abnormalities and a stable laryngeal framework, whose airway patency has been confirmed by CT can be conservatively managed. Conservative management consists of a minimum of a 24-hour admission to a high-dependency unit, with regular observations, serial flexible nasoendoscopy, and use of humidified oxygen. A mixture of oxygen and helium should be on standby in case respiratory embarrassment develops. The patient's head is elevated to reduce further edema, and corticosteroids are administered if the patient presents within 24 hours of injury. All patients are prescribed a proton pump inhibitor, and, if the laryngeal mucosa has been breached, they are also given prophylactic broad-spectrum antibiotics.

Patients with more significant injuries require surgical intervention. The optimal timing of repair is a subject of

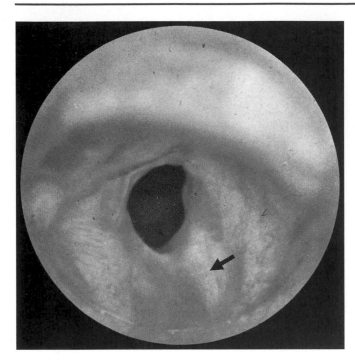

Figure 27.3 Posttraumatic laryngeal stenosis.

debate and in polytrauma patients, laryngeal surgery may need to be coordinated with other surgeries. We aim to repair all laryngeal injuries within 12 hours of presentation, and are reluctant to accept delays beyond 24 hours. Delays in treatment can lead to granulation and scar tissue formation, which can progress to laryngeal stenosis (**Fig. 27.3**), a difficult surgical problem to subsequently correct.

All patients who are not managed conservatively should undergo a microlaryngoscopy, tracheoscopy, direct pharyngoscopy, and direct esophagoscopy. In a proportion of patients, definitive endolaryngeal treatment can be undertaken endoscopically. Hematomas can be drained, mucosal and selected vocal cord lacerations can be repaired, and dislocated cricoarytenoid joints can be reduced. If there have been extensive injuries to opposing laryngeal mucosal surfaces, stents or keels can also be deployed endoscopically to prevent adhesions.[28]

The main indications for open repair are unstable or comminuted laryngeal fractures, cricotracheal separation, detachment of the anterior commissure, or extensive mucosal disruption. For open exploration, a transverse neck incision is placed over the cricoid, and subplatysmal flaps are elevated. Strap muscles are separated in the midline and retracted. In a proportion of patients with unstable laryngeal fractures but with minimal or endoscopically treatable endolaryngeal injuries, a thyrotomy can be avoided. Repair of the anterior commissure, or significant endolaryngeal injuries, is achieved through an anterior vertical laryngofissure. However, a paramedian fracture close to the midline may also be used. Hematomas are evacuated and mucosa tears repaired with 5–0 or 6–0 absorbable sutures. Mucosal loss can often be reconstructed with local mucosal

flaps and in particular, posterior commissure injuries can and should be reconstructed with piriform fossa or supraglottic mucosa to prevent laryngeal stenosis. The anterior margins of the vocal folds are attached to the anterior limit of the thyroid cartilage or its outer perichondrium using a slow-absorbing monofilament suture. It is very important to re-establish the appropriate height of the vocal folds to optimize voice outcomes. Thyroid cartilage fractures are repaired using permanent or resorbable miniplates. Even in the older patient, the cricoid arch does not fully calcify and can be repaired using suture material alone.

The indications for stenting are controversial because the need for endolaryngeal support needs to be considered against the potential for further mucosal injury. Our primary indication for stenting is significant framework comminution. Stents can also be used to prevent anterior commissure webbing in cases of bilateral vocal fold epithelial loss. We prefer to use soft silastic stents for this purpose to minimize further mucosal injury and foreign body reaction associated with the use of stents fashioned from endotracheal tubes. Endolaryngeal stents are commercially available but can also be fashioned from the vertical limb of a silastic T-tube that is over sewn at the top. The stent is held in place with a 2–0 Prolene suture through the anterior stent, laryngeal ventricles and knotted over the larynx following closure of the laryngofissure. The stent is removed endoscopically 10 to 14 days later. The securing suture can be cut flush with the endoluminal airway or removed via a small neck incision.

Vocal cord mobility can usually be determined during preoperative flexible laryngoscopy. Cricoarytenoid joint mobility can be assessed preoperatively, but definitive assessment of joint mobility requires microlaryngoscopy and instrumentation. Vocal cord immobility due to cricoarytenoid joint dislocation can often be managed with endoscopic manipulation and reduction. Recurrent laryngeal nerves can be severed in penetrating trauma or during cricotracheal separation, or crushed during laryngeal trauma. Only if a complete palsy is confirmed should exploration of the affected nerve be considered. Anatomically intact nerves should be allowed to regenerate. Where possible, severed nerves should be repaired in a tension-free manner. If this is not possible, then a cable graft using the greater auricular or sural nerve should be considered. The other option is to consider ansa cervicalis to recurrent laryngeal repair. Nerve repairs do not restore the intricate motor function of the larynx, but may provide sufficient muscle tone to improve vocalization.

During surgery for cricitracheal separation, a tracheotomy is fashioned or moved to a healthy part of the lower trachea before re-anastomosis. During the surgery, a small reinforced endotracheal tube is placed through the tracheotomy for ventilation and is replaced with a small tracheotomy tube at the end of the procedure. The repair begins with the posterior anastomosis using a combination of 3–0 absorbable and nonabsorbable sutures working toward the anterior trachea (**Fig. 27.4**). All knots are extraluminal and the sutures run

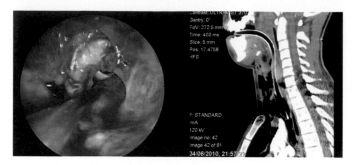

Figure 27.4 Endoscopic and computed tomographic appearances of cricotracheal separation.

through the submucosal plane. Avascular and damaged tissue is resected. If there is an associated crush injury to the trachea, a temporary soft silastic stent may need to be placed in the lumen before anastomosis. In cases of massive laryngeal injury with significant tissue loss, partial or total laryngectomy may be indicated, although this is rare in civilian practice.[22]

Any repairs to the vocal folds should be followed by strict voice rest for 48 to 72 hours. A nasogastric tube should be inserted at the time of surgery and should remain in situ until the safety of swallowing is confirmed. All patients with mucosal tears should be placed on antireflux therapy and prophylactic antibiotics. The patient is nursed in head-up position to minimize edema and standard tracheotomy care is provided. Early ambulation is encouraged. Stents are removed at 10 to 14 days and the patient is decannulated. Regular endoscopic examinations are undertaken, and granulation tissue is removed to prevent long-term scarring. In patients with cricotracheal separation, the neck is kept in flexion for 7 days postoperatively to prevent traction on the anastomosis. A large monofilament suture from the submental skin to the anterior chest skin, placed at the time of surgery, may be necessary for the first few postoperative days. The tracheotomy can be removed at 7 days and the airway stent can be removed endoscopically at 10 to 14 days.

Sequelae of Laryngeal Trauma

Long-term morbidity may be due to laryngeal stenosis, dysphonia, or aspiration. These long-term injuries may not become apparent for up to 12 months after the initial injury. Vocal cord paralysis should be regularly reviewed for signs of recovery, and in patients with a normal vibratory apparatus structure and unilateral vocal cord paralysis, definitive medialization procedures should only be attempted after 6 to 9 months. In the interim, the voice can be temporarily improved by collagen or fat injection. In cases of bilateral vocal cord palsy causing laryngeal inlet obstruction, consideration should be given to retaining the tracheotomy in preference to performing an early laser arytenoidectomy, in anticipation of return of vocal cord function. Laryngeal stenosis due to posterior commissure or tracheal granulation tissue should be promptly treated with intralesional steroid injections and reduction of granulation tissue. The granulation tissue should not be allowed to mature into a scar, as this is a much more difficult problem to manage.[29] In our experience, the most difficult injuries to manage are laryngeal inlet obliteration followed by interarytenoid scarring or webbing. The treatment of glottic stenosis is almost always a compromise among voice, airway, and swallowing, and gains in one domain are often at the expense of another.

Outcome of External Laryngeal Trauma

This is dependent both on the nature and severity of the original injury, and on whether the injury was promptly recognized and adequately treated. Schaefer and recently Juutilainen et al found that the voice, but not the airway outcome, correlates with the severity of the initial injury as determined by Schaefer's classification system (**Table 27.3**),[5,22] while Bent et al found that intervention within 48 hours was associated with an improved outcome.[16] Delays in intervention can lead to complete laryngotracheal stenosis.

Table 27.3 Outcome of Treating Laryngeal Trauma[5,22]

Group	Voice Outcome			Airway Outcome		
	Good	Fair	Poor	Good	Fair	Poor
Results from Schaefer						
1	20	0	0	20	0	0
2	38	3	0	40	1	0
3	18	3	0	21	0	0
4	22	10	0	31	0	2
Results from Juutilainen et al						
2	12	4	0	16	0	0
3	7	6	0	13	0	0
4	1	3	0	4	0	0

Caustic/Thermal Laryngeal Trauma

Upper aerodigestive tract injury caused by ingestion of caustic substances occurs in 5000 to 15,000 persons in the United States annually and the majority of injuries are caused by ingestion of alkaline substances.[30] The larynx is involved in approximately 40% of cases.[31] Thermal injury to the larynx is a sequela of inhaling superheated air. Inhalation burns occur in 30% of all burn patients, and 20% of patients with inhalation injury have extensive laryngeal injury. A further 7% of patients with inhalation injury have both laryngeal and tracheobronchial injuries.[32]

Ingestion of alkali causes liquefaction necrosis of muscle, collagen, and lipids and creates an injury that worsens with time. By contrast, acids cause coagulation necrosis of the superficial tissues. Caustic substance ingestion is virtually always accidental in children where small amounts of liquids are taken, but are almost always due to attempted suicide in adults and is associated with ingestion of large volumes of liquid.[31] The type of liquid taken varies widely with geography, with alkaline and acid ingestion being more common in the developed and developing countries, respectively.[30,33] Inhalation injury is typically a consequence of fires in closed spaces and causes a six-fold increase in the mortality rate associated with the burn.[32]

Management

All patients with caustic or thermal laryngeal injuries should be admitted for a minimum of 24 hours for airway observation. The first priority is the establishment of a safe airway, followed by cardiovascular resuscitation, as per standard burns care protocols. The presence of facial or body burns and soot in the oral cavity and endoscopic finding of laryngeal edema predict the need for airway intervention.[34] Endotracheal intubation plays an even lesser role in managing these patients, compared with external laryngeal trauma patients. Arévalo-Silva et al found a 100% association between endotracheal intubation and subsequent tracheotomy for airway stenosis in patients with laryngeal injury due to caustic ingestion.[31] The situation with airway management in thermal injuries is somewhat less clear, as there have been reports of increased stenosis rates with tracheotomy, as opposed to intubation, in patients with inhalation injury.[35] However, unless there are strong contraindications to performing a tracheotomy, such as extensive cervical burns, we iterate the view that with glottic stenosis having a far worse prognosis than tracheal stenosis, a possible increase in the rate of post-tracheotomy stomal stenosis is an acceptable trade-off.

If patients are to undergo a microlaryngoscopy, tracheobronchoscopy, or esophagoscopy, then this should be within 24 hours of injury. Beyond this period, edema and ulceration are more marked and instrumentation may exacerbate subsequent problems. The upper aerodigestive tract should be irrigated in cases of caustic injury to remove any residual substances. Further treatment is dependent on the nature and extent of injuries found and the consequences of healing and scarring.

Sequela of Caustic/Thermal Laryngeal Injuries

Caustic and thermal injuries can cause laryngeal and tracheal airway strictures, whose severity is reported to be greater than those associated with postintubation laryngotracheal stenosis[36] with dysphonia being present in as many as 70% of patients with inhalation injuries 16 to 25 years after the initial injury.[37]

Special Considerations in Pediatric External Laryngeal Trauma

The neonatal larynx lies at the level of C3 and descends during the first 3 years of life to its adult position at the level of C6. The pediatric larynx is smaller in absolute and relative dimensions compared with the adult larynx. Furthermore, laryngeal mucosa is less firmly adherent to the cartilaginous framework in infants and children compared with adults. This combination of factors mean that while the pediatric larynx is better shielded and is therefore less liable to injury, if an injury does occur, it is more likely to result in loss of airway due to mucosal edema and hematoma formation.[7,38] Furthermore, it is usually not possible to perform tracheotomies under local anesthetic in children. Therefore, children are managed along the same lines as patients with acute epiglottitis. The surgeon is prepared for an emergency tracheotomy, but in most cases the airway can be secured with an endotracheal tube or ventilating bronchoscope, followed promptly by a tracheotomy under general anesthesia. CT may then be considered before airway reconstruction. As with adult patients, selected, more limited injuries can be managed endoscopically and without tracheotomies.[39]

References

1. Lumb AB. Nunn's Applied Respiratory Physiology. 6th ed. Oxford: Butterworth-Heinemann; 2005
2. Bhojani RA, Rosenbaum DH, Dikmen E, et al. Contemporary assessment of laryngotracheal trauma. J Thorac Cardiovasc Surg 2005;130(2):426–432
3. Gussack GS, Jurkovich GJ, Luterman A. Laryngotracheal trauma: a protocol approach to a rare injury. Laryngoscope 1986;96(6):660–665
4. Jewett BS, Shockley WW, Rutledge R. External laryngeal trauma analysis of 392 patients. Arch Otolaryngol Head Neck Surg 1999;125(8):877–880
5. Juutilainen M, Vintturi J, Robinson S, Back L, Lehtonen H, Makitie AA. Laryngeal fractures: clinical findings and considerations on suboptimal outcome. Acta Otolaryngol 2008;128(2):213–218
6. Minard G, Kudsk KA, Croce MA, Butts JA, Cicala RS, Fabian TC. Laryngotracheal trauma. Am Surg 1992;58(3):181–187

7. Ford HR, Gardner MJ, Lynch JM. Laryngotracheal disruption from blunt pediatric neck injuries: impact of early recognition and intervention on outcome. J Pediatr Surg 1995;30(2):331–334, discussion 334–335

8. Close DM. Traumatic avulsion of the larynx. J Laryngol Otol 1981;95(11):1157–1158

9. Graham J, Dick R, Parnell D, Aitken ME. Clothesline injury mechanism associated with all-terrain vehicle use by children. Pediatr Emerg Care 2006;22(1):45–47

10. Maxeiner H, Bockholdt B. Homicidal and suicidal ligature strangulation—a comparison of the post-mortem findings. Forensic Sci Int 2003;137(1):60–66

11. Rejali SD, Bennett JD, Upile T, Rothera MP. Diagnostic pitfalls in sports related laryngeal injury. Br J Sports Med 1998;32(2): 180–181

12. Pennington CL. External trauma of the larynx and trachea. Immediate treatment and management. Ann Otol Rhinol Laryngol 1972;81(4):546–554

13. Nahum AM, Siegel AW. Biodynamics of injury to the larynx in automobile collisions. Ann Otol Rhinol Laryngol 1967;76(4): 781–785

14. Mupparapu M, Vuppalapati A. Ossification of laryngeal cartilages on lateral cephalometric radiographs. Angle Orthod 2005;75(2): 196–201

15. Danic D, Prgomet D, Sekelj A, Jakovina K, Danic A. External laryngotracheal trauma. Eur Arch Otorhinolaryngol 2006;263(3):228–232

16. Bent JP III, Silver JR, Porubsky ES. Acute laryngeal trauma: a review of 77 patients. Otolaryngol Head Neck Surg 1993;109(3, Pt 1):441–449

17. Cohn AM, Larson DL. Laryngeal injury: a critical review. Arch Otolaryngol 1976;102(3):166–170

18. Francis S, Gaspard DJ, Rogers N, Stain SC. Diagnosis and management of laryngotracheal trauma. J Natl Med Assoc 2002;94(1):21–24

19. Harris HH, Ainsworth JZ. Immediate management of laryngeal and tracheal injuries. Laryngoscope 1965;75:1103–1115

20. Harris HH, Tobin HA. Acute injuries of the larynx and trachea in 49 patients. (Observations over a 15-year period). Laryngoscope 1970;80(9):1376–1384

21. Lambert GE Jr, McMurry GT. Laryngotracheal trauma: recognition and management. JACEP 1976;5(11):883–887

22. Schaefer SD. The acute management of external laryngeal trauma. A 27-year experience. Arch Otolaryngol Head Neck Surg 1992;118(6):598–604

23. Shaia FT, Cassady CL. Laryngeal trauma. Arch Otolaryngol 1972;95(2):104–108

24. Schaefer SD. Primary management of laryngeal trauma. Ann Otol Rhinol Laryngol 1982;91(4, Pt 1):399–402

25. Hoffman JR, Mower WR, Wolfson AB, Todd KH, Zucker MI. National Emergency X-Radiography Utilization Study Group. Validity of a set of clinical criteria to rule out injury to the cervical spine in patients with blunt trauma. N Engl J Med 2000;343(2):94–99

26. Fuhrman GM, Stieg FH III, Buerk CA. Blunt laryngeal trauma: classification and management protocol. J Trauma 1990;30(1): 87–92

27. Lee WT, Eliashar R, Eliachar I. Acute external laryngotracheal trauma: diagnosis and management. Ear Nose Throat J 2006;85(3):179–184

28. Mace A, Sandhu GS, Howard DJ. Securing tracheal stents: a new and simple method. J Laryngol Otol 2005;119(3):207–208

29. Nouraei SAR, Singh A, Patel A, Ferguson C, Howard DJ, Sandhu GS. Early endoscopic treatment of acute inflammatory airway lesions improves the outcome of postintubation airway stenosis. Laryngoscope 2006;116(8):1417–1421

30. Erdoğan E, Eroğlu E, Tekant G, et al. Management of esophagogastric corrosive injuries in children. Eur J Pediatr Surg 2003;13(5): 289–293

31. Arévalo-Silva C, Eliashar R, Wohlgelernter J, Elidan J, Gross M. Ingestion of caustic substances: a 15-year experience. Laryngoscope 2006;116(8):1422–1426

32. Nottet JB, Duruisseau O, Herve S, et al. Inhalation burns: apropos of 198 cases. Incidence of laryngotracheal involvement [in French]. Ann Otolaryngol Chir Cervicofac 1997;114(6):220–225

33. Ramasamy K, Gumaste VV. Corrosive ingestion in adults. J Clin Gastroenterol 2003;37(2):119–124

34. Madnani DD, Steele NP, de Vries E. Factors that predict the need for intubation in patients with smoke inhalation injury. Ear Nose Throat J 2006;85(4):278–280

35. Lund T, Goodwin CW, McManus WF, et al. Upper airway sequelae in burn patients requiring endotracheal intubation or tracheostomy. Ann Surg 1985;201(3):374–382

36. Gaissert HA, Lofgren RH, Grillo HC. Upper airway compromise after inhalation injury. Complex strictures of the larynx and trachea and their management. Ann Surg 1993;218(5):672–678

37. Casper JK, Clark WR, Kelley RT, Colton RH. Laryngeal and phonatory status after burn/inhalation injury: a long term follow-up study. J Burn Care Rehabil 2002;23(4):235–243

38. Myer CM III, Orobello P, Cotton RT, Bratcher GO. Blunt laryngeal trauma in children. Laryngoscope 1987;97(9):1043–1048

39. Elmaraghy CA, Tanna N, Wiet GJ, Kang DR. Endoscopic management of blunt pediatric laryngeal trauma. Ann Otol Rhinol Laryngol 2007;116(3):192–194

28 Management of Benign Laryngotracheal Stenosis in Adults

Guri S. Sandhu and S. A. Reza Nouraei

The larynx, trachea, and bronchi form the conduit between the external environment and the lungs through which respiratory gases are transported and pulmonary secretions are expectorated. The principle function of the larynx is to protect the airway from aspiration during swallowing, but the larynx is also involved with phonation and the Valsalva maneuver. The narrowest sites of the adult airway are the larynx and trachea (**Fig. 28.1**).

Upper airway stenosis can have a significant impact on the quality of life and sometimes on life itself. Abnormal narrowing of the laryngotracheal complex causes breathlessness, especially during physical activity. Retention of pulmonary secretions may lead to lung infection or collapse. Laryngeal stenosis can interfere with phonation and a dysfunctional larynx can affect swallowing safety. Due to medical advances, more patients are surviving periods of ventilation on intensive care units (ICUs).[1,2] As a consequence, the incidence of laryngotracheal injury is probably increasing but remains unknown.

Poiseuille law

$$R = \frac{8nl}{\pi r^4}$$

- *R* = resistance
- *n* = viscosity
- *l* = length
- *r* = radius

In laminar airflow, airway resistance is dictated by the diameter of the airway and by the density of the inspired gas (Poiseuille law). Because of the fourth power in the denominator, resistance increases rapidly as diameter decreases. However, an area of airway stenosis also produces turbulence, which adds to resistance, but cannot easily be calculated.

During inspiration, the intrathoracic airways expand along with the expanding lungs. However, the extrathoracic trachea will have a reduced lumen during inspiration because the intraluminal pressure is lower than atmospheric. The reverse happens during expiration. A variable obstruction of the airway also changes size with breathing. Hence, an extrathoracic variable tracheal stenosis will limit inspiration, whereas an intrathoracic variable lesion will limit expiration. A fixed obstruction, whether intrathoracic or extrathoracic, will limit peak airflow on inspiration and expiration in equal proportions and produce a characteristic flow volume loop (**Fig. 28.2**).[3] The exact physiological causes of dyspnea are not known; however, the extra work of breathing, altered afferent input from the respiratory tract, and the tendency toward carbon dioxide retention must play a role.

Pediatric laryngotracheal stenosis is a well-researched area of medicine and treatments include airway augmentation with rib grafts as well as tracheal and cricotracheal resections. Adult laryngotracheal stenosis has been poorly researched and the surgical options include tracheostomy, tracheal resection, or cricotracheal resection.[4] Some surgeons continue to use primary cartilage grafts to augment the adult airway. There has been little appreciation of the fact that there is a high incidence of ischemic necrosis of primary rib graft in adult patients.[5] Furthermore, the quality and quantity of rib cartilage that can be harvested diminishes with age.[5] Pediatric airway stenosis nearly always involves the subglottis[6] and most commonly is due to prolonged endotracheal intubation. However, the lesional anatomy, anatomical sites, and pathologies behind adult laryngotracheal stenosis differ greatly from the pediatric group.

The most widely used grading system to describe the degree of airway stenosis is the Myer-Cotton grading system,[7] which refers to the surface area of the stenosis (**Fig. 28.3**) as opposed to the size of the patient's airway. This grading system was developed to help decision making in pediatric airway surgery with respect to conservative or surgical treatments. In pediatrics, a decannulation is deemed a successful outcome and in the adult population, the outcomes are often graded as "excellent," "good," "satisfactory," "failure," or "death" with little mention of swallowing or voice outcomes.

Table 28.1 illustrates the etiologies in 400 consecutive adult patients treated for benign airway stenosis by the National Centre for Airway Reconstruction in the United

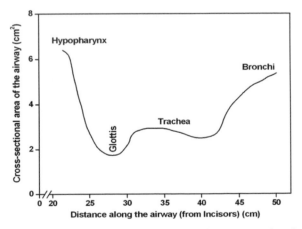

Figure 28.1 The narrowest site in the adult airway is the glottis followed by the trachea.

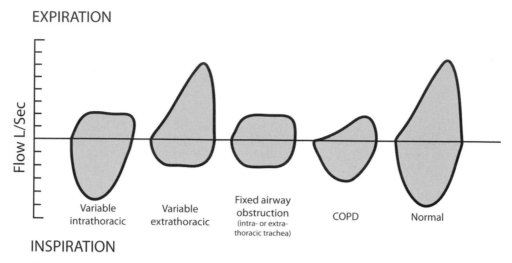

EXPIRATION

Flow L/Sec

Variable intrathoracic

Variable extrathoracic

Fixed airway obstruction
(intra- or extra-thoracic trachea)

COPD

Normal

INSPIRATION

Figure 28.2 Patterns of flow volume loops[3]—these graphically depict the rate of airflow on the *y*-axis and the total volume expired (above) inspired (below) on the *x*-axis. The patient is asked to take the deepest breathe, apply the mouth to the device, and breathe out as hard as possible and for as long as possible. This is followed by a maximum and rapid inspiration. COPD, chronic obstructive pulmonary disease.

Classification	From	To
Grade I	No Obstruction	50% Obstruction
Grade II	51% Obstruction	70% Obstruction
Grade III	71% Obstruction	99% Obstruction
Grade IV	No Detectable Lumen	

Figure 28.3 Myer-Cotton grading system for pediatric subglottic stenosis.

Kingdom. Of the relative etiological factors, more than half the cases of adult laryngotracheal stenosis were due to a period of ventilation on an ICU. The incidence of stenosis in patients who were ventilated with endotracheal tubes or converted earlier to tracheostomies was very similar, only the site of the injury differed. Early tracheostomy did, however, reduce the incidence of damage to the vocal folds and their mobility. Unlike pediatric laryngotracheal stenosis, which almost always affects the subglottis, in the adult population, one-third of the patients had stenosis of the cervical trachea. Nearly half of the adult patients had airway compromise due to other disease processes such as Wegener granulomatosis, sarcoidosis, and idiopathic subglottic stenosis (ISS).

The male larynx differs little in size from that of the female larynx until puberty. The adult male larynx

Table 28.1 Four hundred consecutive adult referrals with laryngotracheal stenosis

- 48% Acquired laryngotracheal stenosis
  - 34.75% Subglottic stenosis
  - 13.25% Tracheal stenosis
- 14.75% Bilateral vocal cord mobility impairment
  - 8.75% Nerve injury
  - 4.75% Scar/fixation
  - 1.25% Rheumatoid arthritis
- 11.25% Wegener granulomatosis
- 9.75% Idiopathic subglottic stenosis
- 5.5% Supraglottic stenosis (2.5% sarcoid, 3.0% other)
- 3.25% Previous papillomatosis treatment
- 3.25% Glottic web
- 2.0% Tracheomalacia (1.25% relapsing polychondritis)
- 1.0% Amyloidosis
- 0.75% Vascular lesion
- 0.5% Subglottic stenosis congenital

undergoes significant growth and the adult female larynx undergoes a lesser degree under the influence of the hormones responsible for secondary sexual characteristics. The adult male larynx averages 44 mm in length and the adult female larynx averages 36 mm.[8] The anteroposterior length in the adult male averages 41 mm, and 26 mm in the adult female. Contrary to traditional teaching, the diameter of the trachea relates to height regardless of sex (**Fig. 28.4**), both in children and adults.[9]

The trachea is a tube that spans between the lower border of the cricoid cartilage of the larynx, at the level of the sixth cervical vertebra, and the carina at the level

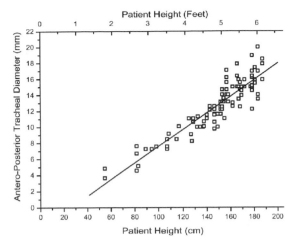

Figure 28.4 Graph showing relationship between height and tracheal diameter (*adapted from* reference 9).

of the sternal angle. At the carina, the trachea divides to give rise to the right and left main bronchi. In the adult, the trachea varies between 10 and 13 cm in length and in the adult is composed of approximately 20 c-shaped cartilaginous rings that are connected by fibrous bands and covered by respiratory mucosa. Posteriorly, the tracheal wall is composed of a flat fibromuscular structure that spans between the arms of the C and contains the unpaired trachealis muscle.[10] The trachealis constricts the trachea during a cough allowing the high velocity passage of air during a cough.

Surgery and Anesthesia for Patients with Airway Compromise

Endoscopic airway assessment is performed by respiratory physicians, thoracic surgeons, and otolaryngologists. Pulmonologists and thoracic surgeons are trained to use both flexible and rigid bronchoscopes. Flexible bronchoscopy is usually performed in the spontaneous breathing and sedated patient who has had topical anesthetic applied to the upper aerodigestive tract. This technique allows assessment of the dynamic airway, the trachea, and bronchi with the ability to perform the full spectrum of interventions. However, with a flexible bronchoscope placed through a narrow stenosis, the patient's airway becomes obstructed. Similarly, attempted dilatation of an airway stenosis leads to temporary airway obstruction. The rigid ventilating bronchoscope (**Fig. 28.5**) requires the patient to be paralyzed and ventilated by a face mask or endotracheal tube until the bronchoscope is inserted. For assessment of the airway beyond an area of stenosis, the bronchoscope has to be forced through the stenosis. This has the effect of dilating the stenosis, but it also causes stripping of the mucosa in a longitudinal fashion.

Neither flexible bronchoscopy nor rigid bronchoscopy allows prolonged access or endoscopic surgery on the larynx or subglottis.

Suspension laryngoscopy is performed routinely by otolaryngologists for access to the supraglottic and glottic larynx. Laryngologists are also comfortable operating on the subglottis via the microscope or rigid endoscopes. The advantages of the microscope are binocular vision, depth of field, and superior axial illumination and it also allows two hands free for instrumentation. Also, the laser can be used with a "line-of-sight" technique through a micromanipulator attached to the microscope. Many otolaryngologists still use the ventilating bronchoscope for tracheal or bronchial assessment and surgery. Suspension laryngoscopy allows the use of both optical rigid endoscopes and flexible bronchoscopes to access the airway. The advantages are that the patient is paralyzed and the full spectrum of rigid instrumentation, dilators, lasers, and stents can be inserted and used with relative ease. As the patient is ventilated using a supraglottic jetting technique, lasers can also be used without the risk of airway fires (**Fig. 28.6**).

Pediatric airway surgery performed by an otolaryngologist differs in that the child is usually breathing spontaneously and oxygen or a combination of oxygen and an anesthetic gas is delivered by a nasotracheal tube withdrawn into the hypopharynx. Endoscopes and instrumentation can then be passed through the glottis to access the trachea and bronchi. This type of prolonged spontaneous breathing technique is not possible in an adult patient. Adults tend to lighten from anesthesia much quicker with the associated risk of laryngospasm. Also, access to the larynx in an adult is much easier in a paralyzed patient.

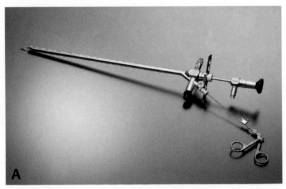
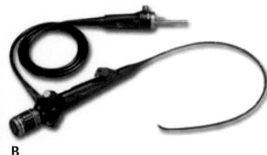

Figure 28.5 (A) A rigid ventilating bronchoscope and (B) a flexible bronchoscope.

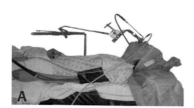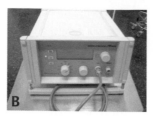

Figure 28.6   (A) Suspension laryngoscopy and (B) mistral (Acutronic, Switzerland) automated high-frequency jet ventilator.

The senior author (G.S.S.) prefers a technique of suspension laryngoscopy and supraglottic jet ventilation via a cannula attached to the laryngoscope (**Fig. 28.6**). **Fig. 28.7** demonstrates the differing views of the glottis in the same patient having supraglottic jet ventilation, subglottic jet ventilation, and a microlaryngoscopy endotracheal ventilating tube.

The jetting is delivered at high frequency (up to 100 jets per minute) using an automated device called Mistral (Acutronic, Switzerland). This device has built-in safety that sets an alarm if either the delivery of the jet or the return of gas is obstructed in the airway. No incidence of a pneumothorax has been reported when using this device in adult patients in our department over the past 10 years. This amounts to nearly 10,000 procedures. Pneumothorax has been reported when using jet ventilation delivered by a "manual jet" 'Sanders type' device.[11] This is probably related to the fact that the delivery of the anesthetic agents is less well controlled and there is no safety cut-out mechanism.

Tracheobronchial Stenting

Charles Thomas Stent was a British dentist in the late 19th century. He developed dental impression material that was used as a template to support skin grafts for repair of oral trauma. Initially the term "stent" was used to describe artificial structures for preserving the viability and function of tissue. Today, the term is used to describe devices for maintaining the patency of tubular structures, including the tracheobronchial tree. Early experience of stents was gained through their use in the biliary tree, esophagus, urinary tract, and blood vessels. There has also been a proliferation of devices for airway stenting. There are currently a variety of silicone and expandable metal stents. The metal stents can be uncovered, covered, or partially covered (hybrid).

Wire stents tend to be covered with polyurethane, although Teflon sheeting is used in some designs. The next generation of stents will be reabsorbable or bioengineered in other ways, negating the need for subsequent removal.

In benign and malignant disease, stents have been used to palliate the effects of large airway obstruction caused by extrinsic compression, endoluminal disease, or loss of cartilaginous support. Indications in benign disease include long length stenoses, failed previous repair, patient comorbidities that restrict reconstructive surgery, or patient preference. Stents are also used temporarily following airway surgery.

The first airway stent was a metal alloy stent described by William Hankins of St Louis, United States, in 1952.[12] However, there were problems related to repeated obstruction and migration of this stent, which led to the development of the silicone T-tube, first used by Montgomery in the 1960s.[13] The T limb prevented migration of the endoluminal tube. In 1982, Westaby et al described their modification of this silicone stent, which included a bifurcation at the lower end, allowing stenting of the trachea and both bronchi.[14] In the 1990s, Dumon produced the first dedicated endobronchial silicone stent.[15] Current metal stents tend to be made from steel or nitinol (a titanium and nickel alloy with a memory) wire mesh. The Gianturco metal stent is an uncovered stainless steel mesh stent and was first described in 1986.[16]

Although patients with metal stents enjoy immediate palliation of symptomatic tracheal stenosis, metal stents are associated with a high incidence of obstruction with granulation.[17] They are also susceptible to metal fatigue and fracture over time. Based on personal experience and a review of the literature,[18] the authors recommend that uncovered or hybrid metal stents should only be used in a select group of patients with a short life expectancy. If not removed within the first few weeks of deployment, they become a permanent fixture in the airway (**Fig. 28.8**).

Silicone stents also have complication rates, ranging from 21.5%[19] to 42%.[20] There is a high incidence of bacterial colonization of all stents, which can lead to granular tissue formation,[21,22] the most common organisms being *Staphylococcus aureus* and *Pseudomonas aeruginosa* in most series. The difficulty in culturing the airway and stents by conventional flexible or rigid bronchoscopy is that the passage of these devices introduces contamination from oral and pharyngeal secretions. Our study was unique in that we

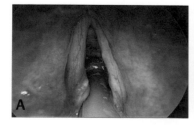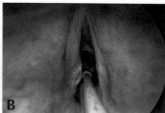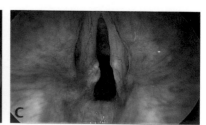

Figure 28.7   Picture demonstrates the improving access to the posterior glottis and subglottis when ventilating with a (A) microlaryngoscopy endotracheal tube, (B) subglottic jetting catheter, and (C) supraglottic jetting.

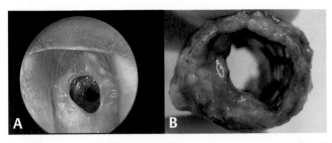

Figure 28.8 A partially uncovered (hybrid) wire stent inserted in the airway to deal with a benign postintubation stenosis has caused worse damage to the airway (A) and had to be removed via laryngotracheal fissure and sharp dissection (B).

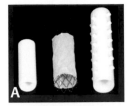
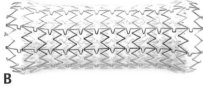

Figure 28.10 Various tracheal stents. Cut length of silastic T-tube (A left), partially covered wire stent (A middle), Dumon (Novatech, Cedex, France) silastic stent (A right), Aero expanding wire (Merit, Utah, USA) stent[23] covered with polyurethane (B).

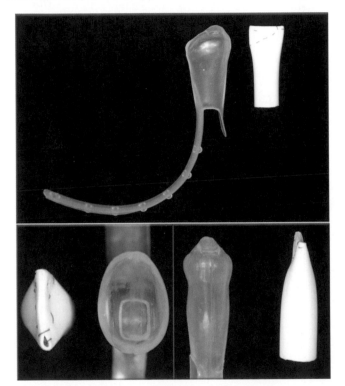

Figure 28.9 Two types of laryngeal stents. These have to be closed superiorly to prevent aspiration. Eliachar (Hood Laboratories, Pembroke, MA, USA) stent and over-sewn silastic T-tube (white).[3]

used suspension laryngoscopy and an apneic technique for "clean" removal of the stent before starting supraglottic jet ventilation[21] in a paralyzed patient.

The senior author (G.S.S.) has more than 12 years of experience of using tracheobronchial stents of all designs. It is widely accepted that wire stents have a higher incidence of granulation formation, especially at their ends. Some authors report that silicone stents have a higher incidence of mucus plugging than wire stents (**Fig. 28.9**).[17] However, this experience largely relates to the use of stents in the bronchi. In the upper trachea, bio fouling and mucus plugging are much greater in wire stents than in silicone stents. This may be due to the relative lower humidity in this area. The incidence of stent migration is widely reported as being higher in the subglottis than in the remainder of the tracheobronchial tree. The reason for this appears to be due to the fact that the

subglottis is a fixed structure, which is narrower than the trachea, especially with the expansion allowed by trachealis. Hence, there is a natural tendency for stents to be pushed down. Stents placed high into the subglottis also run the risk of damaging the vocal folds and causing granulation in this area. There is very little data on migration rates of different tracheobronchial stents. Our unit has, for over 15 years, been using the vertical limb of a silicone T-tube as a stent (**Fig. 28.10**, A left). Different diameters of T-tubes are available and can be cut to a suitable length and are placed in the airway under general anesthesia and suspension laryngoscopy. The stent is held in place with a suture through the tissues of the neck (**Fig. 28.11**), which is buried under the skin.[24]

In our series, migration of this type of stent, following failure of the suture, occurred in 2:200 cases (1%) without detriment to the patient. This review included patients in whom the stent was left in for more than a year. This is the lowest migration rate of any endoluminal stenting device. The added advantage of using this stenting technique is that it is not reliant for its fixation on firm adherence to the tracheal wall. As a result, ciliary action continues to take place between the stent and the tracheal wall. This limits the degree of mucus plugging.

Insertion of Tracheobronchial Stents

Silicone stents usually have to be placed under general anesthesia, using a ventilating rigid bronchoscope. The team uses a technique of suspension laryngoscopy with supraglottic jet ventilation and placement of a silicone stent with rigid stent forceps. Visualization is assisted by a 0-degree, 30-cm Hopkins optical endoscope, which is 4 mm in diameter or a flexible bronchoscope. Wire stents come preloaded in delivery devices and can be passed parallel to a flexible bronchoscope in a spontaneously breathing, sedated patient, or using fluoroscopic screening techniques. Wire stents can also be inserted under general anesthesia. Stent removal is easiest using a general anesthetic technique. This allows the use of rigid biopsy or grasping forceps to firmly grip the stent even if embedded in granulation. Uncovered wire stents that have been in place more than 3 months will usually require an open surgical approach for removal.[17]

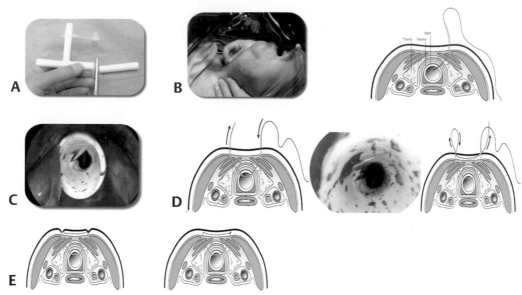

Figure 28.11   Securing an endoluminal silastic stent.[24] The stent is cut from a length of silastic T-tube (A) positioned in the airway using suspension laryngoscopy (B). A monofilament suture with a large needle is used to secure the stent as shown (C, D). The ends bury themselves within a few days (E). For stent removal, the suture is divided endoscopically and removed through a small incision in the neck.

Postoperative Care of Tracheobronchial Stents

All patients with stents are prescribed saline nebulizers daily. Carbocysteine can be added in those patients in whom there is evidence of mucus plugging. There is no research evidence to support the use of any of these measures.

Etiology of Adult Postintubation Laryngotracheal Stenosis

In 1950, anesthesiologist, Peter Safar, established the concept of "advanced support of life," keeping patients sedated and ventilated in an intensive care environment. During the polio epidemic in Copenhagen, Denmark, in 1952 (where paralyzed patients had to be ventilated for prolonged period), Bjorn Ibsen set up the first Intensive Care Unit (ICU).[25] This led to an ever widening use of mechanical ventilation to treat respiratory failure. These iatrogenic lesions provided a whole new field of endeavor for surgeons. In the 1960s, scores of papers appeared in Europe and North America, describing surgical resection of postintubation strictures. Prevention of postintubation injury quickly became a priority once the origin of these lesions was evident. Initially, high-pressure cuffs were used and risked ischemic injury to the mucosa and necrosis of the cartilage of the trachea. Carroll et al in 1969 recommended a cuff with a large volume and low pressure, which only resulted in small increases in tracheal wall pressure with overinflation.[26] Although the incidence of postintubation airway stenosis in post-ICU patients is unknown and can only be approximated between 1 and 4%,[27–30] a significant early injury is evident in 47% of patients.[31] This is despite the use of these high-volume, low-pressure cuffs on endotracheal and tracheostomy tubes (**Fig. 28.12**). This is the only paper in the literature where

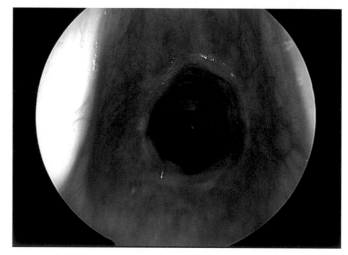

Figure 28.12   Demonstration of an early postintubation airway stenosis.

the trachea has been examined at the time of endotracheal tube removal. Unfortunately, it does not make the definition of "significant injury" clear.

The anatomical and pathological differences between stomal and cuff stenoses and other postintubation injuries were described at this time by Pearson et al and Grillo. They also stressed the importance of allowing florid inflammation to subside before the surgical correction.[32–35] They demonstrated that surgical resection and anastomosis produced better results than repeated dilatation, steroid injection, or cryotherapy. The results of treating postintubation stenosis with resection by the same authors achieved an 87.5% "cure" in 200 patients in 1992. The definition of "cure" appears to include patients with a suboptimal airway. Couraud et al reported a 96% success rate in 217 patients in 1994, and Grillo et al cited a 94% success in

503 patients in 1995.[4,36,37] They also described the correction of postintubation stenosis involving the subglottic area as being more difficult than lesions of the trachea. The etiology of postintubation stenosis injuries was initially unclear. At first it was thought to be due to irritation from the materials from which tubes and cuffs were made.[38] Later it became clear that pressure necrosis from tubes and cuffs leading to circumferential injury and contracture was the principal explanation.[39]

The risk factors for laryngotracheal stenosis following a period of ventilation on the ICU include sizing of endotracheal tubes, excessive lateral cuff pressure due to poor cuff pressure monitoring, hypotension, local infection, duration of intubation, use of steroids and other causes of reduced patient immunity, patient movement and agitation, tracheostomies, and bilateral injuries of posterior vocal cords. The majority of patients ventilated on ICUs do not appear to develop airway stenosis. Although there are many etiological factors, patients who tend to scar excessively following injury may self-select for airway stenosis; however, there is no clinical study to support this.

With respect to endotracheal tubes, modern tubes are of a high volume and low pressure, design to reduce the risk of airway injury. To prevent ischemic damage, the cuff should not exceed a pressure greater than the capillary perfusion pressure of the mucosa. The mean capillary blood pressure is approximately 20 mm Hg. This is 27.2 cm H_2O pressure.[40] The recommendation is that the cuff inflation pressure, of a ventilation tube, should not exceed 30 cm. Seegobin and van Hasselt[41] studied four types of large-volume, low-pressure cuff types. Following periods of endotracheal intubation, photographs were taken of the circumferential trachea at the site of cuff contact. Photographs were taken for varied cuff pressures after a period of 15 minutes. The conclusion of the study was that lateral wall pressures above 30 cm of water compromise mucosal capillary blood flow leading to pressure necrosis of the adjacent mucosa and eventually the cartilage.

The other risk factors for laryngotracheal injury in a ventilated patient on the ICU probably include gastric reflux, infection, coexisting health problems (such as diabetes mellitus and arteriopathy), and altered immunity as part of the stress response. There is, however, no research to support these as potential risk factors.

Posttracheostomy stenosis had been described as early as 1886 when Colles found four strictures in 57 patients treated for diphtheria.[42] In the senior author's (G.S.S.) series of 400 adult patients with benign laryngotracheal stenosis, the incidence of airway stenosis from endotracheal tubes was approximately the same as the incidence from tracheostomies. Damage to vocal fold anatomy and impairment of vocal cord mobility are more common with endotracheal tubes.[43,44] Surgical management of bilateral vocal fold immobility is always a compromise between voice and airway. There is very little evidence supporting early tracheostomy on ICUs.[45] The TracMan study was a multicenter UK study designed to look at the timing, morbidity, and mortality associated with tracheostomies on ICUs. Although the trial phase of this multicenter study took place in 2004, the main phase of the study failed to progress. Although this thesis cannot comment on the morbidity and mortality associated with early versus late tracheostomy, following review of the 400 patients in the database, some conclusions can be reached. There is a real risk of damage to the normal function of the glottis and vocal folds, which exists with endotracheal intubation that does not occur in patients with a tracheostomy. As the surgical results of restoration of impaired glottic function remain suboptimal, early tracheostomy would minimize the risk of glottis stenosis and bilateral vocal fold mobility impairment.

Surgery for Laryngotracheal Stenosis

The Rig Veda noted that the trachea could reunite "when the cervical cartilages are cut across, provided they are not entirely severed." This description dates from circa 2000 BC. The earliest description of surgery for laryngotracheal stenosis was provided by L. von Schroetter in Vienna, Austria, in 1871. He described two techniques. The first involved the use of metal "olives" after placement of a tracheostomy. The second procedure was dilatation of the airway with hard rubber bougies delivered through the mouth.[46,47] In 1885, O'Dwyer in New York[48] described similar techniques of dilatation that became used widely in the United States. Gluck and Zeller in 1881 demonstrated healing after end-to-end tracheal anastomosis in dogs and believed that the technique could be applied in man.[49] Primary anastomosis of the trachea after limited resection for posttraumatic stenosis was performed in man by Kuster in 1886.[50] Nowakowski in 1909[51] described complex methods of repair of cervical tracheal defects and through cadaver studies placed the limit of tracheal resection at 3 to 4 cm. This was following cadaveric studies. It was many years later before Conley successfully resected the second and third tracheal rings for scar in 1953 with primary end-to-end anastomosis.[52] In 1968, Grillo and Mulliken[53] reported the length of trachea that could be resected for postintubation stenosis at 4.5 cm (~7.2 rings). He discovered that the length that could be resected in older patients was progressively shorter because of the reduced elasticity between the cartilaginous rings. He further demonstrated that it would be possible, with additional maneuvers involving release of pulmonary ligaments and suprahyoid laryngeal release, to resect a further 2 cm.[53]

Open approaches for the treatment of subglottic stenosis can be traced as far back as the late 1800s and early 1900s. Killian in Germany described an operation referred to as "laryngotracheostomy."[47] A vertical skin incision and a median vertical fissure of the larynx and trachea were created. A fistula was maintained and progressively larger, soft rubber tubes were inserted through the tracheostomy site. There is also a description in the German literature in 1896[54] describing the use of rib cartilage graft in a two-stage procedure to close an open tracheal wound. These original papers were essentially case reports but modifications of these techniques are still used in modern airway surgery.[55]

In 1927, M. F. Arbuckle[27] in St Louis described his experience with three children who had been treated unsuccessfully with repeated intubations after a diphtheria throat infection. The larynx and subglottis were exposed after a median vertical incision through the skin and the airway. Arbuckle excised all visible scar tissue and placed a skin graft over the denuded area within the lumen of the airway. The graft was held in place with a rubber balloon attached inferiorly to a string that was brought out through the tracheotomy. He also described a similar technique with a balloon that was held by a stay suture from the outside, transfixing the larynx, graft, and balloon. In each case, the balloon was removed after 8 days.

Schmiegelow[56] from Copenhagen described, in 1927, a surgical technique which he said he had been using since 1910. Via a laryngotracheal fissure, he entirely removed any structures or scar tissue encroaching on the lumen such that it appeared normal in size. He then placed a rubber drain slightly wider than the lumen, fixed into position using silver wire through the soft tissues and skin of the neck. This "stent" was left in place for several weeks or months.

Before the 1930s, the majority of stenoses of the airway resulted from infections and inflammatory processes. Often this was exacerbated by iatrogenic injuries from surgery. In 1921, Chevalier Jackson[57] from Philadelphia, PA, United States, cautioned against the placement of a "high tracheotomy," which he described as on or near the cricoid cartilage. LeJeune and Owens[58] from New Orleans, LA, United States, noted in 1935 that 90% of their cases of laryngotracheal stenosis were caused by disease or trauma. They advocated complete dissection of all scar, granulation, cartilage, and osseous tissues via laryngofissure and application of a skin graft over a stent—their argument being that primary tissue healing where there is skin approximation produces less scar tissue than healing by secondary intention. Jackson in his article of 1936[46] stated that all cases of congenital or acquired stenosis of the larynx were curable. He also stated that the wearing of a canula (tracheotomy) would dominate the entire life of a person and create an inferiority complex. Jackson favored the placement of elastic rubber core molds that changed weekly and slowly increasing in size. These rubber stents were placed above the tracheotomy. Jackson admonished the cutting of the cricoid cartilage even in laryngeal atresia as "it is the only complete ring in the airway." Some of the principles described by Jackson are part of modern laryngology teaching.

In 1938, Edward Looper from Baltimore, Maryland, United States, described the use of the hyoid bone as an autologous material for grafting in airway reconstruction. He described it as being advantageous over the use of rib or ear cartilage.[59] This is the first reference to cartilaginous graft tissue for airway reconstruction. In addition to performing the first tracheal resection in 1953, John Conley of New York[52] summarized several techniques for treatment of subglottic stenosis. He performed a laryngofissure,

removed all scar tissue, and placed a split skin graft, over a petroleum jelly gauze, over a foam rubber sponge. He also mentioned that autologous cartilage could be used to assist in reconstructing the tubular form of the trachea. He did not discuss specific cases, but the ideas are in use in pediatric airway reconstruction today.[60]

In 1971, Grahne of Helsinki[61] continued to completely remove scar tissue, but described a hole placed through an Aboulker stent to accommodate a metal tracheostomy tube. This stent was left in place for 4 months. By the 1970s, the principal cause of airway stenosis was no longer infectious diseases, high tracheostomies, or surgical dilatations. The principal cause then was a period of prolonged ventilation using an endotracheal tube. In 1972, Fearon and Cotton in Toronto[62] published an experimental procedure where thyroid cartilage was used to augment an anteriorly split thyroid cartilage in a monkey. They also demonstrated that there was no inhibition of laryngeal growth following this. In 1974, Evans and Todd in London[63] reported the use of rib cartilage in laryngotracheoplasty, but favored a castellated laryngofissure to expand the airway over a piece of rolled silastic sheet used as a stent for 6 weeks. Cotton in Cincinnati (Ohio, United States) in 1978[55] described in detail laryngotracheal reconstruction (LTR) with an anterior costal cartilage graft. Later, in 1984, Cotton[64] published a series of 100 cases of LTR in children over a decade. He emphasized that the stenosis should be mature before undertaking open surgery. In 1985, Fearon and McMillin in Toronto, Ontario, Canada,[65] described cricoid resection and thyrotracheal anastomosis in primates. They demonstrated that there was no interference with normal laryngeal growth following this. Ranne et al in Kansas City (MO, United States) are credited with the first cricoid resection in patients,[66] published in 1991. This procedure, originally described by Pearson et al,[67] was adopted by Monnier et al in Switzerland, who subsequently published their series in 1993.[68] Robin Cotton's group in Cincinnati, when considering an open procedure for subglottic stenosis, primarily perform anterior and posterior augmentations. In only 15% of cases, usually those that have failed augmentation surgery, do they consider cricotracheal resection.

One other technique, originally described by Herberhold et al,[69] was the use of preserved tracheal allografts. These held the promise of being able to treat long-segment tracheal stenosis in children and adults without the need for immunosuppression. These grafts consisted of chemically treated cadaveric tracheas to remove donor cells and antigenicity. The simplicity of the technique was the ability to tailor the size and shape of the tissue to suit the patient's requirements. However, like other teams[70,71] our unit discovered that, following an intense inflammatory response lasting several weeks, these grafted tracheas were replaced in time by host scar tissue. When the technique worked, it appeared to do so if the scar tissue retained the size and shape of the original graft. Publications by Herberhold et al did not give detailed follow-up data to allow full appreciation of the long-term results.

Resection of the damaged airway had become the "gold standard" for treating laryngotracheal stenosis in adults at the start of this research. Grillo[59] had the largest experience of this technique in adult patients and most other publications were case series. He achieved "successful" outcomes in the majority of his patients; however, the possibility of bias based on patient selection cannot be ruled out. These results are all the more difficult to interpret as there were no standardized and validated outcome measures in widespread use. As Abraham Maslow,[72] a psychologist, wrote in 1966, "it is tempting, if the only tool you have is a hammer, to treat everything as if it were a nail."

Endoscopic Approach to Postintubation Subglottic and Tracheal Stenosis

In clinical practice, the majority of patients with postintubation upper airway stenosis have mature fibrotic airway scars with minimal evidence of ongoing airway inflammation. These patients typically have had an intubation episode in the relatively distant past and some of them have been treated for "adult onset asthma" for some time before the diagnosis is secured. Less commonly, patients are referred within a few weeks of extubation with airway symptoms during the active fibroinflammatory phase of tracheal injury (**Fig. 28.13**).

These two presentations occur at different times within the natural history of the same disease process. The early phase of the postintubation airway stenosis is characterized by mucosal ulceration and perichondritis followed by the formation of exophytic granulation tissue. As healing progresses, granulation tissue is gradually replaced with mature fibrotic tissue and the wound contracts giving rise to the classical picture of mature airway scar (**Fig. 28.14**). It has been shown

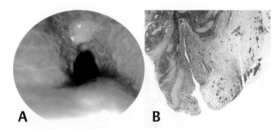

Figure 28.13 (A) Endoscopic and (B) histological views of acute airway granulation.

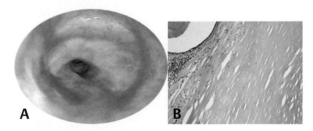

Figure 28.14 (A) Endoscopic and (B) histological view of "mature" airway scar.

that inflammatory conditions in the airway do respond to intralesional steroids.[30] Using suspension laryngoscopy and supraglottic jet ventilation, up to 3 mL of methylprednisolone acetate (40 mg/mL) can be injected into the stenosis. Radial cuts are then made into the stenosis with the carbon dioxide laser (8 to 10 W continuous) delivered through the microscope using a line-of-sight technique. The lesion is then dilated using a pulmonary balloon dilator to the size of the adjacent normal airway. With more mature and fibrotic lesions, intralesional steroids are of limited value. In these cases, radial cuts into the lesion are followed by balloon dilatation and topical mitomycin-C application may be considered. Endoscopic surgery is repeated every 3 to 4 weeks. Patients whose lesions prove recalcitrant to endoscopic therapy, and this usually became evident by the third procedure, should be treated with open laryngotracheal reconstruction or tracheal resection techniques. Also, where there is collapse and damage to the laryngotracheal cartilaginous structure, open surgical techniques should be considered, as endoscopic techniques are likely to fail. **Fig. 28.15** shows the overall success rate of the endoscopic approach to airway stenosis ($n = 62$) of 72%. Patients with a body mass index of greater than 45 failed endoscopic airway surgery.[73]

Endoscopic Tracheoplasty for Treating Tracheostomy-Related Airway Stenosis

A less common variant of postventilation tracheal stenosis is seen in a small number of tracheostomy patients. This is

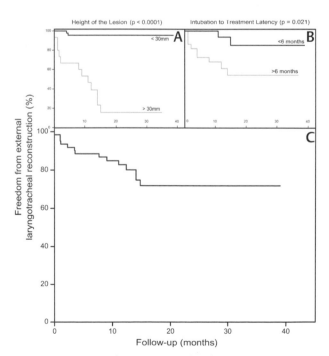

Figure 28.15 Actuarial success rate of endoscopic surgery to treat postintubation tracheal stenosis (log-rank analysis). (A) Likelihood of endoscopic success as a function of the height of lesion. (B) Likelihood of success as a function of time from intubation to first treatment. (C) Overall success rate of endoscopic surgery.[73]

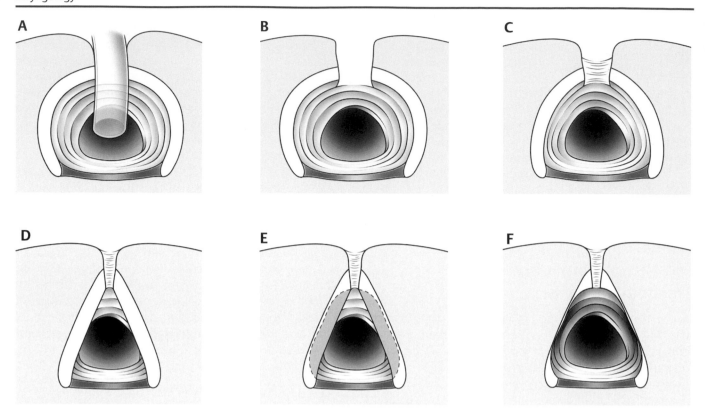

Figure 28.16 Formation of "lambdoid" deformity (A) of trachea. On decannulation, excessive scar contracture at the stoma draws in remnant tracheal cartilage rings (B–D). These encroaching cartilage rings can be ablated with a CO_2 laser (E) to produce a near normal airway (F).

caused by overresection or fracturing of anterior tracheal rings during tracheostomy. At decannulation, there is scarring and contracture at the stoma site, which draws in the lateral ring remnants as a result of the wound contracture leading to a "lambda-shaped" stenotic deformity and airway compromise. The lesion usually extends over 1 to 2 tracheal rings with normal proximal and distal trachea.[74] The trachealis is not involved and there is usually a small anterior bridge not contributing to the stenosis (**Fig. 28.16**).

Tracheal resection and anastomosis has been recommended for this condition,[59] but this is a major operation with associated morbidity and a small mortality rate.

The lesion can be treated using a CO_2 laser, delivering 8 to 10 W continuously, deployed through a micromanipulator attached to the microscope using a "line-of-sight" technique. The proximal and distal trachea is used as a guide to the limits of the resection and the collapsed cartilage is vaporized (**Fig. 28.17**). The resection can extend to the tracheal fascia if necessary. A pulmonary balloon dilator may be used to expand the airway. The mucosa over the trachealis and the apex of the Lambda must be preserved because a circumferential injury with the laser will lead to further stenosis.

The patient can be discharged home the following day with a 1-week course of a broad-spectrum antibiotic. The airway is reassessed under anesthesia at 3 to 4 weeks. Any residual cartilage or granulation, encroaching into the airway, is removed. It is unusual for a patient to require more

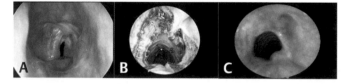

Figure 28.17. Picture demonstrates a posttracheotomy "lambdoid" deformity, (A) before, (B) immediately post-laser, and (C) 4 weeks later.

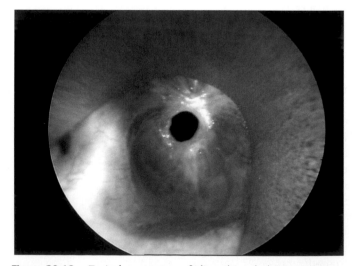

Figure 28.18. Typical appearance of idiopathic subglottic stenosis.

than three endoscopic procedures.[74] In such cases, tracheal resection should be considered.

Table 28.2   Diagnostic criteria for idiopathic subglottic stenosis

Clinical features	Serum biochemistry
<ul><li>Female patient (males very rare)</li><li>No history of laryngotracheal injury<ul><li>No endotracheal intubation or tracheotomy/no occurrence of exertional dyspnea within 2 years of intubation/tracheotomy</li><li>No thyroid/anterior neck surgery</li><li>No neck irradiation</li><li>No caustic or thermal injuries</li><li>No significant anterior neck trauma (blunt or penetrating)</li></ul></li><li>No history of autoimmunity<ul><li>Negative history for vasculitis, formally ascertained through a vasculitis-specific systemic enquiry and semiquantified using the Birmingham Vasculitis Activity Scale</li><li>No history to suggest sarcoidosis or amyloidosis</li></ul></li></ul>	<ul><li>Negative titers for:<ul><li>Angiotensin-converting enzyme</li><li>Antinuclear antibody</li><li>Rheumatoid factor</li><li>Antineutrophil cytoplasmic antibody</li></ul></li></ul> **Gross lesion morphology**<ul><li>The stenosis must include the subglottis</li></ul>**Histopathology**[a]<ul><li>Exclusion of other pathological entities (e.g., tumors, vasculitides, and amyloidosis)</li><li>Fibrosis restricted to lamina propria with normal perichondrium/cartilage</li><li>Mixture of granulation and fibrosis with a prominence of keloidal fibrosis</li></ul>

[a]This is established with a deep endoscopic biopsy at the time of first treatment.

Idiopathic Laryngotracheal Stenosis

Idiopathic subglottic stenosis (ISS) is a rare, slowly progressive, fibroinflammatory process of unknown cause, which leads to narrowing of the airway in the subglottic region and usually involves the first and second tracheal rings. This form of airway stenosis should strictly be called laryngotracheal stenosis, as it involves the proximal trachea and extends up to the glottis (**Fig. 28.18**).

It occurs predominantly in women postpuberty, but it has also been reported in males.[75–79] During the period of this research, the team have treated 50 patients with this condition. Only one of these is male. All the patients are Caucasian and of European origin. The diagnosis is one of exclusion and our criteria for making this diagnosis are included in **Table 28.2**. In each case, the antineutrophil cytoplasmic antibody (ANCA) and angiotensin-converting enzyme tests have to be repeated at intervals, as neither test is 100% sensitive. Tissue for histology is also sent at each surgical procedure (**Fig. 28.19**).

Unfortunately, seven of the women in the series were treated for asthma for many years and were finally intubated for supposed asthma that had proven refractory to medical treatment. At the point of extubation, they were then diagnosed with postintubation airway stenosis. An assumptive diagnosis of ISS was made in these patients based on the history, anatomy of the lesion, and the fact

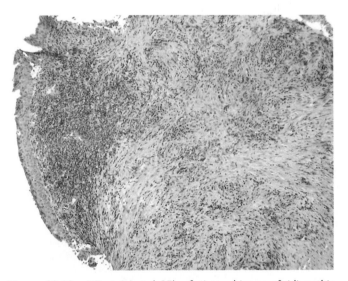

Figure 28.19. HE staining (x25) of tissue biopsy of idiopathic subglottic stenosis. Respiratory epithelium (left) with stroma consisting of acute and chronic inflammation (polymorphs, histiocytes, and plasma cells) and fibrosis.

that tests for other causes of airway stenosis had proven negative. In addition, these patients were ventilated for very short periods, making the diagnosis of postintubation laryngotracheal stenosis unlikely. Each of the 50 patients in this series has had histological tissue sent for analysis (**Fig. 28.19**) and the majority of patients have had this tissue tested for estrogen and progesterone markers. All have proven negative. Although Valdezand Shapshay[77] proposes a link with estrogen, his group did not isolate estrogen receptors in the tissue that they analyzed. Most series[75–79] describe an initial assessment of the airway stenosis under anesthesia with management using some form of dilatation.

Other groups have undertaken endoscopic procedures using local mucosal flaps,[80] while others have explored the use of mitomycin-C[77] and steroid injections. None of these have proven therapeutic benefits. Care must, however, be taken because patients with ISS have a highly reactive airway and injudicious attempts at endoscopic laser photo resection of the stenosis, pushing rigid bronchoscopes through, or stenting will almost invariably produce aggressive scar formation that can wholly close up the airway (**Fig. 28.20**). Similarly, long-term tracheostomy is not a solution, as the airway above the tracheostomy will scar and close down and cause aphonia. The reason for the hyperreactivity of the airway in these patients is unknown. The disease does not affect or infiltrate the adjacent cartilaginous framework of the airway.[81] Embryologically, there does not appear to be any developmental significance to this anatomical site, although it is an area of intense immune activity. **Table 28.3** illustrates all the published case series that included more than 15 patients compared with our figures.

The approach varies from cricotracheal resection to repeated endoscopic procedures. The majority of our patients have elective endoscopic airway surgery once or twice a year as described below. This technique can also be applied to patients presenting for the first time with this condition, to treat the associated dyspnea. Examination under anesthesia, using suspension laryngoscopy, supraglottic jet ventilation, and rigid endoscopes, allows for the dimensions of the lesion to be determined. Up to 3 mL of methylprednisolone acetate is injected into the lesion using an appropriate needle. The use of this steroid is unproven and its use is based purely on the fact that there is an inflammatory component to the lesion. Three or four radial incisions are made into the lesion using the carbon dioxide laser set at 8 to 10 W (**Fig. 28.21**). This laser is deployed through a micromanipulator attached to the operating microscope. (It does not seem appropriate to use a KTP laser to treat ISS because it causes deeper tissue

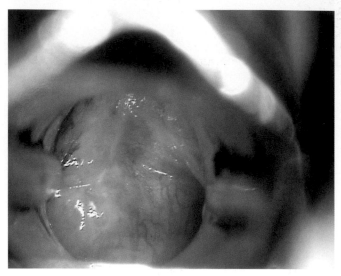

Figure 28.20 Complete stenosis of the glottis extending to the tracheostomy in a patient treated aggressively for idiopathic subglottic stenosis.

penetration and more aggressive collateral tissue injury when compared with a CO_2 laser.) Following these radial cuts, the lesion is dilated using a pulmonary balloon dilatation system and the lesion is dilated to 15 to 16 mm. A deep tissue biopsy is taken at this stage using microcup forceps and hemostasis is achieved using topical adrenaline applied with a neurosurgical patty soaked in 1:1000 adrenaline.

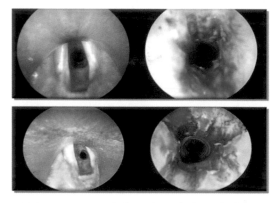

Figure 28.21 Two cases of idiopathic subglottic before treatment (left) and after steroid injection, laser, and balloon dilatation (right).

Table 28.3 Review of the reported clinical series in the literature with more than 15 patients with idiopathic subglottic stenosis

Authors	No. of patients	No. of patients treated	Period (years)	Endoscopically treated patients	No. of open-neck procedures	No. of failed open-neck procedures
Dedo and Catten[78]	52	50	30	50	7	7
Grillo et al[4,76]	65	65	31	2	65	6
Giudice et al[79]	30	30	17	30	5	5
Valdez and Shapshay[77]	16	14	12	14	2	0
Benjamin et al[75]	15	15	15	12	1	4
Sandhu et al (2011)	55	55	7	45	10	0

Grillo[76] et al published a series of 73 patients whom he had treated with cricotracheal resection. Only 65 of these patients turned out to have likely ISS. He had six failures in this series of cricotracheal resection. Dedo and Catten published a series of 52 patients,[78] 7 of whom were treated with cricotracheal resection and all failed. No other group has had a series as large as Grillo, nor have they been able to duplicate his success rate with cricotracheal resection. Our approach to open surgery differs from the orthodoxy of cricotracheal resection and anastomosis. The reason is that ISS is primarily a mucosal disease that overlies healthy perichondrium and cartilage.[81] In addition, no one has been able to duplicate the excellent cure rates reported by Grillo's group using cricotracheal resection. There is concern that cricotracheal resection in a condition that predominantly affects females is likely to leave these patients with "male-type" voices after the surgery.[82] Moreover, cricotracheal resection conceptually treats this condition as a benign neoplasm, and in our series, the disease often extends up to the glottis (**Fig. 28.22**) and it is difficult to conceive how a resection could be performed within millimeters of the vocal folds without leaving damage in this area.

With our technique, a laryngofissure with posterior cricoid split is performed. The majority of the stenosed mucosa is removed and a piece of costal cartilage is placed as a "spacer" to expand the posterior cricoid split (as for the open management of dense interarytenoid scar tissue; **Fig. 28.23**). A closed laryngeal stent, covered with a

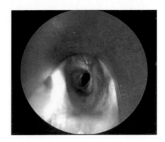

Figure 28.22 Typical appearance of idiopathic subglottic stenosis extending up to the vocal folds.

superficial skin graft (similar to **Fig. 28.24**), is held in place with a single, strong, monofilament suture. A temporary tracheostomy is required because there is no airway through the larynx once the laryngofissure is closed. Two weeks later, the stent is removed endoscopically, followed by the tracheostomy. Keratinocytes colonize the parts of the airway where the diseased mucosa was excised and inhibit restenosis. Keratosis is generally not a problem and can be managed with segmental, staged, lasering.

Bilateral Vocal Cord Mobility Impairment

Bilateral vocal fold palsy or bilateral vocal fold immobility are both terms commonly used to describe the lack of movement of both vocal folds. The terms do not, however, include cases

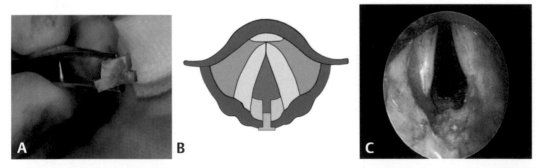

Figure 28.23 Posterior rib graft (as a "spacer") is the only solution (A) to separating thick interarytenoid scar. Case from **Figure 28.31**, following successful treatment (B). Centre illustration demonstrates position of cartilage (C).

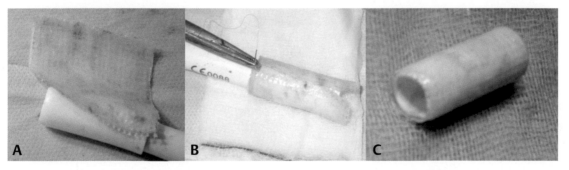

Figure 28.24 Superficial skin graft, with epidermal surface in contact with paraffin-gauze sheet (A), draped over a silastic stent and sutured in place (B). The finished composite stent is used for laryngotracheal reconstruction (C). This covered stent is associated with a reduced foreign body response and keratinocytes have fibroinhibitory properties.[83]

where there is reduced mobility rather than immobility. The term bilateral vocal cord mobility impairment (BVCMI) is more accurate and preferred, as it includes cases were there may be partial recovery or some degree of motion in at least one of the vocal folds. The analysis of the cases in the series is part of a future research project, but some of the preliminary findings are included in this thesis. It is quite clear that there are three mechanisms of injury:

1. Bilateral denervation (thyroid surgery or neck and chest malignancy)
2. Cricoarytenoid joint fixation (rheumatoid arthritis or trauma)
3. Interarytenoid scarring (postintubation)

The management of bilateral vocal fold mobility impairment remains controversial and unsatisfactory. In the authors' experience that the majority of current techniques lead to a compromise between voice, airway, and swallowing. Bilateral recurrent laryngeal nerve injuries leave the vocal folds in the paramedian position and patients suffer with significant shortness of breath and demonstrate stridor. They often end up with a tracheostomy in the acute situation. Various techniques have been described to manage this problem and these include laser to the posterior vocal fold or arytenoid and suture lateralization of the vocal folds. Various reinnervation techniques have been described, which include ansa cervicalis to recurrent laryngeal nerve, ansa to thyroarytenoid neuromuscular pedicle, and hypoglossal to recurrent laryngeal nerve as well as various muscle nerve pedicle procedures. Most of these techniques lead to synkinesis and work best with unilateral cord palsies in restoring voice.[84] More promising techniques, as yet unpublished and pioneered by Professor Jean-Paul Marie in France, involve a technique of mobilizing one division of the phrenic nerve or accessory phrenic nerve and anastomosing it to the posterior cricoarytenoid muscle. This manages to produce abduction on inspiration in the more successful cases. Other groups have looked at reanimation of the paralyzed human larynx with implantable electrical stimulation devices.[85] These techniques are, however, in very early stage clinical trials. The patients in this series have, to date, been managed by a unilateral or a bilateral laser partial arytenoidectomy as shown in **Fig. 28.25**.

The partial arytenoidectomy is performed very posteriorly into the body of the arytenoid cartilage, on the one side initially, and can be repeated in the opposite arytenoid if necessary. All patients need to be pre-assessed for baseline swallowing function. This technique has been successful in decannulating all patients with bilateral recurrent laryngeal nerve palsies and improving respiratory function in the others. However, the price paid by the patient is a breathy quality to the voice. This very posterior technique has the advantage that the whole vocal fold does not become lateralized as in techniques where the vocal process of the arytenoid is lasered or where a suture lateralization is employed. Further research needs to be undertaken in this area to compare quality of voice and improvement in respiratory function using different surgical techniques. Unfortunately, the numbers of these cases are very small and rather than being referred to specialist centers, are managed by surgeons in their individual hospitals.

The second type of injury leading to BVCMI is fixation of the cricoarytenoid joints. In this series, there were several cases where this was related to rheumatoid arthritis affecting the cricoarytenoid joints. Fixation of the cricoarytenoid joint does occur as a result of trauma leading to dislocation or subluxation of the cricoarytenoid joint. This generally occurs as a result of attempts at airway intubation, direct laryngoscopy, or blunt laryngeal trauma. The incidence of these injuries is very small[43] and described at approximately 0.1% of tracheal intubations. Bilateral subluxation and fixation as a result of trauma is even more unusual (case reports only). The management of bilateral fixed cricoarytenoid joints is similar to that of recurrent laryngeal nerve palsy in that a laser arytenoidectomy can be performed unilaterally or bilaterally depending on the symptoms. It is even more important to assess swallowing difficulties in these patients, as connective tissue disorders often lead to problems with the cervical spine and consequently impact on swallowing. **Figure 28.26** demonstrates a laser arytenoidectomy in a patient with fixation of the cricoarytenoid joints due to rheumatoid arthritis. **Figure 28.26** (center) shows degeneration material exuding out of the cricoarytenoid joint during the laser procedure.

The third cause of fixation of the arytenoids relates to interarytenoid scarring. This is mostly a postintubation finding. There were cases in this series where vocal process granulomas coalesce to form adhesions between

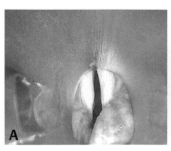
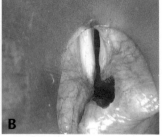

Figure 28.25 Right laser arytenoidectomy procedure for grade I BVCMI (before laser, A; and after laser, B).

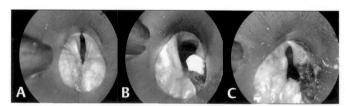

Figure 28.26 Grade II BVCMI. Right laser arytenoidectomy performed (before treatment, A); degenerative material from cricoarytenoid joint (B); after treatment (C).

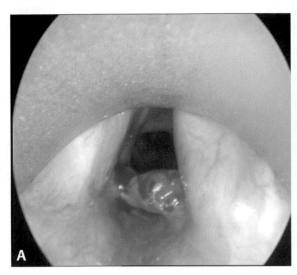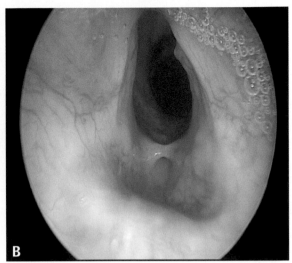

Figure 28.27 (A) Vocal granulation tissue formed as a result of endotracheal intubation coalescing. If undivided this will become a mature scar tissue (B) and lead to ankylosis of cricoarytenoid joints.

the arytenoids, but sparing the interarytenoid mucosa (**Fig. 28.27**).

In the case of **Fig. 28.27** (left), this adhesion can simply be divided and normal vocal fold function will return. If this granular injury is allowed to mature such as in **Fig. 28.27** (right), then there will be ankylosis of the cricoarytenoid joint and even division and balloon dilatation will not restore vocal fold function, and the compromise between voice and airway remains as in the cases described above. In the cases of interarytenoid scarring, distinction must be made between early granular inflammatory (**Fig. 28.28**) injury (grade III) and mature scar tissue between the arytenoids (grade IV).

Management of grade 1 and grade 2 injuries has already been described. Grade 3 injuries present early and usually demonstrate a granular inflammatory injury between the arytenoids (**Fig. 28.29**). This must be treated with steroid injection, gentle reduction of granulation tissue,

mitomycin-C topical application, and balloon expansion of the posterior glottis at 2 to 3 weekly intervals to prevent mature scar formation between the arytenoids.

It is evident that grade 3 injuries are the type least frequently seen. **Figure 28.30** shows a thin web of interarytenoid scarring, which could be treated by division with a sickle knife, balloon dilatation, and then mitomycin-C application. This procedure, if repeated at 3 to 4 weekly intervals, may produce resolution of this injury.

The majority of the mature interarytenoid scar cases are thicker and more fibrotic as demonstrated in **Fig. 28.31**, which shows an attempt at a large laser arytenoidectomy, with subsequent reformation of the scar and narrowing of the posterior glottis (**Fig. 28.31**, right).

The only technique that the senior author has (G.S.S.) been able to use successfully in managing this type of dense posterior interarytenoid scar is to perform an anterior laryngofissure and posterior cricoid split, dividing this scar and separating it with a piece of costal cartilage (**Fig. 28.23**) as a temporary spacing device. This provides separation of the posterior scar tissue so that recurrent interarytenoid scar and contracture do not recur.

In a large number of cases, this piece of cartilage is resorbed and cannot be considered as a reliable augment. Fortunately, the glottic aperture enlarges and patients can be decannulated. More research needs to be done in the area of bilateral vocal fold mobility impairment and this is a potential project for the future. Currently, all efforts must be made at prevention and it is therefore recommended that ICUs consider early tracheostomy in patients who are potentially going to be ventilated for more than 1 week. Early intervention with steroids and mitomycin-C in grade 3 lesions also needs to be promoted. The future management of grade 1 lesions probably lies in laryngeal pacing or novel reinnervation techniques. The management of grade 2 and 4 lesions will, for the time being, be an unsatisfactory compromise between voice and airway.

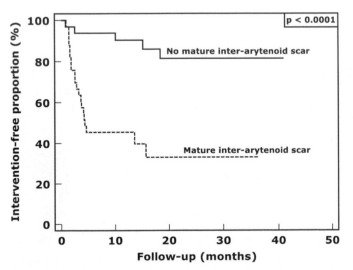

Figure 28.28 Difference in the treatment of mature interarytenoid scar versus non-mature scar (granulation).

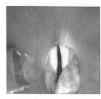

Grade I – CAJs mobile/no scar

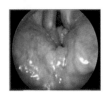

Grade II – CAJs fixed/no scar

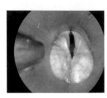

Grade III – Early granular/inflammatory injury between the arytenoids

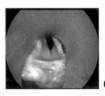

Grade IV – Mature scar between arytenoids (thin/thick)

Figure 28.29   Grading of bilateral vocal fold mobility impairment. Grade I: CAJs mobile/no scar; Grade II: CAJs fixed/no scar; Grade III: early granular/inflammatory injury between the arytenoids; Grade IV: mature scar between arytenoids (thin/thick). CAJs, cricoarytenoid joints.

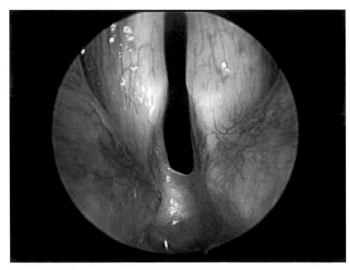

Figure 28.30   Thin interarytenoid scar.

Laryngotracheal Compromise Due to Inflammatory Diseases

Wegener's granulomatosis is a multisystem inflammatory disease with an underlying vasculitis involving small and medium size vessels. There is associated granuloma formation and necrosis (**Fig. 28.32**), and the condition classically involves the upper and lower respiratory tracts and the kidneys.

Wegener's granulomatosis is believed to have been first described in 1931 by Klinger[86] who reported a patient with destructive sinusitis, nephritis, and disseminated vasculitis. In 1936, Wegener clearly defined the disease as a distinct clinical and pathological entity.[87] A Scottish otolaryngologist, Peter McBride,[88] may in fact have been the first to describe the condition in 1897 in the *British Medical Journal* in an article entitled "Photographs of a case of rapid destruction of the nose and face."

More than 80% of patients with Wegener's granulomatosis experience rhinological morbidity and 20 to 40% experience otological morbidity at some point during their lives.[89] Seventeen to 23% of patients with Wegener's granulomatosis develop a subglottic stenosis.[90] This subglottic inflammation and narrowing does not uniformly respond to systemic immunosuppressives and may persist despite adequate disease control in other organ systems.[90] Sometimes, localized subglottic stenosis may occasionally be the only presentation of Wegener's granulomatosis. This type of focal disease may make it difficult to justify the use of systemic corticosteroids and cytotoxic drugs.

The diagnosis of Wegener's granulomatosis is often made on clinical presentation when a patient has had the

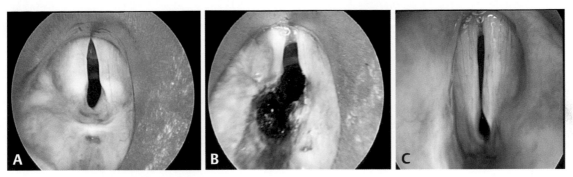

Figure 28.31   Thick interarytenoid scar (A), extended laser arytenoidectomy and scar division (B), and unfortunately the scar tissue quickly reforms (C).

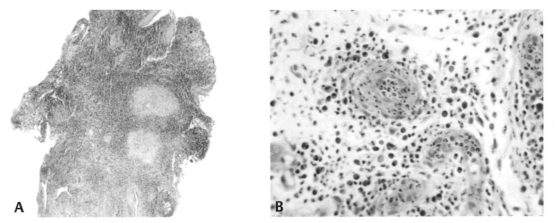

Figure 28.32   HE stain pathology slides of Wegener granulomatosis. (A), slide (x25) of respiratory mucosa showing granulomas. (B), slide (x200) showing vessels in respiratory epithelium with acute inflammatory infiltrate (vasculitis).

appropriate symptoms for a prolonged period of time. In addition to the otolaryngological manifestations already mentioned, patients usually also have involvement of the lungs and kidneys and there may be an element of renal failure.

The presence of a positive ANCA test may aid in the diagnosis, but positivity is not conclusive and negative ANCA results are not sufficient to reject the diagnosis. A definitive diagnosis of Wegener's granulomatosis can be made by a biopsy of suspicious lesions (demonstrating granulomatous inflammation) in conjunction with positive serological analysis (**Fig. 28.32**). However, it must be recognized that up to 20% of patients with untreated active Wegener granulomatosis lack cANCA[91] or may show positivity later on in the disease history.

Intralesional corticosteroid injections, radiate lesion cuts, and dilatation will treat the majority of new stenoses involving the larynx trachea, and bronchi due to Wegener's granulomatosis.[92] The use of tracheostomies and long-term stents can lead to airway complications which are difficult to treat.[4,93]

Laryngotracheal Sarcoidosis

Cesar Boeck of Christiania, Denmark, was the first to use the word "sarcoid" and describe the multisystem nature of the disease in 1899.[94,95] He mentioned the clinical similarity to a previous case described by Jonathan Hutchinson of London in 1898 as Mortimer's Malady where a female patient, Mrs. Mortimer, had generalized skin lesions and swelling of the bridge of the nose. Sarcoidosis has a world-wide distribution and can affect any race, ethnicity, gender, or age group. Typically, it is found in patients aged 20 to 40 years and has a female-to-male ratio of 2:1, and has a predilection for black African Americans.[95] Otolaryngological involvement occurs in <3% of cases and can occur in isolation as the only initial presenting symptom or can represent progression of this systemic disease.[96] Laryngeal pathology is often overlooked and many authors have suggested that if actively sought, a high incidence would be found. Laryngeal sarcoidosis thus has a variable incidence reported between 1 and 5%.[97–99]

The pathophysiology behind sarcoidosis remains obscure and numerous infectious, chemical, or occupational agents have been postulated as inducing disease. Abnormal autoimmune mechanisms are seen in sarcoidosis such as the inability to mount or maintain delayed-type hypersensitivity reactions.[100] This forms the basis for a negative tuberculin test that is characteristically seen. Current hypotheses propose sarcoidosis to occur in generally susceptible individuals through alterations in immune responses after exposure to various "triggering" agents.

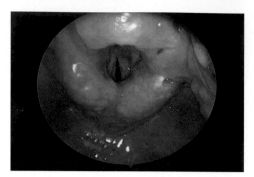

Figure 28.33 Showing diffuse swelling of the supraglottic larynx typical of sarcoidosis.

The diagnosis of sarcoidosis depends on the presence of typical clinical features and noncaseating granulomatous inflammation on biopsy of an affected organ with the exclusion of other known causes of granulomas, including tuberculosis, leprosy, syphilis, and fungal disease.

Anatomically, laryngeal sarcoid has a predilection for the supraglottic region, particularly the epiglottis, aryepiglottic folds, and arytenoids (**Fig. 28.33**).

The macroscopic appearance of the supraglottis is diffusely thick, edematous and characteristically pale or pink in color. These features are considered pathognomonic for this condition.[97] Although exophytic, polypoidal, nodular, and granulating lesions have been described, these are less common.[99] Isolated involvement of the glottis is exceedingly rare.[101] This may be explained by the paucity of lymphatics draining the glottis. Sarcoidosis is a disease of the reticuloendothelial system.[102] Decreased vocal cord mobility is a feature seen with diffuse laryngeal invasion. True vocal cord paralysis can also occur as a result of perineural invasion or multiple cranial nerve polyneuritis.[97] Laryngeal disease tends to progress slowly with a relapsing and remitting course. The disease may ultimately "burn out" in later stages. Symptoms are recognized when granulomatous lesions are present; however, they may persist despite remission, due to subsequent fibrosis.

Traditionally, high-dose systemic steroids have been recommended as the first-line treatment of laryngeal sarcoid.[105] Surgery, such as endoscopic laser reduction, has been used as a last resort where conservative therapy has failed. Our technique for managing laryngeal sarcoidosis has led to a reduction or cessation of systemic steroids and decannulation in the majority of cases.[103]

The procedure is performed under general anesthesia using suspension laryngoscopy and a supraglottic or subglottic high frequency jet ventilation technique. The larynx and airway are visualized using a combination of microscope and a rigid endoscope.

A biopsy of the laryngeal lesion is routinely performed for histology and microbiological studies (**Fig. 28.34**). Up to 3 mL of methylprednisolone acetate, at a concentration of 40 mg/mL, is injected at multiple sites into the lesion using a standard microlaryngoscopy injection needle. The end point of injection should produce almost complete blanching

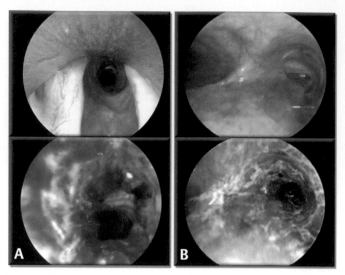

Figure 28.34 (A) Intraoperative results of treating a tracheal lesion. (B) Intraoperative results of treating a bronchial lesion. The white streaks are displaced methylprednisolone.

of the lesion. Following infiltration, the lesion is reduced using the carbon dioxide laser at a continuous setting of 8 to 10 W. Intralesional steroids help control localized disease in the medium to long term; however, immediate airway improvement is achieved through lesional volume reduction using the laser. The laser is delivered via a micromanipulator attached to the microscope. Any pedunculated lesions encroaching into the airway are excised with a small arc using the laser. It is important not to create a circumferential injury in or around the laryngeal inlet as this has the potential for stenosis through scarring. Multiple narrow pits are created with the CO_2 laser, separated by approximately 2 mm, and extending to the depth of the lesion. This "pepper pot" pattern is mucosa sparing but reduces the volume of the disease both immediately and as healing takes place by scarring and contracture (**Fig. 28.35**). Most patients require on average of two treatments (range 1 to 4) separated by 3 to 4 weeks.

Mitomycin-C

Mitomycin-C, a potent antibiotic derived from the *Streptomyces caespitosus* bacteria, can modify wound healing at the molecular level and has been used to interfere with postsurgical scar formation. Available since the 1960s as a systemic chemotherapeutic agent in the treatment of solid tumors, mitomycin-C was first applied topically for the treatment of superficial bladder tumors. Later, ophthalmologists pioneered its use in preventing scar tissue after surgery. It was first reported in the ENT literature for the treatment of tracheal scarring after tracheal reconstruction in a small case series.[104] The mechanism of the drug's anticellular action has not been definitively characterized. It is known to be a prodrug that is activated into toxic forms that produce oxygen-free radicals creating DNA strand breaks. Mitomycin-C also induces apoptosis in fibroblast cells.[105]

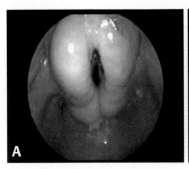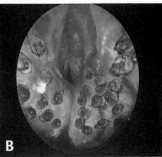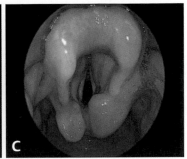

Figure 28.35 Endoscopic views of laryngeal sarcoid. (A) Preoperative and (C) 3 weeks postsurgery. (B) Perioperative view demonstrating appearance after steroid injection and "pepper-pot" laser photoreduction.

Several randomized prospective animal studies have shown impressive results in prevention of postoperative glottic and subglottic stenosis following surgery to the airway.[106–109] Its use in airway surgery has become fairly routine, despite no randomized controlled trials proving its efficacy. It is used in various concentrations and durations of application because optimum guidelines have not been firmly established. Its use in the airway in the United States is for 0.4 mg/mL concentration, although some units have used higher concentrations (0.6 mg/mL). Philippe Monnier (Lausanne, Switzerland) has used mitomycin at a concentration of 2 mg/mL applied topically for 2 minutes. At one time, it was used routinely by the authors, but no discernible difference in symptom-free intervals was apparent when comparing endoscopic surgery before mitomycin and after mitomycin. There is also concern expressed regarding the long-term consequences of having used mitomycin for benign disease.

Future of Laryngotracheal Stenosis Management

The repair of long lengths of airway defects remains a major problem for clinicians. Up to 6 cm of trachea can be resected[59] in an adult with primary anastomosis. The repair of tracheas beyond this length or where there has been failed previous resective surgery has proven difficult. Tissue engineering and tracheal allotransplantation are two techniques that are being explored and hold promise for the future. Similarly, laryngeal transplantation may be the solution to restore the airway where this organ is damaged beyond repair.

Advances in biotechnology may provide the solution to difficult problems such as long length tracheal replacement and tracheomalacia. Biocompatible and biointegratable scaffolds that mimic the mechanical properties of tracheal cartilage could be used to provide shape of muscle flaps for use as tracheal replacements. Biointegratable stents could be an even simpler solution for the management of airway stenosis.

Until these technologies are proven and widely available, prevention of laryngotracheal airway compromise is essential. This does not just mean the early recognition and treatment of associated diseases but also an understanding of the risk factors for airway injury in the ICU. This requires appropriate sizing of endotracheal and tracheostomy tubes, monitoring cuff pressures, and early change to tracheostomies in patients destined for prolonged ventilation.

References

1. Williams TA, Dobb GJ, Finn JC, Webb SA. Long-term survival from intensive care: a review. Intensive Care Med 2005;31(10):1306–1315

2. Intensive Care National Audit & Research Centre. United Kingdom; 2011; Available at: www.icnarc.org

3. Sandhu GS, Howard DJ. Acquired laryngopharyngeal stenosis. In: Rubin J, Sataloff R, Korovin G, eds. Diagnosis and treatment of Voice Disorders. 3rd ed. Abingdon, UK: Plural Publishing; 2006

4. Grillo HC, Donahue DM, Mathisen DJ, Wain JC, Wright CD. Postintubation tracheal stenosis. Treatment and results. J Thorac Cardiovasc Surg 1995;109(3):486–492, discussion 492–493

5. Schultz-Coulon HJ, Stange T, Neumann A. The risks of autogenous cartilage grafting in laryngotracheal reconstruction in adults [in German]. HNO 2011;59(1):45–54

6. Cotton RT. The problem of pediatric laryngotracheal stenosis: a clinical and experimental study on the efficacy of autogenous cartilaginous grafts placed between the vertically divided halves of the posterior lamina of the cricoid cartilage. Laryngoscope 1991; 101(12, Pt 2; Suppl 56)1–34

7. Myer CM III, O'Connor DM, Cotton RT. Proposed grading system for subglottic stenosis based on endotracheal tube sizes. Ann Otol Rhinol Laryngol 1994;103(4, Pt 1):319–323

8. Grey H. Anatomy of the Human Body. 20th ed. Philadelphia, PA: Lea & Febiger (bartleby.com); 2000

9. Griscom NT, Wohl ME. Dimensions of the growing trachea related to body height. Length, anteroposterior and transverse diameters, cross-sectional area, and volume in subjects younger than 20 years of age. Am Rev Respir Dis 1985;131(6):840–844

10. Shapshay S, Valdez T. Laser therapy for tracheobronchial lesions. In: Grillo H, ed. Surgery of the Trachea and Bronchi. Hamilton: BC Decker Inc; 2003:719–734

11. Hardy MJ, Huard C, Lundblad TC. Bilateral tension pneumothorax during jet ventilation: a case report. AANA J 2000;68(3):241–244

12. Harkins WB. An endotracheal metallic prosthesis in the treatment of stenosis of the upper trachea. Ann Otol Rhinol Laryngol 1952;61(3):663–676

13. Montgomery WW. T-tube tracheal stent. Arch Otolaryngol 1965;82:320–321

14. Westaby S, Jackson JW, Pearson FG. A bifurcated silicone rubber stent for relief of tracheobronchial obstruction. J Thorac Cardiovasc Surg 1982;83(3):414–417

15. Dumon JF. A dedicated tracheobronchial stent. Chest 1990;97(2): 328–332

16. Wallace MJ, Charnsangavej C, Ogawa K, et al. Tracheobronchial tree: expandable metallic stents used in experimental and clinical applications. Work in progress. Radiology 1986;158(2): 309–312

17. Ranu H, Madden BP. Endobronchial stenting in the management of large airway pathology. Postgrad Med J 2009;85(1010):682–687

18. de Mello-Filho FV, Antonio SM, Carrau RL. Endoscopically placed expandable metal tracheal stents for the management of complicated tracheal stenosis. Am J Otolaryngol 2003;24(1):34–40

19. Dumon J, Cavaliere S, Diaz-Jimenez J. Seven-year experience with the Dumon prosthesis. J Bronchol. 1996;3:6–10

20. Wood DE, Liu YH, Vallières E, Karmy-Jones R, Mulligan MS. Airway stenting for malignant and benign tracheobronchial stenosis. Ann Thorac Surg 2003;76(1):167–172, discussion 173–174

21. Nouraei SAR, Petrou MA, Randhawa PS, Singh A, Howard DJ, Sandhu GS. Bacterial colonization of airway stents: a promoter of granulation tissue formation following laryngotracheal reconstruction. Arch Otolaryngol Head Neck Surg 2006;132(10):1086–1090

22. Noppen M, Piérard D, Meysman M, Claes I, Vincken W. Bacterial colonization of central airways after stenting. Am J Respir Crit Care Med 1999;160(2):672–677

23. George PJ, Irving JD, Mantell BS, Rudd RM. Covered expandable metal stent for recurrent tracheal obstruction. Lancet 1990;335(8689): 582–584

24. Mace A, Sandhu G, Howard D. Securing tracheal stents: a new and simple method. J Laryngol Otol 2005;119(3):207–208

25. Szmuk P, Ezri T, Evron S, Roth Y, Katz J. A brief history of tracheostomy and tracheal intubation, from the Bronze Age to the Space Age. Intensive Care Med 2008;34(2):222–228

26. Carroll R, Hedden M, Safar P. Intratracheal cuffs: performance characteristics. Anesthesiology 1969;31(3):275–281

27. Arbuckle M. Cicatricial laryngo-trachea stenosis treated successfully by an open operation and skin graft. Trans Am Laryngol Rhinol Otol Soc 1927;33:450–452

28. Healy GB. Subglottic stenosis. Otolaryngol Clin North Am 1989;22(3):599–606

29. Lund T, Goodwin CW, McManus WF, et al. Upper airway sequelae in burn patients requiring endotracheal intubation or tracheostomy. Ann Surg 1985;201(3):374–382

30. Lorenz RR. Adult laryngotracheal stenosis: etiology and surgical management. Curr Opin Otolaryngol Head Neck Surg 2003;11(6): 467–472

31. Esteller-Moré E, Ibañez J, Matiñó E, Ademà JM, Nolla M, Quer IM. Prognostic factors in laryngotracheal injury following intubation and/or tracheotomy in ICU patients. Eur Arch Otorhinolaryngol 2005;262(11):880–883

32. Deverall PB. Tracheal stricture following tracheostomy. Thorax 1967;22(6):572–576

33. Grillo HC. The management of tracheal stenosis following assisted respiration. J Thorac Cardiovasc Surg 1969;57(1):52–71

34. Pearson FG, Goldberg M, da Silva AJ. Tracheal stenosis complicating tracheostomy with cuffed tubes. Clinical experience and observations from a prospective study. Arch Surg 1968;97(3): 380–394

35. Couraud L, Chevalier P, Bruneteau A, DuPont P. Le traitement des stenoses tracheales apres tracheotomie. Ann Chir Thorac Cardiovasc 1969;8:351–357

36. Bisson A, Bonnette P, el Kadi NB, et al. Tracheal sleeve resection for iatrogenic stenoses (subglottic laryngeal and tracheal). J Thorac Cardiovasc Surg 1992;104(4):882–887

37. Couraud L, Jougan J, Velly J, Klein C. Stenoses iatrogenes de la voie respiratoire. Evolution des indications therapentiques. Ann Chir Thorac Cardiovasc 1994;48:277–283

38. Cooper JD, Grillo HC. The evolution of tracheal injury due to ventilatory assistance through cuffed tubes: a pathologic study. Ann Surg 1969;169(3):334–348

39. Andrews MJ, Pearson FG. Incidence and pathogenesis of tracheal injury following cuffed tube tracheostomy with assisted ventilation: analysis of a two-year prospective study. Ann Surg 1971;173(2):249–263

40. Nordin U. The trachea and cuff-induced tracheal injury. An experimental study on causative factors and prevention. Acta Otolaryngol Suppl 1977;345(Suppl):1–71

41. Seegobin RD, van Hasselt GL. Endotracheal cuff pressure and tracheal mucosal blood flow: endoscopic study of effects of four large volume cuffs. Br Med J (Clin Res Ed) 1984;288(6422):965–968

42. Colles CJ. On the stenosis of the trachea after tracheotomy for croup and diphtheria. Ann Surg 1886;3(6):499–507

43. Tadié J-M, Behm E, Lecuyer L, et al. Post-intubation laryngeal injuries and extubation failure: a fiberoptic endoscopic study. Intensive Care Med 2010;36(6):991–998

44. Colton House J, Noordzij JP, Murgia B, Langmore S. Laryngeal injury from prolonged intubation: a prospective analysis of contributing factors. Laryngoscope 2011;121(3):596–600

45. Griffiths JR, Barber VS, Morgan L, Young JD. Systematic review and meta-analysis of studies of the timing of tracheostomy in adult patients undergoing artificial ventilation. BMJ 2005;330(7502):1243–1248

46. Jackson C. Stenosis of the larynx with special reference to curative with core moulds. Trans Am Laryngol Rhinol Otol Soc 1936;42:12–24

47. Winslow J. Reports of cases illustrating our progress in the surgical management of chronic stenosis of the larynx and trachea. Trans Am Laryngol Assoc 1909;31:177–190

48. O'Dwyer. New York Med Journal. 1885 Aug 8.

49. Gluck T, Zeller A. Die prophylactische resektion der trachea. Arch Klin Chir 1881;26:427–436

50. Kuster E. Uber narbige stenosen der trachea. Zentralbl Chir 1886;13:759–760

51. Nowakowski K. Beitrag zur tracheoplastik. Arch Klin Chir. 1909;90:847–861

52. Conley JJ. Reconstruction of the subglottic air passage. Ann Otol Rhinol Laryngol 1953;62(2):477–495

53. Mulliken JB, Grillo HC. The limits of tracheal resection with primary anastomosis: further anatomical studies in man. J Thorac Cardiovasc Surg 1968;55(3):418–421

54. Koenig F. Berl Klin Wochenschr 1896;51

55. Cotton R. Management of subglottic stenosis in infancy and childhood. Review of a consecutive series of cases managed by surgical reconstruction. Ann Otol Rhinol Laryngol 1978;87(5, Pt 1):649–657

56. Schmiegelow E. Stenosis of the larynx: a new method of surgical treatment. Arch Otolaryngol 1927;9(5):473–493

57. Jackson C. High Tracheotomy and other errors the chief cause of chronic laryngeal stenosis. Surg Gynecol Obstet 1921;32:392–398

58. LeJeune F, Owens N. Chronic laryngeal stenosis. Ann Otol Rhinol Laryngol 1935;44:354–363

59. Grillo H. Postintubation stenosis. In: Grillo H, ed. Surgery of the Trachea and Bronchi. Hamilton: BC Decker Inc; 2003:301–331

60. Cotton RT, Gray SD, Miller RP. Update of the Cincinnati experience in pediatric laryngotracheal reconstruction. Laryngoscope 1989;99(11):1111–1116

61. Grahne B. Operative treatment of severe chronic traumatic laryngeal stenosis in infants up to three years old. Acta Otolaryngol 1971;72(1):134–137

62. Fearon B, Cotton R. Surgical correction of subglottic stenosis of the larynx. Preliminary report of an experimental surgical technique. Ann Otol Rhinol Laryngol 1972;81(4):508–513

63. Evans JN, Todd GB. Laryngotracheoplasty. J Laryngol Otol 1974;88(7):589–597

64. Cotton RT. Pediatric laryngotracheal stenosis. J Pediatr Surg 1984;19(6):699–704

65. Fearon B, McMillin B. Cricoid resection and thyrotracheal anastomosis. Ann Otol Rhinol Laryngol 1985;94:131–133

66. Ranne R, Lindley S, Holder T, Ashcraft K, Sharp R, Amoury R. Relief of an anterior subglottic stenosis by cricoid resection: an operation for the difficult case. J Pediatr Surg 1991;26(3):255–258, discussion 258–259

67. Pearson FG, Cooper JD, Nelems JM, Van Nostrand AW. Primary tracheal anastomosis after resection of the cricoid cartilage with preservation of recurrent laryngeal nerves. J Thorac Cardiovasc Surg 1975;70(5):806–816

68. Monnier P, Savary M, Chapuis G. Partial cricoid resection with primary tracheal anastomosis for subglottic stenosis in infants and children. Laryngoscope 1993;103(11, Pt 1):1273–1283

69. Herberhold C, Stein M, Bierhoff E, Kost S. Tracheal reconstruction with preserved tracheal homograft—new aspects [in German]. Laryngorhinootologie 1999;78(1):54–56

70. Grillo HC, McKhann CF. The acceptance and evolution of dermal homografts freed of viable cells. Transplantation 1964;2:48–59

71. Jacobs JP, Elliott MJ, Haw MP, Bailey CM, Herberhold C. Pediatric tracheal homograft reconstruction: a novel approach to complex tracheal stenoses in children. J Thorac Cardiovasc Surg 1996;112(6):1549–1558, discussion 1559–1560

72. Maslow A. The Psychology of Science: A reconnaissance. New York: Harper & Row; 1966

73. Nouraei SAR, Ghufoor K, Patel A, Ferguson T, Howard DJ, Sandhu GS. Outcome of endoscopic treatment of adult postintubation tracheal stenosis. Laryngoscope 2007;117(6):1073–1079

74. Nouraei SAR, Kapoor KV, Nouraei SM, Ghufoor K, Howard DJ, Sandhu GS. Results of endoscopic tracheoplasty for treating tracheostomy-related airway stenosis. Clin Otolaryngol 2007;32(6):471–475

75. Benjamin B, Jacobson I, Eckstein R. Idiopathic subglottic stenosis: diagnosis and endoscopic laser treatment. Ann Otol Rhinol Laryngol 1997;106(9):770–774

76. Grillo HC, Mark EJ, Mathisen DJ, Wain JC. Idiopathic laryngotracheal stenosis and its management. Ann Thorac Surg 1993;56(1):80–87

77. Valdez TA, Shapshay SM. Idiopathic subglottic stenosis revisited. Ann Otol Rhinol Laryngol 2002;111(8):690–695

78. Dedo HH, Catten MD. Idiopathic progressive subglottic stenosis: findings and treatment in 52 patients. Ann Otol Rhinol Laryngol 2001;110(4):305–311

79. Giudice M, Piazza C, Foccoli P, Toninelli C, Cavaliere S, Peretti G. Idiopathic subglottic stenosis: management by endoscopic and open-neck surgery in a series of 30 patients. Eur Arch Otorhinolaryngol 2003;260(5):235–238

80. Dedo HH, Sooy CD. Endoscopic laser repair of posterior glottic, subglottic and tracheal stenosis by division or micro-trapdoor flap. Laryngoscope 1984;94(4):445–450

81. Mark EJ, Meng F, Kradin RL, Mathisen DJ, Matsubara O. Idiopathic tracheal stenosis: a clinicopathologic study of 63 cases and comparison of the pathology with chondromalacia. Am J Surg Pathol 2008;32(8):1138–1143

82. Smith ME, Roy N, Stoddard K, Barton M. How does cricotracheal resection affect the female voice? Ann Otol Rhinol Laryngol 2008;117(2):85–89

83. Garner WL. Epidermal regulation of dermal fibroblast activity. Plast Reconstr Surg 1998;102(1):135–139

84. Aynehchi BB, McCoul ED, Sundaram K. Systematic review of laryngeal reinnervation techniques. Otolaryngol Head Neck Surg 2010;143(6):749–759

85. Zealear DL, Billante CR, Courey MS, et al. Reanimation of the paralyzed human larynx with an implantable electrical stimulation device. Laryngoscope 2003;113(7):1149–1156

86. Klinger H. Grenzformen der periarteritis nodosa. Frankf Z Pathol 1931;42:455

87. Wegener F. Uber generalisierte, septische Gefasserkrankungen. Verhandlungen der Deutschen pathologischen Gessellschaft. 1936;29:202–10

88. Friedmann I. McBride and the midfacial granuloma syndrome. (The second 'McBride Lecture', Edinburgh, 1980). J Laryngol Otol 1982;96(1):1–23

89. Srouji IA, Andrews P, Edwards C, Lund VJ. Patterns of presentation and diagnosis of patients with Wegener's granulomatosis: ENT aspects. J Laryngol Otol 2007;121(7):653–658

90. Langford CA, Sneller MC, Hallahan CW, et al. Clinical features and therapeutic management of subglottic stenosis in patients with Wegener's granulomatosis. Arthritis Rheum 1996;39(10):1754–1760

91. Seo P, Stone JH. The antineutrophil cytoplasmic antibody-associated vasculitides. Am J Med 2004;117(1):39–50

92. Nouraei SAR, Obholzer R, Ind PW, et al. Results of endoscopic surgery and intralesional steroid therapy for airway compromise due to tracheobronchial Wegener's granulomatosis. Thorax 2008;63(1):49–52

93. McCaffrey TV. Management of laryngotracheal stenosis on the basis of site and severity. Otolaryngol Head Neck Surg 1993;109(3, Pt 1):468–473

94. Black JI. Sarcoidosis of the nose. Proc R Soc Med 1973;66(7):669–675

95. Newman LS, Rose CS, Maier LA. Sarcoidosis. N Engl J Med 1997;336(17):1224–1234

96. Judson MA, Baughman RP, Teirstein AS, Terrin ML, Yeager H Jr. Defining organ involvement in sarcoidosis: the ACCESS proposed instrument. ACCESS Research Group. A Case Control Etiologic Study of Sarcoidosis. Sarcoidosis Vasc Diffuse Lung Dis 1999;16(1):75–86

97. Devine KD. Sarcoidosis and sarcoidosis of the larynx. Laryngoscope 1965;75:533–569

98. Krespi YP, Mitrani M, Husain S, Meltzer CJ. Treatment of laryngeal sarcoidosis with intralesional steroid injection. Ann Otol Rhinol Laryngol 1987;96(6):713–715

99. Ellison DE, Canalis RF. Sarcoidosis of the head and neck. Clin Dermatol 1986;4(4):136–142

100. Gallivan GJ, Landis JN. Sarcoidosis of the larynx: preserving and restoring airway and professional voice. J Voice 1993;7(1):81–94

101. Yanardağ H, Enoz M, Papila I, Uygun S, Caner M, Karayel T. Upper respiratory tract involvement of sarcoidosis in the Turkish population. Otolaryngol Head Neck Surg 2006;134(5):848–851

102. Dean CM, Sataloff RT, Hawkshaw MJ, Pribikin E. Laryngeal sarcoidosis. J Voice 2002;16(2):283–288

103. Butler CR, Nouraei SAR, Mace AD, Khalil S, Sandhu SK, Sandhu GS. Endoscopic airway management of laryngeal sarcoidosis. Arch Otolaryngol Head Neck Surg 2010;136(3):251–255

104. Ward RF, April MM. Mitomycin-C in the treatment of tracheal cicatrix after tracheal reconstruction. Int J Pediatr Otorhinolaryngol 1998;44(3):221–226

105. Cable B, Pazos G, Brietzke S, et al. Topical mitomycin therapy in the paediatric airway: state of the art. Oper Tech Otolaryngol. 2002;13:57–64

106. Eliashar R, Eliachar I, Esclamado R, Gramlich T, Strome M. Can topical mitomycin prevent laryngotracheal stenosis? Laryngoscope 1999;109(10):1594–1600

107. Roediger FC, Orloff LA, Courey MS. Adult subglottic stenosis: management with laser incisions and mitomycin-C. Laryngoscope 2008;118(9):1542–1546

108. Smith ME, Elstad M. Mitomycin C and the endoscopic treatment of laryngotracheal stenosis: are two applications better than one? Laryngoscope 2009;119(2):272–283

109. Rahbar R, Valdez TA, Shapshay SM. Preliminary results of intraoperative mitomycin-C in the treatment and prevention of glottic and subglottic stenosis. J Voice 2000;14(2):282–286

29 Outcome Assessment in Laryngotracheal Stenosis

S.A. Reza Nouraei and Guri S. Sandhu

Laryngotracheal stenosis refers to abnormal narrowing of the central air passages from the supraglottic larynx to the carina and proximal main bronchi.[1] It is caused by a heterogeneous group of diseases that have in common between them the ability to impair airflow and mucociliary clearance and in a smaller number of cases, swallowing and phonation also. The most common benign cause of this condition is intubation-related airway injury, followed by Wegener granulomatosis and idiopathic subglottic stenosis.[1]

Although most cases of laryngotracheal stenosis clinically present in a similar way with exertional dyspnea and chronic stridor, the disease entities that cause these symptoms are very different. The ability to restore a prosthesis-free airway capable of meeting the ventilatory demands of the patient is therefore more determined in the long term by the natural history of the underlying disease process being treated than by the ability of an intervention to acutely improve breathing by restoring lumen dimensions. In patients with supraglottic and laryngeal stenosis, restoration of the ventilatory conduit needs also to be balanced against the risk of damaging phonatory and/or swallowing mechanisms. These factors need to be carefully considered when assessing and treating patients with this condition.

Outcome assessment is essential in determining safety and success of different treatment strategies used within and between centers. This chapter begins by discussing initial patient assessment and treatment goal setting and goes on to highlight a multidimensional paradigm for assessing outcome in laryngotracheal stenosis.

Initial Patient Assessment and Treatment Goal Setting

The aims of initial assessment are to establish or confirm the diagnosis, to identify disease-specific risk factors and prognostic variables, to set realistic treatment goals in partnership with the patient, and to establish an initial management plan (**Fig. 29.1**).

Medical History

Assessment begins by eliciting general and disease-specific symptoms (**Table 29.1**). Many patients with laryngotracheal stenosis will have been initially misdiagnosed and treated for presumed "resistant" bronchopulmonary diagnoses. It

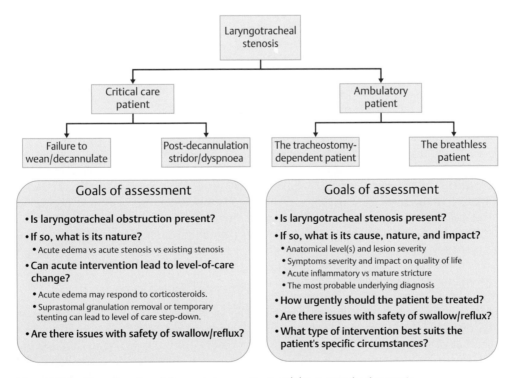

Figure 29.1 Overall approach for assessing a patient with laryngotracheal stenosis.

Table 29.1 Initial Assessment of a Patient with Suspected Laryngotracheal Stenosis

- Most common symptoms of laryngotracheal stenosis
  - Breathlessness
  - Stridor (inspiratory/expiratory/biphasic)
  - Reduced effort tolerance
  - Recurrent chest infections
  - Dysphonia
  - Dysphagia
  - Hemoptysis
  - Cough
  - Throat or chest pains
  - Difficult intubation
  - Chronic tracheostomy dependency
  - Failed extubation
  - Prolonged weaning
- Prediagnosis treatments
  - Date symptoms first noted
  - Initial diagnoses established and treatments given
- Is there a history of endotracheal intubation or tracheostomy?
  - No history of intubation
  - Only minor history of intubation for short (< 1 h) surgery)
  - Significant history of intubation (long surgery/mechanical ventilation)
- If there is a history of significant intubation, then the following additional information needs to be ascertained

Indication for intubation:	[General medical/surgical/trauma/neurological]
Date of intubation:	
Intubation setting:	[Surgery/intensive care]
Duration of intubation:	[h/d]
Agitation in ICU:	[Yes/No]
Use of vasopressors in ICU:	[Yes/No]
Multiple re-intubations:	[Yes/No]
Endotracheal tube size:	[Size]
Tracheostomy in ICU:	[No/Yes: percutaneous/Yes: surgical]
Tracheostomy tube size:	[Size and type]
Decannulation:	[Yes/No]
Decannulation date:	[Date]

d, day; h, hours.

is important therefore to try and obtain a clear time line of when symptoms were first noted as well as dates when initial diagnoses were made and treatments given.

Over half of all cases of laryngotracheal stenosis are caused by intubation-related airway injuries. Obtaining a detailed intubation history is therefore mandatory (**Table 29.1**). The second common cause of benign laryngotracheal stenosis is vasculitis-related airway stenosis, most commonly secondary to Wegener granulomatosis. Vasculitis symptoms need therefore to be specifically sought and if there is known or suspected vasculitis, then disease activity needs to be quantified. We use the Birmingham Vasculitis Activity Score (BVAS) for this purpose.[2]

Another factor which significantly impacts on treatment success is safety of swallowing, especially in supraglottic and laryngeal cases where laryngotracheal reconstruction may itself impact upon safety of swallowing, and in patients with neurological swallowing impairment where lumen restoration may lead to the development or worsening of chronic aspiration. Symptoms of chronic aspiration need therefore to be specifically sought and documented. A global assessment of patient function and ventilatory demands helps determine the most appropriate extent of reconstructive surgery.

Physical Examination

Physical examination for laryngotracheal stenosis consists of a general medical examination, an ear-nose-throat (ENT) examination, and a directed examination of the supraglottis and larynx with flexible endoscopy. Patient's weight and height also needs to be noted. A body mass index > 40 significantly reduces the likelihood of treatment success.[3]

Stridor cannot reliably be elicited through auscultation during quiet breathing. It requires the patient to forcefully inspire and expire through the mouth and the clinician to auscultate over the trachea. Flexible nasoendoscopy aims to detect any obstructive supraglottic lesions, vocal fold movements, and any evidence of impaired swallowing such as hypopharyngeal pooling of secretions. If there are any concerns regarding safety of swallow, then a video fluoroscopy should be performed. A subglottic stenosis can sometimes be viewed with a flexible nasoendoscope, but this is not a reliable tool. In our practice all patients receive an examination under general anesthesia under suspension laryngoscopy and as such we do not place great reliance on outpatient tracheobronchoscopy. Outpatients tracheobronchoscopy, provided that it is done with topical laryngotracheal anesthesia and with video recording to allow detailed examination and photodocumentation of findings, is however a valid alternative method of visualizing the laryngotracheal complex.

Evaluating the Intensive Care Patient

Within intensive care settings, a patient with obstructive laryngotracheal edema or acute or pre-existing stenosis may manifest with failure to wean or decannulate or post-extubation stridor. Many cases of extubation failure or stridor are due to acute laryngotracheal edema and are successfully managed with systemic corticosteroid therapy.[4] ENT assessment is often reserved for refractory or acutely life-threatening cases. The aim of this assessment is to distinguish between laryngeal swelling and obstructive granulation tissue formation (**Fig. 29.2**) or structural

laryngotracheal deformities to determine whether minimally invasive surgery can help with critical care step-down and the degree of urgency of such treatment[5] and whether the patient is likely to require post-discharge follow-up.

The newly developed stenosis manifesting following decannulation represents a particularly hazardous clinical scenario in that a newly developed stenosis may acutely compromise an airway that is no longer protected in a patient whose diminished physiological reserve immediately following critical illness predisposes them to rapid decompensation which may readily prove fatal. A standard flexible nasoendoscopy is not an inadequate examination, and detailed visualization of the airways from the supraglottic larynx to the carina either endoscopically or radiologically is mandatory to rule out an acute stenosis or obstructive laryngotracheal edema. A flow-volume loop examination in cooperative patients is also highly desirable in these cases.

Outcome Assessment in Laryngotracheal Stenosis

Under physiological conditions it is the performance of the cardiovascular system and not the respiratory system that limits exercise capacity. The principal objective of laryngotracheal reconstruction is therefore long-term restoration of a prosthesis-free airway whose reconstructed dimensions do not constrain the ventilatory demands of the patient while maintaining good phonation and a safe swallow. The four domains in which treatment *efficacy* can be assessed are anatomy, physiology, symptoms, and quality of life. Systematic documentation of occurrence and severity of disease or treatment-specific complications is also critical for assessing treatment efficacy (**Table 29.2**).

Treatment *durability* can be assessed by measuring the intertreatment interval, but this can only be meaningfully done for individual pathological disease processes. For example, idiopathic subglottic stenosis and Wegener granulomatosis are intrinsically recurrent disease processes. Deciding between what "treatment failure" is and what is treatment for recurrence of an intrinsically recurrent disease can therefore be difficult. By contrast, intubation-related airway stenosis is in most cases a nonrecurrent disease process that can be expected to be "cured" by surgery. Post-treatment recurrence in the intubation-related stenosis can therefore be considered a true treatment failure.

Assessment of Airway Anatomy

The most commonly used system for assessing stenosis anatomy is the Myer-Cotton grading system.[6] This system is based on the degree of cross-sectional lumen encroachment. Grade I lesions encroach in between 0 and 50% of the lumen, grade II lesions obstruct between 51 and 70% of the lumen, grade III lesions obstruct between 71 and 99%, and grade IV lesions cause total lumen obliteration. This system was initially developed for assessing the subglottis in children,

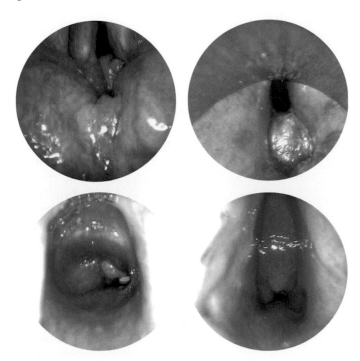

Figure 29.2 Examples of acute intubation-related obstructive airway injuries.

Table 29.2   Disease-Specific Complications in Laryngotracheal Stenosis

- Nature of complication
  - ○ Wound/stent-suture infection
  - ○ Deep neck sepsis
  - ○ Aspiration pneumonia
  - ○ Chest infection
  - ○ Major vessel injury
  - ○ Pressure sore
  - ○ Pneumothorax
  - ○ Hemothorax
  - ○ Respiratory arrest/acutely life-threatening event
  - ○ Stent fracture or migration
  - ○ Significant sudden worsening of symptoms requiring admission
  - ○ Bleeding
  - ○ Severe pain
  - ○ Unplanned admission for medical therapy (steroids, mucolytics, etc.)
  - ○ Sedation withdrawal
  - ○ Other
- Severity grading for complications
  - ○ 0: No adverse event
  - ○ 1: Mild adverse event (minor no specific intervention)
  - ○ 2: Moderate adverse event (minimal intervention)
  - ○ 3: Severe and undesirable adverse event (significant symptoms)
  - ○ 4: Life-threatening or disabling adverse event (need for intensive care or invasive procedures)
  - ○ 5: Death related to adverse event

but has since been expanded to encompass tracheal lesions in both children and adults. More recently, Freitag et al proposed a more detailed descriptive system for assessing the nature and extent of tracheobronchial stenoses (**Fig. 29.3**).[7]

In 1992, McCaffrey proposed a different system which was based on the site of involvement.[8] McCaffrey divided stenoses into four groups based on the length of the lesion and on whether or not the glottis was involved (**Fig. 29.4**). The classification was validated against actuarial time to decannulation.

In our experience the four key prognostic factors are the nature of the underlying disease process, presence of acute fibroinflammatory stenoses as opposed to mature fibrotic strictures (**Fig. 29.5**), site of the stenosis, and in particular whether the glottis is involved, and vertical height of the lesion (**Fig. 29.6**).[3,9] Details of our approach to anatomical airway assessment are provided in **Table 29.3**.

Some years ago we developed a system for quantitative endoscopy to determine the precise degree of luminal obstruction as an assessment method and an outcome measure.[10] There had been previous and subsequent efforts by other workers to achieve the same objective and in particular, the computed tomography-based "laryngotracheal profile" by Kiesler et al provides a most eloquent approach to assess airway dimensions (**Fig. 29.7**).[11–13]

We have, however, subsequently found detailed assessment of cross-sectional airway anatomy to be unnecessary and have reverted to using the Myer-Cotton

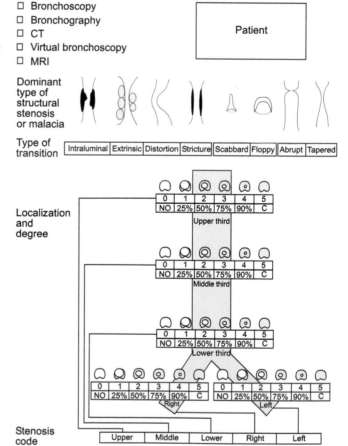

Figure 29.3   Freitag system for documentation of stenosis severity.

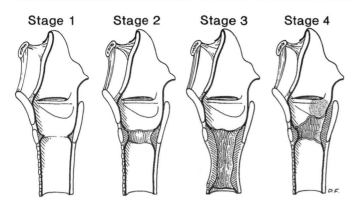

Figure 29.4 McCaffrey system of laryngotracheal stenosis classification.

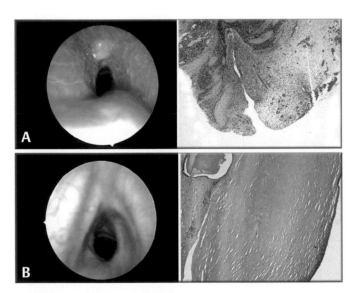

Figure 29.5 Endoscopic and histological appearances of tracheal stenosis. (A) Left panel: The "cobblestone" endoscopic appearance of acute airway granulation. Right panel: Histological appearance of acute airway granulation tissue overlying respiratory epithelium at ×250 magnification. (B) Left panel: Endoscopic appearance of a "mature" airway scar. Right panel: Histological appearance of a mature airway scar at ×250 magnification, showing hyalinized paucicellular fibrotic stroma, overlain with flattened respiratory epithelium and overlying a seromucinous gland. These appearances are characteristic of a chronic airway scar.

Source: Nouraei SA, Singh A, Patel A, Ferguson C, Howard DJ, Sandhu GS. Early endoscopic treatment of acute inflammatory airway lesions improves the outcome of postintubation airway stenosis. Laryngoscope 2006;116(8):1417–1421. Printed with permission.

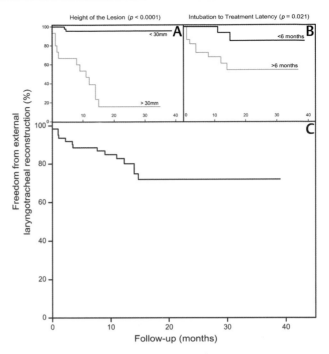

Figure 29.6 Actuarial success rate of endoscopic surgery to treat postintubation tracheal stenosis (log-rank analysis). (A) Likelihood of endoscopic success as a function of height of the lesion. (B) Likelihood of endoscopic success as a function of time from intubation to first treatment. (C) Overall success rate of endoscopic surgery.[3]

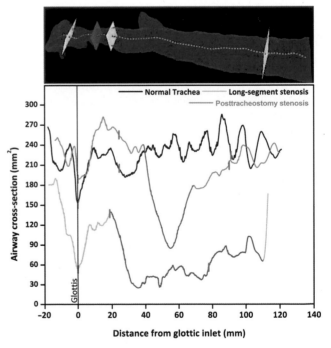

Figure 29.7 Laryngotracheal profile in one normal patient and two patients with laryngotracheal stenosis.[13]

system (**Table 29.3**). The reason for this is the nonlinear relationship between the degree of cross-sectional stenosis and symptoms. It has long been known that most patients are asymptomatic or minimally symptomatic for prolonged period but suddenly develop severe clinical symptoms and need to be operated on urgently.

The reason for the sudden switch, as opposed to linear worsening of symptoms as the stenosis grows, is the fact that pressure drop across a stenosis does not become significant in lesions of up to 70% but thereafter, flow-dependent drop in pressure becomes exponentially greater with small additional impairments in lumen diameter.[14] As such,

Table 29.3 Anatomical Assessment of Laryngotracheal Stenosis

Site of the stenosis (>1 can be present)[a]	Anatomical severity of the stenosis (subglottis, trachea, and bronchi)
• Supraglottis • Glottis • Subglottis • Trachea • Carina • Right main bronchus • Left main bronchus • Distal bronchi: unilateral • Distal bronchi: bilateral	For glottis (type of lesion causing obstruction) • Anterior web • Vocal fold mobility impairment • Complex or total laryngeal stenosis For subglottis, trachea, and carina • Distance from vocal folds to lesion (cm) • Vertical height of the lesion (cm)
Nature of impediment to airflow (supraglottis, subglottis, trachea, carina, bronchi) • Lumen stenosis: acute and granular • Lumen stenosis: mature stricture • Lumen stenosis: other/malignant • Extrinsic airway compression • Airway malacia • Traumatic airway rupture • Airway fistula • Hemoptysis • Pulmonary collapse/recurrent infections	Percentage of cross-section obstruction[a] For bronchi Percentage of the length of bronchus stenosed Percentage of cross-section obstruction
Nature of impediment to airflow (glottis) • Neurogenic: bilateral vocal fold palsy • Cricoarytenoid joint ankylosis (e.g., rheumatoid arthritis) • Interarytenoid scar: fresh granular interarytenoid scar • Interarytenoid scar: <50% of interarytenoid height • Interarytenoid scar: >50% of interarytenoid height	Anatomical severity of the stenosis (supraglottis) For supraglottis (site[s] involved) • Pharyngeal wall	• Arytenoids • False cords	• Epiglottis | • Aryepiglottic folds

[a]This value would then need to be converted into a "Myer-Cotton grade." 0–50%: Grade 1; 51–70%: Grade 2; 71–99%: Grade 3; 100%: Grade 4.

patient symptoms and flow physiology are better guides to the need to intervene than precise knowledge of lesion cross-sectional anatomy, which, in our practice, obviates the need to assess precise lumen cross-section.

Assessment of Airway Physiology

Physiological measurements are the cornerstone of noninvasive outcome assessment in laryngotracheal stenosis. The two main classes of physiological assessment are flow and effort physiology.

Flow Physiology

Basic spirometry, that is, the measurement of forced expiratory volume in 1 second (FEV1), forced vital capacity (FVC), and peak expiratory flow rate (PEFR), is the simplest way of assessing outcome in airway stenosis. PEFR in particular, being affected by the total tracheobronchial resistance, is sensitive to changes in lumen dimensions (**Fig. 29.8**).

The flow-volume loop is the mainstay of diagnosis and monitoring in patients with laryngotracheal stenosis. The flow-volume loop maneuver begins from total lung capacity as a maximum effort expiration of the forced vital capacity,

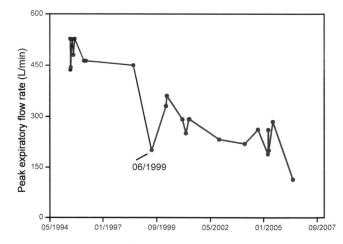

Figure 29.8 Serial peak flow measurements in a patient with Wegener granulomatosis before and after development and recurrences of subglottic stenosis.

which is then proceeded by a maximum effort inspiration back to total lung capacity (**Fig. 29.9**).

From a diagnostic perspective, flow-volume loop can distinguish between obstructive and restrictive lung

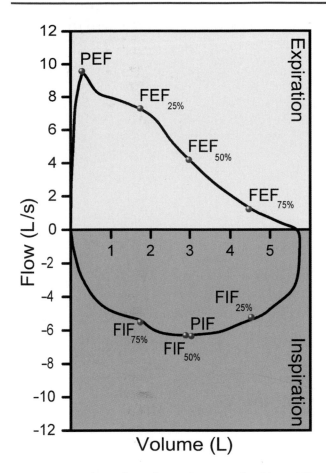

Figure 29.9 Flow-volume loop of a normal subject. PEF, peak expiratory flow; PIF, peak inspiratory flow; FEF, forced expiratory flow; FIF, forced inspiratory flow at 25%, 50%, and 75% of vital capacity.

diseases, can characterize airway obstruction as upper airway or lower airway, and can separate upper airway obstruction into fixed obstruction, variable extrathoracic obstruction, and variable intrathoracic obstruction (**Fig. 29.10**).

From a monitoring perspective, flow-volume loop is highly sensitive to stenosis severity (**Fig. 29.11**) and can be used to quantify treatment response (**Fig. 29.12**).

Overall tracheobronchial tree resistance can be measured in a whole-body plethysmogram and added airway resistance as the stenosis can be directly but invasively measured by concomitantly measuring airflow and trans-stenosis pressure changes using an oesophageal balloon. These latter highly specialist tests are not widely available and have not gained popularity in routine physiological assessment of these patients.

Effort Physiology
The net effect of the presence of an upper airway stenosis is to place a limit on the performance of the respiratory system, and this clinically manifests as exertional dyspnea and effort intolerance. It is therefore more closely related to patient symptoms and potentially therefore provides a more patient-related outcome measure than measurement of flow restriction. Measures such as the Shuttle test or the 6-minute walk test are more subjective and operator-dependent than flow measurements and are therefore more difficult to standardize and interpret. We have recently begun using cardiopulmonary exercise testing (CPET) as a method of assessing integrated exercise tolerance (**Fig. 29.13**), but its efficacy remains at this time unproven.

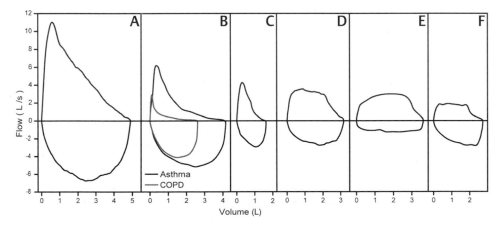

Figure 29.10 Flow-volume loops in health and disease. (A) Flow-volume loop in a healthy subject. (B) Flow-volume loops in asthma and chronic obstructive pulmonary disease. Patients with bronchopulmonary obstructive disease have normal inspiratory flow-volume loops, but an abnormal expiratory profile characterized by early drop in expiratory flow rate is caused by air trapping. (C) Patients with pulmonary fibrosis have normal flow-volume loop shapes but both lung volumes and flow rates are significantly reduced. (D) A fixed stenosis which does not move with respiration, like a fibrotic lesion which is restricted to the region of the cricoid cartilage, impairs inspiration and expiration equally and causes a "fixed" obstructive pattern. Variable stenoses are mobile. During inspiration, negative extrathoracic tracheal pressure tends to worsen a mobile extrathoracic stenosis while improving an intrathoracic mobile lesion. The reverse is true during expiration. As such, a mobile extrathoracic lesion has a greater impact on inspiratory airflow (E), while a mobile intrathoracic lesion has a greater impact on expiratory flow (F).

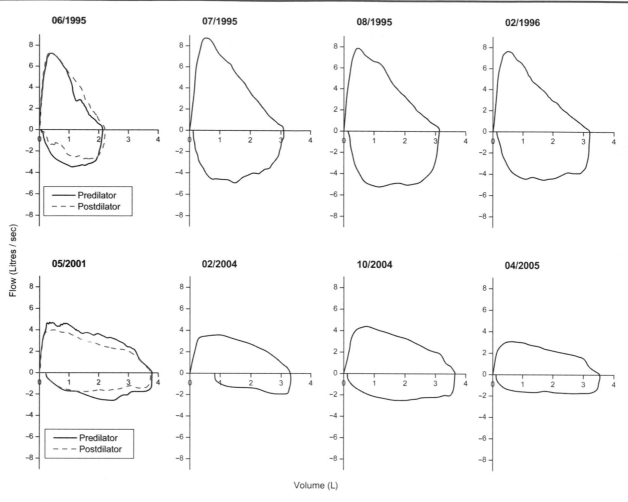

Figure 29.11 Flow-volume loop examinations in a patient with Wegener granulomatosis before and following development of a relapsing-remitting pattern of vasculitis-associated subglottic stenosis.

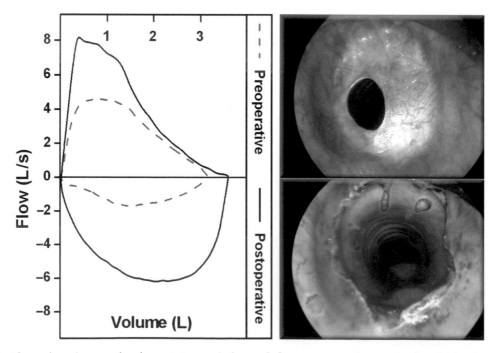

Figure 29.12 Flow-volume loops and endoscopic images before and after treatment of an acquired tracheal web.

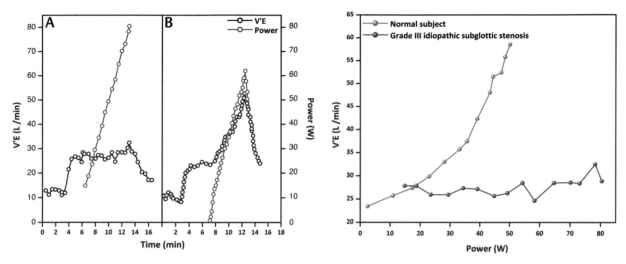

Figure 29.13 Ventilation rate (V'E) against time and exercise power in an incremental exercise cardiopulmonary exercise protocol. There is a failure for V'E to rise to match the increased workload demands of the exercise leading to perception of dyspnea (left panel A). By contrast, in a normal subject ventilation rises to match the increased demand imposed by exercise. Right panel (B) shows failure of ventilation to match additional imposed workload demand in the same patients.

Assessment of Disease-Specific Symptoms and Quality of Life

Patient-related outcome measures (PROMs) are increasingly important in assessing patient's experience and are used to assess treatment efficacy and outcome. Their inherently "subjective" nature has led to some clinical reluctance to adopt them as "scientific" disease outcome measures. In our opinion, however, laryngotracheal stenosis lends itself well to assessment by PROMs. The reason for this is that its primary clinical manifestation, exertional dyspnea, is a perceptual or psychophysical symptom and the additional domains of airway status, voice, and swallowing can likewise be assessed on ordinal scales.

We have proposed the use of the Airway-Dyspnea-Voice-Swallow (ADVS) ordinal scale as a way of summarizing airway status (**Table 29.4**).[15] The dyspnea domain of the ADVS scale is the Medical Research Council Dyspnea grade which we have validated as a disease-specific outcome measure for laryngotracheal stenosis.[16]

It is important to note that dyspnea can be measured using one of several scales, including the Borg scale, oxygen cost diagrams (OCD), and Mahler's Baseline/Transitional Dyspnea Indices (BDI/TDI).[17] The Borg scale provides a measure how breathless the patient actually feels, while the MRC and BDI/TDI scales measure the degree of effort intolerance resulting from dyspnea.

There are also more detailed scales for assessing the degree of respiratory symptoms and disability. Examples include AQ-20,[18] St George's Respiratory Questionnaire, and the Clinical Chronic Obstructive Pulmonary Disease (COPD) Questionnaire.[19] We have formally validated the Clinical COPD Questionnaire (www.ccq.nl) as a disease-specific outcome measure for adult laryngotracheal stenosis.[20] One of the advantages of using the Clinical COPD Questionnaire is the fact that its minimum clinical important difference (MCID) in respiratory disease has been established. A change of 0.4 or more in the overall scale represents a significant clinical change, and this can be used in outcome studies in much the same way as has been established in lower airway disease.[21] Voice and swallowing functions are assessed using the 10-item version of the Voice Handicap Index (VHI-10)[22] and Eating Assessment Tool-10 scale for oropharyngeal dysphagia,[23] respectively. More detailed assessments of voice or swallowing are only performed if specifically indicated.

Assessment of Treatment Durability

Treatment durability can be determined in several ways. Decannulation (an A1 or A2 airway) has been the traditional marker of treatment success, but as almost all patients are eventually decannulated it is not very discriminating. Decannulation time as an actuarial variable has been used to assess treatment effectiveness. Outcome can also be defined as time to attainment of a prosthesis-free airway (an A1 airway), and time to its attainment has also been used as an outcome measure. If treatment intention has been to manage a patient endoscopically, then freedom from open cervico-mediastinal surgery can be used either as a binary or actuarial variable. Outcome of treating intrinsically recurrent disease processes such as Wegener granulomatosis or idiopathic subglottic stenosis can be assessed by time to first recurrence as an actuarial variable, but more appropriately, as rate of intervention which can then be compared with parametric or nonparametric statistics depending on the normality of its distribution.

Table 29.4   Adult Airway-Dyspnea-Voice-Swallow System

Airway status		Dyspnea	
Score	Description	Score	Description
A$_1$	No airway prosthesis	D$_1$	I get short of breath only on strenuous exercise
A$_2$	Intraluminal airway prosthesis in situ	D$_2$	I get short of breath when hurrying on the level or up a slight hill
A$_3$	Tracheostomy/T-tube dependent, patient voices	D$_3$	I walk slower than people of the same age on the level because of breathlessness, or have to stop for breath when walking at my own pace on the level
A$_4$	Tracheostomy/T-tube dependent, patient does not voice	D$_4$	I stop for breath after walking 100 yards or after a few minutes on the level
A$_5$	Death as a direct complication of airway disease	D$_5$	I am too breathless to leave the house
Voice		**Swallowing**	
Score	Description	Score	Description
V$_1$	I have had no problems with my voice	S$_1$	I have been able to eat and drink normally
V$_2$	I have had some problems with my voice. For example: The sound of my voice may vary throughout the day I have had some difficulty being heard/understood in loud environments	S$_2$	I have been able to eat a normal diet but with some difficulty. For example: I have occasionally had to cough to clear my throat I find some foods more difficult than others to swallow It takes me longer to finish a meal than it does people around me I tend sometimes to cough when I drink liquids quickly
V$_3$	I have quite a rough voice. I find making voice effortful and have significant difficulties being heard/understood in loud environments	S$_3$	I have had significant swallowing difficulties. For example: I have tended to cough to clear my throat, or do a double swallows during most meals I tend to eat soft or pureed foods that are easier to swallow. It takes me much longer to finish a meal than most people Drinking fluids, frequently makes me cough
V$_4$	I can only produce a weak voice/whisper despite my best efforts, and have difficulty being heard/understood in normal conversation or on the telephone	S$_4$	My swallowing is a serious problem/is seriously abnormal. For example: My diet consists almost entirely of semiliquid/liquidized foods I need to take a significant amount of the fluids I drink as thickened fluids I take regular dietary supplements -or-I receive a proportion of my diet through a stomach tube (gastrostomy tube)
V$_5$	I have no voice	S$_5$	I am unable to swallow. I take all of my nutrition through a stomach tube (PEG)

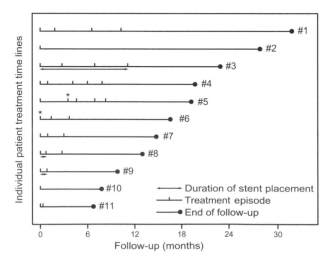

Figure 29.14   An example of a treatment time line plot.[24]

The time line plot is a simple way of visually presenting a series of up to 30 patients (**Fig. 29.14**).[24]

Pediatric Airway Outcome Assessment

Pediatric subglottic stenosis has traditionally been classified based on the Myer-Cotton system. Decannulation has been the primary outcome measure for assessing treatment success. Young children cannot undergo lung function testing and techniques and in children with a tracheostomy rhinomanometry has been adopted as a way of measuring suprastomal airway resistance to predict decannulation success.[25] We have recently adopted the ADVS system for the pediatric population (**Table 29.5**) and have developed a pediatric airway PROM (**Table 29.6**) which as yet remains unvalidated.[26]

Table 29.5   Pediatric Airway-Dyspnea-Voice-Swallow System

Airway
- A_1 Prosthesis-free airway
- A_2 Internal stent in situ
- A_3 Tracheostomy in situ, patient voices
- A_4 Tracheostomy in situ, patient does not voice

Dyspnea
- D_1 No age-appropriate dyspnea-related limitation on exercise or activities
- D_2 Dyspnea *and/or* stridor on moderate physical exertion (e.g., crying, running, playing with other children)
- D_3 Dyspnea *and/or* stridor on mild physical exertion (e.g., feeding, crawling, or walking at normal pace)
- D_4 Dyspnea *and/or* stridor at rest

Voice
- V_1 Normal voice
- V_2 Voice not normal but easily understood by others
- V_3 Weak / breathy voice that is not easily understood by others
- V_4 No voice

Swallow
- S_1 Normal feeding/eating and drinking
- S_2 Swallow not normal but the child manages to thrive without the need for dietary modification(s) and/or supplementation
- S_3 Swallow abnormal and the child needs dietary modification(s) and/or supplementation
- S_4 Dependent on feeding tube

Table 29.6   Patient-Related Outcome Measure for Pediatric Laryngotracheal Stenosis

On average during the past week how often...	Never	Hardly ever	A few times	Several times	A great many times	All of the time
	0	1	2	3	4	5
...was the child's breathing noisy?						
...was the child short of breath at rest?						
...was the child short of breath during mild physical activities (such as feeding, crawling, or walking)?						
...was the child short of breath during more strenuous physical activities (such as crying, running, climbing stairs, or playing with other children)?						
...did the child cough when not eating, drinking, or being fed?						
...did the child cough/choke during feeding/eating or drinking?						
...did the child refuse to feed/have food?						
...did the child have special dietary supplements (such as special formula milk or food supplements)?						
...was the child able to eat or drink without the aid of a feeding tube?						
...did the child have an abnormal cry or a hoarse voice?						
...did the child have difficulty being heard in loud environments?						
...did the child have difficulty being heard in quiet environments?						
...did the child lose his or her voice completely and was not able to verbally communicate?						

Note: This questionnaire should be completed by a parent or guardian.
How to calculate scores:
Total score: (Item 1 + Item 2 + Item 3...+ Item 13)/6.5.
Airway domain: (Item 1 + Item 2 + Item 3 + Item 4 + Item 5)/2.5.
Voice domain: (Item 10 + Item 11 + Item 12 + Item 13)/2.
Swallow domain: (Item 6 + Item 7 + Item 8 + Item 9)/2.

Current and Future Issues Concerning Outcome Assessment in Laryngotracheal Stenosis

Although the Clinical COPD Questionnaire provides questions on general well-being, there are not as yet any suitably sized formal studies of health utility and quality of life using a generic quality of life instrument such as the Short Form 36 (SF-36) or EuroQol (Eq. 5D) scales in this patient group. This means that Quality-Adjusted Life Years (QALY) and cost per QALY values have not yet been established.

There is also work to be done to develop and standardize dyspnea-related effort physiology. We have begun work on using CPET as a way of achieving this objective, but the findings are still at their infancy.

Moreover and more fundamentally, current methodologies are aimed at measuring the impact of an obstructive stenosis on patient physiology, symptomatology, and quality of life. This leaves assessment of patients whose lesion has been bypassed with a tracheostomy or who have long-term indwelling stents or T-tube inadequately addressed. A substantial body of work should be done to develop and validate outcome instruments to encompass both stenosed and bypassed airways and to combine the three domains of airway, voice, and swallowing symptoms within a single disease-specific PROM for laryngotracheal stenosis.

References

1. Lorenz RR. Adult laryngotracheal stenosis: etiology and surgical management. Curr Opin Otolaryngol Head Neck Surg 2003;11(6):467–472
2. Suppiah R, Mukhtyar C, Flossmann O, et al. A cross-sectional study of the Birmingham Vasculitis Activity Score version 3 in systemic vasculitis. Rheumatology (Oxford) 2011;50(5):899–905
3. Nouraei SAR, Ghufoor K, Patel A, Ferguson T, Howard DJ, Sandhu GS. Outcome of endoscopic treatment of adult postintubation tracheal stenosis. Laryngoscope 2007;117(6):1073–1079
4. Jaber S, Jung B, Chanques G, Bonnet F, Marret E. Effects of steroids on reintubation and post-extubation stridor in adults: meta-analysis of randomised controlled trials. Crit Care 2009;13(2):R49
5. Colt HG, Harrell JH. Therapeutic rigid bronchoscopy allows level of care changes in patients with acute respiratory failure from central airways obstruction. Chest 1997;112(1):202–206
6. Myer CM III, O'Connor DM, Cotton RT. Proposed grading system for subglottic stenosis based on endotracheal tube sizes. Ann Otol Rhinol Laryngol 1994;103(4 Pt 1):319–323
7. Freitag L, Ernst A, Unger M, Kovitz K, Marquette CH. A proposed classification system of central airway stenosis. Eur Respir J 2007;30(1):7–12
8. McCaffrey TV. Classification of laryngotracheal stenosis. Laryngoscope 1992;102(12 Pt 1):1335–1340
9. Nouraei SAR, Singh A, Patel A, Ferguson C, Howard DJ, Sandhu GS. Early endoscopic treatment of acute inflammatory airway lesions improves the outcome of postintubation airway stenosis. Laryngoscope 2006;116(8):1417–1421
10. Nouraei SAR, McPartlin DW, Nouraei SM, et al. Objective sizing of upper airway stenosis: a quantitative endoscopic approach. Laryngoscope 2006;116(1):12–17
11. Doolin EJ, Strande L. Calibration of endoscopic images. Ann Otol Rhinol Laryngol 1995;104(1):19–23
12. Dörffel WV, Fietze I, Hentschel D, et al. A new bronchoscopic method to measure airway size. Eur Respir J 1999;14(4):783–788
13. Kiesler K, Gugatschka M, Sorantin E, Friedrich G. Laryngo-tracheal profile: a new method for assessing laryngo-tracheal stenoses. Eur Arch Otorhinolaryngol 2007;264(3):251–256
14. Brouns M, Jayaraju ST, Lacor C, et al. Tracheal stenosis: a flow dynamics study. J Appl Physiol 2007;102(3):1178–1184
15. Nouraei SAR, Nouraei SM, Upile T, Howard DJ, Sandhu GS. A proposed system for documenting the functional outcome of adult laryngotracheal stenosis. Clin Otolaryngol 2007;32(5):407–409
16. Nouraei SAR, Nouraei SM, Randhawa PS, et al. Sensitivity and responsiveness of the Medical Research Council dyspnoea scale to the presence and treatment of adult laryngotracheal stenosis. Clin Otolaryngol 2008;33(6):575–580
17. Mahler DA, Wells CK. Evaluation of clinical methods for rating dyspnea. Chest 1988;93(3):580–586
18. Hajiro T, Nishimura K, Jones PW, et al. A novel, short, and simple questionnaire to measure health-related quality of life in patients with chronic obstructive pulmonary disease. Am J Respir Crit Care Med 1999;159(6):1874–1878
19. van der Molen T, Willemse BW, Schokker S, ten Hacken NH, Postma DS, Juniper EF. Development, validity and responsiveness of the Clinical COPD Questionnaire. Health Qual Life Outcomes 2003;1:13
20. Nouraei SAR, Randhawa PS, Koury EF, et al. Validation of the Clinical COPD Questionnaire as a psychophysical outcome measure in adult laryngotracheal stenosis. Clin Otolaryngol 2009;34(4):343–348
21. Kocks JW, Tuinenga MG, Uil SM, van den Berg JW, Ståhl E, van der Molen T. Health status measurement in COPD: the minimal clinically important difference of the clinical COPD questionnaire. Respir Res 2006;7:62
22. Deary IJ, Webb A, Mackenzie K, Wilson JA, Carding PN. Short, self-report voice symptom scales: psychometric characteristics of the voice handicap index-10 and the vocal performance questionnaire. Otolaryngol Head Neck Surg 2004;131(3):232–235
23. Belafsky PC, Mouadeb DA, Rees CJ, et al. Validity and reliability of the Eating Assessment Tool (EAT-10). Ann Otol Rhinol Laryngol 2008;117(12):919–924
24. Nouraei SAR, Kapoor KV, Nouraei SM, Ghufoor K, Howard DJ, Sandhu GS. Results of endoscopic tracheoplasty for treating tracheostomy-related airway stenosis. Clin Otolaryngol 2007;32(6):471–475
25. Kearns DB, Albert DM, Choa DI, Wickstead M, Bailey CM, Evans JN. Functional assessment of the paediatric laryngeal airway. Clin Otolaryngol Allied Sci 1990;15(1):53–58
26. Nouraei SAR, Koury EF, Sandhu GS. A proposed system for documenting the functional outcome of paediatric laryngotracheal stenosis. Clin Otolaryngol 2011;36(3):284–286

Section F

Miscellaneous Topics

30 Laryngopharyngeal Reflux—Reflux beyond the Esophagus: Pathophysiology, Diagnosis, and Treatment

Cathal Coyle and Rishi Talwar

Reflux of gastric contents not only causes the commonly presenting symptoms of heartburn and dyspepsia but is also responsible for a surprisingly wide range of extraesophageal symptoms and conditions. The reflux of gastric contents, including acid, pepsin, and bile, principally manifests as gastroesophageal reflux disease (GERD). However, reflux of gastric contents can also occur beyond the upper esophageal sphincter (UOS) and penetrate the upper aerodigestive tract. At this point, it can be responsible for a host of symptoms and conditions that are collectively known as atypical manifestations of GERD, also known as extraesophageal reflux (EOR) or laryngopharyngeal reflux (LPR). Awareness of EOR/LPR is relatively high within the ENT community and understanding of the condition is increasing within primary care.[1]

Gastroesophageal reflux (GOR) is a normal physiological phenomenon that occurs in most people, particularly after meals.[2] This reflux, called physiological reflux, is characterized by a short duration of reflux episodes, infrequency during sleep, and lack of damage to the esophageal mucosa and does not normally cause symptoms.[3] In contrast, GERD is a condition that develops when the reflux of stomach contents causes troublesome symptoms and/or complications. Exactly where GERD begins along the continuum, from physiological reflux at one end to complicated esophagitis at the other, may be problematic.[4] According to the recent Montreal definition and classification of reflux disease, the manifestations of GERD are divided into esophageal and extraesophageal syndromes, with extraesophageal syndromes divided into established and proposed associations.[5] The rationale for this terminology was that clinicians may need to define and classify patients based on differing amounts of information.

GOR is very common. We all reflux and approximately 20% of the adult population has reflux symptoms at least once a week,[6,7] with almost 10% of the adult population experiencing symptoms on a daily basis. Furthermore, it is estimated that up to 10% of patients visiting otolaryngology clinics have reflux-related disease and up to 55% of patients with hoarseness have reflux into the pharynx.[8,9] Thus, reflux is considered one of the most important factors causing inflammation in the upper aerodigestive tract.

In the literature, several different terms have been used to describe reflux that passes beyond the UOS. The term *LPR* was first introduced by Jamie Koufman in 1991[8] to describe the backflow of gastric contents that reaches

pharyngeal and laryngeal areas. Subsequently, terms such as gastropharyngeal reflux, esophagopharyngeal reflux, and silent reflux have been used synonymously. All of these may be considered part of EOR, which is reflux anywhere beyond the UOS, including, for example, the sinus, oral cavity, and middle ear, the difference being that only symptoms or findings associated with the larynx and pharynx are considered when talking about LPR.

History

Although the initial reports are from the beginning of the 20th century,[10,11] the clinical importance of reflux for laryngeal lesions was first noticed in 1968 when Cherry and Margulies published their study on contact ulcer patients.[12] In their study, reflux was diagnosed by barium swallow and cinefluoroscopy, methods that have since been superseded. Öhman et al[13] reported the first series of laryngeal patients evaluated for reflux disease with modern diagnostic methods, that is, with esophageal manometry and 24-hour pH monitoring. Eventually, Wiener et al[14] introduced the pioneering study on dual-probe pH monitoring, where the pharyngeal probe was "piggy-backed" onto the esophageal probe and positioned into the hypopharynx, enabling pH measurements to be taken in the upper aerodigestive tract. Since then, there have been several studies implicating acid injury as a contributing factor to upper and lower airway symptoms.[15–18]

Mechanisms of Laryngopharyngeal Reflux

GOR is necessary for LPR to occur, but not all episodes of GOR are associated with LPR. Owing to effective peristaltic motility and esophageal clearance mechanisms, salivary and esophageal gland secretions, as well as the tone of the UOS, the upper aerodigestive tract is well protected against reflux under physiological conditions.[19,20] It has been speculated that the UOS function is defective in subjects with LPR. Some investigators have noted elevated UOS pressures in patients with reflux laryngitis, while others have found normal resting pressures. Shaker and his group[21] have extensively studied the mechanisms of reflux above the UOS and found that it occurred in three different circumstances.

A major mechanism of reflux into the pharynx was belching, which causes transient complete UOS relaxation, allowing gastric contents from the esophagus to reach the larynx and the pharynx. Additionally, spontaneous LPR could also be detected when the UOS pressure dropped transiently to approximately 10 to 25 mm Hg (low residual UOS pressure). Finally, when the esophagus contained residual acid in the supine position, swallowing could predispose to LPR.

The results concerning esophageal motility in patients with LPR have been controversial. Some researchers have found ineffective peristaltic contractions with abnormal distal clearance times in patients with LPR, whereas others have found no significant difference in esophageal clearance times compared with patients with GERD. At least secondary peristalsis seems to be preserved in patients with posterior laryngitis (PL).[22]

Physiologically normal levels of GOR can lead to LPR in a subset of patients. In healthy individuals, these events would not be accompanied by classic symptoms of reflux, such as heartburn and regurgitation, and would therefore not be reported. It is the patient with LPR symptoms, in the absence of classic reflux symptoms, which makes the diagnosis sometimes counterintuitive and difficult to connect to the reflux of gastric content in the first place.

Liquid, Gas, or Gas–Liquid Matrix?

The notion that reflux may be something other than a liquid bolus is a recent phenomenon and is still more theoretical than proven. It originates from the detection of acid in the pharynx and pepsin in the saliva as well as in the exhaled breath condensate of patients with suspected LPR. The presence of these substances (*refluxate*) in areas so distantly removed from the stomach is more conceivable if they were in an aerosol form rather than in a liquid bolus rising from the stomach.

Refluxate as an aerosol has numerous implications. First, it more plausibly explains the occurrence of refluxate deep in the lungs[23,24] and in the middle ear (in otitis media with effusion[25] where bile acids have also been identified[26]). Second, liquid refluxate almost certainly has higher concentrations of acid and pepsin, but an aerosol would carry these injurious agents further into the upper aerodigestive tract. Third, their presence verifies that refluxate has reached these areas. When in excess and in the correct clinical circumstances, the findings are arguably diagnostic of LPR. Lastly, it highlights a key therapeutic need, namely the development of treatments to more successfully reduce pepsin in the refluxate.

Antireflux Mechanisms

The esophageal defensive system preventing GOR will of course prevent LPR. The major elements of the antireflux mechanisms are the tone of the lower esophageal sphincter (LOS) and the diaphragm. The right crus of the diaphragm supports the LOS in its barrier function by physically encircling it and acting as a mechanical support, particularly during physical exercise.[19] Four factors are known to contribute to esophageal luminal acid clearance; two of these, gravity and esophageal peristalsis, handle refluxate bolus clearance and, after effective bolus clearance, the other two, salivary and esophageal gland secretions, handle refluxate acid clearance.[19] The third line of the defense mechanism consists of epithelial resistance.

However, there are other "response mechanisms" that become activated after certain stimulation and may prevent reflux into the upper aerodigestive tract. According to Shaker and Hogan, distension of the esophagus or pressure stimulation of the pharyngeal wall may result either in fortification of the UOS barriers (esophago-UOS, pharyngo-UOS, and laryngo-UOS contractile reflexes) or closure of the glottis (esophagoglottal and pharyngoglottal closure reflexes).[27] In addition, there are other reflexes included among the response mechanisms (such as pharyngeal swallow and secondary peristalsis induced by pharyngeal liquid stimulation and esophageal distension by refluxate) that result in pharyngeal and esophageal volume clearance. These further reduce the chance of refluxate contact with the tracheal, bronchial, and glottal structures.

Pathophysiology

There are several theories for how reflux causes laryngeal pathology or pharyngeal and laryngeal symptoms. The *microaspiration* theory implies a direct acid–pepsin injury to the larynx and surrounding tissues.[12] The stomach normally secretes acid at a pH of 1.5 to 2. This contrasts with the luminal pH of the pharynx and larynx, where pH is roughly neutral (pH 7).[28] Consequently, pharyngeal pH decreases dramatically when LPR occurs. In addition to acidic pH levels, substances that can contribute to the noxious quality of the refluxate include pepsin, bile salts, pancreatic enzymes, bacteria, and bacterial products. Unlike the esophagus, the laryngeal structures are not rinsed with saliva, so small amounts of gastric contents are probably capable of producing injury to the respiratory epithelium. The microaspiration theory is supported by experimental studies, which show that minute amounts of acid and pepsin applied several times a week were capable of inducing subglottic lesions in dogs.[8] Moreover, in vitro studies on laryngeal fibroblasts have shown that acid and pepsin together demonstrate considerable synergy, initiating the production of proteins involved in wound repair and angiogenesis.[29]

According to the *trauma* theory, the mere entry of gastric acid is not sufficient to produce or maintain injuries but that some additional factor is necessary for mucosal lesions to appear. This theory is supported by other animal studies, which found that the application of acid and pepsin was insufficient to break down the mucosal barrier on the vocal processes of the arytenoids.[8] One may hypothesize that LPR only results in laryngeal injury as a result of comorbidity or when acting together with other risk factors for laryngitis, such as vocal abuse or concomitant viral infection.[30]

Finally, the *esophageal–bronchial reflex* theory suggests that acid in the distal esophagus stimulates vagally mediated reflexes, resulting in chronic repetitive throat clearing and coughing,[31] which may lead to laryngeal symptoms and lesions. Furthermore, gastric contents in the pharynx irritate the mucosa locally, which may also alter laryngeal behavior. A combination of these mechanisms may be present in the same patient.

Effect of Pepsin on Epithelial Cells

Based on esophageal and laryngeal biopsies from patients with LPR compared with healthy individuals, Johnston et al made three key observations: pepsin adhered to epithelial cells, was endocytosed, and led to internal cell derangements.[32-35] Pepsin was found on the surface of laryngeal epithelial cells in LPR patients but not in healthy individuals.[32] The absence in healthy individuals is not surprising because significant reflux had previously been excluded by esophageal physiological measurements.

In its active form, pepsin (a proteolytic enzyme) damages intercellular connective proteins and also intracellular proteins concerned with defense. Inactive pepsin is taken up within the cells by endocytosis via a competitive receptor-mediated mechanism and is apparent in vesicles situated in the Golgi system.[33] This endocytosis is unanticipated as it seems unlikely that receptors specific for pepsin are present in laryngeal tissues. Apparently, such receptors provide some other function but when exposed to pepsin, they transport the enzyme into the cells. When cells were exposed to human pepsin 3B at pH 7.4, a level at which the enzyme is inactive, several major alterations happened, affecting the inner cell structure and function.[34] The Golgi system has a pH of approximately 5.5 and together with its associated endosomes processes large molecules such as proteins and receptors through its mildly acidic environment. The supposition is that the changes result from reactivation of the inactive pepsin inside the cell. The cells distend and structural damage to the mitochondria and Golgi system became evident on electron microscopy within an hour, and damage was amplified by 12 hours. The early damage was accompanied by increased expression of seven genes concerned with cell stress and toxicity, including specific heat shock proteins. Late changes were accompanied by the diminished expression of 18 other stress genes.

The evidence strongly argues for the following chain of events: inactive pepsin is endocytosed, is activated within the cells, and causes cell damage. This induces oxidative stress and the accumulation of free radicals, which damage mitochondria and may lead to cell death.[36] In the assay used, the cells were only exposed once to pepsin, thereby modeling what might occur with a single episode of LPR. Although damaged, the cells were still viable at 12 hours, but with recurring exposure, as would be likely in persistent LPR, the damaged cells may not survive.[34]

Investigations and Diagnosis

The definition of pathological LPR is uncertain because pharyngeal reflux also occurs in healthy subjects and we are missing normative data from different age groups and do not know the impact of age on LPR. Esophageal symptoms and mucosal damage have traditionally been related to acid reflux episodes with pH less than 4.[2,37] This limit is based on experimental studies that have shown a correlation between pain and the pH of infused material in the esophagus. Its clinical usefulness has also been verified in relation to the development of reflux esophagitis. Hence, the same limit of acid reflux has been applied to pharyngeal reflux disease.

Pharyngeal reflux is typically quantified by counting the total number of events or by calculating the percentage time of acid exposure. Some consider even one single pharyngeal reflux episode abnormal,[8] while others suggest that 4 to 18 acid exposure episodes to the pharynx may be normal.[38,39] Nevertheless, simply counting the number of reflux episodes may be insufficient, owing to the varying duration of exposure. An average pharyngeal reflux episode in asymptomatic people lasts 6 seconds,[40] whereas patients with PL have an average length of 30 seconds.[15] In addition, according to Oelschlager et al,[40] the longest pharyngeal acid exposure in healthy controls was 19 seconds, while exposure times as long as 16 minutes have been measured in PL patients.[41]

In recent meta-analyses, LPR events were demonstrated in 10 to 30% of asymptomatic normal adults,[42,43] but acid exposure times (AETs) in normal subjects were very low (between 0.00 and 0.01%).[42] It is nonetheless evident that there is an overlap in the occurrence of pharyngeal reflux between healthy controls and patients with LPR disease.[43]

One area of controversy is that pepsin has been shown to retain its activity at pH 5 to 6, suggesting that a threshold of pH 5 is also of importance when assessing the clinical presence of reflux.[44] This pharyngeal, weak acidic reflux seems to be due mainly to regurgitation of more acidic material, which is then presumably buffered by saliva and secretions from the esophageal glands before reaching the hypopharynx. Another cause might be regurgitation of weakly acidic gastric contents. The frequent postprandial occurrence suggests this to be a combined effect of transient lower esophageal sphincter relaxation (TLESR) events triggered by gastric distension and the nonuniform intragastric buffering effect of food. Moreover, weakly acidic reflux may also be expected in patients treated with proton pump inhibitors (PPIs) since these drugs shift the gastric pH toward a less acidic mean value.[45] Anderson et al have published normative data for pharyngeal reflux at pH 5.[46] They found that pharyngeal pH 5 reflux episodes occurred in 91% of healthy controls with a median AET of 0.1%, and the upper limit of normality was 1.5%.

Barium swallow is no longer routinely used to diagnose reflux disease, although it still has a significant function if structural changes, such as achalasia, are suspected. The *Bernstein acid perfusion test* has also fallen out of favor, but has been used recently in research into reflux-related cough. Upper gastrointestinal endoscopy is helpful in the identification of GERD but is regularly normal in patients with LPR. Esophageal manometry has not been routinely used in the diagnosis of LPR but is required to establish the position of UOS and LOS. This directs the accurate positioning and spacing of electrodes for pH monitoring and is valuable in the measurement of esophageal dysmotility, which may be contributing to symptoms.

The *24-hour dual-channel pH monitoring*, with electrodes placed at the distal esophagus and the UOS, has been the major basis for the diagnosis of LPR.[47] Single-channel pH monitoring can help diagnose GERD but is not as useful in the diagnosis of LPR, as the damaging component may be aerosol or a nonacid composition. Many authors believe that any episode of reflux reaching the pharynx is abnormal, while others consider that more than four episodes in 24 hours are necessary to establish a diagnosis. More recently, multichannel intraluminal impedance measurement has been coupled with pH monitoring (MII-pH) and may improve diagnostic accuracy, particularly for weakly acidic or nonacidic reflux events.[48] Both procedures are invasive, involving the transnasal insertion of a catheter, costly to carry out, and poorly tolerated by a large number of patients. The procedures require patients to reduce or stop their antireflux medication for a period of time preceding the investigations and therefore can result in an exacerbation of symptoms. However, for patients in whom surgery for LPR is indicated, physiological verification of the condition by pH monitoring or MII-pH is usually necessary.

A noninvasive test that allows rapid results would be very helpful in patient management.[49] One noninvasive procedure that has recently become available (Peptest, RD Biomed Limited, Hull, United Kingdom) uses a *pepsin immunoassay* applied within a lateral flow device for sampling pharyngeal secretions. If pepsin is detected, then the patient probably suffers from LPR.[50] An additional minimally invasive procedure involves monitoring airway pH in the pharynx to detect aerosolized reflux (Restech, Respiratory Technology Corp., San Diego, California, United States).[51] In ventilated patients, measurement of pH in exhaled breath condensate may also be helpful.[52] One study has shown that in patients with cough related to LPR, which did not respond to standard medication, some patients were found to be positive for *Helicobacter pylori* and improved subsequent to eradication.[53] Although compelling, it must be remembered that even though LPR is a potential cause of laryngopharyngeal inflammation, it is by no means the solitary cause. If there is any clinical suspicion whatsoever, then neoplasia must first be excluded.

Symptoms

The diagnosis of LPR begins with the patient's history. Symptoms reported to be related to LPR are tabulated in **Table 30.1**. The most common symptoms from the upper aerodigestive tract associated with LPR are *hoarseness*, *globus* sensation, *throat clearing*, and *coughing*.[8,15,16] In addition, symptoms such as sore throat, laryngospasm, and choking sensation are related to LPR, but they are less studied. A diagnosis based purely on the history is challenging because all these symptoms are unspecific and common in several other laryngeal disorders.

Belafsky et al[54] developed the Reflux Symptom Index, a self-administered nine-item questionnaire to help categorize the severity of LPR (see **Table 30.2**). Heartburn and regurgitation, which are typical symptoms of GERD, are absent in 50% of patients with LPR[15,55] for reasons previously described.

The most frequent laryngeal finding associated with LPR is PL that occurs in up to 70% of LPR patients.[8,15,17] It is characterized by edema or hypertrophy and sometimes erythema and hyperemia on the posterior aspect of the glottis. Sometimes the inflammation reaches up to the medial surface of the arytenoid cartilages. Some authors use the terms PL and reflux laryngitis interchangeably. However, reflux laryngitis encompasses wider changes in the mucosa, not only in the posterior glottis. Other changes often associated with LPR are vocal granuloma[56] and pseudosulcus (subglottic edema producing a double-edged appearance).[16] Of patients with pseudosulcus, 60 to 90% have LPR, while 65% of granuloma patients are LPR positive.

The clinician must not forget that the most severe laryngeal diseases associated with reflux are laryngeal carcinoma and posterior glottic or subglottic stenosis. There is also some controversy regarding the sensitivity of the above-mentioned laryngeal findings. Some of this is certainly due to the problems with diagnostic tests in pharyngeal reflux. Despite

Table 30.1 Symptoms Reported to Be Related to Laryngopharyngeal Reflux

- Chronic cough
- Chronic throat clearing
- Excessive throat mucous
- Chronic dysphonia/hoarseness
- Intermittent dysphonia/hoarseness
- Vocal fatigue
- Globus
- Voice breaks
- Postnasal drip
- Intermittent airway obstruction
- Chronic airway obstruction
- Wheezing

Table 30.2   Reflux Symptom Index (RSI)

Circle the appropriate response							
Within the last MONTH, how did the following problems affect you?	**0 = No problem 5 = Severe problem**						
Hoarseness or a problem with your voice	0	1	2	3	4	5	
Clearing your throat	0	1	2	3	4	5	
Excess throat or postnasal drip	0	1	2	3	4	5	
Difficulty swallowing food, liquids, or pills	0	1	2	3	4	5	
Coughing after you ate or after lying down	0	1	2	3	4	5	
Breathing difficulties or choking episodes	0	1	2	3	4	5	RSI
Troublesome or annoying cough	0	1	2	3	4	5	
Sensation of something sticking in your throat or a lump in your throat	0	1	2	3	4	5	
Heartburn, chest pain, indigestion, or stomach acid coming up?	0	1	2	3	4	5	
							Max score: 45

Adapted from reference 54.

Notes: Validated self-completed questionnaire. ≥ 10 considered clinically significant and ≥ 13 is diagnostic.

these limitations, laryngoscopy continues to be an important tool in the evaluation of LPR. Moreover, a summary of these findings on fiberoptic examination of the larynx has been tabulated and ranked by Belafsky et al in the Reflux Finding Score (RFS) (see **Table 30.3**).[57] However, the RFS has been criticized for its high levels of interobserver variability.

Impact of Reflux on Health-Related Quality of Life

GERD is a disorder associated with substantial reductions in health-related quality of life (HRQL).[58] Nevertheless, the consequences of LPR on HRQL have not yet been extensively studied. A recent report from Carrau et al shows that LPR has a significant negative impact on the lives of patients.[59] According to their study, HRQL of the patients with LPR was significantly lower than that of the US general population

and that LPR had a more significant impact on patients' social functioning and vitality than GERD. Other studies have shown significantly reduced social activities[60] with an adverse social life as a result of illness and significant increase in psychological distress, with more anxiety in comparison with healthy controls.[61]

Treatment

Treatment of LPR consists primarily of dietary and lifestyle advice for all patients, pharmacotherapy for many, and surgery reserved for the extremely resistant patients. There is currently no consensus algorithm or guidelines within the United Kingdom for the diagnosis and management of LPR.

Diet and lifestyle advice have been shown to be very helpful in the management of LPR. Patient information leaflets, an explanation of LPR, and how to manage it are

Table 30.3   Reflux Finding Score

Pseudosulcus/Subglottic Edema	2 Present			
Ventricular obliteration	2 Partial		4 Complete	
Erythema/hyperemia	2 Arytenoids (only)		4 Diffuse	
Vocal cord edema	1 Mild	2 Moderate	3 Severe	4 Polypoid
Diffuse laryngeal edema	1 Mild	2 Moderate	3 Severe	4 Obstructing
Posterior commissure hypertrophy	1 Mild	2 Moderate	3 Severe	4 Obstructing
Granuloma/granulation	2 Present			
Thick mucus	2 Present			

RFS, reflux finding score.

Adapted from reference 57.

Notes: Fiberoptic examination of the larynx with scores for the above features. Maximum score = 26 and ≥ 5 is significant.

now considered standard within various ENT and speech and language therapy departments, many of which work as specialist voice clinics. The core principles consist of avoiding fatty foods, fizzy drinks, and citrus fruit juices. Food should be avoided within 3 hours of going to sleep. Smoking should be stopped and alcohol, especially spirits, should be reduced. Patients susceptible to supine reflux benefit from using extra pillows or propping up the head of the bed, and sleeping on the left side rather than the right may reduce the tendency to reflux. Vigorous exercise such as jogging or circuit training may also exacerbate symptoms. Obesity and tight clothing also increase intra-abdominal mechanical pressure, leading to an increased likelihood of reflux.[49] A reflux advice session from trained speech and language therapists may improve compliance with antireflux medication, and voice therapy for those patients with hoarseness can improve outcomes.

Alginate reflux suppressants (e.g., Gaviscon Advance) have been shown to be effective in the management of LPR symptoms, either alone[62] or in combination with PPIs.[63] They are commonly mistaken as antacid preparations, but the majority have no antacid properties and actually work by forming a buoyant mechanical barrier between the stomach content and the esophagus, thereby preventing reflux per se as opposed to treating one component of the refluxate, as PPIs do for acid. They are also a nonsystemic medication. Alginates should be given after each meal and last thing at night. Nothing should be taken by mouth after the night-time dose, so patients should be advised to brush their teeth and drink some water before taking the alginate.

H_2-*receptor antagonists* (e.g., ranitidine) have mainly been superseded by PPIs, which are a more potent medication for blocking gastric acid secretion, although they may have a role in patients who experience nocturnal acid breakthrough despite twice-daily PPIs.[49]

All *PPIs* (e.g., lansoprazole) act for merely 12 to 14 hours and only work on activated proton pumps. These pumps are activated by the smell, taste, and sight of food via vagal-, histamine-, and gastrin-mediated pathways. Thus, if used for the treatment of LPR, twice-daily dosing is required to give full 24-hour protection, and timing of use is essential and should be given before meals due to their mechanism of action. A period of 2 to 3 months is necessary to establish benefit from the medication. There has been controversy regarding the use of PPIs in LPR,[64] and long-term use is not recommended.[65] Most patients require treatment for approximately 6 months and should be progressively stepped down and weaned off the drug to reduce the likelihood of rebound acid hypersecretion.[66] It must also be reiterated that acid is not the only component of the refluxate and pepsin has been implicated in laryngeal damage in LPR patients, so prevention of reflux per se may be more effective in treating LPR than acid suppression alone. PPIs are at best an indirect treatment for LPR, helping to reduce the activity of pepsin. Presently, there are no drugs available that directly affect pepsin, but alginates may be effective in reducing the amount of refluxate, and therefore pepsin, reaching the larynx and even the esophagus.[49]

Prokinetic agents (e.g., domperidone and metoclopramide) can be helpful in GERD, particularly when dysmotility is an issue, but they are generally not useful in LPR.

Newer agents that protect against TLESR are in development, including $GABA_\beta$ agonists[67] and metabotropic glutamate receptor 5 antagonists.[68] In the longer term, the majority of patients can manage their condition by dietary and lifestyle changes, supplemented by an alginate-based reflux suppressant[49] and/or twice-daily PPIs.

A small number of patients either fail to respond to medical treatment or require long-term high-dose PPIs to control their symptoms. If it is confirmed following investigations that LPR is present, after 24-hour dual-channel pH monitoring or MII-pH, then laparoscopic fundoplication has anecdotally been found to be effective.[49] Antireflux surgery for GERD provides good results in the majority of patients who are selected for this operation. Since GOR is at the root of both GERD and LPR, it is appealing to suppose an antireflux operation will also give analogous benefits in LPR. There are indeed anecdotal instances where surgery has helped individual patients, but as yet this cannot be generalized, for there are substantial differences between the two conditions. There are as yet no specific selection criteria with which to identify those with LPR who are likely to benefit from surgery.[36] The development of such criteria for GERD and the optimization of antireflux surgery have advanced during the past two decades of the 20th century. It is likely to take several years for a similar position to be reached for the surgical treatment of LPR.[36]

Conclusion

LPR is frequently diagnosed within ENT clinics. Most patients are treated on the basis of a clinical diagnosis, with invasive investigations being set aside for patients where the diagnosis is in doubt or treatment proves complicated. New less invasive techniques (e.g., Peptest and Restech) may become increasingly valuable in clinical practice. The majority of cases respond to dietary and lifestyle modification, followed by medical therapy, with only a small proportion requiring antireflux surgery.

References

1. Dettmar P, Strugala V. Diagnosis and drug treatment of extraoesophageal reflux. Prescriber 2008;19(13–14):15–20
2. Demeester TR, Johnson LF, Joseph GJ, Toscano MS, Hall AW, Skinner DB. Patterns of gastroesophageal reflux in health and disease. Ann Surg 1976;184(4):459–470
3. Galmiche JP, Janssens J. The pathophysiology of gastro-oesophageal reflux disease: an overview. Scand J Gastroenterol Suppl 1995;211: 7–18
4. Quigley EM. 24-h pH monitoring for gastroesophageal reflux disease: already standard but not yet gold? Am J Gastroenterol 1992;87(9):1071–1075

5. Vakil N, van Zanten SV, Kahrilas P, Dent J, Jones R; Global Consensus Group. The Montreal definition and classification of gastroesophageal reflux disease: a global evidence-based consensus. Am J Gastroenterol 2006;101(8):1900–1920, quiz 1943

6. Locke GR III, Talley NJ, Fett SL, Zinsmeister AR, Melton LJ III. Prevalence and clinical spectrum of gastroesophageal reflux: a population-based study in Olmsted County, Minnesota. Gastroenterology 1997;112(5):1448–1456

7. Nilsson M, Johnsen R, Ye W, Hveem K, Lagergren J. Prevalence of gastro-oesophageal reflux symptoms and the influence of age and sex. Scand J Gastroenterol 2004;39(11):1040–1045

8. Koufman JA. The otolaryngologic manifestations of gastroesophageal reflux disease (GERD): a clinical investigation of 225 patients using ambulatory 24-hour pH monitoring and an experimental investigation of the role of acid and pepsin in the development of laryngeal injury. Laryngoscope 1991;101(4, Pt 2; Suppl 53):1–78

9. Koufman JA, Amin MR, Panetti M. Prevalence of reflux in 113 consecutive patients with laryngeal and voice disorders. Otolaryngol Head Neck Surg 2000;123(4):385–388

10. Coffin LA. The relationship of upper airway passages to diseases of gastrointestinal tract. Ann Otol Rhinol Laryngol 1903;12:521–526

11. Jackson C. Contact ulcer of the larynx. Ann Otol Rhinol Laryngol 1928;37:227–230

12. Cherry J, Margulies SI. Contact ulcer of the larynx. Laryngoscope 1968;78(11):1937–1940

13. Öhman L, Olofsson J, Tibbling L, Ericsson G. Esophageal dysfunction in patients with contact ulcer of the larynx. Ann Otol Rhinol Laryngol 1983;92(3, Pt 1):228–230

14. Wiener GJ, Koufman JA, Wu WC, Cooper JB, Richter JE, Castell DO. Chronic hoarseness secondary to gastroesophageal reflux disease: documentation with 24-h ambulatory pH monitoring. Am J Gastroenterol 1989;84(12):1503–1508

15. Ylitalo R, Lindestad PA, Ramel S. Symptoms, laryngeal findings, and 24-hour pH monitoring in patients with suspected gastroesophago-pharyngeal reflux. Laryngoscope 2001;111(10):1735–1741

16. Belafsky PC, Postma GN, Koufman JA. The association between laryngeal pseudosulcus and laryngopharyngeal reflux. Otolaryngol Head Neck Surg 2002;126(6):649–652

17. Noordzij JP, Khidr A, Desper E, Meek RB, Reibel JF, Levine PA. Correlation of pH probe-measured laryngopharyngeal reflux with symptoms and signs of reflux laryngitis. Laryngoscope 2002;112(12):2192–2195

18. Jaspersen D, Kulig M, Labenz J, et al. Prevalence of extra-oesophageal manifestations in gastro-oesophageal reflux disease: an analysis based on the ProGERD Study. Aliment Pharmacol Ther 2003;17(12):1515–1520

19. Orlando RC. Pathogenesis of gastroesophageal reflux disease. Am J Med Sci 2003;326(5):274–278

20. Schreiber S, Garten D, Sudhoff H. Pathophysiological mechanisms of extraesophageal reflux in otolaryngeal disorders. Eur Arch Otorhinolaryngol 2009;266(1):17–24

21. Shaker R, Dodds WJ, Hogan WJ, Arndorfer R, Hofmann C, Dent J. Mechanisms of esophago-pharyngeal acid regurgitation. Gastroenterology 1991;100(5):A241

22. Ulualp S, Toohill RJ, Shaker R. Secondary esophageal peristalsis is preserved in patients with posterior laryngitis. Gastroenterology 1998;114(4):G1291

23. D'Ovidio F, Mura M, Tsang M, et al. Bile acid aspiration and the development of bronchiolitis obliterans after lung transplantation. J Thorac Cardiovasc Surg 2005;129(5):1144–1152

24. Ward C, Forrest IA, Brownlee IA, et al. Pepsin like activity in bronchoalveolar lavage fluid is suggestive of gastric aspiration in lung allografts. Thorax 2005;60(10):872–874

25. Tasker A, Dettmar PW, Panetti M, Koufman JA, Birchall JP, Pearson JP. Reflux of gastric juice and glue ear in children. Lancet 2002;359(9305):493

26. Klokkenburg JJ, Hoeve HL, Francke J, Wieringa MH, Borgstein J, Feenstra L. Bile acids identified in middle ear effusions of children with otitis media with effusion. Laryngoscope 2009;119(2):396–400

27. Shaker R, Hogan WJ. Reflex-mediated enhancement of airway protective mechanisms. Am J Med 2000;108(Suppl 4a):8S–14S

28. Feldman M, Friedman LS, Sleisenger MH, eds. Sleisenger & Fortran's Gastrointestinal and liver disease. 7th ed. Philadelphia, PA: Saunders; 2002:715–731

29. Ylitalo R, Baugh A, Li W, Thibeault S. Effect of acid and pepsin on gene expression in laryngeal fibroblasts. Ann Otol Rhinol Laryngol 2004;113(11):866–871

30. Ford CN. Evaluation and management of laryngopharyngeal reflux. JAMA 2005;294(12):1534–1540

31. Ing AJ, Ngu MC, Breslin AB. Pathogenesis of chronic persistent cough associated with gastroesophageal reflux. Am J Respir Crit Care Med 1994;149(1):160–167

32. Johnston N, Knight J, Dettmar PW, Lively MO, Koufman J. Pepsin and carbonic anhydrase isoenzyme III as diagnostic markers for laryngopharyngeal reflux disease. Laryngoscope 2004;114(12):2129–2134

33. Johnston N, Wells CW, Blumin JH, Toohill RJ, Merati AL. Receptor-mediated uptake of pepsin by laryngeal epithelial cells. Ann Otol Rhinol Laryngol 2007;116(12):934–938

34. Johnston N, Wells CW, Samuels TL, Blumin JH. Pepsin in nonacidic refluxate can damage hypopharyngeal epithelial cells. Ann Otol Rhinol Laryngol 2009;118(9):677–685

35. Johnston N, Dettmar PW, Lively MO, et al. Effect of pepsin on laryngeal stress protein (Sep70, Sep53, and Hsp70) response: role in laryngopharyngeal reflux disease. Ann Otol Rhinol Laryngol 2006;115(1):47–58

36. Bardhan KD, Strugala V, Dettmar PW. Reflux revisited: advancing the role of pepsin. Int J Otolaryngol 2012;2012:646901

37. Sifrim D. Acid, weakly acidic and non-acid gastro-oesophageal reflux: differences, prevalence and clinical relevance. Eur J Gastroenterol Hepatol 2004;16(9):823–830

38. Smit CF, Tan J, Devriese PP, Mathus-Vliegen LM, Brandsen M, Schouwenburg PF. Ambulatory pH measurements at the upper esophageal sphincter. Laryngoscope 1998;108(2):299–302

39. Bove M, Ruth M, Cange L, Månsson I. 24-H pharyngeal pH monitoring in healthy volunteers: a normative study. Scand J Gastroenterol 2000;35(3):234–241

40. Oelschlager BK, Quiroga E, Isch JA, Cuenca-Abente F. Gastroesophageal and pharyngeal reflux detection using impedance and 24-hour pH monitoring in asymptomatic subjects: defining the normal environment. J Gastrointest Surg 2006;10(1):54–62

41. Ulualp SO, Roland PS, Toohill RJ, Shaker R. Prevalence of gastroesophagopharyngeal acid reflux events: an evidence-based systematic review. Am J Otolaryngol 2005;26(4):239–244

42. Merati AL, Lim HJ, Ulualp SO, Toohill RJ. Meta-analysis of upper probe measurements in normal subjects and patients with laryngopharyngeal reflux. Ann Otol Rhinol Laryngol 2005;114(3):177–182

43. Joniau S, Bradshaw A, Esterman A, Carney AS. Reflux and laryngitis: a systematic review. Otolaryngol Head Neck Surg 2007;136(5):686–692

44. Sifrim D. Acid, weakly acidic and non-acid gastro-oesophageal reflux: differences, prevalence and clinical relevance. Eur J Gastroenterol Hepatol 2004;16(9):823–830

45. Lind T, Rydberg L, Kylebäck A, et al. Esomeprazole provides improved acid control vs. omeprazole In patients with symptoms of gastro-oesophageal reflux disease. Aliment Pharmacol Ther 2000;14(7):861–867

46. Anderson O, Ylitalo R, Finizia C, Bove M, Magnus R. Pharyngeal reflux episodes at pH 5 in healthy volunteers. Scand J Gastroenterol 2006;41(2):138–143

47. Postma GN. Ambulatory pH monitoring methodology. Ann Otol Rhinol Laryngol Suppl 2000;184:10–14

48. Blondeau K, Tack J. Pro: impedance testing is useful in the management of GERD. Am J Gastroenterol 2009;104(11):2664–2666

49. Pearson JP, Parikh S, Orlando RC, et al. Review article: reflux and its consequences—the laryngeal, pulmonary and oesophageal manifestations. Conference held in conjunction with the 9th International Symposium on Human Pepsin (ISHP) Kingston-upon-Hull, UK, 21-23 April 2010. Aliment Pharmacol Ther 2011; 33(Suppl 1):1–71

50. Strugala V, McGlashan JA, Watson MG, Morice AH, Granier B, Dettmar PW. Detection of pepsin using a non-invasive lateral flow test for the diagnosis of extra-oesophageal reflux—results of a pilot study. Gut 2007;56(Suppl 111):A212

51. Sun G, Muddana S, Slaughter JC, et al. A new pH catheter for laryngopharyngeal reflux: normal values. Laryngoscope 2009;119(8):1639–1643

52. Strugala V, Dettmar PW, Morice AH. S1895 detection of pepsin in sputum and exhaled breath condensate: could be a useful marker for reflux-related respiratory disease? Gastroenterology 2009;136(5, Suppl 1):A-287

53. Talaat M, Gad MS, Magdy EA, Aggag SM, Nour YA. *Helicobacter pylori* infection and chronic, persistent cough: is there an association? J Laryngol Otol 2007;121(10):962–967

54. Belafsky PC, Postma GN, Koufman JA. Validity and reliability of the reflux symptom index (RSI). J Voice 2002;16(2):274–277

55. Wo JM, Koopman J, Harrell SP, Parker K, Winstead W, Lentsch E. Double-blind, placebo-controlled trial with single-dose pantoprazole for laryngopharyngeal reflux. Am J Gastroenterol 2006;101(9):1972–1978, quiz 2169

56. Ylitalo R, Ramel S. Extraesophageal reflux in patients with contact granuloma: a prospective controlled study. Ann Otol Rhinol Laryngol 2002;111(5 Pt 1):441–446

57. Belafsky PC, Postma GN, Koufman JA. The validity and reliability of the reflux finding score (RFS). Laryngoscope 2001;111(8):1313–1317

58. Revicki DA, Wood M, Maton PN, Sorensen S. The impact of gastroesophageal reflux disease on health-related quality of life. Am J Med 1998;104(3):252–258

59. Carrau RL, Khidr A, Crawley JA, Hillson EM, Davis JK, Pashos CL. The impact of laryngopharyngeal reflux on patient-reported quality of life. Laryngoscope 2004;114(4):670–674

60. Cheung TK, Lam PK, Wei WI, et al. Quality of life in patients with laryngopharyngeal reflux. Digestion 2009;79(1):52–57

61. Siupsinskiene N, Adamonis K, Toohill RJ. Quality of life in laryngopharyngeal reflux patients. Laryngoscope 2007;117(3):480–484

62. McGlashan JA, Johnstone LM, Sykes J, Strugala V, Dettmar PW. The value of a liquid alginate suspension (Gaviscon Advance) in the management of laryngopharyngeal reflux. Eur Arch Otorhinolaryngol 2009;266(2):243–251

63. Strugala V, Dettmar PW. Alginate in the treatment of extra-esophageal reflux. In: Johnston N, Toohill RJ, eds. Effects, Diagnosis and Management of Extra-Esophageal Reflux. New York, NY: Nova Science Publishers Inc.; 2010:145–168

64. Karkos PD, Wilson JA. Empiric treatment of laryngopharyngeal reflux with proton pump inhibitors: a systematic review. Laryngoscope 2006;116(1):144–148

65. The National Institute of Clinical Excellence (NICE) Dyspepsia Guidelines. Management of dyspepsia in adults in primary care. Clinical Guideline 17. August 2004

66. Gillen D, Wirz AA, Ardill JE, McColl KEL. Rebound hypersecretion after omeprazole and its relation to on-treatment acid suppression and *Helicobacter pylori* status. Gastroenterology 1999;116(2):239–247

67. Boeckxstaens GE, Beamont H, Hatlebakk J, et al. Efficacy and tolerability of the novel reflux inhibitor, AZD3355, as an add-on treatment in GERD patients with symptoms despite proton pump inhibitor therapy. Gastroenterology 2009;136(Suppl):M1875

68. Keywood CGA, Wakefield M, Tack J. A proof of concept study evaluating the effect of ADX10059, a metatropic glutamate receptor-5 negative allosteric modulator, on acid exposure and symptoms in gastro-esophageal reflux disease. Gut 2009;59:1192–1199

31 Pediatric Laryngology: Diagnosis and Treatment of Congenital Anomalies

Yogesh Bajaj and Ben Hartley

The pediatric larynx is different from the adult larynx in size, shape, and position. The main functions of the larynx are providing breathing passage, prevention of aspiration, and voice production. As a result, the laryngeal anomalies present with symptoms related to these functions.

Laryngomalacia

Laryngomalacia or "floppy larynx" is the most common congenital anomaly of the pediatric larynx. It is the most common cause of stridor in young children. Nearly 50 to 75% of stridor in children in the general population can be attributed to laryngomalacia.[1] It is characterized by collapse of the supraglottic structures on inspiration. The spectrum of presentation of disease, progression, and outcomes varies. Some children have a mild stridor with no consequences, while others can have feeding difficulties or severe airway compromise.[2]

There are three theories of etiology.

1. Immature cartilage has been proposed but histopathology has demonstrated normal cartilage, and the absence of laryngomalacia in premature infants makes this unlikely.
2. A neuromuscular imbalance has been suggested. This may explain laryngomalacia in children with neurological disease but is unlikely to be the explanation in normal children.
3. A variant in normal anatomy that leads to progressive collapse over the early weeks of life before growth and increased rigidity lead to a reduction in symptoms. This seems most likely.

Most of the published literature suggests that the affected infants are likely to be male and term pregnancies in Caucasians. African-American infants of all gestational ages may be at risk and low birth weight may be a stronger predictor of laryngomalacia regardless of patients' gender and ethnicity.[3]

Gastroesophageal reflux disease contributes to feeding difficulties. Medical comorbidities, especially neurological abnormalities, heart disease, and associated anomalies contribute to disease severity and affect surgical outcomes.

Various classification systems have been proposed but offer little contribution to the clinical management. They are essentially descriptive. Three abnormalities are present to a greater or lesser degree: tightly curled epiglottis, short aryepiglottic folds, and prolapsing arytenoids (**Fig. 31.1**).

The history is highly suggestive of the diagnosis of laryngomalacia in most of the cases. These children usually present with an inspiratory stridor within the first 2 weeks of life. The stridor varies with position of the child and level of activity. The stridor is worse with crying and feeding and in supine position. On examination, subcostal retraction indicates severe obstruction and pectus excavatum indicates chronic obstruction. Severe cases may be associated with feeding difficulty, failure to thrive, intermittent complete obstruction, or cardiac failure.[4] The stridor usually increases in severity over the initial few months, being at its worst at 6 months of age. This improves and resolves gradually. The possibility of synchronous lesions should not be overlooked as 27% of the children presenting to a tertiary referral center with laryngomalacia can have synchronous airway anomalies.[5]

Most of the children with laryngomalacia have mild symptoms and do not require surgical intervention. The symptoms usually begin at 2 weeks of age and are at its worst by 6 months of age and then plateau and gradually start resolving. The majority of these will resolve spontaneously by 18 to 24 months. Children with reflux disease have improvement in their symptoms with antireflux medications.

Nearly 20% of children with laryngomalacia have airway or feeding symptoms severe enough to need surgical management. Children with severe disease and no other comorbidities should be offered aryepiglottoplasty and have good outcomes. Others with multiple medical comorbidities could be offered aryepiglottoplasty, but do not have good outcomes. Supraglottoplasty (**Fig. 31.2A, B**) encompasses any

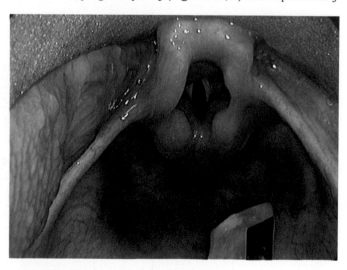

Figure 31.1 Endoscopic view of laryngomalacia.

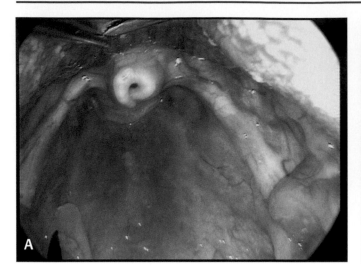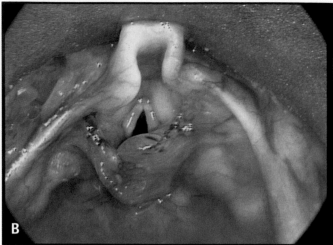

Figure 31.2   Endoscopic view of a child with laryngomalacia (A) before supraglottoplasty and (B) immediately after supraglottoplasty.

surgical procedure to modify flaccid obstructing supraglottic structures. The position and extent of the surgical excision is adapted to fit the individual patient's anomaly. Complications of the procedure include supraglottic stenosis, aspiration, dysphagia, and lower respiratory infections. Very rarely tracheostomy is required for severe cases of collapse of the supraglottis.

Clinical Pearls

- Laryngomalacia is the most common cause of stridor, but every stridor in a child is not laryngomalacia.
- Airway endoscopy should be performed early if there are any odd features in the history.
- Aryepiglottoplasty is a good surgical treatment, but the excision needs to be conservative to minimize complications.

Saccular Cyst/Laryngocele

The saccule is a pouch arising from the anterior end of the laryngeal ventricle. Saccular cyst or a laryngocele is an abnormal dilatation of the saccule. It is usually filled up with air and mucus.

A saccular cyst can be congenital or acquired. Its lumen is isolated from the interior of the larynx and it does not contain air. These features differentiate it from a laryngocele. A saccular cyst is also submucosal and is covered with normal mucous membrane. These cysts usually are secondary to developmental failure of patency of opening of the saccule or occlusion of the opening secondary to inflammation, trauma, or any other lesions. Two types of saccular cysts are lateral and anterior. The lateral saccular cyst extends posterosuperiorly into the false cord and aryepiglottic fold. The anterior cyst extends medially and posteriorly and protrudes into the laryngeal lumen.

A laryngocele can be internal or external. Internal laryngocele is confined to the interior of the larynx and

extends into the false cord and aryepiglottic fold. An external laryngocele extends laterally into the neck through the thyrohyoid membrane. Laryngoceles can also be congenital or acquired.

The presenting symptoms in these conditions are usually intermittent hoarseness and worsening dyspnea with crying. Other symptoms include weak cry or aphonia or inspiratory stridor.

Diagnosis is confirmed by airway endoscopy or magnetic resonance imaging (MRI) scan if indicated.

Treatment includes aspiration or excision or deroofing of the cyst. External approach for excision is considered if endoscopic approach is unsuccessful.

Vocal Cord Paralysis

Vocal cord paralysis in infants is the third most common cause of congenital stridor after laryngomalacia and congenital subglottic stenosis. It can be unilateral or bilateral. Bilateral cord palsy can be secondary to other congenital anomalies, that is, myelomeningocele, Arnold-Chari malformation, and hydrocephalus. This is the result of raised intracranial pressure.

Acquired vocal fold paralysis of one or both cords can follow a surgical procedure for tracheoesophageal fistula, neck surgery, or cardiothoracic surgery. The paralysis can also follow an external injury (strangulation and road traffic accident) or internal injury (endotracheal intubation or esophageal stethoscope.

Children with bilateral vocal cord palsy present with inspiratory stridor, which is usually high pitched. This is because of the paradoxical movement of vocal cords being further adducted during inspiration as a result of negative intrathoracic pressure, rather than expected abduction. During expiration, the paralyzed vocal cords abduct passively. Unilateral vocal cord palsy has more subtle symptoms such as coughing, choking, aspiration, breathy voice, and weak cry. These children only rarely will have stridor.

Both unilateral vocal cord paralysis and bilateral vocal cord paralysis need to be investigated, including detailed examination of the airways. Unless the cause is obvious from the history, because of the possibility of congenital cardiac or central nervous system anomalies, cardiology opinion (with echocardiogram) and a neurology opinion (with MRI of the brain) is essential. For unilateral palsy with no obvious cause, computed tomography scan from the skull base to the diaphragm is indicated in older children to exclude neoplasia.

Diagnosis of vocal cord palsy can be made by awake flexible laryngoscopy or laryngoscopy under general anesthesia. It is essential to differentiate paralysis from immobility due to anterior webbing, posterior glottic scarring, or cricoarytenoid joint fixation or an infiltrative lesion. Some centers perform ultrasound to diagnose/confirm cord palsy. Flow volume loops give an objective assessment of the degree of airway obstruction in bilateral cord palsy. Up to 45% of the patients may have other coexisting airway pathologies, so a formal airway endoscopy is essential.

Vocal cord paralysis in children usually resolves spontaneously within 6 to 24 months. If the recovery does not happen within 2 to 3 years, the chances of improvement are remote. The majority of children with unilateral and at least 50% with bilateral cord palsy can be managed conservatively. Surgical options for younger children include tracheostomy to bypass the obstruction caused by the paralyzed cords. Any operations on the vocal folds for bilateral paralysis are deferred until the child is at least 3 to 4 years of age to allow time for natural recovery. Any procedure to improve the airway is likely to have an adverse effect on the quality and volume of the voice. Surgical procedures are chosen on individual patient basis. Tracheostomy on its own gives the child a safe airway and does not affect the vocal cords and the potential of a good voice; however, it has the morbidities associated with it. Other surgical techniques focus on enlarging the glottic airway. The techniques include arytenoidectomy,[6] lateralization suture, cordectomy, and laser cordotomy.[7] In severe cases, laryngotracheal reconstruction with a posterior graft is an option. For unilateral paralysis, to reduce the aspiration and strengthen the voice, the options are of vocal cord injection or rarely thyroplasty.

Clinical Pearls

- Children with vocal cord palsy should have a full airway assessment to rule out any additional pathology.
- Surgical treatments to improve the airway do carry a small risk of worsening the voice.

Laryngeal Webs

Laryngeal webs are usually congenital. The majority of these are glottic, with an extension into the subglottis.

Children with a glottic web would usually present with voice change ranging from hoarseness to aphonia. The voice is usually high pitched. They can also present with varying degrees of airway obstruction depending on the extent of webbing. The glottic webs are classified according to Cohen's classification:

- Type I: Anterior web involving up to 35% of glottis. Symptoms include mild hoarseness and minimal airway obstruction.
- Type II: Anterior web involving 35 to 50% of glottis. The web may be thin or thick with subglottic extension. Symptoms include hoarse voice and some degree of airway obstruction.
- Type III: Anterior web involving 50 to 75% of glottis. Usually a thick glottic web with subglottic extension. Symptoms include airway obstruction and a weak voice.
- Type IV: Anterior web involving 75 to 90% of glottis with subglottic extension. Symptoms are severe airway obstruction and aphonia.

Posterior glottic webs are usually acquired as a result of scarring. An endotracheal tube sitting on the interarytenoid area long term can lead to chronic irritation that leads to scarring and web formation.

Subglottic webs on its own are much rarer than glottic web. These may be classified as congenital subglottic stenosis and managed accordingly. Glottic webs with subglottic extension or subglottic web have an associated abnormal elliptical-shaped cricoid ring.

Supraglottic webs are very rare. They may represent fusion of the false cords usually anteriorly. They may be asymptomatic or cause airway obstruction depending on the severity.

Suspicion of a web is raised with the history. The diagnosis is confirmed by a formal airway endoscopy under general anesthesia (**Fig. 31.3**). The thickness and extent of the web are confirmed by palpation.

Congenital laryngeal atresia is an acute emergency at birth and needs tracheostomy immediately. If the child survives, treatment is complicated because of grossly abnormal airway and multilevel stenosis.

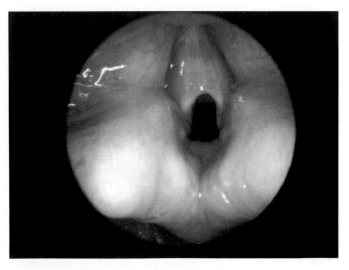

Figure 31.3 Endoscopic view of a laryngeal web.

Table 31.1 Grading of Stenosis according to Endotracheal Tube Size

Patient age		ID 2.0	ID 2.5	ID 3.0	ID 3.5	ID 4.0	ID 4.5	ID 5.0	ID 5.5	ID 6.0
Premature		40								
		58	30							
0–3 mo		68	48	26						
3–9 mo	No detectable lumen	75	59	41	22					
9 mo to 2 y		80	67	53	38	20				
2 y		84	74	62	50	35	19			
4 y		86	78	68	57	45	32	17		
6 y		89	81	73	64	54	43	30	16	
	Grade IV	Grade III				Grade II		Grade I		

Adapted from reference 10.
mo, month(s); y, year(s).

Management is tailored according to the severity of the symptom and the extent and thickness of the web. Type I glottic web if asymptomatic can be managed conservatively. The other option is of incision and balloon dilatation to improve the voice. Similarly, type II glottic webs can be managed by incision and balloon dilatation, but may need repeat endoscopic procedures, and the final results are not very good. The ideal treatment for grade II, grade III, and grade IV webs is laryngotracheal reconstruction with an anterior cartilage graft.[8] This treats both the glottic web and the associated congenital subglottic stenosis that is almost invariably present. Grades II and III should be aimed to be done as a single-stage procedure. Children with grade IV web might have a pre-existing tracheostomy and can be done as a two-stage procedure. Isolated posterior glottic webs can be treated with incision and balloon dilatation and, if unsuccessful, with laryngotracheal reconstruction with posterior graft. Children with multilevel stenosis will ultimately need a reconstruction tailor-made to their pathology.

Clinical Pearls

- Laryngeal webs usually have a thick subglottic component in addition to the obvious glottic component.
- Incision of the web does not have good results and tends to reformation of the web.
- Open reconstruction has good results.

Congenital Subglottic Stenosis

Congenital subglottic stenosis is the second most common cause of stridor in children after laryngomalacia.[9] This is due to defective canalization of the cricoid cartilage. This can be an isolated pathology or maybe associated with pathology in the glottis, supraglottis, or trachea. This is usually associated with a thickened elliptical cricoid cartilage and/or excess submucosal tissue.

The presenting symptoms include airway obstruction with biphasic stridor. The typical presentation is with episodes of recurrent croup starting in children younger than 1 year of age. The child might be asymptomatic apart from these episodes, which result from further airway narrowing after an upper respiratory tract illness on top of the underlying subglottic stenosis.

Diagnosis is confirmed at a formal airway endoscopy under general anesthesia. The assessment of the degree of stenosis is done objectively by checking the size of endotracheal tube the stenosis accepts with a leak on positive pressure. This is measured against the age-appropriate endotracheal tube for that child, and the stenosis is graded accordingly[10] as shown in **Table 31.1**.

Congenital subglottic stenosis on endoscopy examination is seen as an elliptical narrowing rather than circular (**Fig. 31.4**). This is as a result of the elliptical cricoid cartilage. The lumen is virtually normal anteroposteriorly, but narrow side to side.

Treatment varies from cricoid split to laryngotracheal reconstruction with anterior and/or posterior grafts or

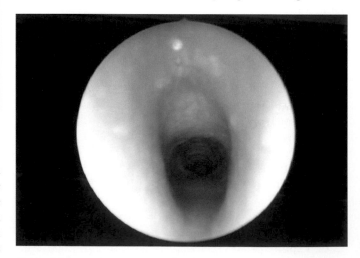

Figure 31.4 Endoscopic view of congenital subglottic stenosis.

partial cricotracheal resection for more severe stenosis. Endoscopic dilatation and laser resection are not advisable as they are ineffective in expanding a thickened ring of cricoid cartilage. Tracheostomy can be performed as a temporary measure for severely compromised airway.

Cricoid split is essentially a decompression operation. Diagnosis of exclusive subglottic stenosis should be confirmed. Any other associated pathology of the glottis (including vocal cord paresis), trachea, and bronchi should be ruled out. The neonate should weigh a minimum 1500 g and must have an adequate pulmonary reserve with no ventilatory support required 10 days before surgery. The oxygen requirement should be less than 30%. There should be no acute respiratory infection, congestive cardiac failure, or hypertension. The procedure is usually performed through a horizontal neck incision. The cricoid cartilage, lower half of the thyroid cartilage, and first two tracheal rings are divided in the midline. After the split, the child is intubated with an age-appropriate endotracheal tube. The endotracheal tube is left in place for 4 to 7 days when an extubation is attempted under steroid cover.

Clinical Pearls

- Congenital subglottic stenosis needs to be managed conservatively as far as possible.
- Cricoid ring needs to be split surgically for good outcomes.

Laryngeal Clefts

Laryngeal cleft is a congenital deficiency in the posterior laryngeal wall in the midline, extending to various degrees into the trachea. Laryngeal clefts are rare congenital anomalies and were first described in 1792 by Richter. The incidence is 1 in 10,000 to 20,000 births. Laryngeal clefts result from a failure of fusion of the posterior cricoid lamina and development of the tracheoesophageal septum.[11] Laryngeal clefts can be associated with tracheal agenesis or other congenital anomalies.[12] Laryngeal clefts can be seen in children with G syndrome, Opitz-Frias syndrome, and Pallister-Hall syndrome. Other associations include esophageal atresia with or without tracheoesophageal fistula, cleft lip and palate, congenital heart disease, gastrointestinal and genitourinary anomalies, and other midline anomalies such as hypospadias. Varying severity of reflux disease is universally seen in all children with laryngeal cleft.

Presenting symptoms of laryngeal cleft include aspiration and breathing difficulties. Aspiration during feeds results in choking and coughing bouts. The child might have a weak or absent cry. Inspiratory stridor can be present as a result of supraglottic structures collapsing into the laryngeal inlet. Expiratory stridor results if the child has significant tracheomalacia.

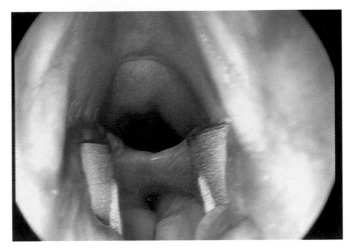

Figure 31.5 Endoscopic view showing laryngeal cleft type II.

Diagnosis of laryngeal cleft is suspected if there is a history of airway obstruction, aspiration, and weak voice. Videofluoroscopy will confirm aspiration. The diagnosis of laryngeal cleft is confirmed on a formal diagnostic airway examination under general anesthesia (**Fig. 31.5**). Careful examination of the interarytenoid and posterior larynx is required to assess the full extent of the defect, using a blunt probe. Also detailed examination of tracheobronchial tree is done to look for tracheoesophageal fistula or tracheobronchomalacia.

Laryngeal clefts are classified according to the length of the cleft in the posterior laryngeal wall as follows:

- Type I: Cleft extends down to vocal cords, not involving the cricoid.
- Type II: Cleft extends below the vocal cords into the cricoid, but not through the whole length of the cricoid.
- Type III: Cleft extends through the whole length of the cricoid, into the cervical trachea (**Fig. 31.6**).
- Type IV: Cleft extends into the thoracic trachea and may reach up to the carina.

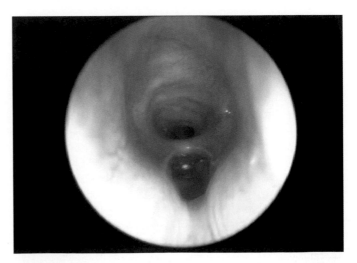

Figure 31.6 Laryngeal cleft type III.

Management of the laryngeal cleft is guided by the extent of the cleft. Type I laryngeal clefts can be managed by endoscopic repair.[13] If there is no evidence of aspiration clinically or on videofluoroscopy, the child can be managed conservatively. Surgical closure is clearly indicated if the child has definite aspiration.

Before any surgical intervention, gastroesophageal reflux needs to be managed adequately either medically or by Nissen fundoplication if required. Other congenital anomalies may be usually associated and should be looked for.

Type II clefts can be managed conservatively, by endoscopic[14] or open surgical repair.[13] Open surgical repair involves midline full laryngofissure to open the laryngeal framework for exposure and repair. Temporary tracheostomy is performed lower down for ventilation during the procedure. The margins of the cleft are excised under direct vision. The repair is performed in two separate layers, esophageal mucosal layer and tracheal mucosal layer. Some surgeons use fascia or muscle in between these two layers. The operation can be performed as a two-stage procedure if the child had a tracheostomy previously, which can be decannulated at a later date. The operation can also be done as a single-stage procedure, with the child kept intubated on the intensive care unit for 3 to 4 days after the operation.

Type III clefts will nearly always need an open surgical procedure because of the extent of the cleft.[15] The operation can be done as a single-stage or a two-stage procedure if the child had a tracheostomy previously. Usually a gastrostomy and Nissen fundoplication are required to control the reflux reliably.

Type IV clefts are very rare and only few children survive. The repair is done jointly with cardiothoracic surgeons as the exposure for repair needs midline sternotomy. Also the oxygenation during the operation is performed by an extracorporeal membrane oxygenation ECMO circuit or cardiopulmonary bypass.

Clinical Pearls

- Laryngeal cleft should be suspected in children with recurrent aspiration.
- Endoscopic or open surgical closure has good outcomes.

Subglottic Hemangioma

Subglottic hemangioma is a potentially life-threatening condition. It presents with stridor during the first few weeks or months of age.[16] Usually the child will present with a biphasic stridor and a normal cry.[17] The male to female ratio is reported as 1:2.[18] Nearly 50% of patients with a subglottic hemangioma display associated cutaneous hemangiomas, but only 1 to 2% of children with a cutaneous hemangioma also have a subglottic hemangioma. The diagnosis is confirmed on a laryngoscopy examination under general anesthesia. The classical appearance is an asymmetrical bluish/pinkish submucosal swelling in the subglottis (**Fig. 31.7**).

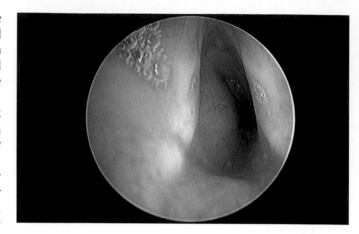

Figure 31.7 Endoscopic view of subglottic hemangioma.

The treatment options for large subglottic hemangiomata include steroids, laser ablation, open excision, tracheostomy, and more recently propranolol.[16,19] These lesions almost always eventually involute spontaneously, but the time course for involution is unpredictable, and tracheostomy may be required for several years.[18,20]

Steroids have been used as the mainstay of medical treatment for many years, but are associated with side effects from prolonged use.[21] Propranolol has been used more recently as a medical treatment for infantile hemangiomata[22] including subglottic hemangiomata.[23] Carbon dioxide laser treatment, although effective, carries a significant risk of subglottic stenosis. A policy of "wait and watch" can only be employed for hemangiomas with minor symptoms. A tracheostomy does not influence the natural course of the hemangioma and usually must remain in place for several years. Moreover, a tracheostomy has considerable consequences for general and speech development, is associated with respiratory tract infections, and has a mortality rate of 1 to 2%. Open surgical excision has been reported to be successful in several series.[19] Open surgical excision involves a midline laryngofissure approach followed by submucosal dissection and excision of the hemangioma covered by a temporary tracheostomy (**Fig. 31.8**). This is

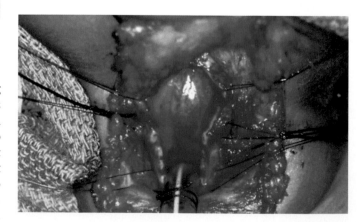

Figure 31.8 Open surgical excision of subglottic hemangioma via the laryngofissure approach.

usually done as a single-stage procedure with postoperative intubation for a few days. Propranolol has recently been used by various authors for subglottic hemangioma with good results.

Clinical Pearls

- Propranolol should be tried as the first-line medical treatment, but the treatment is prolonged and needs regular monitoring.
- Surgical excision has good results and is a one-stop treatment.
- Laryngomalacia is the most common congenital anomaly of the pediatric larynx and is the most common cause of stridor in young children. Children with severe disease and no other comorbidities should be offered aryepiglottoplasty and have good outcomes.
- Congenital subglottic stenosis is the second most common cause of stridor in children. Treatment varies from cricoid split to laryngotracheal reconstruction with anterior and/or posterior grafts or partial cricotracheal resection for more severe stenosis.
- Vocal cord paralysis in infants is the third most common cause of congenital stridor. Both unilateral vocal cord paralysis and bilateral vocal cord paralysis need to be investigated, including detailed examination of the airways. The majority of children with unilateral and at least 50% with bilateral cord palsy can be managed conservatively.
- Saccular cyst or a laryngocele is an abnormal dilatation of the saccule. A saccular cyst can be congenital or acquired. Treatment includes aspiration or excision or deroofing of the cyst.
- Laryngeal webs are usually congenital; the majority of these are glottic with an extension into the subglottis. Ideal treatment for severe webs is laryngotracheal reconstruction with an anterior cartilage graft.
- Laryngeal cleft is a congenital deficiency in the posterior laryngeal wall in the midline, extending to various degrees into the trachea. Treatment is usually endoscopic or open surgical repair.

References

1. Holinger PH, Johnson KC, Schiller F. Congenital anomalies of the larynx. Ann Otol Rhinol Laryngol 1954;63(3):581–606
2. Thompson DM. Laryngomalacia: factors that influence disease severity and outcomes of management. Curr Opin Otolaryngol Head Neck Surg 2010;18(6):564–570
3. Edmondson NE, Bent JP III, Chan C. Laryngomalacia: the role of gender and ethnicity. Int J Pediatr Otorhinolaryngol 2011;75(12):1562–1564
4. Zalzal GH, Anon JB, Cotton RT. Epiglottoplasty for the treatment of laryngomalacia. Ann Otol Rhinol Laryngol 1987;96(1 Pt 1):72–76
5. Gonzalez C, Reilly JS, Bluestone CD. Synchronous airway lesions in infancy. Ann Otol Rhinol Laryngol 1987;96(1 Pt 1):77–80
6. Worley G, Bajaj Y, Cavalli L, Hartley B. Laser arytenoidectomy in children with bilateral vocal fold immobility. J Laryngol Otol 2007;121(1):25–27
7. Bajaj Y, Sethi N, Shayah A, et al. Vocal fold paralysis: role of bilateral transverse cordotomy. J Laryngol Otol 2009;123(12):1348–1351
8. Wyatt ME, Hartley BE. Laryngotracheal reconstruction in congenital laryngeal webs and atresias. Otolaryngol Head Neck Surg 2005;132(2):232–238
9. Holinger LD, Holinger PC, Holinger PH. Etiology of bilateral abductor vocal cord paralysis: a review of 389 cases. Ann Otol Rhinol Laryngol 1976;85(4 Pt 1):428–436
10. Myer CM III, O'Connor DM, Cotton RT. Proposed grading system for subglottic stenosis based on endotracheal tube sizes. Ann Otol Rhinol Laryngol 1994;103(4 Pt 1):319–323
11. Pezzettigotta SM, Leboulanger N, Roger G, Denoyelle F, Garabédian EN. Laryngeal cleft. Otolaryngol Clin North Am 2008;41(5):913–933, ix
12. Holinger LD, Volk MS, Tucker GF Jr. Congenital laryngeal anomalies associated with tracheal agenesis. Ann Otol Rhinol Laryngol 1987;96(5):505–508
13. Thiel G, Clement WA, Kubba H. The management of laryngeal clefts. Int J Pediatr Otorhinolaryngol 2011;75(12):1525–1528
14. Rahbar R, Chen JL, Rosen RL, et al. Endoscopic repair of laryngeal cleft type I and type II: when and why? Laryngoscope 2009;119(9):1797–1802
15. Kubba H, Gibson D, Bailey M, Hartley BE. Techniques and outcomes of laryngeal cleft repair: an update to the Great Ormond Street Hospital series. Ann Otol Rhinol Laryngol 2005;114(4):309–313
16. Wiatrak BJ, Reilly JS, Seid AB, Pransky SM, Castillo JV. Open surgical excision of subglottic hemangioma in children. Int J Pediatr Otorhinolaryngol 1996;34(1–2):191–206
17. McGill TJ. Vascular anomalies of the head and neck. In: Wetmore RF, Muntz HR, McGill TJ, eds. Pediatric Otolaryngology. New York, NY: Thieme Medical Publishers; 2000:87–100
18. Brodsky L, Yoshpe N, Ruben RJ. Clinical-pathological correlates of congenital subglottic hemangiomas. Ann Otol Rhinol Laryngol Suppl 1983;105:4–18
19. Bajaj Y, Hartley BEJ, Wyatt ME, Albert DM, Bailey CM. Subglottic haemangioma in children: experience with open surgical excision. J Laryngol Otol 2006;120(12):1033–1037
20. Pierce MK. Subglottic hemangiomas in infants. A presumptive clinical test for diagnosis. Ann Otol Rhinol Laryngol 1962;71:1057–1062
21. George ME, Sharma V, Jacobson J, Simon S, Nopper AJ. Adverse effects of systemic glucocorticosteroid therapy in infants with hemangiomas. Arch Dermatol 2004;140(8):963–969
22. Buckmiller LM, Munson PD, Dyamenahalli U, Dai Y, Richter GT. Propranolol for infantile hemangiomas: early experience at a tertiary vascular anomalies center. Laryngoscope 2010;120(4):676–681
23. Truong MT, Perkins JA, Messner AH, Chang KW. Propranolol for the treatment of airway hemangiomas: a case series and treatment algorithm. Int J Pediatr Otorhinolaryngol 2010;74(9):1043–1048

32 Pediatric Laryngology: Diagnosis and Treatment of Acquired Disorders of the Larynx

Yogesh Bajaj and Ben Hartley

Subglottic Stenosis

Subglottic stenosis is one of the common causes of airway obstruction in children. Subglottis extends from the inferior surface of the true vocal cords up to inferior margin of the cricoid cartilage.[1] The diameter of the normal subglottic lumen is 4.5 to 5.5 mm in a full-term infant and 3.5 mm in a premature infant. The diameter of subglottis less than 4 mm in a full-term infant is considered narrow.

Subglottic stenosis can be classified on the basis of etiology into congenital or acquired. Other classifications are based on the characteristics, for example, soft or hard stenosis and degree of stenosis.

Congenital subglottic stenosis is by definition when there is no apparent cause for the stenosis, for example, trauma or prolonged intubation. This has been discussed in detail in the congenital anomalies of larynx (Chapter 31). Acquired subglottic stenosis patients have a history of prolonged intubation or laryngeal trauma. Vast majority (90%) of acquired stenosis are secondary to prolonged endotracheal intubation.[2] The incidence of subglottic stenosis after intubation in children ranges from 0.9 to 8.3%. The incidence of acquired subglottic stenosis following neonatal intubation is reported as less than 1%[3] and is usually a result of prolonged endotracheal intubation.

Prolonged endotracheal intubation is well tolerated in neonatal age group as the cricoid cartilage is relatively immature.[4] As the child grows, the cricoid cartilage becomes more fibrous and rigid, and as a result, the larynx becomes less tolerant of the intubation in older children. Ischemic injury occurs if the pressure exerted by the endotracheal tube is greater than the capillary pressure. Ischemia leads to edema, pressure necrosis, and finally ulceration of the mucosa. These ulcerations eventually heal up by forming granulation tissues and eventually scarring causing subglottic stenosis.

The factors that predispose to the development of subglottic stenosis include gastroesophageal reflux; shape and size of larynx (congenital subglottic stenosis); duration of intubation; size of endotracheal tube; repeated intubations; traumatic intubation; sepsis; systemic factors (malnutrition, hypoxemia); chronic inflammatory disorders; external laryngeal injury; chemical and thermal injury; and benign or malignant neoplasms (papillomas, hemangiomas). The use of a large-diameter endotracheal tube even for a short period can lead to ischemic ulceration and scarring. Poor fixation of the tube allowing movement also causes injury.

Measures taken to prevent subglottic stenosis include use of an uncuffed tube placed via a nasal route that reduces potential tube movement to a minimum. Injury to the airway is less likely with a small tube that allows a small leak on positive pressure ventilation. Good nursing care and hygiene are paramount.[5]

Symptoms of acquired subglottic stenosis include biphasic stridor, with a normal cry/voice. In an intubated child, the presentation is usually failure to extubate or accepting smaller than age-appropriate tube. Signs include increased work of breathing and use of accessory muscles of respiration.

Subglottic stenosis is evaluated by a direct laryngotracheobronchoscopy examination under a general anesthetic (**Figs. 32.1** to **32.3**). A complete assessment of the airway is required to confirm the suspected diagnosis and to rule out any coexisting tracheobronchial pathology. The exact diameter of the stenosis is measured by passing various sizes of endotracheal tubes and graded using the Myer-Cotton grading system for the stenosis.[6] In addition, an assessment is made of the length of the stenosis and if it is a soft or firm stenosis. The assessment of the degree of stenosis is performed objectively by checking the size of endotracheal tube the stenosis accepts with a leak on positive pressure. This is measured against the age-appropriate endotracheal tube for that child, and the stenosis is graded accordingly[6] as shown in **Table 32.1.**

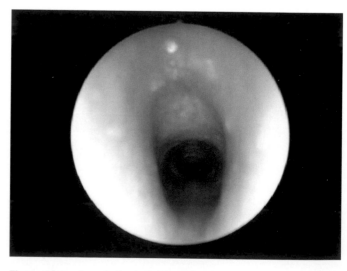

Figure 32.1 A grade II subglottic stenosis.

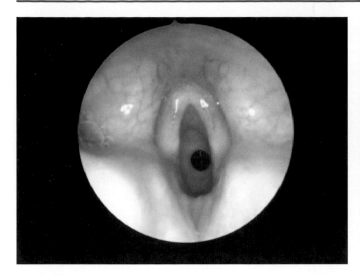

Figure 32.2   A grade III subglottic stenosis.

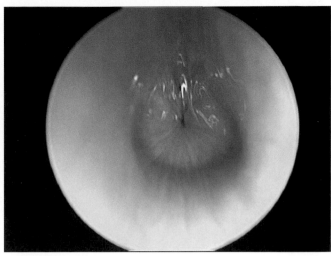

Figure 32.3   A grade IV subglottic stenosis.

The management of subglottic stenosis depends on the severity, location, and type (soft/firm) of stenosis. Surgery is the primary treatment modality via either an open or an endoscopic approach. Grade I stenosis can be managed simply under the watchful eye of a qualified surgeon. Grade II stenosis can be treated by endoscopic procedures, that is, incision ± balloon dilatation. Endoscopic procedures may need to be repeated on a regular basis. If endoscopic management is not successful, then open procedure may be required. Grade III and IV stenosis will require open procedures.

The two most common open procedures are laryngotracheal reconstruction (LTR) and partial cricotracheal resection (CTR). LTR involves splitting the cricoid cartilage and expanding the framework with a cartilage graft. Partial CTR involves segmental excision of the stenotic segment, preserving the posterior cricoid plate, and an end-to-end anastomosis.[7] The management of pediatric airway reconstruction has changed considerably since its introduction in the 1970s.

Surgical correction of subglottic stenosis was first attempted by Negus,[8] using laryngofissure and dermal grafting in adults. Rethi[9] reported splitting the cricoid ring anteriorly and posteriorly in adults. Aboulker[7] (1966) introduced a stent that could be wired into the tracheostomy tube. Grahne[10] first described the application of the Rethi procedure to children. Doig et al[11] reported using a cartilage graft positioned in an anterior cricoid split to expand the cricoid ring, and then Evans and Todd[12] described laryngotracheoplasty, which involved splitting the trachea and cricoid using a castellated incision and re-suturing it in an open manner over a stent. Cotton, unaware of Doig's publication in the German literature,

Table 32.1   Grading of Stenosis According to Endotracheal Tube Size

Patient age (years)		ID 2.0	ID 2.5	ID 3.0	ID 3.5	ID 4.0	ID 4.5	ID 5.0	ID 5.5	ID 6.0
Premature	No detectable lumen	40								
		58	30							
0–3/12		68	48	26						
3–9/12		75	59	41	22					
9/12–2		80	67	53	38	20				
2		84	74	62	50	35	19			
4		86	78	68	57	45	32	17		
6		89	81	73	64	54	43	30	16	
	Grade IV	Grade III			Grade II		Grade I			

The Myer-Cotton grading system: Grade I, <50% obstruction; Grade II, 51–70% obstruction; Grade III, 71–99% obstruction; Grade IV, no detectable lumen.

separately introduced the LTR with cartilage grafting (1978) after earlier animal work with Fearon[13] and developed it into the preferred technique for framework expansion. In the 1970s and 80s, laryngotracheoplasty and LTR were the main surgical procedures, and Cotton & Evans[2] reported a 5-year follow-up of LTR in children. The next development was single-stage LTR, using an endotracheal tube as an airway and stent.[14,15] Monnier et al[16] published the first series of successful CTRs in children.

In general, LTR with costal cartilage grafting is the mainstay of surgical management for grade II and mild-grade III subglottic stenosis. Mild stenosis can be treated with an anterior graft and isolated posterior scarring or stenosis with a posterior graft. Severe stenosis needs both anterior and posterior grafts. In general, LTR is a less complex and extensive procedure than CTR, because tracheal mobilization is not required. For grade IV stenosis and severe grade III stenosis, the preferred option is CTR. By definition, in a two-stage LTR, the tracheostomy tube is kept in place at the conclusion of the procedure, and the patient is decannulated several weeks later. The single-stage LTR allows immediate decannulation at the time of the reconstruction, or avoidance of tracheostomy altogether.

LTR with autologous cartilage grafts has been demonstrated to be an effective and reliable technique for the surgical management of subglottic stenosis. Good results have been reported from many different institutions around the world.[17–20] Generally, the two-stage LTR is advocated in children with complex multilevel stenosis, significant neurological deficits, significant lung disease, or cases where reintubation is anatomically difficult (e.g., craniofacial anomalies).[21] Some authors perform two-stage LTR in cases with severe stenosis,[19,22] although many others advocate partial CTR in selected cases with grade III/IV subglottic stenosis where the disease is separated from the glottis by an adequate margin.[7,23]

Pediatric airway stenosis presents with varying degrees of severity and significant comorbidities. The choice of operation for reconstructing the airway must be considered carefully by the surgeon depending upon which modality is considered likely to achieve safe and expeditious surgical reconstruction in each individual patient.

The final results of LTR are generally expressed in terms of decannulation rates. Most of the patients who have a tracheostomy undergo surgery primarily to get rid of the tracheostomy, and thus decannulation does become an important outcome measure. For those patients who did not have a tracheostomy before the LTR, the outcomes were based on the improvement in their symptoms and the airway endoscopy findings before and after the procedure.

Clinical Pearls

- The incidence of acquired subglottic stenosis is increasing as more preterm children are surviving with history of prolonged intubation at some stage.
- The treatment needs to be tailored to the individual patients' symptoms and severity of the stenosis.

Acute Laryngotracheobronchitis

Acute laryngotracheobronchitis or "croup" is one of the common inflammatory conditions of the pediatric airway. This accounts for a nearly 90% of acute infections leading to respiratory distress.[24] Croup is associated with an upper respiratory infection and is more common in winter. Most of the children are between 6 months and 3 years of age at presentation. Of all children, 3 to 5% would have had one episode of croup in their lifetime, and of these 5% will continue to have recurrent episodes of croup.[25]

The underlying etiology is subglottic edema following an upper respiratory tract infection. Children with recurrent croup might have an underlying congenital subglottic stenosis. This is primarily a viral illness caused by parainfluenza (types I and II), respiratory syncytial virus, and influenza A and B. On the basis of history and examination findings, the diagnosis of croup is clinical. The child has coryzal symptoms in association with a brassy cough. The child usually has a hoarse voice and a biphasic stridor. X-ray of neck anteroposterior view demonstrates a "steeple" sign indicating narrowing in the subglottis (**Fig. 32.4**).

Treatment of croup is aimed at reducing inflammation in the airway and improving symptoms. Single dose of oral corticosteroid is the first-line treatment for croup.[26] This has been reported in a meta-analysis of randomized controlled trials that this reduces return to hospital rates and rates of admission to the hospital. In addition, it has been shown that a dose of dexamethasone 0.15 mg/kg is as effective as a larger dose. Steroids act by reducing the capillary endothelial permeability, decreasing mucosal edema, stabilizing the lysosomal membranes, and decreasing the inflammatory reaction. Nebulized adrenaline provides symptomatic relief

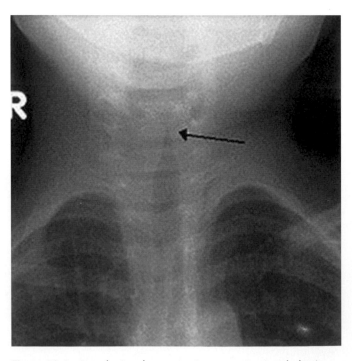

Figure 32.4 Steeple sign demonstrating narrowing in subglottis.

in the moderate to severe cases.[26] Nebulized adrenaline causes vasoconstriction of the subglottic edema and provides transient symptomatic relief till the systemic steroids start having their effect. Limited data suggest that heliox may have some role in refractory cases, though data on efficacy of humidified oxygen are lacking.[27] If treatment with steroids and adrenaline fails, then the child is taken to the operating theater for endoscopy and intubation to confirm the diagnosis and secure the airway.

> **Clinical Pearls**
>
> - Croup is managed medically in the majority of cases.
> - Recurrent croup warrants a detailed airway examination to look for an underlying subglottic stenosis.

Acute Epiglottitis

Acute epiglottitis or supraglottitis is a fulminant infection of the supraglottic larynx. The etiology is supraglottic edema secondary to a bacterial infection. The most common causative organism used to be *Haemophilus influenzae* type B (HIB), but since the HIB vaccine, other pathogens such as *Candida albicans*, *H. parainfluenzae*, and *Staphylococcus aureus* are the common causative organisms now. The supraglottic edema leads to pain on swallowing and respiratory distress. The common age at presentation varies from 1 to 5 years though the child can get supraglottitis at any age.

The child usually presents with symptoms of upper respiratory infection and odynophagia. On examination, the child looks toxic, pale, and is drooling. Usually, the child is sitting up, leaning forward with mouth open and drooling, and has a hot potato voice. As the inflammation progresses, the child will have symptoms of respiratory distress, including stridor and muffled voice.

The diagnosis is on clinical basis. The child should not be distressed by attempting intraoral examination or IV cannulation and should be allowed to be comforted by parents. The child should not be sent for an X-ray, though the classical appearance on a lateral view of the neck is a "thumbprint sign." The child should be given humidified oxygen, and the senior most ENT surgeon and an anesthetist should be contacted. The child should be taken directly to the operating theater to confirm the diagnosis and secure the airway. The child is anesthetized, and the diagnosis is confirmed at direct laryngoscopy (**Fig. 32.5**). Once the diagnosis is confirmed, the child is intubated using an introducer or an endotracheal tube over a rigid endoscope. If intubation fails, then need to proceed to tracheostomy. The child needs to be treated with high-dose cephalosporins. Steroids are added to the treatment to help reduce the edema. Extubation is attempted when the swollen epiglottis has subsided and there is a leak around the tube.

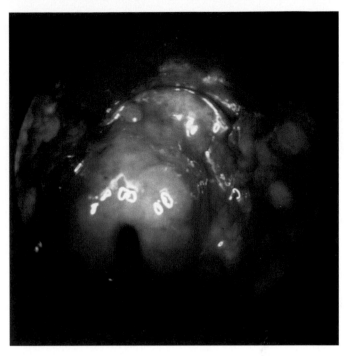

Figure 32.5   Acute epiglottitis.

> **Clinical Pearls**
>
> - Acute epiglottitis in a child should be managed by an experienced ENT surgeon and anesthetist in an operation theater setting.
> - Treatment is medical, with high-dose antibiotics and steroids.

Recurrent Respiratory Papillomatosis

Recurrent respiratory papillomatosis (RRP) is a disease characterized by the development of papillomas in the respiratory tract. It is caused by human papilloma virus (HPV) subtypes 6 and 11. Maternal genital warts have been implicated in the development of RRP, but exact relationship has not been established. Usually, earlier onset disease is more aggressive. More aggressive disease is associated with HPV 11 rather than with HPV 6 subtype.[28]

The presenting symptoms are persistent hoarseness and various degree of airway obstruction. The diagnosis is confirmed at a formal airway assessment under a general anesthetic. The papillomas usually arise within the larynx, specifically the true vocal cords, false cords, subglottis, and the laryngeal surface of the epiglottis (**Figs. 32.6** and **32.7**). They may be spread to areas beyond the airways, that is, palate, tonsils, nasopharynx, nasal cavities, pharynx, and esophagus.

HPV has a specific affinity for squamous epithelial tissue. HPV DNA integrates in the basal epithelial layer within the epithelial transition zones in the airway, at the junction of the squamous and ciliated epithelium. The virus proliferates

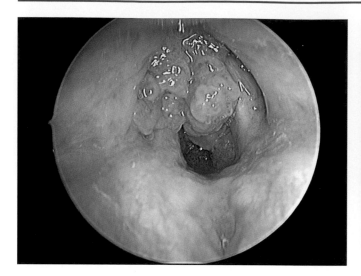

Figure 32.6 Extensive papillomas in the larynx.

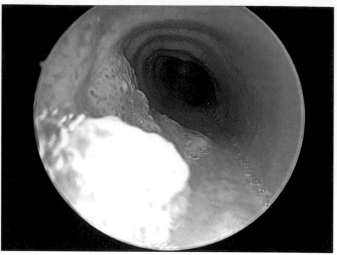

Figure 32.7 Papillomas in the trachea.

and stimulates the growth of the overlying epithelial layers, resulting in papilloma formation. Histology examination of these papillomas appears as exophytic projection of keratinized, stratified squamous epithelium overlying a fibrovascular core.

The course of the disease is unpredictable. Although spontaneous remission is possible, pulmonary spread and malignant transformation has been reported in severe cases. Healthy cells within the respiratory tract may harbor latent virus particles, which explains the tendency of papillomas to recur after an apparent resolution of the disease.[29] For some of the patients, the disease involutes around the time of puberty, which led to the belief that hormonally induced alterations of the immune system may be responsible for involution of the disease.[30]

The management of this condition is still challenging, as no specific definitive treatment exists. Surgical excision aims to provide an adequate airway and to improve and maintain the voice. Recommended surgical treatments include removal with cold steel instruments, use of carbon dioxide laser, or excision using a microdebrider which is the gold standard at present. Laser excision vaporizes the papillomas precisely, whereas with repeated procedures, the same procedure results in more scarring in the larynx when compared with cold steel excision using a microdebrider. In addition, as the microdebrider works on the principle of suction and excision, the potential of virus spread/inoculation is reduced.

RRP usually remains localized to the larynx, but may become aggressive and spread beyond the larynx into rest of the airway. The papillomas can extend into the trachea and bronchi as well as spread to involve lung parenchyma. Squamous cell carcinomas can arise in children with long-standing RRP.

Adjuvant therapies should be considered if the child needs surgical excisions at very short intervals. Intralesional cidofovir can be used at the base of the lesion after the papilloma has been excised.[31]

Recent development of vaccine against HPV could be effective in treating RRP in addition to preventing HPV infections. It is possible that the vaccine may decrease the prevalence of HPV disease in women and subsequently decrease the incidence of RRP in children. There is no evidence at present that existing patients with RRP will benefit with the vaccine or not.

Clinical Pearls

- Prolonged hoarse voice in a child warrants an airway endoscopy to rule out papillomas or other airway conditions.
- Excision using a laryngeal microdebrider is the gold standard for respiratory papillomatosis.
- Tracheostomy should be avoided as far as possible in children with papillomas.
- Subglottic stenosis is one of the common causes of airway obstruction in children. A complete assessment of the airway is required to confirm the suspected diagnosis and rule out any coexisting tracheobronchial pathology.
- The management of subglottic stenosis depends on the severity, location, and type (soft/firm) of stenosis. Surgery is the primary treatment modality via either an open or an endoscopic approach. The two most common open procedures are LTR and partial CTR.
- Acute laryngotracheobronchitis or "croup" is one of the common inflammatory conditions of the pediatric airway. Single dose of oral corticosteroid is the first-line treatment for croup.
- If croup fails to respond to steroids and adrenaline, then the child is taken to operating theater for endoscopy and intubation to confirm the diagnosis and secure the airway.

- Acute epiglottitis or supraglottitis is a fulminant infection of the supraglottic larynx. The child should be taken directly to the operating theater to confirm the diagnosis and secure the airway.
- RRP is caused by HPV subtypes 6 and 11.
- The management of respiratory papillomas is challenging, as no specific definitive treatment exists. Surgical excision aims to provide an adequate airway and to improve and maintain the voice.

References

1. Holinger PH, Johnson KC, Schiller F. Congenital anomalies of the larynx. Ann Otol Rhinol Laryngol 1954;63(3):581–606
2. Cotton RT, Evans JN. Laryngotracheal reconstruction in children. Five-year follow-up. Ann Otol Rhinol Laryngol 1981;90(5 Pt 1):516–520
3. Ratner I, Whitfield J. Acquired subglottic stenosis in the very-low-birth-weight infant. Am J Dis Child 1983;137(1):40–43
4. Hawkins DB. Hyaline membrane disease of the neonate prolonged intubation in management: effects on the larynx. Laryngoscope 1978;88(2 Pt 1):201–224
5. Cotton RT, Myer CM III. Contemporary surgical management of laryngeal stenosis in children. Am J Otolaryngol 1984;5(5):360–368
6. Myer CM III, O'Connor DM, Cotton RT. Proposed grading system for subglottic stenosis based on endotracheal tube sizes. Ann Otol Rhinol Laryngol 1994;103(4 Pt 1):319–323
7. Hartley BEJ, Cotton RT. Paediatric airway stenosis: laryngotracheal reconstruction or cricotracheal resection? Clin Otolaryngol Allied Sci 2000;25(5):342–349
8. Negus VE. Treatment of chronic stenosis of the larynx with special reference to skin grafting. Ann Otol Rhinol Laryngol 1938;47:891–901
9. Rethi A. An operation for cicatrical stenosis of the larynx. J Laryngol Otol 1953;70:283–296
10. Grahne B. Operative treatment of severe chronic traumatic laryngeal stenosis in infants up to three years old. Acta Otolaryngol 1971;72(1):134–137
11. Doig C, Eckstein HB, Waterston DJ. The surgical treatment of laryngeal and subglottic obstruction in infancy and childhood. Z Kinderchir Grenzgeb 1973;12:299–303
12. Evans JNG, Todd GB. Laryngo-tracheoplasty. J Laryngol Otol 1974;88(7):589–597
13. Fearon B, Cotton RT. Surgical correction of subglottic stenosis of the larynx. Prelimenary report of an experimental surgical technique. Ann Otol Rhinol Laryngol 1972;81(4):508–513
14. Cotton RT, Myer CM III, O'Connor DM, Smith ME. Pediatric laryngotracheal reconstruction with cartilage grafts and endotracheal tube stenting: the single-stage approach. Laryngoscope 1995;105(8 Pt 1):818–821
15. Seid AB, Pransky SM, Kearns DB. One-stage laryngotracheoplasty. Arch Otolaryngol Head Neck Surg 1991;117(4):408–410
16. Monnier P, Savary M, Chapuis G. Partial cricoid resection with primary tracheal anastomosis for subglottic stenosis in infants and children. Laryngoscope 1993;103(11 Pt 1):1273–1283
17. Cotton RT. Management of subglottic stenosis in infancy and childhood. Review of a consecutive series of cases managed by surgical reconstruction. Ann Otol Rhinol Laryngol 1978;87 (5 Pt 1):649–657
18. Cotton RT, O'Connor DM. Paediatric laryngotracheal reconstruction: 20 years' experience. Acta Otorhinolaryngol Belg 1995;49(4): 367–372
19. McQueen CT, Shapiro NL, Leighton S, Guo XG, Albert DM. Single-stage laryngotracheal reconstruction: the Great Ormond Street experience and guidelines for patient selection. Arch Otolaryngol Head Neck Surg 1999;125(3):320–322
20. Zalzal GH. Treatment of laryngotracheal stenosis with anterior and posterior cartilage grafts. A report of 41 children. Arch Otolaryngol Head Neck Surg 1993;119(1):82–86
21. Gustafson LM, Hartley BEJ, Liu JH, et al Single-stage laryngotracheal reconstruction in children: a review of 200 cases. Otolaryngol Head Neck Surg 2000;123(4):430–434
22. Agrawal N, Black M, Morrison G. Ten-year review of laryngotracheal reconstruction for paediatric airway stenosis. Int J Pediatr Otorhinolaryngol 2007;71(5):699–703
23. Rutter MJ, Hartley BEJ, Cotton RT. Cricotracheal resection in children. Arch Otolaryngol Head Neck Surg 2001;127(3):289–292
24. Skolnik NS. Treatment of croup. A critical review. Am J Dis Child 1989;143(9):1045–1049
25. Battaglia JD. Severe croup: the child with fever and upper airway obstruction. Pediatr Rev 1986;7(8):227–233
26. Pitluk JD, Uman H, Safranek S. Clinical inquiries. What's best for croup? J Fam Pract 2011;60(11):680–681
27. Brown JC. The management of croup. Br Med Bull 2002;61:189–202
28. Wiatrak BJ, Wiatrak DW, Broker TR, Lewis L. Recurrent respiratory papillomatosis: a longitudinal study comparing severity associated with human papilloma viral types 6 and 11 and other risk factors in a large pediatric population. Laryngoscope 2004;114(11 Pt 2, Suppl 104)1–23
29. Abramson AL, Steinberg BM, Winkler B. Laryngeal papillomatosis: clinical, histopathologic and molecular studies. Laryngoscope 1987;97(6):678–685
30. Corbitt G, Zarod AP, Arrand JR, Longson M, Farrington WT. Human papilloma virus (HPV) genotypes associated with laryngeal papilloma. J Clin Pathol 1988;41(3):284–288
31. Mandell DL, Arjmand EM, Kay DJ, Casselbrant ML, Rosen CA. Intralesional cidofovir for pediatric recurrent respiratory papillomatosis. Arch Otolaryngol Head Neck Surg 2004;130(11):1319–1323

33 Tracheostomy

Shalini Arulanandam and Jeevendra Kanagalingam

History

Tracheostomy is an ancient operation designed to relieve upper airway obstruction and prevent death by asphyxiation. The aim of the procedure is to create a hole in the anterior wall of the trachea to help patients breathe—bypassing any obstruction in the airway at the level of the larynx or above.

The word *tracheostomy* is derived from Greek words *trachea* for windpipe and *stoma* for mouth. The correct term for the operation should be *tracheotomy*, as the Greek suffix *tomo* means *to cut*. The word tracheotomy first appeared in print in 1649, but was not commonly used until a century later when it was introduced by the German surgeon Lorenz Heister in 1718.[1]

The early days of tracheostomy were dogged by controversy, as many reputable physicians such as Hippocrates were opposed to the operation because of its high mortality and morbidity rate. Although there are several documentations of surgeons performing tracheotomies as lifesaving procedures from the 1500s, it was not until 1825 when Bretonneu reported a successful tracheotomy in a 5-year-old girl with diphtheria did the operation regain its popularity. Trousseau later reported 200 cases of tracheotomy for diphtheria—giving legitimacy to the operation—despite only 50 of his cases surviving the operation!

In the early days, tracheostomies were often performed "high," entering the trachea via the larynx, thereby dividing the cricoid cartilage. This led to laryngeal stenosis. A "low" tracheostomy (entering the trachea directly) was discouraged as dividing the thyroid isthmus was frowned upon. In 1923, Chevalier Jackson of Pittsburgh recognized that dividing the cricoid led to stenosis. He described placement of the tracheostomy below the first tracheal ring and the necessary meticulous aftercare. Due to his contributions, mortality from tracheostomy plummeted from 25% to 1 or 2%, and he is rightfully regarded as the father of the modern tracheostomy.[2]

Indications and Contraindications

There are really only three indications for a tracheostomy: upper airway obstruction, prolonged ventilation, and tracheobronchial toilet.

Upper Airway Obstruction

As diphtheria is no longer a major scourge, fewer emergent tracheostomies are performed for upper airway obstruction. The most common causes for upper airway obstruction requiring a tracheostomy would be neoplasm of the larynx, pharynx, or other sites in the neck; head, maxillofacial, or neck trauma; and neck abscesses and neurological conditions such as bilateral vocal cord paralysis (**Table 33.1**). Even in these situations, intubation is often possible, and tracheostomy then becomes an elective procedure. Complex head and neck surgery often begins with an elective tracheostomy, as upper airway obstruction is anticipated postoperatively.[3]

In pediatric patients, the most common indications for tracheostomy are subglottic stenosis, bilateral vocal cord paralysis, congenital airway malformations, and tumors.[4]

Prolonged Ventilation

Today, the most common indication for tracheostomy is for patients who require prolonged ventilation. This enables patients on mechanical ventilation to be extubated and potentially reduces the duration of an intensive care unit (ICU) admission. There is much debate as to when a tracheostomy should be performed in an intubated patient. Recent reviews have shown that whether a tracheostomy is performed early (within 10 days of intubation) or late (after 10 days of intubation) does not have an impact on the patients' mortality in hospital or morbidity from pneumonia, beyond reducing their ICU stay.[5,6]

Ideally, however, because of the risk of irreversible damage to glottic mucosa from an endotracheal tube (ETT), a patient should have an elective tracheostomy if he is unlikely to be extubated within 7 days of intubation. There is an oft-quoted dictum attributed to Moser "the time to do a tracheostomy is when you first think of it" which has much truth in it.

Tracheobronchial Toilet

In patients in whom the cough reflex is poor, saliva is chronically aspirated with retention of mucus in the tracheobronchial tree; thus, tracheostomy allows for suctioning and tracheobronchial "toilet." It is important to note that tracheostomy per se does not obliterate the risk of aspiration. Indeed, some patients may aspirate as a result of a tracheostomy. Therefore, aspiration is not in itself an indication for tracheostomy if a patient can cough adequately and clear their secretions.

There are very few absolute contraindications to a tracheostomy when the indication for one is clear. The method of tracheostomy however depends on many factors – both anatomical and physiological—and percutaneous dilatational tracheostomy (PDT) may be contraindicated in certain circumstances[7] (**Table 33.2**).

Table 33.1   Common Causes of Upper Airway Obstruction Requiring Tracheostomy in Adults and Children

Adult	Pediatric

• Neoplasm
  ○ Larynx
  ○ Thyroid
  ○ Other neck sites
• Trauma
  ○ Head
  ○ Maxillofacial
  ○ Neck
• Infection
  ○ Neck abscesses
  ○ Tetanus
• Others
  ○ Neurological
  ○ Foreign body aspiration
	• Congenital
	  ○ Subglottic stenosis
	  ○ Bilateral vocal cord paralysis
	  ○ Congenital airway malformations
	  ○ Craniofacial syndromes
	  ○ Laryngeal clefts
	  ○ Lymphovascular abnormalities
	• Acquired
	  ○ Subglottic stenosis
	  ○ Tumors
	• Laryngomalacia

A large goiter that overlies the length of the cervical trachea, large anterior neck veins, or a "high-riding" innominate artery are reasons to avoid a PDT and perform a conventional surgical tracheostomy. Imaging, either by ultrasound or computed tomography, is often useful when there is concern about anomalous anatomy.

Coagulopathy is another perennial concern particularly if this cannot be corrected. Some surgeons would prefer PDT in this instance, as the shorter cut skin edges bleed less and undissected tissue planes allow for better tamponade. High ventilating pressures too are a concern when performing a tracheostomy, as the risk of surgical emphysema and pneumothorax is substantial. It is often advisable to delay tracheostomy in these patients until ventilating pressures are reduced.

Recent reports have shown that in many conditions previously thought to be contraindications for PDT such as obesity, burns to the neck, and emergency airway situations, PDT may be safely performed given that the necessary precautions are taken.[8-10]

Advantages and Disadvantages

The advantages of tracheostomy over noninvasive ventilation (e.g., a tight-fitting face mask) or an ETT are obvious. A tracheostomy reduces the anatomical dead space of the upper airway by approximately 150 mL or 50%. This reduces the work of breathing, airway resistance, peak inspiratory pressures, and intrinsic or auto positive end-expiratory pressures (PEEP) substantially.[11] Improvements in ventilator synchronization and triggering, as well as better clearance of secretions may facilitate earlier weaning off the ventilator.[8] A tracheostomy tube is less irritating to the upper airway than an ETT and allows tracheostomized patients to be unsedated and more alert. It also allows patients to eat and talk—albeit with a speaking valve.

Table 33.2   Contraindications to Percutaneous Dilatational Tracheostomy

* Age less than 8 y
* Gross distortion of neck anatomy
  * Hematoma
  * Enlarged thyroid
  * Tumor
  * High innominate artery
* Acute airway obstruction requiring emergency airway
  * Obesity with short neck obscuring landmarks
  * Medically uncorrectable bleeding diatheses
    - PT or APTT more than 1.5 times normal range
    - Platelets less than 50,000
    - Bleeding time more than 10 min
  * PEEP more than 20 cm of water
  * Soft tissue infections at the puncture site

y, year(s); PT, prothrombin time; APTT, activated partial thromboplastin time, min, minute(s); PEEP, positive end-expiratory pressures.

There are, however, disadvantageous physiological changes in a tracheostomized patient. Airflow bypasses the nose and throat where humidification and warming normally occur. Unfiltered, dry and cold air enters the trachea directly, stimulating the proliferation of mucus-producing goblet cells and disrupting normal mucociliary clearance, hence the excessive mucus that is produced soon after a patient has a tracheostomy. This mucus can cause plugging of the lower bronchioles or form crusts that may obstruct the larger airways. Over time, the normal respiratory mucosa of the trachea undergoes squamous metaplasia.[12]

Evidence is divided on whether the presence of a tracheostomy tube impairs the mechanism of swallowing and therefore increases the risk of aspiration. It was initially thought that a tracheostomy tube may impair swallowing by splinting the larynx and preventing the normal upward excursion of the larynx. The presence of an inflated tracheostomy tube cuff, or a one-way valve (such as the Passy-Muir valve that allows some air to be directed into the larynx and pharynx for speech production) may also impede the stimulation of subglottic pressure receptors, thus impairing a specific segmental swallowing reflex.[13,14] There is, however, no evidence that tracheostomy increases aspiration or laryngeal penetration.[15]

The loss of a cough reflex following tracheostomy is to be expected as patients cannot generate high intrathoracic tracheal pressures to initiate a cough. This impedes their ability to clear the secretions. When secretions are copious soon after tracheostomy, suctioning is necessary to clear these secretions. Eventually, patients develop an effective cough, and secretions lessen, making suctioning no longer necessary.

Methods

Surgical Tracheostomy

A surgical tracheostomy is performed in either an elective, urgent, or emergent manner. It is the safest way to secure an airway and is occasionally lifesaving.

Patient positioning is critical to facilitating a smooth procedure. A head support and shoulder roll allow for neck extension and good exposure of the trachea. The surgeon should palpate the surgical landmarks, for example, the sternal notch, the cricoid cartilage, and the anterior border of sternocleidomastoid muscles and mark these out. It is also advisable to feel for the carotid arteries and a high-riding innominate artery. If there is any doubt, an ultrasound scan may shed light on any anomalies.

A skin crease incision is made halfway between the cricoid cartilage and sternal notch. The length of this incision very much depends on the experience of the surgeon and the depth of subcutaneous tissue overlying the trachea. Typically, incisions are 2 to 4 cm.

Infiltration with epinephrine is advisable. In the awake patient, the use of a dental syringe with a mixture of a local anesthetic and epinephrine is best. Infiltration should proceed down to the trachea gradually. Finally, pass the needle into the tracheal lumen and infiltrate liberally while getting the patient to cough. This maneuver ensures good tracheal anesthesia.

A good surgical assistant is crucial in performing a surgical tracheostomy. Retraction of tissues during the procedure eases the surgery. Ensure that the theater staff, including the anesthetist, is prepared before commencing the operation. In particular, check that the correct tracheostomy tube is available.

Begin by making a transverse skin incision with a blade, and deepen this to the subplatysmal plane using monopolar diathermy. Lift the skin flaps for no more than 2 cm superiorly and inferiorly. In many patients, the platysma is absent in the midline and only present in the lateral-most aspect of the incision. A self-retaining retractor is then placed to hold the skin flaps apart. The superficial investing layer of deep cervical fascia is then divided in the midline and deepened to expose the strap muscles. The strap muscles can then be retracted laterally to expose the isthmus of the thyroid gland (**Fig. 33.1**).

Conventionally, the isthmus of thyroid gland is mobilized, clamped, divided, and transfixed—revealing the trachea beneath. However, in many patients, division and ligation of the thyroid isthmus is unnecessary if a plane can be created between the upper border of the thyroid isthmus and the cricoid cartilage. The pretracheal fascia tightly binds the thyroid gland to the trachea. This needs to be divided to reveal the cartilaginous rings of the trachea.

Once exposure is adequate and hemostasis secured, theater staff and the anesthetist should be warned that the surgeon is about to enter the trachea. In an awake patient, a further intratracheal infiltration of local anesthesia ensures that the patient does not cough when the trachea is incised.

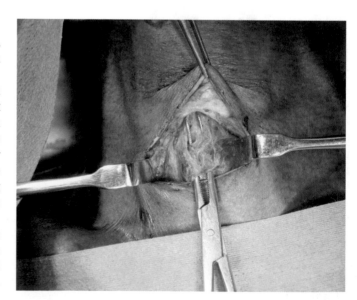

Figure 33.1 Retraction of strap muscles laterally to expose the trachea in the midline.

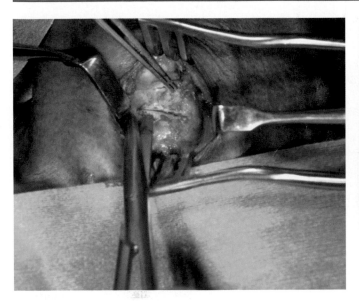

Figure 33.2 The Bjork flap is an inferiorly based ∪-shaped flap that is stitched to the skin.

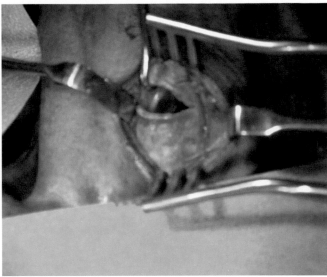

Figure 33.3 The tip of the endotracheal tube that is being withdrawn can be seen through the incision made in the trachea, before the insertion of the tracheostomy tube under direct vision.

To avoid airway fires, diathermy is no longer used at this point. The patient is ventilated on low flow oxygen, and the ETT is passed inferiorly to ensure that the cuff is not inadvertently ruptured when the trachea is entered.

The trachea is best entered between the second and third tracheal rings. Some surgeons prefer removing a window of cartilage, whereas others simply make a generous transverse incision (**Fig. 33.2**).

The "Bjork" flap, which is an inferiorly based flap in the anterior tracheal wall, was designed to aid tube changes. The tip of the flap is sutured to skin, creating a passage into the tracheal lumen. Occasionally, this suture is disrupted during a tube change, and the tip of the new tracheostomy tube pushes the flap into tracheal lumen, obstructing the airway.

Whichever the method, it is best to devise a routine for this part of the procedure with a set sequence of instruments. The author's own preference is as follows: a blade to incise the trachea, Metzenbaum scissors to widen the incision, a cricoid hook—inserted into the incision, turned 90 degrees so that the hook faces superiorly then gently retracted (or the use of tracheal dilators if available), suction to clear any mucus or blood from the trachea, then insertion of the tracheostomy tube in a smooth gentle manner. To facilitate this, lay items such as blade, scissors, cricoid hook, or tracheal dilators, suction, and tracheostomy tube on the patient's chest in this order. In the intubated patient, the anesthetist should be asked to deflate the cuff of the ETT and withdraw it once the tracheal lumen is entered (**Fig. 33.3**).

The first tracheostomy tube to be inserted should be a cuffed, nonfenestrated tube—either single or double lumen. This allows for positive pressure ventilation and minimizes air leak and surgical emphysema due to the fenestration. The tube should be secured both with tapes or ties and sutures to the skin. Tie these snugly; enough to allow two fingers to

pass underneath them. In patients who have had major head and neck surgery with free tissue transfer reconstruction, tapes are contraindicated as these may affect flow in the microvascular anastomoses.

Pediatric Tracheostomy

Tracheostomy in a neonate, infant, or child is challenging in terms of the surgical anatomy of the procedure, the psychosocial implications of living with a tracheostomy, and the aftercare.

The anatomical differences in the child extend beyond the relative difference in size. The hyoid bone and laryngeal cartilages are situated higher in the neck of a child than in the adult. These are difficult to palpate, particularly as there is a pre-tracheal fat pad that overlies these structures. The innominate artery and left brachiocephalic vein often run high in the superior mediastinum. Neck extension draws these vessels and the apices of the lung into the neck and places them at risk in a "low" tracheostomy. The recurrent laryngeal nerves run lateral to the trachea and are more prone to injury with lateral dissection than in the adult.

The surgical steps of a pediatric tracheostomy commence with appropriate positioning to ensure some extension but not hyperextension. Following infiltration, a horizontal incision is made approximately one finger breath above the suprasternal notch. Superficial fat is best removed to expose the strap muscles. Separation in the midline should expose the thyroid isthmus. The isthmus can often be retracted superiorly, making division and transfixion unnecessary.

Two monofilament stay sutures are then placed on either side of the planned vertical tracheotomy that runs from the second to the fourth tracheal ring. It is important

Table 33.3 Comparison of Endotracheal Tube, Tracheostomy Tube, and Bronchoscope Size Relative to Age and Estimated Tracheal Diameter

Age	Tracheal Diameter (mm)	Bronchoscope Size	ETT Size (*Portex*)	Shiley Tracheostomy Tube Inner Diameter (size)	Outer Diameter
Premature neonates	4–5	2.0	2.5	3.0	4.5
<1 mo	5–6	2.5	3.0	3.0	4.5
1–6 mo	5–7	3.0	3.5	3.5	5.2
6–18 mo	6–8	3.5	4.0	4.0	5.9
18 mo to 3 y	7–9	4.0	4.5	4.5	6.5
3–6 y	8–10	4.5	5.0	5.0	7.1
6–9 y	9–13	5.0	6.0	5.5	7.7
9–12 y	10–13	6.0	7.0	6.0	8.3
>12 y	> 13	6.0	8.0	6.5	9.0

ETT, endotracheal tube; mo, month(s); y, year(s).

to spend time choosing the appropriate tracheostomy tube that is compatible. **Table 33.3** is a quick reference to aid the surgeon—matching age, estimated tracheal diameter, ETT size, bronchoscope size, and inner and outer diameters of a *Shiley* tracheostomy tube.[16,17] In children, it is not necessary to use a cuffed tube. The subglottic trachea is narrow and this prevents an air leak when un-cuffed tubes are used.

Once the tracheostomy tube is inserted and secured with tapes, the monofilament stay sutures should be marked "left" and "right" and taped to the chest with instructions written on the tape warning against their removal. Should the tracheostomy tube be inadvertently dislodged, the stay sutures allow the clinician to both draw the trachea to the skin, and splay open the vertical tracheotomy.

Percutaneous Dilatational Tracheostomy

Percutaneous dilatational tracheostomy (PDT) refers to a bedside procedure that is performed on intubated patients in an ICU. The procedure was first described in 1955 but gained popularity in 1985 when Pasquale Ciaglia introduced serial dilators. These days, PDT is often performed with endoscopic or bronchoscopic guidance. The procedure is best performed in slim individuals with a prominent and palpable trachea. A preoperative ultrasound scan is often useful in detecting any anomalous vessels or an enlarged thyroid gland. Contraindications to percutaneous tracheostomy are discussed earlier in this chapter.

The method is based on the *Seldinger* technique to create a passage into the trachea which is then either serially dilated or gradually dilated using a single tapered horn-like dilator. This creates a passage into the tracheal lumen into which a tracheostomy tube is passed.

Percutaneous dilatational tracheostomy is a well-established and common procedure. Its proponents point to a smaller incision, less tissue dissection, lower wound infection rates, and lower costs as the key benefits. Although there are many studies comparing open surgical tracheostomy (OST) with PDT, these are largely nonrandomized, and hence some bias is present as more difficult patients are usually referred for OST. One trial that randomized ICU patients into bedside PDT and bedside OST groups found a low complication rate for both OST and PDT, whereas patients who did not meet the criteria for the bedside procedures and hence had OST in the operating room were three times more likely to have complications such as pneumothorax, major hemorrhage, and airway loss.[18] A recent meta-analysis by Higgins and Punthakee[19] demonstrated no significant difference when comparing overall complications in OST and PDT, with a trend toward favoring percutaneous method. Despite its substantial popularity, PDT does have limitations and risks. In Higgins and Punthakee's meta-analysis, the percutaneous method was associated with a higher incidence of decannulation and obstruction.

Complications

Tracheostomy is a safe procedure but still carries a risk of complications that varies between 5 and 40%.[20] The most commonly occurring complications are postoperative hemorrhage, tube obstruction, and tube displacement. **Table 33.4** summarizes the complications that can arise intraoperatively, in the postoperative period, and after decannulation. Death occurs in 0.5 to 1.6% of patients following a tracheostomy and is most often a consequence of tube displacement.[21]

Hemorrhage is by far the most common complication following a tracheostomy. Often, this is limited to oozing of the surgical wound. It is best to correct any coagulopathy and cease antiplatelet medication for 7 to 10 days preoperatively.

Table 33.4 Complications of Tracheostomy

Stage	Complications
Intraoperative	Hemorrhage (minor or major)
	Wrong placement of tracheostomy tube
	Pneumothorax/pneumomediastinum
	Esophageal perforation
	Airway fire
	Injury to the laryngeal cartilage
	Air embolism
	Apnea
Postoperative (tube in situ)	Tube obstruction
	Accidental decannulation
	Air leak
	Subcutaneous emphysema
	Secondary hemorrhage including tracheoinnominate fistula
	Wound infection
	Skin ulceration or pressure sores from tracheostomy tube
	Tracheal necrosis or ulcers
	Tube migration
	Dysphagia/aspiration
	Ventilator-associated pneumonia
	Tracheoesophageal fistula

Meticulous surgical techniques, such as oversewing the divided ends of the thyroid isthmus, ligating the anterior thyroid veins, and minimizing unnecessary dissection laterally, contribute to better hemostasis.

Should hemorrhage occur postoperatively, inflate the cuff of the tracheostomy tube, elevate the head of the patient, and administer high flow oxygen before attempting to arrest the hemorrhage. Bleeding can be from around the tracheostomy or from within the tracheal lumen. Oozing from the edge of the surgical wound can be addressed by packing with adrenaline-soaked ribbon-gauze or alginate dressings. If these measures fail to arrest the bleed, then it may be necessary to re-explore the neck in the operating theater. It is best to decannulate the patient and intubate orally to allow for a thorough inspection of the wound.

Late complications after tracheostomy may be related to placement of the tube, leaving the tube in place for a prolonged period of time, or abnormal healing of injured tracheal mucosa in contact with the tip or the cuff of the tube. Laryngopharyngeal reflux and pooled inflammatory secretions above the tracheostomy cuff can further aggravate mucosal injury.[22]

Three to twelve percent of tracheostomized patients develop stomal stenosis that ultimately requires surgical intervention. Prevention includes limiting the size of the tracheal defect created, prevention of mechanical irritation and traction on the trachea by using swivel adaptors and ventilator tubing support, meticulous stoma care and the use of prophylactic antibiotics to prevent chondritis.

Significant stenosis may be treated with bronchoscopic dilation and laser excision, with tracheal stenting or resection reserved for severe cases.[23]

Tracheo-innominate fistulae, though rare (<1%), have an almost 100% mortality rate. The full-blown hemorrhage usually occurs within 3 to 4 weeks of tracheostomy and is sometimes heralded by a smaller gush of fresh blood from the tracheostomy. The innominate artery crosses the trachea at approximately the ninth tracheal ring and can be eroded into by the tube when there is too low a placement of tracheostomy (below the third tracheal ring), excessive movement of the trachea, or tracheal necrosis caused by a combination of increased cuff pressure and chondritis.

Aspiration has been noted in various studies in 30 to 83%[24] of patients on tracheostomy, and may be related to compression of the esophagus by the tracheostomy cuff. It is recommended that all newly tracheostomized patients undergo a swallowing assessment before commencing oral feeds.[22]

Types of Tracheostomy Tubes

Cuffed and Noncuffed Tubes

A cuffed tube is used to maintain a closed circuit loop for ventilation. A cuff can also be used to protect the airway, such as when the patient has significant bleeding from the upper aerodigestive tract. The cuff should be inflated just enough to allow minimal air leak, and cuff pressure should be checked twice a day to maintain cuff pressure within a range of 20 to 25 mm Hg. When the patient is using a speaking valve, the cuff should be deflated. The disadvantage of cuffed tubes is a higher risk of pressure necrosis of the trachea and of granulation formation. Pediatric tracheostomy tubes are usually cuffless to reduce the risk of subsequent tracheal stenosis.

Fenestrated and Unfenestrated Tubes

Fenestrations refer to holes in the lumen of the tube that allow airflow to be directed to the oro- and nasopharynx. They reduce the work of breathing, and assist in weaning off the tracheostomy and in phonation. However, it is more difficult to ventilate a patient with a fenestrated tracheostomy tube; hence, an unfenestrated tube is preferred for the first placement of the tube and for patients on mechanical ventilation (although an un-fenestrated inner tube may be used as an interim measure). The fenestrations also pose a risk of aspiration of oral and gastric contents in patients with poor cough reflexes.

Single and Double Lumen Tubes

A single lumen tube decreases airway resistance by maximizing the inner diameter of the tube. However, the lumen can get blocked easily and the tube must be changed every 5 to 7 days. Double lumen tubes have an inner cannula that can be removed for cleaning, allowing a period of up to 29 days between tube changes. The presence of the inner cannula reduces the internal diameter of the tube by 1 to 1.5 mm.

Special Tubes

Extra-length tubes may have extra horizontal length or extra vertical length. Tubes with extra horizontal length are useful for patients with deep-set tracheas such as obese patients, or those with distorted neck anatomy from infection, tumor, or edema, whereas those with extra vertical length are useful for those with tracheal stenosis or granulations, or tracheomalacia. Patients with spinal abnormalities such as scoliosis or kyphosis may also benefit from these tubes. Some have adjustable flanges to allow bedside adjustments, although frequent adjustments are not recommended due to the risk of accidental decannulation and potential failure of the locking mechanism of the tubes.[25]

Some tubes have a built-in tubing to allow for suctioning of secretions that accumulate above the cuff in the subglottis. These are believed to reduce the risk of microaspirations and ventilator-associated pneumonia.[26]

Talking tracheostomy tubes, for example, Shiley Phonate (Nellcor, Pleasanton, California, United States) and Portex Trach Talk Blue Line (Smith Medical, Saint Paul, Minnesota, United States) enable phonation with an inflated cuffed tube.

Care of the Tracheostomized Patient

Care of the tracheostomized patient, whether by nursing staff or by home caregivers, is labor-intensive and requires considerable training in many aspects, including the following:

- Suctioning of secretions from the tracheostomy as often as required, in a sterile manner and without causing trauma to the airway.
- Changing and cleaning of the inner cannula every 8 hours.
- Uncuffing and cuffing of the tube to the required cuff pressure.
- Management of the humidification equipment.
- Change of dressing and tapes and prevention of pressure sores and infection.
- Reinsertion of the tracheostomy in the case of decannulation.
- How to recognize and act in emergencies such as tube occlusion.

The following equipment is recommended for routine care of a tracheostomized patient:

- Suction tubing, suction catheters, gloves, and a bottle of sterile water changed daily for cleaning of the catheters.
- Humidification equipment.
- Spare tracheostomy tubes of the same size and one size below.
- A clean container to hold spare inner cannulas and the introducer.
- Tracheal dilator.
- Self-inflating bag (e.g., Laerdal bag) and connector for emergency ventilation.
- Gauze and tapes for changing the dressing.

Weaning and Decannulation

Criteria for weaning off tracheostomy include the following[27]:

- Resolution of initial cause of upper airway obstruction.
- Patient is able to maintain adequate gas exchange, without the need for mechanical ventilation. In chronic conditions, such as obstructive sleep apnea and chronic obstructive pulmonary disease, the patient may require supplemental oxygen; however, it is recommended that the FiO_2 be less than 40% before decannulation.
- No sign of deteriorating bronchial infection or excessive secretions.
- Additional criteria include
  ○ presence of a good cough reflex;
  ○ absence of aspiration;
  ○ Glasgow Coma Scale score of above 8.

Methods of decannulation vary between practices. In patients who have been on long-term tracheostomy, examination with flexible nasoendoscopy may be warranted before initiating the decannulation protocol to confirm the resolution of airway obstruction and rule out long-term complications of tracheostomy such as granulations and tracheal stenosis.

Some practitioners perform the "deflated cuff tracheostomy occlusion procedure" as a bedside test before capping of the tracheostomy, where the tracheostomy cuff is deflated and the tracheal tube opening closed with a gloved finger, while observing for signs of respiratory distress and monitoring for oxygen desaturation.

Others advocate changing to cuffless tubes, fenestrated tubes, or downsizing the tracheostomy to allow for more air to pass from the upper airway, before the tracheostomy is capped. The Passy Muir or other speaking valve may also be used instead of a cap; however, it must be noted that as these valves do entrain some air, the ability of a patient to phonate cannot be interpreted as fitness for decannulation. It is important to ensure that nonfenestrated tracheostomy tubes must have their cuffs deflated before "capping" or application of speaking valves, to avoid complete airway obstruction.

Following decannulation, a patient should be closely observed with continuous oxygen saturation monitoring for at least 24 hours. For some patients, a short period of admission may be required. Failure to decannulate may occur in 2 to 5% of patients.[28]

Decannulation before the tract has fully matured, usually between 7 and 10 days, is also not advised as attempted re-insertion in an emergency has a high risk of entering the pretracheal space and anterior mediastinum, with resultant airway obstruction. In the case of accidental decannulation of a fresh tract, orotracheal intubation may be the safest option. A skilled provider may be able to rapidly re-insert the tracheostomy tube using fiber-optic guidance, a pediatric laryngoscope blade to visualize the tract or by passing the tube over a suction catheter (Seldinger technique).

Future Directions

The tracheostomy has come full circle from being a high-risk emergency operation in the early days to one that is more commonly performed electively for prolonged ventilation. As the indications change, there is also compelling evidence that alternatives to the OST, such as the PDT, may have fewer overall complications and may be more cost-effective by releasing operating room time and personnel, and potentially allowing nonsurgeons to perform the procedure at the bedside.[19]

While it is healthy that nonsurgeons develop expertise in PDTs, it is perhaps wise for ENT surgeons to also master the PDT technique to allow for flexibility in choosing the appropriate technique for each patient who requires a tracheostomy, and also to manage complications of PDTs when called upon to do so.

References

1. Rajesh O, Meher R. Historical review of tracheostomy. Internet J Otorhinolaryngol 2006;4(2):doi:10.5580/1178
2. Tucker JA, Reilly BK, Tucker ST, Reilly JS. Pediatric otolaryngology in the United States: Chevalier Jackson's legacy for the 21st century. Otolaryngol Head Neck Surg 2012;146(1):5–7
3. Gilyoma JM, Balumuka DD, Chalya PL. Ten-year experiences with tracheostomy at a university teaching hospital in Northwestern Tanzania: a retrospective review of 214 cases. World J Emerg Surg 2011;6(1):38
4. Corbett HJ, Mann KS, Mitra I, Jesudason EC, Losty PD, Clarke RW. Tracheostomy: a 10-year experience from a UK pediatric surgical center. J Pediatr Surg 2007;42(7):1251–1254
5. Gomes Silva BN, Andriolo RB, Saconato H, Atallah AN, Valente O. Early versus late tracheostomy for critically ill patients. Cochrane Database Syst Rev 2012;3:CD007271
6. Griffiths J, Barber VS, Morgan L, Young JD. Systematic review and meta-analysis of studies of the timing of tracheostomy in adult patients undergoing artificial ventilation. Br Med J 2005;330(7502):1243
7. Blankenship DR, Kulbersh BD, Gourin CG, Blanchard AR, Terris DJ. High-risk tracheostomy: exploring the limits of the percutaneous tracheostomy. Laryngoscope 2005;115(6):987–989
8. Kluge S, Meyer A, Kühnelt P, Baumann HJ, Kreymann G. Percutaneous tracheostomy is safe in patients with severe thrombocytopenia. Chest 2004;126(2):547–551
9. Gravvanis AI, Tsoutsos DA, Iconomou TG, Papadopoulos SG. Percutaneous versus conventional tracheostomy in burned patients with inhalation injury. World J Surg 2005;29(12):1571–1575
10. Ben Nun A, Orlovsky M, Best LA. Percutaneous tracheostomy in patients with cervical spine fractures: feasible and safe. Interact Cardiovasc Thorac Surg 2006;5(4):427–429
11. Diehl JR, El Atrous S, Touchard D, Lemaire F, Brochard L. Changes in the work of breathing induced by tracheostomy in ventilator-dependent patients. AM J Respir Crit Care Med 1999;159(2):393–388
12. Epstein SK. Anatomy and physiology of tracheostomy. Respir Care 2005;50(4):476–482
13. Donzelli J, Brady S, Wesling M, Theisen M. Effects of the removal of the tracheotomy tube on swallowing during the fiberoptic endoscopic exam of the swallow (FEES). Dysphagia 2005;20(4):283–289
14. Gross RD, Mahlmann J, Grayhack JP. Physiologic effects of open and closed tracheostomy tubes on the pharyngeal swallow. Ann Otol Rhinol Laryngol 2003;112(2):143–152
15. Leder SB, Ross DA. Investigation of the causal relationship between tracheotomy and aspiration in the acute care setting. Laryngoscope 2000;110(4):641–644
16. Wetmore RF. Tracheotomy. In: Bluestone CD, Stool SE, Alper CM, Arjmand EM, Casselbrant ML, Dohar JE, Yellow RF (eds). Pediatric Otolaryngology. Philadelphia, PA: Saunders; 2003:1583–1598
17. Behl S, Watt JW. Prediction of tracheostomy tube size for paediatric long-term ventilation: an audit of children with spinal cord injury. Br J Anaesth 2005;94(1):88–91
18. Massick DD, Yao S, Powell DM, et al. Bedside tracheostomy in the intensive care unit: a prospective randomized trial comparing open surgical tracheostomy with endoscopically guided percutaneous dilational tracheotomy. Laryngoscope 2001;111(3):494–500
19. Higgins KM, Punthakee X. Meta-analysis comparison of open versus percutaneous tracheostomy. Laryngoscope 2007;117(3):447–454
20. Miller JD, Kapp JP. Complications of tracheostomies in neurosurgical patients. Surg Neurol 1984;22(2):186–188

21. Stauffer JL, Olson DE, Petty TL. Complications and consequences of endotracheal intubation and tracheotomy. A prospective study of 150 critically ill adult patients. Am J Med 1981;70(1):65–76

22. Epstein SK. Late complications of tracheostomy. Respir Care 2005;50(4):542–549

23. Brichet A, Verkindre C, Dupont J, et al. Multidisciplinary approach to management of postintubation tracheal stenoses. Eur Respir J 1999;13(4):888–893

24. Leder SB. Incidence and type of aspiration in acute care patients requiring mechanical ventilation via a new tracheotomy. Chest 2002;122(5):1721–1726

25. Hess DR. Tracheostomy tubes and related appliances. Respir Care 2005;50(4):497–510

26. Coffman HM, Rees CJ, Sievers AE, Belafsky PC. Proximal suction tracheotomy tube reduces aspiration volume. Otolaryngol Head Neck Surg 2008;138(4):441–445

27. Heffner JE. The technique of weaning from tracheostomy. Criteria for weaning; practical measures to prevent failure. J Crit Illn 1995;10(10):729–733

28. O'Connor HH, White AC. Tracheostomy decannulation. Respir Care 2010;55(8):1076–1081

34 Management of Dysphagia

Jayakumar R. Menon

Swallowing disorders presenting to an ENT outpatient department are not uncommon. However, many patients do not get the attention they deserve. Inadequate understanding of the pathophysiology may probably lead indifference on the part of the physician toward the swallowing problem. In this chapter, we will look at the common swallowing problems that may be encountered by the ENT surgeon. However, a discussion of infective and neoplastic causes is beyond the scope of this chapter.

Anatomy and Physiology of Swallowing

Muscles of the lips and adjacent facial muscles such as buccinators supplied by the facial nerve play major role in the oral stage of swallowing. Muscles of mastication supplied by the trigeminal nerve are the key to the oral preparatory phase. Tongue muscles with innervation from the hypoglossal nerve are indispensible for both oral and pharyngeal stages. Sensations transmitted through nerves, such as lingual, chorda tympani, and glossopharyngeal, are also very important for the normal swallowing act.

Pharynx, with its three constrictor muscles, has to play the most complex of the three stages. Of the three constrictors, inferior constrictor is the most important yet least understood. It has two parts, namely thyropharyngeus and cricopharyngeus. The space between the two is Killain dehiscence—a potential space for herniation. The constrictors are supplied by the pharyngeal plexus, and cricopharyngeus gets innervations from recurrent laryngeal nerve. The interesting part about the cricopharyngeus is the fact that it is in a state of tonic contraction and relaxes only during the act of swallowing. We do not know of a mechanism wherein a muscular relaxation occurring with acetylcholine-mediated nerve stimulation occurs. It is quite possible that some central mechanisms play a role.[1]

Disorders of the Oral Stage

Neurological Causes

Facial palsy will result in improper closing of the lips and inadequate obliteration of the oral vestibule. As a result, part of the food can spill out of the oral cavity and part can get trapped in the vestibule. Bilateral facial palsy will cause even greater problems. Buccinator weakness will result in stasis of food in the oral vestibule. Trigeminal nerve involvement will affect the chewing mechanism and, consequently, the preparatory phase will be compromised.

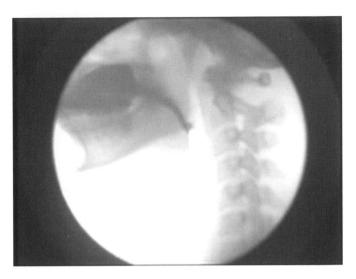

Figure 34.1 Total glossectomy videofluoroscopic picture.

Bilateral hypoglossal palsy can result in severe swallowing problem both at the oral and at the oropharyngeal levels. However, unilateral hypoglossal nerve palsy, unless accompanied by other neurological deficits, rarely produces major swallowing problems.

Iatrogenic Causes

Surgical resection of lips and or tongue can result in significant morbidity of the swallowing mechanism. If commissure of the lips is resected, then morbidity will be even more. Total glossectomy (**Fig. 34.1**) makes the act of swallowing extremely difficult, if not impossible. Partial glossectomy generally does not produce as much dysphagia. Reconstruction procedures also affect the swallowing efficiency. While an optimum-sized flap will obliterate the vacuum created by the surgery and improve the swallowing, a poorly designed over-sized flap will hamper the act of bolus transit. Floor of mouth cancers requires removal of varying degrees of muscles of the floor of mouth as well as part of the mandible. If symphysis menti is resected, then hyomandibular complex will be disrupted resulting in severe swallowing difficulty.[2] Mandibular arch, mylohyoid muscles and raphe, geniohyoid muscles, and hyoid bone constitute the hyomandibular complex. As in the case of glossectomy, here also the type of reconstruction is important for the swallowing outcome. Hard palate resections are the least problematic of the lot as far as the swallowing is concerned. A suitable prosthesis will effectively eradicate any problem with swallowing in these cases.

Diagnosis

Apart from history taking, ENT and neurological examination, watching the act of swallowing is very important. Many a time, it gives the physician not only an idea about the pathophysiology, but also about the possible therapeutic strategies. Videofluoroscopic assessment of the swallowing act with radio opaque substances such as barium or Gastrografin is the most important diagnostic tool in oral dysphagia. Both anteroposterior and lateral views are important in this regard. Tongue muscle dysfunction, stasis of bolus in the vestibule, and their potential corrective strategies can be detected from the fluoroscopy.

Management

Swallowing therapy techniques are the mainstay of treatment in oral dysphagia in vast majority of the cases. There are direct as well as indirect swallowing therapy techniques. Indirect swallowing therapy aims at improving the swallowing function without attempting to feed the patient. Improving the tongue movements, improving the lip closure by strengthening the lips, and maximizing the power of the masticatory muscles are examples of this.[3] Direct swallowing therapy tries to orally feed the patient, with techniques designed to avoid or circumvent the swallowing difficulty experienced by the patient. For example, asking the patient to extend the head and neck while swallowing so that gravity helps to send the bolus down is a direct swallowing therapy technique. Using specially designed spoons or tubes to directly place the food into the pharynx is another direct swallowing therapy technique. Changing the texture of the feeds can solve the problem to a great extent in many cases. Vast majority of the patients having oral dysphagia can be managed satisfactorily with direct or indirect swallowing therapy techniques or both. Some of them however require temporary or permanent nonoral modes of feeding such as nasogastric tube, gastrostomy, or jejunostomy feeding.

Disorders of the Pharyngeal Stage—Oropharyngeal Phase

Neurological Causes

Bilateral hypoglossal paralysis, as we have already seen, will affect the swallowing considerably, both at the oral and oropharyngeal stages. The propulsion of the bolus by the tongue base will not take place, if the tongue is paralyzed. Parkinsonism is a condition that can adversely affect the oropharyngeal and laryngopharyngeal stages of swallowing.[4] Many of these patients show on videofluoroscopy, what is known as the "swing" movement of the tongue. Here, as the bolus reaches the oropharynx, the posterior third of tongue raises and sends the bolus back to the oral cavity. This to and fro movement goes on for a long-time swing—the swing effect during barium swallow videofluoroscopy.

Palatal paralysis, especially bilateral cases, causes incomplete velopharyngeal closure and results in nasal regurgitation. Cerebral palsy children may have drooling of saliva, secondary to reduced frequency of swallowing. In these patients, both oral and oropharyngeal stages may be affected.

Iatrogenic Causes

Surgical resection of the tongue base—unilateral or bilateral—will cause significant swallowing problems. Palatal excisions can cause nasal regurgitation and swallowing difficulty.

Management

Dysphagia due to tongue base paralysis or total glossectomy is one of the most difficult swallowing disorders to correct. By altering the feeding position and using specially designed feeding spoons, this may be partly corrected. Pumping in semisolid diet into the oropharynx with a 50-cc syringe through a polythene cannula is a simple, inexpensive yet efficient mode of feeding these patients. Swallowing problems in parkinsonism respond well to antiparkinsonism treatment. Masako maneuver is the technique wherein patient is asked to protrude the tongue and bite onto it while swallowing.[5] This prevents in coordinate tongue base movements seen in the cases of parkinsonism.

Drooling in cerebral palsy children can be corrected by submandibular duct relocation surgery. In this operation, both submandibular salivary ducts are dissected per orally and are relocated into the tonsillar fossae. This causes the saliva to reach the oropharynx, thus initiating the act of swallowing. The result will be even better, if this is combined with swallowing therapy. The two aspects of swallowing therapy in these patients are (1) to improve the lips closure and (2) to stimulate the swallowing act. The first is done by the button and thread exercise wherein the child is asked to keep a button anchored to a thread, inside the lips, but outside the teeth. The child is encouraged to keep the button in its position with the help of the lips against the pull of the thread, exerted by the child himself or herself. Teaching the child to initiate the act of swallowing on hearing an auditory stimulus or on seeing a visual stimulus is also very useful. This is a sort of conditioning reflex.

For velopharyngeal incompetence, direct swallowing therapy involves swallowing with chin flexed and touching the chest. Pinching the nose tightly while swallowing also is a very useful method. Indirect swallowing therapy techniques for palatal incompetence include palate-strengthening exercises such as blowing balloon. A sphincter pharyngoplasty with a tight velopharyngeal port might help, though it runs the risk of causing snoring.

Disorders of the Laryngopharyngeal Phase

Upper esophageal sphincter (UES) is a key area in swallowing. This is contributed by the inferior constrictor muscle. The upper part is the thyropharyngeus, and the lower part is the cricopharyngeus. The perfect harmony of their contraction and relaxation is a must for smooth swallowing. In resting state, the cricopharyngeus is in a state of tonic contraction. It will relax only when the bolus has passed beyond the thyropharyngeus. During this particular phase, the larynx will close itself, thus avoiding any possibility of aspiration. Once the bolus has passed beyond the cricopharyngeus, the muscle will contract again, and the larynx will reopen for respiration.

For better understanding, laryngopharyngeal pathology may be divided into three groups, though it must be remembered that various permutations and combinations of the three can be present in each patients. They are laryngopharyngeal paralysis, laryngeal incompetence, and cricopharyngeal dysmotility.

Laryngopharyngeal Paralysis

Motor neuron diseases, Parkinsonism, and stroke are known to produce laryngopharyngeal paralysis, which is the condition characterized by the absence of upward movement of the larynx during deglutition. As a result, the larynx remains unprotected, and cricopharynx fails to open.[6] Extensive surgical resection involving the upper neck and the oropharynx also can result in laryngopharyngeal paralysis. Condition is diagnosed by the fact that during the attempted swallow, there is hardly any upward movement of the larynx. Videofluoroscopy confirms the diagnosis. Another useful investigation is flexible endoscopic evaluation of swallowing (FEES). In total laryngopharyngeal paralysis, this will show the entire bolus in the pyriform fossae even after many attempted swallows. This can later enter the laryngeal inlet resulting in coughing and choking episodes. In less severe forms, the amount of food bolus will be reduced after multiple swallow attempts.

Management
This is a difficult condition to treat. Two useful direct techniques in swallowing therapy are (1) Mendelssohn maneuver and (2) chin tuck. Mendelssohn maneuver involves in manually elevating the larynx, while patient attempts to swallow. This procedure results in, at least partially, closing the larynx and opening up the cricopharynx.[7] The chin tuck technique uses extreme flexion of the head, resulting in opening up of the epiglottic angle. The pressure exerted on the trachea and larynx will also partly prevent aspiration. Permanently elevating the larynx by doing a mandibulohyoid suspension also is useful in this condition. Indirect swallowing therapy for this condition is suprahyoid muscle strengthening. Shaker exercise is aimed at this.[8] Patient is asked to lie supine and lift the head off the bed and keep it in that position for as long as he or she can. This is to be performed many times a day.

Laryngeal Incompetence

Hemilaryngeal or total laryngeal paralysis can result in significant aspiration, especially the latter. It is important to note that bilateral recurrent laryngeal nerve palsy alone will not cause significant aspiration. Only when the superior laryngeal nerve or nerves are also involved, aspiration becomes a major problem. Cerebrovascular accidents (CVAs), head injury, and neurosurgical procedures can cause this problem. Laryngeal incompetence will cause the larynx to remain incompletely closed during the pharyngeal stage of swallowing, thus resulting in aspiration.

Management
Hemilaryngeal paralysis causing aspiration is easier to handle. Most of the young patients should be okay with swallowing therapy. For this, supraglottic swallowing technique is very useful. Here, the patient is instructed to swallow after holding the breath.[9] It is important to note that patient should not be asked to take a too deep an inspiration before holding the breath. By doing so, the larynx will descend in the neck, thus keeping the glottis slightly open. Moreover, elevation of the larynx is an important stimulus to open up the cricopharyngeal sphincter. If the incompetence is severe, then super-supraglottic technique may be tried. The difference here is that patient is asked to bear down once breath is being held. It has been found that in super-supraglottic swallow, swallowing time is shorter.

Occasionally, especially in older patients, swallowing therapy alone may not be sufficient. Then, a medialization thyroplasty can help by improving the efficiency of the glottic closure. If there is a big posterior glottis chink or a vertical-level asymmetry of the vocal cords, then an arytenoid rotation also will have to be performed along with the medialization thyroplasty.

Total laryngeal paralysis is a formidable problem. Here, the swallowing takes a back seat, as prevention of fatal aspiration is the more pressing need. Luckily, a cuffed tracheostomy will most often solve the problem. However, occasionally one can come across a patient, who still drowns in his or her own secretions. There are a few surgical options for these patients. Laryngeal diversion is the procedure, wherein larynx and trachea are disconnected from each other. The lower end of the larynx is closed, and the upper end of trachea is brought out as the tracheostomy. Another operation is epiglottic over sew, in which the epiglottis is sutured over the laryngeal inlet as a lid. A third option is the procedure known as glottic closure. Here, the medial edges of the vocal cords are made raw and then sutured to each other. The most definite surgical procedure to prevent aspiration is total laryngectomy, though seldom resorted to. Apart from their efficacy, reversibility of the procedure also has to be taken into consideration, while choosing the procedure. While total laryngectomy is the most efficient in preventing the aspiration, it is also an irreversible procedure. Reversibility is best for epiglottic over sew followed by laryngotracheal diversion and glottis closure.

Cricopharyngeal Dysmotility

By this terminology, it is meant that the cricopharynx does not open up in time, when the bolus reaches it. Even

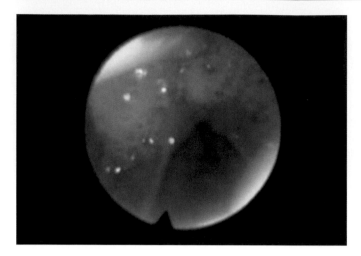

Figure 34.2 Cricopharyngeal dysmotility.

if the larynx is competent, then this condition can result in aspiration. This happens because, the bolus which is still at the level of cricopharynx, finds its way into the larynx, when the glottis open for inspiration. Cricopharyngeal dysmotility is not an uncommon problem in many a patients who suffered CVAs.[10] It is especially common in Wallenberg syndrome (**Fig. 34.2**). Neurosurgeries of the brain stem also can cause this. Surgeries of the hypopharynx and upper esophagus can also result in this condition.

Functional Endoscopic Evaluation of Swallowing

Dynamic assessment of the pharyngeal stage of swallowing can be studied with a flexible rhinolaryngoscope, preferably with a suction channel.[11] A colored food-like jelly is given to the patient to swallow, while the physician does the scopy. Green color gives the best possible contrast. The procedure is performed with patient is sitting position, if possible. It is better not to use any topical anesthesia, as it is likely to adversely affect the swallowing process. First, the scope is gently introduced through the nose and advanced beyond the soft palate, and the tip is positioned just above the epiglottis. The whole of the laryngeal introitus and both pyriform fossae along with the postcricoid region should be clearly visible. Then, the suitably colored food bolus is kept inside the mouth, and patient is asked to swallow. Look for any upward movement of the bolus suggestive of nasopharyngeal regurgitation. Next, look for the fleeting disappearance of the laryngeal introitus from the vision. This suggests that larynx is normally elevating during the act of swallowing. It is the absence of this temporary disappearance of the larynx from the vision, which is sinister. This is suggestive of laryngopharyngeal paralysis. Laryngeal competence is looked for next. Vocal cord movements are assessed. Check whether the food bolus is just entering the laryngeal vestibule (penetration) or passing beyond the true vocal cords (aspiration). Careful assessment of the cough

reflex is carried out at this stage. If patient is having good effective cough, even as food bolus enters the laryngeal vestibule, then it is a good sign. It suggests that, even though patient is having some degree of laryngeal incompetence, the risk of life-threatening aspiration pneumonia is very unlikely. On the contrary, if there is little or no cough even after the food bolus has passed beyond the true vocal cords, then it suggests that patient's life is in grave danger due to the very high possibility of aspiration pneumonia. Next logical step would be watching the pyriform fossae and the postcricoid region. Look for any significant reduction in the amount of the bolus after each attempted swallow. If the amount comes down even by a little bit, then it suggests that cricopharyngeal incompetence is not complete. Also, look for secondary penetration/aspiration. This happens in patients with good laryngeal competence. Due to cricopharyngeal dysmotility, part or most of the food bolus stays in the pyriform fossae and postcricoid region, which spills into the laryngeal introitus, when the glottis opens for inspiration.

Management

Most of these patients, especially those with CVAs tend to recover spontaneously within 6 weeks' time. Almost all of them have problems in swallowing liquids rather than solids. This is due to the fact that liquids with less mass are unable to exert a force to open up the cricopharynx. Due to the same reason, almost all of these patients will be seen spitting out saliva very frequently. Swallowing therapy with Mendelssohn maneuver and supraglottic swallowing technique can help many of these patients. Hot fomentation to the neck to relieve the spasm is advisable. Large, warm, and sour bolus is the best to start swallowing therapy.

Injection of botulinum toxin into each side of cricopharyngeus muscle under electromyography control is useful in patients, not recovering in 6 weeks either spontaneously or with swallowing therapy. Unlike other spastic conditions, it rarely requires subsequent injection. Still refractory cases can be managed by cricopharyngeal myotomy.

It is important to remember that in all these patients a combination of more than one of these UES dysfunction can occur. It is unusual to have a single type of dysfunction alone. Consequently, each one of these patients requires different treatment planning.

Plummer-Vinson Syndrome and Cricopharyngeal Bar

Plummer–Vinson syndrome is characterized by a postcricoid web (**Fig. 34.3**). Dysphagia will be mainly for solids than liquids. Barium swallow and videofluoroscopy will show an anterior bar at the postcricoid level on lateral films. Treatment is by endoscopic dilatation and correction of iron deficiency anemia. The patient has to be under continuous follow-up, because of its premalignant nature. By contrast, cricopharyngeal bar or idiopathic cricopharyngeal spasm is

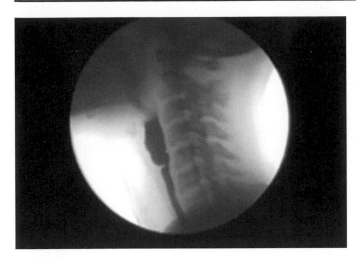

Figure 34.3   Postcricoid web in "Plummer-Vinson syndrome."

the condition, which will affect liquids more than solids.[12] Here, the cricopharyngeal bar will be posterior on lateral view videofluoroscopy barium swallow. The treatment is botulinum toxin injection or cricopharyngeal myotomy. Cervical esophageal webs are also not uncommon. They respond well to dilatation.

Osteophytes

Osteophytes can indent the posterior wall of the pharynx, and esophagus causing dysphagia and occasionally warranting surgical treatment. A lateral view radiograph of the neck and barium swallow videofluoroscopy will clinch the diagnosis, and these can be used to educate, convince, and reassure the patients.

Pharyngeal Pouch

Pharyngeal pouch or Zenker diverticulum is a pulsion diverticulum resulting from coordinated contractions of thyropharyngeus–cricopharyngeus complex.[13] It is more common above the age of 50 and has a slight male preponderance. The typical symptoms include regurgitation of food particles consumed earlier and bad taste in the mouth. Sometimes, a gurgling sound also can be heard while the patient swallows. As the pouch becomes larger, patient will start having symptoms of dysphagia. Occasionally, carcinoma may develop in the pouch. In that case, hoarseness also can occur due to the involvement of the recurrent laryngeal nerve.

Diagnosis is by barium swallow videofluoroscopy. Both lateral and anteroposterior views are needed. In a suspected malignancy, computed tomography scan of neck will give more information regarding the involvement of adjacent structures.

Surgery is the mainstay of treatment. Three options are available. The standard treatment would be excision of the pouch, cricopharyngeal myotomy, and repair of the surgical rent in the pharynx via a left supraclavicular incision. Before the incision, it is a good idea to do hypopharyngoscopy to

clean the pouch of any debris and to pack it with either a colored pack or inflated Foley catheter bulb. This latter step helps in easy identification of the pouch, during the surgical procedure. Postoperatively, the patient is fed through a nasogastric tube till the 10th postoperative day. Oral feeding is resumed after confirming the integrity of the pharyngeal repair with a barium swallow videofluoroscopy after 10 days.

Endoscopic stapling can be performed with Dohlman scope in selected cases. This surgery needs no neck incision, early oral feeding, and very short hospitalization. However, bigger pouches are not amenable to this method of treatment. In very old or unfit patients, diverticuloesophagostomy has been advocated. This is a symptom relieving rather than curative operation.

Conclusion

Deprivation of the ability to eat drink is one of the hardest things to stomach for any patient. Many conditions can adversely affect the complex act of swallowing, with neurological and oncological disorders forming the chunk of them. Understanding the exact pathophysiology will help the physician in charting out ideal diagnostic tests as well as the most appropriate treatment options. Fluoroscopic and endoscopic evaluations of the act of swallowing are the best methods to accurately diagnose these conditions. We may not be able to make all these patients have a three-course dinner. However, the vast majority of them can be made to eat and drink at least some amount of food with various swallowing therapy techniques and few surgical procedures and a sizable proportion of them can get rid of the various feeding tubes they were carrying. That alone makes the specialty a truly gratifying one.

References

1. Shapiro J, Martin S. Disorders of the Upper Oesophageal Sphincter in the Larynx. A Multidisciplinary Approach. St Louis, MO: Mosby; 1996:337–355
2. Murry T, Carrau RL. Swallowing disorders arising from surgical treatment. In: Murry T, Carrau RL, eds. Clinical Management of Swallowing Disorders. 2nd ed. San Diego, CA: Plural Publishing Inc.; 2006;81–96
3. Logemann JA. Therapy for oropharyngeal swallowing disorders. In: Perlman AL, Schulze-Delrieu K, eds. Deglutition and its Disorders. San Diego, CA: Singular Publishing Group; 1997:451–455
4. Bushmann M, Dobmeyer SM, Leeker L, Perlmutter JS. Swallowing abnormalities and their response to treatment in Parkinson's disease. Neurology 1989;39(10):1309–1314
5. Fujiu M, Logemann JA. Effect of a tongue holding maneuver on posterior pharyngeal wall movement during deglutition. Am J Speech Lang Pathol 1996;5:23–30
6. Zaino C. et al The Pharyngeal Sphincter. Springfield, Ill, 1970 Charles c Thomas
7. Ding R, Larson CR, Logemann JA, Rademaker AW. Surface electromyographic and electroglottographic studies in normal subjects under two swallow conditions: normal and during the Mendelsohn manuever. Dysphagia 2002;17(1):1–12

8. Shaker R, Kern M, Bardan E, et al Augmentation of deglutitive upper esophageal sphincter opening in the elderly by exercise. Am J Physiol 1997;272(6 Pt 1):G1518–G1522

9. Donzelli J, Brady S. The effects of breath-holding on vocal fold adduction: implications for safe swallowing. Arch Otolaryngol Head Neck Surg 2004;130(2):208–210

10. Silbiger ML, Pikielney R, Donner MW. Neuromuscular disorders affecting the pharynx. Cineradiographic analysis. Invest Radiol 1967;2(6):442–448

11. Langmore SE, Schatz K, Olson N. Fibreoptic endoscopic evaluation of swallowing safety. Dysphagia 1988;2(4):216–219

12. Ekberg O, Nylander G. Dysfunction of the cricopharyngeal muscle. A cineradiographic study of patients with dysphagia. Radiology 1982;143(2):481–486

13. Cook IJ, Gabb M, Panagopoulos V, et al. Pharyngeal (Zenker's) diverticulum is a disorder of upper esophageal sphincter opening. Gastroenterology 1992;103(4):1229–1235

Section G

Professional Voice

35 Assessment of the Professional Voice: The Three-Part Examination

James Thomas

In most ways, a professional's voice is no different from other individuals. The vocal cords open for the professional to breathe in and they close, air is passed through them and they vibrate to generate sound, just like any other person.

How then is the professional's voice different? By definition, a professional uses his or her voice to earn her living. Consequently, any impairment of the voice risks a corresponding financial instability. The vocal cords are a highly valuable organ for the voice professionals.

Another difference in the professional's voice (and it is a generalization) is that individuals who are innately talkative often seek out and find a profession where they can apply their talkativeness to work for them. Professional voice users, who are then often innately talkative, risk overusing their voice both at work and at play.

A professional voice user is not universally talkative. Occasionally, a very quiet person ends up in an occupation where he is required to use his voice much more than he anticipated. A quiet professional voice user suffers from a different set of problems than the talkative voice professional.

Besides vocal personality, vocal technique may have a significant impact on the voice professional's sound quality. Depending on how vocal cords are used, various impairments in vocal quality may occur.

The following three uses of the voice — overuse, underuse, and improper use — constitute a group of voice disorders that we may label *functional voice disorders*. The label *functional* implies that how the voice is used causes impairment in sound quality. By contrast, when a change in the structure of the vocal cords occurs primarily and causes a change in airflow, we may label this a *structural voice disorder*.

Consequently, while a voice professional is subject to all the same vocal disorders that any individual is, when she complains of hoarseness, she has a higher risk of having a *functional voice disorder* than any other type. An assessment of the professional voice requires an elevated awareness of the potential for a *functional voice disorder*.

First, let us define the terms voice and hoarseness.

Voice

Voice is sound. Sound production is based on physics. All impairment of voice comes down to a physical change in vibration.

In the idealized situation, to make a sound

1. The back of the vocal cords leave the "breathing in" position, moving together until parallel.

2. Tension is applied to the vocal cords as they initially occlude the airway.
3. Air is propelled through them, usually from below.
4. They start flexing open in the middle.
5. Increasing tension causes the cords to snap back closed.

To create pulses of air vibration, steps 4 and 5 repeated (**Fig. 35.1**). The vocal cords oscillate quite rapidly, perhaps 100 to 200 times per second during casual speaking, with smaller cords tending toward faster oscillation. In a set of perfect cords, we could characterize them as

- Being open about half the time and closed about half the time
- Letting air out in measured puffs
- Not leaking air during the closed phase
- Vibrating symmetrically

This creates the sound that we hear, and any single note can be visualized on an oscilloscope as a sine wave—a regular vibration and when we hear it, we hear a musical tone. We can talk about the tone in terms of frequency or vibrations per second. Hertz is a common scientific measurement, which requires the use of logarithms for calculations.

We can also use a scale such as the musical, western chromatic scale to label each tone produced (C3, C3#, D3, D3#, etc.).[a] Each succeeding note is one semitone higher than the previous. This "semi-tone method" for documenting

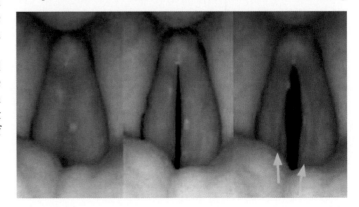

Figure 35.1 Vocal cords vibratory cycle. They are completely closed on the left. They begin to open in the center, and on the right, they have reached maximal opening before they will begin to close again. The mucosal wave can be seen in the right photo as a curved line just lateral to the edge of the vocal cord (arrows). In a video, this line propagates from the margin and moves laterally.

---

[a] Measuring pitch and pitch notation.

the voice visually distributes the sounds into audibly equal intervals without delving into the complexities of the logarithmic Hertz scale.

Hoarseness

Air Leak and Diplophonia

All hoarseness can be described in one of two ways. In the first, the vocal cords do not come together as they should allowing air leak.

Let us call this *husky hoarseness*. The second type of hoarseness is caused by asymmetric vibration. Because there are two vocal cords, when they are not symmetric, they tend to vibrate at two different pitches. A physician would call this sound diplophonia. *Di* means two and *phonia* means voice, so two voices can be heard at once. Usually, because the cords are only slightly out of sync, the diplophonia will be inharmonious, and the perception will be of a rough or gravelly quality. We will call this *rough hoarseness*.

Let us explore these two ideas in more detail

- Husky hoarseness.
- Rough hoarseness.

Whisper

Pure Air Leak

To understand husky hoarseness, it is helpful to think of one of the extreme types of sound production we can make with our larynx: extremely soft sound. We can generate sound in the larynx with the vocal cords in a partially or completely open position—that sound is called a whisper.

Normally, the vocal cords come completely together when making a sound (**Fig. 35.2**). The mid-portion oscillates open and closed.

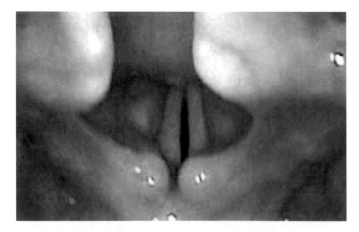

Figure 35.2 During normal sound production, the membranous vocal cords lie parallel to each other and vibrate. Although the back of the vocal cords is hidden from view beneath the arytenoids in the photo, the back of the vocal cords is together. This stroboscopic photo was taken during the open phase of vibration.

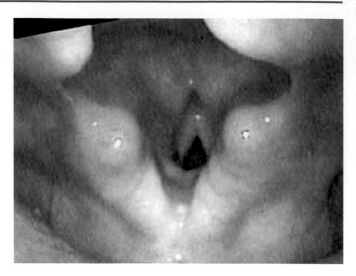

Figure 35.3 In a whisper, the back of the larynx might be open, whereas the membranous vocal cords might be closed such that all the air is forced out through an opening at the posterior end of the vocal cords.

By contrast, in a whisper, the vocal cords do not vibrate (**Fig. 35.3**). The airflow is increased and as it passes a narrowed spot, turbulence is created. Airflow that is turbulent consists of many different pitches simultaneously: white noise. The larynx can narrow the airway in several ways without allowing the vocal cords to vibrate.

This signal, composed of white noise, lacks intensity and cannot be heard well or from very far away. It is not very penetrating. White noise blends with environmental noise.

Conversely, we typically produce voice at a single pitch to generate a strong signal that will stand out against background noise. This is a signal that we modify with vowels and consonants to carry information from one human to the next.

A stage whisper is meant to sound like a whisper, yet the audience needs to hear the speaker. In a stage whisper for a theater production, the vocal cords are allowed to vibrate a little, so that the sound has the character of white noise, but enough vibrations of the vocal cords for the sound to carry into the audience. A stage whisper is really a mixture of a lot of whisper and a little bit of a vibration (**Fig. 35.4**).

In between a whisper (cords not vibrating) and a clear tone (cords completely parallel with all air passing between them), we can have some mix of a pure tone and white noise. The white noise gives the voice a husky quality.

At times, a singer, perhaps a nightclub singer, might wish to add a component of breathiness to her voice to give it a sensual quality. She is adding an intentional gap between the vocal cords to let some air leak out.

So while a whisper is the extreme of turbulent airflow through the larynx, any gap between the vocal cords will add a commensurate degree of turbulence perceived as a huskiness of the voice. We may desire that quality, but if we do not, it is hoarseness.

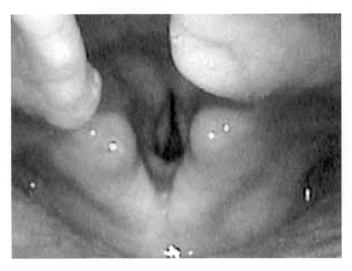

Figure 35.4 In a stage whisper, the membranous vocal cords are held slightly apart such that much of the air exits through the opening behind the vocal cords. However, some air passes between the vocal cords and they vibrate slightly.

Gaps: Huskiness

Remember, under idealized conditions, the posterior portion of the vocal cords moves completely together during voice production, and the vocal cords lie parallel to each other. Air is blown between them, and the vocal cords rapidly open and close, letting out regular pulses of air.

In what ways might the vocal cords incompletely close? There are a couple of characteristic types of gaps that occur between the vocal cords:

- Posterior gap
- Anterior gap
- Central gap
- Split gap
- Timing gap

All of these types of gaps leak air and create a husky hoarseness. Some of these gaps are more common in the professional voice user.

Posterior Gap

If the vocal cords are going from the breathing in, then inverted V-shape toward a parallel position but they stop short of complete closure, this leaves a gap posteriorly (**Fig. 35.5**). One example of this type of gap is muscle tension, where the opening posterior cricoarytenoid (PCA) muscles partially tighten during phonation and hold the cords slightly apart, allowing air to escape between the back portion of the vocal cords.

Anterior Gap

Vocal cord trauma may disrupt the vocal cords where they attach at the front of the larynx (**Fig. 35.6**). If the vocal cords heal slightly apart anteriorly, then air escapes through the front of the vocal cords. This is a very uncommon type of gap.

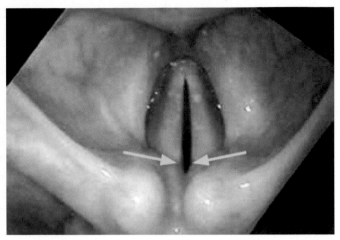

Figure 35.5 Blue arrows lie along the direction of closure and point to the gap remaining between the vocal processes when there is incomplete closure.

Central Gap

If the vocal cord muscles are not exercised regularly by talking, the vocal cord muscles atrophy and can no longer tense to a straight line (**Fig. 35.7**). They remain concave, even when the back of the cords are completely closed. Consequently, a central gap is created.

Aging contributes to this as well. Much like the skin on the face gradually sags with aging, the vocal cords sag with aging as they lose elasticity. Typically, this sagging, or as physicians call it, bowing, is relatively symmetric. There is a nearly oval-shaped gap with pointed ends between the vocal cords. Air leaks out the middle.

Split Gap

Vocal overdoers typically have hefty vocal cord muscles and may have in addition, a callus or swelling on the edge

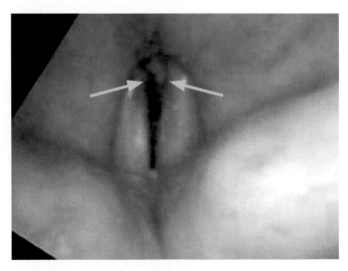

Figure 35.6 Blue arrows point to an anterior opening secondary to scarring after a surgery on the larynx injured the attachment of the vocal cords to the thyroid cartilage.

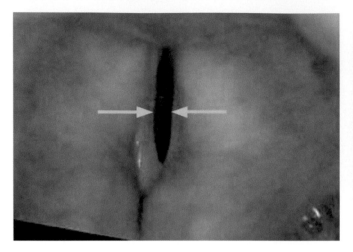

Figure 35.7 At the beginning of sound production, the back of the vocal cords is touched, but the blue arrows point to a large central gap.

of the vibrating portion of the vocal cord (**Fig. 35.8**). This protuberant swelling (or swellings) will touch first as the vocal cords are tensed and leave an opening both anterior and posterior to the swelling. Hence, air will leak from in front of and behind the swellings.

Timing Gap

Anything that makes the vocal cords uneven, particularly tension, can reduce the synchronization of their oscillations (**Fig. 35.9**). With a mild asymmetry, they may oscillate out of phase. Under a strobe light, it will look like they are chasing each other. They may never touch each other and so effectively, even while they are crossing each other's path in the midline, they do so at separate times, so air continuously leaks out. This is a gap created by timing.

If they become slightly more asymmetric, then they may begin to oscillate at different frequencies. Two pitches are created simultaneously. The separate frequencies are

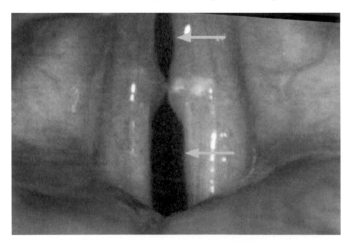

Figure 35.8 Two vocal polyps, slightly different in size, touch before the vocal cords can completely close, allowing air to leak from in front of and behind them (arrows).

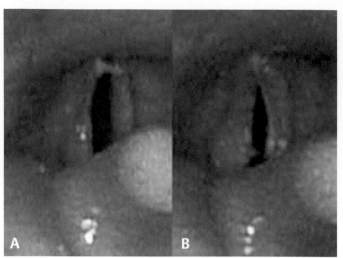

Figure 35.9 The same vocal cords viewed at two moments in time. (A) The right vocal cord is near the midline. (B) The left cord has come to the midline, but the right cord is now lateral.

perceived as roughness. And, in this case, we would actually hear both huskiness and roughness. The huskiness is from the gap. The concept of roughness brings up the other type of hoarseness: roughness due to vocal cord asymmetry.

Asymmetries: Roughness

Asymmetric Tension

When there is an uneven tension from a nerve paresis, the patient unconsciously attempts to compensate by raising her speaking pitch to avoid dyssynchrony. In her lower range where the difference in tension will be more pronounced, at some point, each vocal cord vibrates at a separate pitch (**Fig. 35.10**).

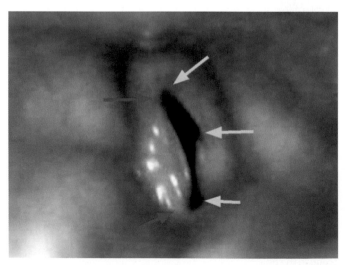

Figure 35.10 Vocal cords oscillating in a wild pattern, because the right side is much looser than the left side at a low pitch. The right cord has two separate wave segments compared with the left cord's single wave.

Producing two separate pitches simultaneously (diplophonia) a patient might say, "I am hoarse" or "My voice is rough at low pitches." A professional might use terms such as roughness, graveliness, or vocal fry to describe this quality. Two pitches, produced simultaneously and sonically competing with each other, are irregular vibrations due to uneven tension.

There are several potential types of unevenness between the vocal cords:

- Asymmetric tension
- Asymmetric mass
- Asymmetric length
- Asymmetric stiffness

Let us explore the different types.

Asymmetric Mass (and Length)

One example demonstrating the effects of asymmetric mass occurs in the patient who yells or screams and suddenly loses his voice (**Fig. 35.11**). In this example case, a hemorrhagic polyp has formed and has blood coursing through it. As he vibrates his vocal cords, the vibrations create a whipping of the polyp back and forth, and the polyp fills with more blood, making this vocal cord heavier and heavier. When the mass between the two vocal cords is different enough, they begin to vibrate separately at different pitches. Hoarseness due to asymmetric mass is most evident at his low pitches.

In the middle of his range, his pitch tends to jump around, and he cannot seem to control it. All of us tighten our vocal cords, as we move up in pitch. At some pitch, the polyp just barely touches the opposite vocal cord. As the pitch where it touches the opposite cord, vibrations are thrown off and the

patient's voice quits, squeaks (the pitch jumps up), or breaks up into roughness. The polyp touching the opposite vocal cord can stop the vibrations completely, split the vibrating cord into two short segments, or throw them completely out of synchrony.

In his upper range with the cords at their tightest, the polyp compresses against the other vocal cord stopping the vibration in the middle, leaving either end to vibrate separately. If the polyp is precisely in the middle, the segments may be the same length (and less than half the length of his vocal cord). They will each vibrate at the same, very high pitch. Effectively he does not have a functional middle range. He can do either low or very high pitches.

If the segments are different lengths, because the polyp is based slightly off the middle of the cord, then we will distinctly hear two different high pitches simultaneously.

In the mid-range, we hear a pitch break, something we normally associate with puberty. The pitch break occurs as the pitch is increased to the point where the polyp just begins to touch the opposite cord. If the vibrations produced by the full cord are suddenly shifted to half the cord, then the pitch jumps up. Alternatively, the touching may be followed by a diplophonia if the touching is light enough to just throw the cords out of sync with each other.

Many people quickly adapt to avoid these pitch breaks. By holding the vocal cords farther and farther apart, the swelling does not touch and disrupt the vibrations. Of course, more air leaks, and a greater huskiness is created by this compensation to avoid the pitch breaks.

Asymmetric Stiffness

Asymmetric stiffness might occur after a vocal cord stripping. If the stripping of one vocal cord removed not only the mucosa (the surface), but also the lubricating layer of the vocal cord, then this stripped vocal cord would be much stiffer than the other vocal cord (**Fig. 35.12**). Consequently, during many

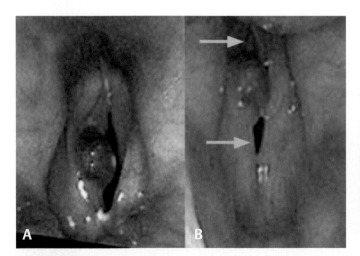

Figure 35.11 At various pitches, we have four types of asymmetries as well as a husky hoarseness: (1) asymmetric mass at low pitches: (in part A, the left vocal cord is heavier than the right because of the blood in the polyp; (2) asymmetric stiffness, the blood filling the polyp reduces the left vocal cord flexibility; (3) asymmetric segment length at high pitches (in part B the front segment is shorter than the rear segment—blue arrows; and (4) huskiness—air leak on either side of the polyp because the cords cannot come together (B—arrows).

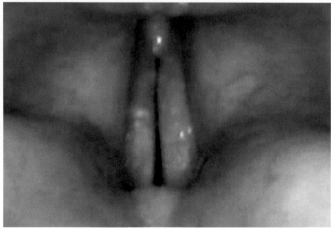

Figure 35.12 The left cord, remaining straight and stiff, is not moving on a stroboscopic examination, whereas the supple right cord oscillates back and forth. The left cord also has a slightly darker hue from the scarring.

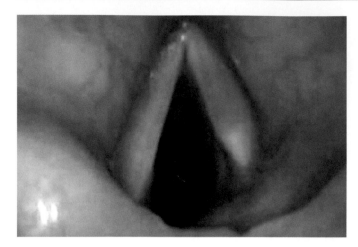

Figure 35.13 The left vocal cord is longer than the right, so something is structurally different between the two sides of the larynx. This length difference means the vocal cords will tend to vibrate at two different pitches when air passes between them.

attempts to make a sound in the mid-range, the more supple cord is trying to oscillate at a different pitch than the stiffer side. We perceive this asymmetric stiffness as roughness.

Asymmetric Length

The vocal cords might be different lengths after a traumatic injury, such as might occur from an endotracheal tube (**Fig. 35.13**).

Asymmetries between the vocal cords, whether in tension, in mass, in length, or in stiffness will tend to cause the vocal cords to go out of sync with each other during vibration. When they do, we will hear two pitches at once. With this double sound or diplophonia, we perceive a rough quality in the voice.

In summary, hoarseness is

- Air leaking between two vocal cords that are not closed—white noise.
- Two different sound sources—cords, which are asymmetric in some sense (mass, length, tension, or stiffness) and vibrating at different pitches, hence diplophonia.
- *Husky hoarseness*: huskiness is a term that can be substituted for air leak.
- *Rough hoarseness*: roughness is a term that can be substituted for diplophonia.
- Disorders may have components of both types of hoarseness.
- Hoarseness is a general term that includes huskiness and roughness.

Talkativeness

When studying with Robert Bastian in 1998, I was introduced to a 7-point scale of talkativeness he had developed (**Fig. 35.14**). It has proved to be an extremely elucidative

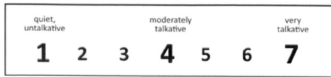

Figure 35.14 A 7-point scale of talkativeness.

vocal test in my voice practice. According to this Likert self-assessment scale (from 1 to 7) sample points define a person as

- 1: an innately quiet person
- 4: a person of average talkativeness
- 7: a person who loves and lives to talk

Interestingly, when presented with a row of numbers 1 through 7; designed so that 4 is the average person, most people can be rather accurate with their self-assessment of talkativeness. A person who can talk until she no longer has any voice at all often rates herself, with a laugh, as an 8 or 10 on the scale. She recognizes the extent of her inner need to talk when asked about it. Much less commonly, a partner will chime in and correct her if she tries to underrate her talkativeness. Most people visiting my office self-rate between 3 and 7.

As a corollary, a person who is a 1 and becomes hoarse, seldom finds that hoarseness is a problem worth seeking treatment for, because he is seldom using his voice very much anyway. He only comes to an office if someone drags him there.

The scale is meant to address personality, not job, though there is a very high correlation between job selection and talkativeness. It is hard to be happy as a midnight watchman if you are a 7. You would need to be on antidepressants just to survive. Most people who are a 7 find great intrinsic rewards participating in occupations such as acting, singing, performing, teaching, preaching, or perhaps just finding a stage to be on. We often, but not always, seek out a job that matches our psychological desire for our degree of innate talkativeness.

This scale is accurate enough that when I reviewed patient charts during my fellowship. I found no patients who had rated themselves a 4 or lower who had vocal cord swellings from overuse.

Using a similar Likert 7-point scale for innate vocal loudness:

- 1 is a soft-spoken person.
- 4 is a person with moderate volume.
- 7 is a person whose voice always projects well.

Volume also has some predictive value for vocal swellings, though not quite as strongly as "talkativeness."

Summary of Voice and Hoarseness

Voice is created by vibration, and voice can be produced only by vibrating structures. In the larynx, the source of vibration is almost always the true vocal cords.

Hoarseness is produced in two different ways: by air leak, or by asymmetric vibrations. Air leak causes a husky hoarseness. Asymmetric vibrations cause a rough hoarseness. Several disorders have both air leak and asymmetric vibrations, perhaps even more than one type of asymmetry.

Air may leak from the front, middle, or back of the vocal cords. The vocal cords may be asymmetric in several different ways: mass, tension, length, stiffness, or timing.

Two personality traits strongly influence vocal cord disorders. Talkativeness is an innate personality trait that puts a person at risk for mucosal lesions. With more vibrations come, an increasing risk of calluses and swellings which typically leads to a mixed rough and husky hoarseness. A lack of talkativeness puts a person at risk for muscle atrophy and typically husky hoarseness and discomfort from muscle compensation.

There is an implicit assumption often made that because voice comes from the larynx, all the examiner has to do is look in the vicinity of the vocal cords and whatever appears on the vocal cords is likely causing the hoarseness. However, mere presence is not sufficient justification to infer cause. The examiner needs to take this one important step further. The examiner must identify specifically what about the vocal cords is causing air leak or asymmetry. Looking for invisible, leaky air is not necessarily intuitive.

Complete Professional Voice User Examination

History

Almost every type of physician–patient interaction begins with a history of the problem. The physician says, "Tell me what happened." The story the patient tells about her problem is the history. In laryngology, three things are accomplished simultaneously during the history. First, this history offers a great many clues about likely types of voice disorders based on when the hoarseness started, simultaneous events at the onset, the duration, etc. Second, the examiner gets to begin hearing the conversational voice for a period of time. Third, the patient highlights preconceived perceptions of her problem that is also important for the physician to address later in the examination.

Talkative people will suffer from a different set of problems than people who are naturally quiet. People who lose their voice suddenly after yelling will have a different problem from those who lose it slowly over time.

The history is the first of a three-part examination: (1) the history, (2) the vocal capabilities testing, and (3) the visual examination.

The simplest first step is to eliminate speech problems. If the volume is loud and clear enough that people can hear the patient, but still not understand the words, then the problem is likely a speech issue. Problems with language are speech issues. Verbal rate and articulation issues are speech issues.

For example, a person with a cleft palate cannot close the palate completely against the back of the throat. Closing the palate completely against the back is required to make certain consonant sounds, otherwise, air leaks out the nose, and those sounds cannot be made. /p/, /t/, /k/ as well as /s/ and /sh/ are typical sounds requiring complete closure of the palate, channeling all of your air out the mouth. If you try to say "Pa, Pa, Pa" with the palate relaxed, air leaks out the nose and you sound to others like you have a cleft palate. From a physician point of view, when I hear this nasal air leakage, I know to look at the palate. I really do not even need to look at the vocal cords. So, hearing the problem directs me where to look.

If the problem is with consonants, vowels, words, and sentences, then the problem is likely not with the vocal cords.

Voice issues should usually involve complaints about pitch, volume, or clarity. Patients may not actually use these words. Volume and roughness qualities are voice issues that nonsingers might typically complain of, and pitch clarity and register are issues singers may more likely notice.

A person might say, in addition to "I am hoarse," something like I cannot get loud enough to be heard in a restaurant (volume problem) or I sound like I have a "frog in my throat" (clarity problem). A singer might say, "I am missing a few notes" (pitch issue).

Vocal Capabilities

Hearing the Voice Problem

Having determined that the problem is with the voice, how do we determine the specific problem and then the cause of that problem? If the vocal cords alter pitch, volume, clarity, and register, ideally, if we can set these parameters constant, then vary only one at time, we will most efficiently find our problem.

Generally, then, the patient does not even need to speak words during an examination of a vocal problem. Technically, singing is far more fruitful for finding a vocal problem than speaking. Perhaps I should say, making various continuous vowel sounds is most helpful, as some people feel they cannot sing. If the examiner can listen to a sound at various volumes and various pitches, then a vocal impairment will be more easily elicited.

Robert Bastian has described this process as vocal capabilities testing. By modifying one parameter at a time, when we hear the problem, we will know quite likely where the problem lies, even before we look at the voice box. Then, when we look, we will not be distracted by the color of the vocal cords, for instance. We will go straight to where the problem should be and find it.

The Vowel /i/

The vowel "e" is most useful for an examination, in phonetic English, /i/ (or /i:/) as in the word feel or bead. This vowel uses the most upright position of the larynx and most open position of the pharynx or throat above the voice box. It makes examination of the vocal cords with an endoscope easier. The /u/ sound is a close second, as in wh<u>o</u> or b<u>oo</u>. The other vowels /æ/, /e/, and /o/ tend to move the tongue and epiglottis back, narrowing the throat and make visualization of the vocal cords more difficult.

Remember, simplify! Pick one vowel and generally stick with it during an examination, so there is one less variable to deal with. Then, put the voice through a series of tests with this vowel. If the patient just says /i/, there may be no obvious hoarseness at one particular pitch or one particular volume, but it may appear at another.

Reading

Record the patient's voice by putting on a headset microphone held out in front of the mouth, requesting the patient read a paragraph from a book out loud in a comfortable voice. Use the same paragraph for every examination. Boring, but when the patient returns in the future, it is very easy to compare the passage. While reading is a mixture of voice and speech, reading does several things for the examiner. Reading relaxes the patient and takes their focus away from the examination.

Second, by listening, the examiner can determine the approximate average-speaking pitch is by matching the voice with a note on the piano. Third, the reading task allows to the examiner to listen and determine whether there are any speech issues.

Maximum Phonation Time

Using the /i/ sound, ask the patient to see how long she can say /i/ on one breath at her comfortable speaking pitch and volume.

This test, the maximum phonation time (MPT), is a rough measure of how completely closed the vocal cords are. The more closed they are, then the less air wasted and the longer the sound can be maintained. As a rough guide, with an MPT of less than 10 seconds duration, most people will complain of being out of breath with talking. Healthy young people can typically go beyond 20 to 30 seconds. There are many variables that affect this test, including lung capacity and vocal strategies used to produce the sound, but the more that the pitch and volume are kept constant, the more the test measures vocal cord approximation.

Vocal Range

Assess the lowest note and the highest note the person is capable of producing, no matter what the volume required, to define the pitch range of the voice. Sometimes, the person has excellent vocal rapport. Playing the notes on a piano, the patient can match the note with her voice. Some people are not so talented, and I will often ask them to glide up or down in pitch and then with my ear try to determine what was the lowest and what was the highest note they were capable of.

Swelling Tests

After obtaining this maximum range, assess the upper and lower ends of the vocal range at the very softest volume the patient can produce. Quite often, this requires some coaching. There are several disorders that impair soft voicing and despite the patient's interest in solving her problem; no one likes to "fail" at a test. This is especially pronounced in singers. Even when they complain that they are missing notes, they try their hardest to avoid sounding "bad" on those notes for the examiner. Coach them to go softer and softer and emphasize that we want to hear when the vocal cords stop vibrating or when their voice sounds bad as that is the purpose of their visit.

One of the easiest ways to determine the upper soft range is to have the patient sing the first four words of the nearly universally known song, "Happy birthday." When singing the words, "Happy birthday to you, between the word "day" and "to" is a melodic interval of a fourth. If no sound comes out on the word "to" or if there is a significant onset delay to the start of vocal cord vibration on that word, then there is some mechanical change in the larynx within this interval of one-fourth. This test can be repeated up or down a note and the point where the voice cuts out denotes the soft cut-off point.

Robert Bastian has termed this test for the soft volume, upper vocal ceiling, the "vocal swelling test." In general, the point at which there is an onset delay signifies the point where a swelling on one vocal cord touches the other vocal cord and stops the vibration, just like putting your finger lightly on a guitar string dampens or stops the vibration. There are some other problems that can be elicited with this test, but more later.

This is often the start of pinpointing the problem.

Volume

Ask the patient to yell robustly, not a scream, but a well-supported yell on the word "hey." This additional stress from increased pressure beneath the vocal cords can cause weak vocal cords to flutter.

The task may allow stiff vocal cords to actually produce sound, when quiet sounds were almost impossible.

Psychogenic problems often show up on this test when the patient hesitates or exaggerates performing this task.

Yelling is a simple task that everyone knows how to do. The important point is to note if the voice is different on this task than it was on the previous tasks.

Vegetative Sounds

Ask the patient to cough, followed by a clearing of her throat. This task can be helpful in sorting out weakness of the glottis or psychogenic problems. For instance, if a patient could whisper only up to this point in the examination, but can produce a robust cough, then the vocal cords have the capacity to come together and generate sound and were likely being held apart with muscle tension up to this point in the examination.

Conclusion

Professional voice users are most frequently affected by *functional voice disorders*. This includes subcategories of mucosal disorders, muscular disorders, and nonorganic disorders.

1. Mucosal lesions come from overuse.
2. Muscular impairment originates in underuse.
3. Nonorganic disorders come from inappropriate vocal technique or use.

The patient's history will orient the examiner toward one of these categories. In particular, using a Likert scale to self-identify talkativeness strongly orients the examiner to the type of problem likely to be found in the professional voice user.

It is helpful to separate speech disorders from voice disorders. Then primarily the vowel /i/ simplifies testing of the voice problem.

Vocal capabilities testing are sufficient to elucidate almost all vocal disorders. At a minimum, these clinical tests will direct the examiner where to look and what task to ask the patient to perform during the third part of an examination, endoscopy with stroboscopy.

Voice is created by vibration and so voice pathology will be present on or between the true vocal cords. When the complaint is hoarseness, the examiner is searching for air leak and irregular vibrations. Air leak is invisible but can be described as white noise and diplophonia. More conceptually we can think of huskiness and roughness.

- Husky hoarseness: A gap between the vocal cords
- Rough hoarseness: An asymmetry between or along the length of the vocal cords.

Endoscopy is the final part of the three-part laryngeal examination, used to confirm or disprove what the patient's history and the examiner's ears have defined as the problem. The examiner identifies gaps and asymmetries by varying the pitch and volume during the endoscopic examination. High pitch with low volume will exacerbate vibration impairment by mucosal lesions. Low pitch and low volume will aggravate problems of weakness such as muscle atrophy from insufficient vocal use.

36 Special Considerations for the Professional Voice User

Nupur Kapoor Nerurkar, Milind V. Kirtane, and Abir K. Bhattacharyya

A professional voice user is anyone whose voice is integral to earning a livelihood. Though singers and actors remain the elite group of professional voice users, teachers, lawyers, physicians, politicians, salespersons, receptionists, and radio jockeys all fall under the umbrella of this increasingly widening group of professional voice users. In today's world, the importance of the role of our voice, in society, is an undisputed fact. It should be borne in mind that treating or restoring a person's voice is often in effect changing or restoring their complete personality.

A voice professional being a vocal athlete is likely to be affected by even slight changes in voice quality. These vocal changes may be due to a plethora of causes ranging from the obvious polyp, nodules, or subepithelial hemorrhage to the more insidious muscle tension dysphonia or laryngeal paresis. Further confounding matters may be the presence of multiple pathologies, not all responsible for the acute discomfort being experienced by the professional voice user. A case in point is a well-established singer, who may present with vocal nodules and a unilateral subepithelial hemorrhage. It is critical to understand that a singer may sing comfortably with nodules and in fact these nodules may be responsible for the singer's characteristic voice. A safe mantra to follow while treating this highly sensitive group of professionals is to always tackle the acute changes first and preferably in a conservative manner. Overenthusiastic treatment to let the singer meet pressing singing commitments may damage the longevity of the voice and it is the duty of the treating physician to explain this gently, but firmly, to the professional voice user. Understanding the anatomy and physiology of phonation is the basis underlying the correct management of professional voice users.

Correct Age to Start Professional Training for Singing

The correct age to begin serious vocal training is controversial. It was felt that waiting till puberty and voice stabilization was safer; however, many singing prodigies have been training seriously since the age of 6 or 7, with no deleterious effects. It seems reasonable to state that children who have vocal aspirations should be permitted to begin training early with a careful watch on any signs of vocal misuse or abuse, thus avoiding permanent pathological changes.

Prolonged Warm-up

When singer complains of the necessity to warm up for an uncharacteristically long time, laryngopharyngeal reflux or vocal fold pathologies on the vibrating edge should be specifically looked for. A singer usually requires 10 to 30 minutes to warm up the voice. Most singers practice for 1 to 2 hours daily. Cooling down exercises are equally important for singers to maintain a good singing voice.

General Health and Environment

Good abdominal muscle tone, respiratory endurance, optimal weight, and a stress-free mind play a role in the quality of our voice.

Adequate hydration of the larynx is of paramount importance, and though eight glasses of water daily has been recommended, the amount may vary in different individuals. A good rule of thumb is to drink adequate water so that the urine is pale.

A nonsmoking, dust-free, and humidified environment is ideal. A dry and smoky environment may cause mucosal irritation and edema resulting in a hoarse voice with vocal fatigue referred to as the "Las Vegas Voice."[1]

Reflux laryngitis is fairly prevalent in the population of singers probably resultant to late night shows occasionally in a smoky environment. Surprisingly, smoking, overeating, drinking, and sleeping on a full stomach are not habits foreign to the singing population.

Good auditory feedback during a show is critical to prevent the singer from the tendency of increasing the vocal intensity of singing in direct response to the background noise. This tendency is referred to as the Lombard effect.[1] Cupping ones ear while singing is an effective way to add 6 to 7 dB to ones perception of voice and is useful in a noisy hall. We often see *qawali* singers (a subgroup in Indian classical singers) cupping one ear and outstretching the other hand. They are attempting to avoid the Lombard effect. For this same reason, hearing loss should not be missed in a singer.

Vocal Abuse and Misuse

Unquestionably, the greatest of all causes of laryngeal disease is the excessive use of one of its normal functions, phonation.
— Chevalier Jackson, 1942

Vocal abuse and misuse in both the singing and speaking voice has to be avoided. A technically correct singer who also happens to be an incessant chatterbox may damage the singing voice eventually. Vocal misuse is commonly due to too much tension on the tongue, neck, or larynx while speaking or singing. Vocal fatigue is a common complaint in such a scenario.

Role of Medication

Antihistamines, given for colds and postnasal drips, are known to cause drying of the mucosa resulting in dryness and laryngeal irritability. Most H1-receptor antagonists have significant anticholinergic effects and need to be avoided before a performance. A good replacement for diphenhydramine is a leukotriene inhibitor such as montelukast.[2]

Decongestants also need to be used with caution due to the drying effect they have on mucous membranes. However, if guaifenesin is present in the decongestant, it counters the drying effect by thinning and increasing the secretions.

Systemic corticosteroids have a huge role in managing many acute emergencies of the singer's vocal folds. Due to a strong anti-inflammatory action, they help in cases of sudden vocal fold edema. However, inhaled corticosteroids produce dryness and should be avoided. Nonsteroidal anti-inflammatory drugs (NSAIDs) should also be avoided, especially just preceding a singing session as their anti-coagulant effect may induce bleeding in the vocal fold.[3,4] Diuretics, many antihypertensive agents, and psychoactive drugs cause a resultant dryness of the larynx.

Menstrual and Endocrine Irregularities

The quality of our voice is dependent on the levels of our sex hormones, namely, estrogen, progesterone, and androgen. Females have all the three hormones, though the testosterone is in a low quantity. Although an excess of testosterone will make the female voice masculine, a small amount is essential to give a libido to the female voice.[5] Males have predominant testosterone, no progesterone, and a low level of estrogen.

In the first half of a female's menstrual cycle, there is abundance of estrogen that helps keep the vocal folds supple, well lubricated with an absence of desquamation of the epithelium. Estrogen promotes the transfer of intravascular fluid to the extra vascular compartment, which gives a better quality to the voice. However, in the second half of the cycle, there is a release of progesterone that causes the vocal folds to get thicker, less lubricated with desquamation of epithelium. Excessive progesterone prevents the return of interstitial fluid to the blood vessels with resultant edema. If the estrogen–progesterone balance is deranged in this second half of the menstrual cycle, some female singers may experience a difficulty in optimal utilization of their performing voice 5 to 6 days before and on the first couple of days of menses. Such singers should be advised to plan stage shows on the 3rd to 20th day of their menstrual cycle.

Pregnancy brings with it a surge of hormones that help keep the vocal folds nicely lubricated giving a sparkly quality to the voice. However, reflux, often associated with pregnancy and loss of breath support, toward the third trimester, interferes with the quality of voice.

Females nearing menopause or several months after stopping hormone replacement therapy may also experience a change in voice. This is more so in thin and lean women as compared with plump women. The reason for this lies in the fact that estrogen is produced by the ovaries, brain, as well as fat cells. A specific gene in our DNA facilitates the transformation of androgens into estrogen in our adipose cells.[5]

A correct balance of the thyroid hormones plays an important role in maintaining a healthy voice. Both hypo- and hyperthyroidism may result in voice changes. Hypothyroidism may often result in a Reinke edema picture and the patient is often lethargic.

Clinical Pearls

- Spend adequate time evaluating a professional voice user. Build a rapport.
- Record voice and stroboscopy findings.
- Educate regarding vocal hygiene, environmental factors, avoiding reflux, and adequate mental and physical rest.
- Female singers may be advised to allocate important singing commitments from 3rd to 20th day of menstrual cycle.
- Avoid antihistamines and NSAIDs before shows.
- Do not shy away from taking a second opinion when in doubt of diagnosis.
- Try to have a basic understanding of various forms of singing and individual artist's requirements.

Aging Voice

As life expectancy is on a steady rise in most countries, the problems faced due to an aging voice (presbyphonia) are also consequently on a rise. Professional voice users are not exempt from life's traumas, which may be in the form of mental stress, pollution, diabetes, cardiovascular diseases, alcohol, and tobacco. Presbyphonia, which is seen at around 80 years of age, is due to atrophy, dryness, and loss of suppleness of the vocal folds.[6] The dryness of the vocal folds is due to atrophy of the mucous glands. The loss of pliability of the vocal folds is following a loss of collagen and elastin fibers in the lamina propria with the remaining fibers become firmer. When an individual with presbyphonia phonates, the vocal folds appear bowed with a spindle-shaped phonatory gap and a weak voice due to air leak. The laryngeal cartilages ossify with age and the vocal fold joints may show signs of arthritis. Due to these anatomical changes, there is a decrease in the intensity of the voice with a narrowing of the vocal range and a drop in pitch. For a singer, these changes may be devastating and difficult to accept.

Vocal Athlete

Professional voice users, especially singers, are vocal athletes. The importance of daily exercise in any athlete's life cannot be exaggerated. There are exceptional singers even at 75 to 80 years of age .These singers have kept their vocal fold muscles healthy by daily vocal training exercises. If the muscles do not receive stimulation, the myofibrils of the striated muscles degenerate, get fibrosed, and replaced eventually by fat cells.[7]

Time Set for Patient Evaluation

While scheduling appointments for singers, it is appropriate to slot double the time one usually would for other patients in the voice clinic. Evaluation of the speaking and singing voice, previous voice recordings, clinical evaluation and discussions regarding management, and expected goals of recovery realistically necessitates 40 minutes or over. It is therefore important to schedule appointments with appropriate time slots to efficiently meet the demands of professional voice users. It is equally important to record voice and stroboscopic findings and involve the speech language pathologist in the decision process.

Vocal Emergencies

Vocal fold subepithelial hemorrhage and mucosal tear are the commonest vocal emergencies seen in singers. Subepithelial hemorrhage is not difficult to diagnose due to the dramatic finding of blood in the subepithelial space (**Fig. 36.1**). However, mucosal tears are seen as an irregular area most commonly on the medial vibrating edge which on stroboscopy is found to be adynamic. When mucosal

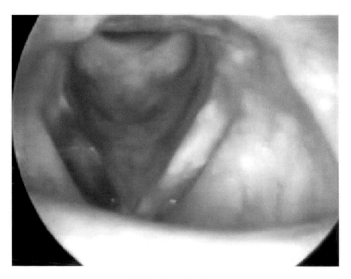

Figure 36.1   Right vocal fold subepithelial hemorrhage.

tears and subepithelial hemorrhage are associated with edema, the superficial lamina propria is very unstable and delicate. Any attempt to perform immediately may result in scar formation, further bleed, and permanent voice damage. However, if the tear or bleed is small and no edema is present, IM steroid injection (5 mg dexamethasone with 100 mg methylprednisolone acetate) acts within an hour allowing immediate performance. Dexamethasone is the most potent corticosteroid and most effective in reducing this type of inflammation.[3] Oral methylprednisolone acts in 24 hours and should be tapered off. The use of NSAIDs and other anticoagulants should be avoided at this time.

Finally, to perform or not in these situations remains a difficult decision made by the singer after being explained the possible consequences by the treating laryngologist.

Nonlaryngeal Surgery

Post-tonsillectomy scarring may create changes in the supraglottic vocal tract and the resonance of the voice, as may any surgery on the palate. The singer's resonance may also change following surgery for nasal polyps. This needs to be carefully discussed with the singer and surgical methods to minimize scarring need to be applied. Thyroid surgery always carries the potential risk of injury to the recurrent and superior laryngeal nerves and cutting the strap muscles in any neck surgery may change the neck tension. In fact, any surgery warranting endotracheal intubation may result in vocal fold paresis, intubation granuloma or trauma and should not be taken lightly in a professional voice user. A safe rule to follow is to use the smallest size of endotracheal tube that the surgery will permit.

When and How to Operate?

Vocal fold surgery performed on a singer and other professional voice users is fraught with anxiety on the part of both the patient and the treating surgeon. All reasonable effort must be made to treat the glottic pathology conservatively; however, this rule holds true for all patients, not just singers. The role of speech therapy cannot be overstated when dealing with vocal fold nodules that may develop very gradually, and in singers, it becomes partially responsible for the singers' characteristic voice quality.

Any professional voice user undergoing surgery is primarily concerned about two things: will they get back a completely normal speaking/singing voice and when can they resume their professional commitments. Tackling these concerns calls for honesty on the treating physicians' part with realistic expectations and possible complications discussed in detail. One way of tackling this is giving one's personal audited complication rate as well as internationally accepted figures. Developing a good rapport with the patient and relatives will almost always avoid misunderstandings and possible litigation.

Before posting for surgery, the postoperative course has to be made clear. Most laryngologists will advise a

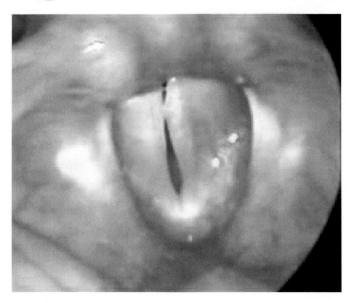

Figure 36.2 Left vocal fold anterior scar with resultant phonatory gap, in a teacher operated for a polyp.

10- to 14-day voice rest followed by a gradual vocalization process with 10 minutes on the first day and doubling the time every day. Normal speaking voice is expected at 4 to 5 weeks postoperatively. Singers are advised not to schedule programs for a period of 3 months. Speech therapy sessions are typically started once the voice rest phase is complete after a laryngoscopic evaluation. A stroboscopic evaluation is performed 4 to 6 weeks postoperatively to look for the return of mucosal wave.

The operating surgeon must be an adequately experienced laryngologist who has a comprehensive understanding of the anatomy and physiology of phonation. The principles of phono-microsurgery are respected at all times, preserving all normal epithelium and superficial lamina propria. Excessive removal of superficial lamina propria may result in a scar with resultant poor postoperative vocal outcomes (**Fig. 36.2**). For benign glottic lesions, a mini-microflap surgery is preferred. The subepithelial infiltration technique (SEIT) of 1 to 2 mL of 1:10,000 saline adrenaline helps provide hemostasis along with a host of other advantages. These include hydrodissection, acting as a heat sink if laser is being used, depth estimation, and a clearer demarcation of margins of the lesion.[8] Postoperative vocal outcome measures were found to be better in patients in whom the SEIT had been used as compared with controls in whom SEIT had not been used for similar glottic lesions operated

by the microflap technique.[9] Optimizing vocal outcomes with phono-microsurgical excision of intracordal vocal fold cysts can be challenging because the cyst often replaces substantial amounts of superficial lamina propria.[10] The possibility of postoperative voice deterioration, however remote, must always be discussed.

Summary

A thorough understanding of the anatomy and physiology of phonation, precise documentation, experience and confidence in performing all types of phono-microsurgery, instruments for diagnosis and treatment of voice disorders, and the teamwork of a speech language pathologist are essential components for developing a good and safe professional voice practice. A good mantra to keep in mind is "do no harm."

References

1. Sataloff RT. Professional voice evaluation. In: Ossoff RH, Shapshay SM, Woodson GE, Netterville JL, eds. The Larynx. Philadelphia, PA: Lippincott Williams & Wilkins; 2003

2. McMillan RM. Leukotrienes in respiratory disease. Paediatr Respir Rev 2001;2(3):238–244

3. Thompson AR. Pharmacological agents with effects on voice. Am J Otolaryngol 1995;16(1):12–18

4. Neely JL, Rosen C. Vocal fold hemorrhage associated with coumadin therapy in an opera singer. J Voice 2000;14(2):272–277

5. Abitbol J. Normal voice maturation: Hormones and age. In: Benninger M, Murry T, eds. The Performer's Voice. San Diego, CA: Plural Publishing; 2006:33–50

6. Von Leden H, Alessi DM. The aging voice. In: Benninger MS, Jacobson BJ, Johnson AF, eds. Vocal Arts Medicine: The Care and Prevention of Professional Voice Disorders. New York, NY: Thieme Medical Publishers; 1994:269–280

7. Malmgren LT, Jones CE, Bookman LM. Muscle fiber and satellite cell apoptosis in the aging human thyroarytenoid muscle: a stereological study with confocal laser scanning microscopy. Otolaryngol Head Neck Surg 2001;125(1):34–39

8. Zeitels SM. Premalignant epithelium and microinvasive cancer of the vocal fold: the evolution of phonomicrosurgical management. Laryngoscope 1995;105(3 Pt 2):1–51

9. Nerurkar N, Narkar N, Joshi A, Kalel K, Bradoo R. Vocal outcomes following subepithelial infiltration technique in microflap surgery: a review of 30 cases. J Laryngol Otol 2007;121(8):768–771

10. Burns JA, Hillman RE, Stadelman-Cohen T, Zeitels SM. Phonomicrosurgical treatment of intracordal vocal-fold cysts in singers. Laryngoscope 2009;119(2):419–422

37 Special Consideration for the Professional Voice User: the UK Perspective

Declan Costello

Professional voice users are those patients who rely on their voices for their livelihoods. This group therefore includes actors, singers, lecturers, teachers, clergy, and lawyers. However, in an increasingly communication-driven world, it also includes call center workers, sales representatives, and other professionals who have to communicate to any significant extent.

This chapter will focus largely on vocal performers and the specific considerations that must be borne in mind in this group.

History

Vocal performers are often exquisitely sensitive about subtle changes in their voices and will be able to pinpoint very precisely the nature of their problem. The consultation should start with an open question allowing the patient to explain their difficulties.

A "standard" history in the voice clinic is covered elsewhere in this volume and will not be rehearsed here. Particularly in singers, the presenting complaint may often be a very subtle problem relating to parts of their range, certain dynamics, or certain vowels.

The *singing style* can have a profound effect on the ability of a performer to sustain their vocal instrument—singing in the musical theater style, for example, has a tendency to be very vocally demanding, with a high "closed quotient" (the vocal folds being closed for a large proportion of the vibratory cycle). The same can be said of many styles of rock and pop singing. In addition, a *change in repertoire* can have a great impact: it is not unusual, for example, for singing students to be required to change their repertoire from one college term to the next. A change of repertoire requires a change in the setup of the laryngeal musculature, and it can lead to vocal problems.

The extent of *vocal training* is an important factor: it is surprising how many young performers have relatively little training and are thrown into rehearsal and performance schedules without adequate preparation. This is particularly true for amateur and semiprofessional performers.

A performer's *schedule of rehearsals and performances* is important: is it not unusual, for example, for a musical theater production to have up to two performances a day for 5 days per week. On the contrary, an opera singer will often perform just on alternate nights. Rehearsal schedules can be very intensive and it is important for the performer to realize that sufficient breaks should be incorporated into their schedule. Rehearsal schedules that are organized by institutions (opera houses, West End shows, etc.) will, on the whole, incorporate sufficient breaks and rests. However, it is often the case that amateur or semiprofessional bands, who have to fit in their rehearsals around other occupations, will have long rehearsals with few breaks.

Some performing roles require *specific vocal demands.* This might include foreign accents, shouting, or other vocal effects. If these gestures are unfamiliar to the performer, or if they are to be sustained for a whole performance, they can lead to unhelpful muscle tension patterns and even vocal fold phonotrauma.

Most performers are aware of the importance of *warming up* their voices. Warming-up regimes vary from performer to performer, but the aim is to prepare the voice for the performance to follow: for many, this will involve humming exercises, sirening (a glissando sliding of the voice from low to high), and singing scales and arpeggios. These warm-ups should not (at least initially) be performed at full vocal intensity. The aim, as with an athlete warming up before a race, is to encourage blood flow to the muscles, and to encourage flexibility in the muscles and other structures of the vocal tract.

Psychological issues are often a major factor in the vocal problems of professional performers. Major life events such as relationship difficulties, bereavement, and changes in circumstances (e.g., moving away from home) can have a profound impact on the patient's psychological well-being, and their vocal problems may be a subtle manifestation of this sort of strain. Delicate and tactful questioning is required to elucidate these factors without suggesting that the problems are "all in the mind" of the patient.

Finally, one must ask the question "why are you here now?" This is an important point, because the patient may volunteer that they feel that they are going to lose their job; they may be concerned about a run of performances next week; or they may be concerned about their ability to get on stage tonight. The approach to the treatment of each of these scenarios is very different.

Much of the performer's *working lifestyle* revolves around late nights, meals late in the evening, and much travelling. All of these can lead to fatigue and, in particular late meals, can exacerbate any problems with laryngopharyngeal reflux.

In addition, *social lifestyle* factors can exacerbate a performer's problems. Young performers in particular think little of socializing several nights each week. Noisy restaurants and clubs require large vocal demands that can significantly hinder their ability to perform to the best of their abilities.

Voice Evaluation

It is very frequently the case that the normal conversational spoken voice in a vocal professional will be unaffected. As discussed above, the vocal professional will more frequently present with subtle problems relating to a certain aspect of their performing voice. This only become manifest when they perform the passage in question.

Therefore, it may be useful to ask the patient to demonstrate the particular vocal difficulties they are experiencing by performing part of a song or speech that they find particularly problematic. Detailed evaluation in terms of objective acoustic analysis (jitter, shimmer, noise-to-harmonic ratio, etc.) is less frequently required.

Laryngeal Examination

Palpation of the neck will reveal any neck masses or lymphadenopathy. It will also highlight any muscular tenderness.

Stroboscopic examination of the vocal folds is mandatory: it is only with the benefit of high-quality videostroboscopic equipment that one will gain sufficient detail of the mucosal surfaces of the vocal folds to be able to exclude subtle pathology. Fiberoptic or mirror examination of the larynx is no longer acceptable mode of examination in vocal professionals.

Stroboscopic examination can be performed either with a rigid endoscope (70 or 90 degrees) or with a chip-tip (distal-chip) flexible endoscope. The details of stroboscopy are discussed elsewhere in this volume, but it is worth bearing in mind the biomechanics of examination in each situation: rigid endoscopy requires the patient's neck to be slightly extended, and for the tongue to be forcibly protruded. The endoscope can then be advanced over the tongue and the vocal folds examined. Needless to say, this is a very "unphysiological" position in which to be phonating. In general, it is only possible to elucidate an "ee" vowel in this position.

By contrast, with the chip-tip endoscope passed through the nose, the performer can sing and speak almost as normal. A wide variety of vocal gestures can be performed, including those specific gestures that are causing the performance problems. This is particularly helpful when muscle tension is believed to be a feature. On the contrary, the images achieved with the distal-chip flexible endoscopes are not quite as good as the rigid views. Different vocal problems may call for different examination techniques, or sometimes both.

Feedback

A crucial part of the consultation with a vocal professional is the explanation of the findings. It is imperative to take time to explain the laryngeal images, so the patient can understand (and engage with) the plan of management.

Management

It is self-evident that the management of the patient will be governed by the pathology (or lack of it) found in the examination. However, other factors will come into play, and a selection of scenarios may help expand on this:

- A 22-year-old student at a performing arts academy is having problems with her voice. She is a music theater singer, and typically becomes hoarse after a few performances. When she rests her voice for a few days, her voice returns, but she runs into similar difficulties when she starts another run of shows. She usually has to sing in one show each day for a week at a time. Examination shows soft vocal fold nodules in the usual locations.
  - In this situation, one must explain that vocal fold nodules will often resolve with speech and language therapy and with the assistance of a good singing teacher.
- Consider the same student again. She is now 25 years old and is having similar difficulties to those she experienced 3 years previously. She has seen two laryngologists in recent years and has had extensive speech therapy and voice coaching. In spite of this, she is having the same problems of vocal fatigue and inability to complete a run of shows. In fact, she now becomes fatigued after just five performances.
  - This is now a difficult situation. She appears to have instituted all of the necessary changes and is still not able to perform to the required standard. Of particular concern is that she is not, at the moment, being required to perform as frequently as a full-time performing professional: if she were in a professional cast, she would be expected to perform up to twice per day for 5 or more days per week. The clinician should have a frank discussion with her about this, and consider either surgical excision of her nodules or a change in her performing regime/style.
- A 27-year-old professional opera singer asks for an urgent consultation: he has a performance tonight, but was having difficulties during last night's performance, and his voice has not "felt right" today. The performance tonight is the last one for several weeks. There is no problem with his singing voice and there are no other features in the history of concern. Examination shows mildly edematous vocal folds but no focal pathology and no evidence of hyperemia.
  - Given that tonight's performance is his last for some time and that there is no evidence of vocal fold hemorrhage or hypervascularity, it would probably be reasonable to consider a single dose of a corticosteroid to help reduce some of the laryngeal inflammation. It would be important to review the patient in the days after the performance to ensure that the inflammation has settled.

- A 26-year-old rock singer is in the middle of a tour in the United Kingdom. After last night's concert, his voice was markedly hoarse, and he has requested an urgent laryngeal evaluation. He has a further 15 shows to perform in the next 3 weeks, and his management team accompany him to his consultation. They are extremely keen to avoid cancelling any shows. Stroboscopic examination shows hemorrhage of the left vocal fold, with blood tracking under the whole length of the mucosal surface.
  - You are duty bound to advice absolute voice rest and that the rest of the shows are cancelled. Vocal fold hemorrhage of this type can be catastrophic for a performer, and it is imperative that the voice is rested to attempt to avoid the formation of scar tissue.

Section H

New Frontiers

38 Laryngeal Transplantation

D. Gregory Farwell and Martin A. Birchall

The intricacy and complexity of the human voice is unique in the animal world. In social settings, our ability to interact verbally is critical to maintaining a sense of normalcy and optimizing quality of life. As our modern communication-centered society becomes less dependent upon manual labor, our ability to effectively vocalize is increasingly essential in maintaining gainful employment. In patients who have undergone laryngectomy or have a severely dysfunctional larynx and have lost their ability to speak, many techniques have been developed to restore voice. These include vibratory speech via an electrolarynx, esophageal speech, or tracheoesophageal puncture. While these methods are successful in allowing most patients to communicate, the voice produced is often abnormal in clarity, volume, and duration. In multiple studies, these changes in voice have been shown to variably impact quality of life.[1–3]

Rather than replacing the complicated larynx with a mechanized vibratory source or a mucosal shunt for a vibrating air column, the transplantation of a larynx offers the potential for physiological return of function. Replacing a dysfunctional or lost larynx with a transplanted larynx has been the goal of surgeons for over 40 years. Starting with the work in dogs by Silver et al[4,5] and the reported transplantation of an avascular human laryngeal graft in 1969 by Kluyskens and Ringoir,[6] the field of laryngeal transplantation was born. Questionnaire studies have shown that patients would be willing to trade the side effects of immunosuppressant medication to experience restoration of normal speech.[7] Over the past four decades, tremendous work has been performed in animal models culminating in two successful North American larynx transplants and several reported transplants in South America.[8–13]

History

In 1966, Silver et al first published their work on laryngeal transplantation in dogs, and in their 1970 article, they described 48 canine laryngeal transplants.[4,5] Several key observations came out of their work. First, all nonimmunosuppressed organs rejected at a microscopic level in 6 to 7 days. On a macroscopic level, rejection was visible in 7 to 8 days after transplant. This rejection was manifested by early edema, friability, and gray-yellow exudates followed by necrosis and cartilage exposure. Additional observations included the short time of ischemia tolerated by the nonperfused larynx. No perfusate was utilized and revascularization that took longer than 45 minutes was associated with ischemic necrosis.

In 1969, Kluyskens and Ringoir reported the first human larynx transplant after performing a laryngectomy in a 62-year-old man with larynx cancer. The organ was not revascularized but placed in a "wrap" of the recipient's perichondrium to encourage revascularization. Postoperatively, there was ischemic necrosis noted on biopsy. Due to the severity of the cancer, they were unable to wait for a perfectly cross-matched donor. The donor organ transplanted was of the same blood type (O+) but only matched 3 of the other 10 antigens tested. Despite immunosuppression with prednisone, azathioprine, actinomycin-C, and antilymphocyte serum, the graft suffered rejection episodes as demonstrated by edema and partial necrosis. This early rejection was rescued by additional immunosuppression. The patient was able to have the nasogastric tube removed at 70 days, and leave the hospital at 3 months before succumbing to aggressive recurrent cancer at 8 months posttransplant.[6] This poignant demonstration of the relationship of immunosuppression to cancer dramatically curbed the enthusiasm for this procedure.

While human transplantation was abandoned for nearly 30 years, experimental work on laryngeal transplant continued in animal models. Additionally, rapid evolution of the field of solid organ transplantation resulted in dramatic improvements in our understanding of immunology, immunosuppression, and graft tolerance. The successful transplantation of vascularized rat larynges was described in 1992 and 1994 by Strome's group at the Cleveland Clinic.[10,11] Work on canine laryngeal preservation by Kevorkian et al[9] demonstrated the ability to extend cold ischemia time and improve graft survival in a large mammalian model. More recently, a porcine model was developed to evaluate revascularization and the immunological response to transplantation.[12] These animal models advanced our understanding of the technical caveats of laryngeal transplantation and the immunosuppression necessary for graft survival.

Blood Supply

Successful larynx transplantation requires adequate blood supply and drainage. The blood supply to the larynx was beautifully described by Pearson in 1975.[14] This blood supply is variable but follows a general pattern of a superior and inferior blood supply off the superior thyroid and inferior thyroid arteries, respectively. The superior laryngeal artery usually branches from the superior thyroid artery and enters the thyrohyoid membrane.[15] An inferior laryngeal artery branches from the inferior thyroid artery to supply the posterior and cricoid region. Often a posterior inferior vessel is noted coming off the inferior thyroid. These branches also supply the membranous trachea and esophagus and provide another source of blood supply to the subglottis and posterior trachea. As any thyroid surgeon knows, there are also multiple vascular communications between the thyroid gland and the ligament of Berry and the underlying larynx and trachea. The inferior thyroid artery is an important contributor to the vascularity of the trachea.[16] As many laryngeal transplant candidates are also deficient in tracheal length, this is a critical attribute of the inferior thyroid artery.

The venous system of the larynx is much less understood and studied. In Pearson's study, a general pattern of veins following the arteries was demonstrated. The inferior laryngeal veins drained into the middle thyroid veins toward the jugular veins, whereas other inferior veins drained into the thyroid isthmus and inferior thyroid veins.[14]

Innervation

The innervation of the larynx has been widely studied and comprehensively described elsewhere in this book. The superior laryngeal nerve provides sensation to the majority of the glottic and supraglottic larynx after branching off of the vagus. Additionally, it supplies motor innervation to the cricothyroid muscle through its external laryngeal nerve branch. The recurrent laryngeal nerve provides subglottic sensation and motor innervations to the rest of the larynx. The recurrent laryngeal nerve typically bifurcates into an abductor and adductor branch before entering the larynx. This provides the opportunity to selectively reinnervate the larynx. However, it is increasingly clear that the innervation of the larynx is far more complex than the superficial description above. There is robust communication between these two main nerves through the nerve of Galen connecting the recurrent laryngeal nerve and superior laryngeal nerve in up to 81% of larynges.[17] Denervation injuries demonstrate variable disability and healing. Similarly, reinnervation procedures have demonstrated less predictable results than surgeons would like. This unpredictable behavior has frustrated laryngologists and may be explained by variable neural anatomy including intralaryngeal branching and neural communications described above.[18]

Transplantation Results

Building on their significant animal research, Strome and colleagues performed the first vascularized laryngeal transplant in 1998.[8] This patient had lost the function of his larynx from a motorcycle accident 20 years ago. He was aphonic, anosmic, and suffered from ageusia by report. After unsuccessful reconstructive attempts, he underwent laryngeal transplantation. Microvascular anastomoses were performed between both recipient and donor superior thyroid arteries. Venous anastomoses were performed between the donor jugular vein and the recipient facial vein on the right side and the middle thyroid veins on the left side. Microneurorrhaphies were performed between both superior laryngeal nerves and the right recurrent laryngeal nerve. Electromyography (EMG) was performed on the transplanted larynx 4 years after transplantation demonstrating innervations of bilateral cricoarytenoid and thyroarytenoid muscles.[19] The intensity of EMG activity was only slightly reduced on the left side despite having only performing microneurorrhaphy on the right side.

His posttransplant course has been remarkable.[20] After not speaking for 20 years, he was able to start an occupation as a motivational speaker posttransplant. He has suffered two episodes of rejection. The first was at 15 months and a second episode occurred 5 years after the transplant. Both episodes were rapidly treated with steroids resolving the laryngeal edema and restoring his voice. Approximately 9 years posttransplant, his left vocal fold developed persistent edema thought to represent chronic rejection. At 11 years posttransplant, he developed right vocal fold edema which was treated with Solu-Medrol (methylprednisolone sodium succinate for injection; Pfizer; Distributed by Pharmacia & Upjohn Co., Division of Pfizer Inc., NY, United States).

According to a report in 2002,[21] a second larynx transplant was performed in Medellin, Columbia. According to verbal presentations and the Internet reports, the transplant has been followed by others, but the exact number is unclear. A technical report describes a total of 25 trachea and larynx donors of which 12 larynges were discarded. No references in the medical literature discuss the functional results of these transplants, so unfortunately little is known of their outcomes.[13,21] The most recent reported laryngeal transplant was performed by our group at University of California, Davis (UC Davis), California, United States, in 2010. The results of this are being published at the time of writing this chapter. The patient was a 51-year-old woman who had received a previous kidney–pancreas transplant for diabetes-induced renal failure. As a complication of her renal failure, she had suffered intubation injury resulting in complete laryngeal and tracheal stenosis. Despite attempts at laryngotracheal repair, she remained tracheotomy dependent with a 100% laryngeal stenosis. She underwent successful transplantation with a modification of the technique described by Strome et al.[8]

Revascularization was achieved with three arterial microvascular anastomoses between the right sided donor and recipient superior thyroid arteries and bilateral donor inferior thyroid arteries to both recipient transverse cervical arteries. The brachiocephalic vein capturing the venous drainage from both the superior and inferior portions of the right thyroid was anastomosed to the right jugular vein and the left superior thyroid vein was anastomosed to the recipient left jugular vein. A functional reinnervation was attempted with microneurorrhaphies between the donor and recipient superior laryngeal nerves bilaterally. The right donor recurrent laryngeal nerve was anastomosed to the right recipient recurrent laryngeal nerve, but the left donor recurrent nerve was split into the adductor and abductor branches. The adductor branch was anastomosed in an end-to-side anastomosis to the left phrenic nerve and the remainder of the recurrent laryngeal nerve (abductor contribution) was anastomosed to the ansa cervicalis. Postoperatively, she has done well with no rejection documented to date. Functionally, she is talking for the first time in a decade and despite significant and persistent dysphagia, she was able to have her gastrostomy tube removed and obtain a full oral diet at 13 months posttransplant.

The edema present during the rejection episodes of the Cleveland patient has made the tracheotomy a safety issue. Both patients have ended up with vocal folds in a near-midline position with limited volitional abduction. For these reasons, both the Cleveland and the UC Davis patients have kept their tracheotomy for control of their airway.

Challenges

Immunosuppression remains the dominant obstacle to organ transplantation. As Silver et al demonstrated in his canine experiment, without appropriate immunosuppression, the body will ultimately reject the organ.[5] Clearly the majority of experience in transplant immunosuppression is in "simple" solid organs, such as the kidney, liver, heart, lung, and pancreas, where the organ is a relatively homogeneous structure with a limited number of tissue and cell types. The larynx belongs to a family of organs known as composite tissue transplants due to the multitude of tissue types inherent in the organ. This family of organs includes hands, upper extremities, lower extremities, face, and abdominal wall. While limited data exist, it appears that these composite grafts are subject to both acute and chronic rejection. By far, the most frequent composite transplantation has been the hand. In this group, 85% have demonstrated acute rejection.[22,23] After hand transplant, rejection often appears at the epithelium, with a rash. This may explain why in the Cleveland larynx transplant patient, edema of the mucosa was the first presenting sign. Little is known how chronic rejection will manifest in these grafts, but the first hand graft loss to chronic rejection occurred in 2009.

After solid organ transplantation, several other complications may occur including opportunistic infections, malignancies, graft-versus-host disease, and medication side effects.[24] Most decisions on immunosuppression in composite tissue transplantations are extrapolated from the experience with solid organ transplantation. As such, it is expected that similar risks will exist. In hand transplant patients, opportunistic infections have occurred in 63.6%, while 50% of patients have suffered metabolic complications.[23,25,26] With improvements in immunosuppressive agents and regiments, future efforts are being directed toward minimizing immunosuppression and working toward immunotolerance.[27] In hand transplants, because of the ability to watch the most antigenic component of this transplant (skin), they have been able to achieve extremely high 1-year survival, as they can diagnose and rescue rejection early. While more accessible than implanted organs, the larynx is still less accessible than the skin for monitoring of rejection. To date, both the Cleveland and UC Davis groups have utilized clinical parameters, such as hoarseness and endoscopic findings of edema, as clues to possible rejection necessitating biopsy. When present in the Cleveland patient, Solu-Medrol rescue was utilized with resolution of the signs and symptoms present. Additional research will be needed to further characterize signs and symptoms of rejection that will aid early detection and treatment.

The risks of immunosuppression remain the biggest ethical concern to more widespread use of this exciting transplantation option. Immunosuppression has been reported to increase the risk of cancer three to five times and the neoplasms tend to behave more aggressively than their counterparts in immunocompetent hosts.[28-30] As such, the risks of laryngeal transplantation must be carefully weighed against the potential benefits of the transplantation. This is especially poignant in the most numerous candidates for the procedure, laryngectomy patients. As most laryngectomees have had their larynx removed for tobacco-induced laryngeal cancer, the risk of locoregional cancer recurrence or tobacco-induced secondary malignancies must be strongly weighed in the risk–benefit ratio of the transplantation.

Functional Results

Functional results are hard to interpret with only two comprehensively described transplants. From an airway perspective, both have retained their tracheotomy. Both patients have ended up with vocal folds near the midline with minimal abduction on respiration. Concern for edema from rejection episodes, viral illness, and exercise intolerance has limited enthusiasm for decannulation.

Certainly, voice results have been very acceptable for both North American patients. The inability to utilize laryngeal speech makes communication difficult. Not only is it hard for the patient to communicate but it is also more difficult for the "listener" of the conversation to comprehend alaryngeal speech. This may lead to shorter, infrequent, and less in-depth conversations. As social beings, humans are at risk for social isolation and depression.[31] Despite the challenges of a tracheostomy, both larynx transplant recipients were extremely satisfied with the restitution of laryngeal speech and noted improvement in social acceptance and integration.

That being said, the success of laryngeal reinnervation must be described as modest at best. While there is evidence of reinnervation in both patients,[19] there is evidence of synkinesis and little or no volitional movement. Despite an attempt at selective abductor and adductor reinnervation of the UC Davis patient, to date, this potential has not been realized. As previously described, there are several theories on why this remains such a challenge. As demonstrated in the Cleveland Clinic patient, despite a unilateral recurrent laryngeal nerve microneurorrhaphy, there is bilateral reinnervation. As proposed in the article by Hydman and Mattsson, the anastomosis between the superior and recurrent laryngeal nerves may explain this synkinetic result.[18] Additionally, neural sprouting from the pharyngeal plexus and adjacent cervical nerves may explain some of the reinnervation findings. Until surgeons are better able to understand and manipulate selective reinnervation, this will remain an important obstacle to functional reinnervation and optimal laryngeal function. Novel and exciting approaches to treating bilateral vocal fold paralysis including laryngeal pacing hold promise and will hopefully improve our techniques in this regard.[32]

Patient Factors

Despite the challenges enumerated above, when given a hypothetical option of laryngeal transplantation, a significant number of laryngectomy patients would still choose a laryngeal transplant.[33,34] In a cohort of laryngectomy patients from the United Kingdom, patients were asked a series of hypothetical questions on their willingness to accept a transplant. In the best scenario, 75% of patients would wish for the procedure if it were "completely safe." That dropped significantly in the direst scenario of "significant risk to your life whilst in hospital." However, 19% of patients would still choose the procedure under that scenario.[33] A similar study of French patients demonstrated that 49% of their patients would accept the transplant if it was "simple and without danger" and 31% would still accept transplantation after a comprehensive discussion of the risks and possible adverse outcomes of the procedure.[34] These numbers speak to the compelling desire of patients to be able to speak in a normal fashion.

The individual questions in these studies are very illustrative and serve as a backdrop for decisions regarding the optimal patients for future transplantations. In the study by Buiret et al,[34] only 16% would accept transplantation if it meant a permanent tracheostomy and importantly, only 1% would accept a permanent gastrostomy as a trade-off for voice. It is clear from these questions that an individualized and comprehensive discussion must take place between the transplant surgeon and patient regarding the risks and possible benefits of the procedure. Both reported transplant patients will likely have a permanent tracheostomy for airway protection. Until improvements in laryngeal reinnervation occur,[35] it is highly probable that future transplant recipients will need to accept that fate. The UC Davis patient had a much delayed swallowing rehabilitation necessitating enteral feeding for more than 1 year. While she had other medical comorbidities that might have contributed to her delayed swallowing rehabilitation, it is likely that other transplant candidates will also have risk factors for dysphagia including previous trauma, radiation, or past surgery. As such, a candid discussion must take place between the surgeon and patient on the potential for trading a new voice for problems in swallowing. Additionally, the need for lifelong immunosuppression and its inherent side effects and risks must play a prominent role in the preoperative consultation.

Conclusion

Laryngeal transplantation is an exciting component of a rapidly changing field of composite tissue transplantation. Future work will undoubtedly result in better immunosuppression regimens and improvement in our ability to functionally rehabilitate these patients. As such, it is an option to consider for very select patients with severely dysfunctional larynges or laryngectomy patients who are at low risk for tumor recurrence or secondary malignancies. Laryngeal transplantation offers the potential for giving patients their voice back. Careful patient selection and counseling will ensure this transformative surgery available to the most appropriate patients.

References

1. Clements KS, Rassekh CH, Seikaly H, Hokanson JA, Calhoun KH. Communication after laryngectomy. An assessment of patient satisfaction. Arch Otolaryngol Head Neck Surg 1997;123(5):493–496
2. Kazi R, De Cordova J, Kanagalingam J, et al. Quality of life following total laryngectomy: assessment using the UW-QOL scale. ORL J Otorhinolaryngol Relat Spec 2007;69(2):100–106
3. Vilaseca I, Chen AY, Backscheider AG. Long-term quality of life after total laryngectomy. Head Neck 2006;28(4):313–320
4. Silver CE, Liebert PS, Som ML. Orthotopic transplantation of the dog larynx. Surg Forum 1966;17:466–468
5. Silver CE, Rosen RG, Dardik I, Eisen H, Schwibner BH, Som ML. Transplantation of the canine larynx. Ann Surg 1970;172(1):142–150
6. Kluyskens P, Ringoir S. Follow-up of a human larynx transplantation. Laryngoscope 1970;80(8):1244–1250
7. Buiret G, Rabilloud M, Combe C, Paliot H, Disant F, Céruse P. Larynx transplantation: laryngectomees' opinion poll. Transplantation 2007;84(12):1584–1589
8. Strome M, Stein J, Esclamado R, et al. Laryngeal transplantation and 40-month follow-up. N Engl J Med 2001;344(22):1676–1679
9. Kevorkian KF, Sercarz JA, Ye M, Kim YM, Hong KH, Berke GS. Extended canine laryngeal preservation for transplantation. Laryngoscope 1997;107(12, Pt 1):1623–1626
10. Strome S, Sloman-Moll E, Samonte BR, Wu J, Strome M. Rat model for a vascularized laryngeal allograft. Ann Otol Rhinol Laryngol 1992;101(11):950–953
11. Strome M, Wu J, Strome S, Brodsky G. A comparison of preservation techniques in a vascularized rat laryngeal transplant model. Laryngoscope 1994;104(6, Pt 1):666–668
12. Gorti GK, Birchall MA, Haverson K, Macchiarini P, Bailey M. A preclinical model for laryngeal transplantation: anatomy and mucosal immunology of the porcine larynx. Transplantation 1999;68(11):1638–1642
13. Duque E, Duque J, Nieves M, Mejía G, López B, Tintinago L. Management of larynx and trachea donors. Transplant Proc 2007;39(7):2076–2078
14. Pearson BW. Laryngeal microcirculation and pathways of cancer spread. Laryngoscope 1975;85(4):700–713
15. Vázquez T, Cobiella R, Maranillo E, et al. Anatomical variations of the superior thyroid and superior laryngeal arteries. Head Neck 2009;31(8):1078–1085
16. Salassa JR, Pearson BW, Payne WS. Gross and microscopical blood supply of the trachea. Ann Thorac Surg 1977;24(2):100–107

17. Naidu L, Ramsaroop L, Partab P, Satyapal KS. Galen's "anastomosis" revisited. Clin Anat 2012;25(6):722–728

18. Hydman J, Mattsson P. Collateral reinnervation by the superior laryngeal nerve after recurrent laryngeal nerve injury. Muscle Nerve 2008;38(4):1280–1289

19. Lorenz RR, Hicks DM, Shields RW Jr, Fritz MA, Strome M. Laryngeal nerve function after total laryngeal transplantation. Otolaryngol Head Neck Surg 2004;131(6):1016–1018

20. Knott PD, Hicks D, Braun W, Strome M. A 12-year perspective on the world's first total laryngeal transplant. Transplantation 2011;91(7):804–805

21. Medellin, pionera en trasplantes. Transplante de laringe. http://altair.udea.edu.co Accessed Sep 2011

22. Gonzalez RN, Gorantla VS, Breidenbach WC. Complications after hand transplantation: osteonecrosis of the hips [Abstract]. J Reconstr Microsurg 2006; 22:A012

23. Petruzzo P, Lanzetta M, Dubernard JM, et al. The international registry on hand and composite tissue transplantation. Transplantation 2010;90(12):1590–1594

24. Dunn DL. Problems related to immunosuppression. Infection and malignancy occurring after solid organ transplantation. Crit Care Clin 1990;6(4):955–977

25. Lanzetta M, Petruzzo P, Margreiter R, et al. The International Registry on Hand and Composite Tissue Transplantation. Transplantation 2005;79(9):1210–1214

26. Breidenbach W, Ravindra K, Buell J. Update on the American hand transplant experience: five hand transplants performed at Louisville [Abstract]. Presented at: American Transplant Congress; May 30–June 3, 2009; Boston, MA

27. Schneeberger S, Gorantla VS, Hautz T, Pulikkottil B, Margreiter R, Lee WP. Immunosuppression and rejection in human hand transplantation. Transplant Proc 2009;41(2):472–475

28. Pollard JD, Hanasono MM, Mikulec AA, Le QT, Terris DJ. Head and neck cancer in cardiothoracic transplant recipients. Laryngoscope 2000;110(8):1257–1261

29. Preciado DA, Matas A, Adams GL. Squamous cell carcinoma of the head and neck in solid organ transplant recipients. Head Neck 2002;24(4):319–325

30. First MR, Peddi VR. Malignancies complicating organ transplantation. Transplant Proc 1998;30(6):2768–2770

31. Devins GM, Stam HJ, Koopmans JP. Psychosocial impact of laryngectomy mediated by perceived stigma and illness intrusiveness. Can J Psychiatry 1994;39(10):608–616

32. Kwak PE, Friedman AD, Lamarre ED, Lorenz RR. Selective reinnervation of the posterior cricoarytenoid and interarytenoid muscles: an anatomical study. Laryngoscope 2010;120(3):463–467

33. Potter CP, Birchall MA. Laryngectomees' views on laryngeal transplantation. Transpl Int 1998;11(6):433–438

34. Buiret G, Rabilloud M, Combe C, Paliot H, Disant F, Céruse P. Larynx transplantation: laryngectomees' opinion poll. Transplantation 2007;84(12):1584–1589

35. Mueller AH. Laryngeal pacing for bilateral vocal fold immobility. Curr Opin Otolaryngol Head Neck Surg 2011;19(6):439–443

39 Recent Advances in Laryngology and Laryngology Research

Taranjit Singh Tatla and Samit Majumdar

The technological revolution witnessed toward the end of the last millennium has exploded into a new evolutionary era for the 21st century, which holds great promise for global health care delivery and patient care. Our everyday lives are being transformed through developments in fiberoptics technology allowing faster broadband, multimedia telecommunications, as well as more powerful computers facilitating advanced software processing and extraordinarily large digital data management.

Medical research has sought to harvest new technological tools in this fertile climate providing promise for innovative, newer methods for disease diagnosis and management. In good tradition, laryngological research has kept abreast of developments and indeed, on many fronts, continues to pioneer and lead the way providing direct and obvious health care improvements. Multidisciplinary research collaborations, crossing geographical as well as disciplinary boundaries, linking public health care providers, academic institutions, and industrial partners, are allowing fusion of ideas and visions with realization of new technological applications in both laryngeal disease diagnostics and therapeutics.

Recent advances have been particularly significant in digital endoscopic imaging of the larynx; adjunctive endoscopic imaging modalities; molecular biomarkers in the context of understanding laryngeal disease processes, diagnosis, and treatment; laser technology in laryngeal surgery; and transoral robotic surgery extending to the larynx. All areas are poised for significant further research and adoption of innovative applications, which may be accelerated still further by emerging nanotechnology applications.

Advances in Endoscopic Imaging Systems for Laryngology

Observations from examination of the human larynx with dental mirrors were first published over 150 years ago[1] and there has been an enormous development in laryngeal imaging since then. Multiple fiber bundle imaging was first described by Hopkins and Kapany[2] from work done at Imperial College London, United Kingdom. Use of the "Hopkins" rigid glass rod with side illumination has since revolutionized minimal access surgery applications across the surgical spectrum, not least in laryngology. Flexible fiberoptic imaging has developed along the same principles of coherent light bundles transmitting image information from a distal illuminated object and image clarity has progressively improved with technological developments including the arrival of analogue charge-coupled device (CCD) and more recent complementary metal-oxide-semiconductor (CMOS) camera image sensors, which have been incorporated into the distal tip of endoscopes to allow high definition, high resolution, still and video digital imaging.

Camera stack systems are produced by several manufacturers, with a variety of advanced imaging techniques for more detailed examination of the larynx, providing the potential for objective measurements of voice quality and vocal cord function, as well as adjunctive diagnostic information of tissue structure and nature.[3-5]

Video-stroboscopic evaluation has gained popularity over the past 25 years among laryngologists and speech pathologists, providing qualitative and quantitative data on vocal cord function, both in the presence and absence of vocal cord pathology.[6] Subtle diagnostic information missed by the unaided, naked eye, provides extra information to assist in further management and response to treatment. Video strobokymography has emerged[7] to build upon the limitations of simple video stroboscopy, providing quantitative measures of motion and geometry of vocal folds, allowing objective information for planning treatment and monitoring progress over time. Video strobokymograms illustrate a temporal image log of cord appearance and behavior, composed of multiple lines of interest from successive recorded frames of stroboscopic digital video images. To create a kymogram, one (and always the same) line perpendicular to the glottis axis is taken from each image and together combined into a new image showing the time course of fold vibrations (**Fig. 39.1**). The wave of the mucous membrane and a clear open–close phase is recognizable allowing quantitative calculations in the context of observing cord function in health and disease.[8] With the new generation video kymographic and high-speed larynx imaging systems, two CCD sensors are used to provide simultaneously a high-definition color laryngoscopic image and a high-speed kymographic image for clinical vocal fold examination.[9]

XION Medical (Xion GmbH, Berlin, Germany) has developed an innovative digital video archiving and evaluation system, which is user-friendly, facilitating ready digital data archiving for modern electronic record keeping. Images and video from different patient episodes can be compared on adjacent windows on the same screen allowing more objective comparison of changes in laryngeal appearance temporally. With increasing and larger number patient datasets being established, in the context of accepted high-speed laryngeal imaging clinical protocols and the

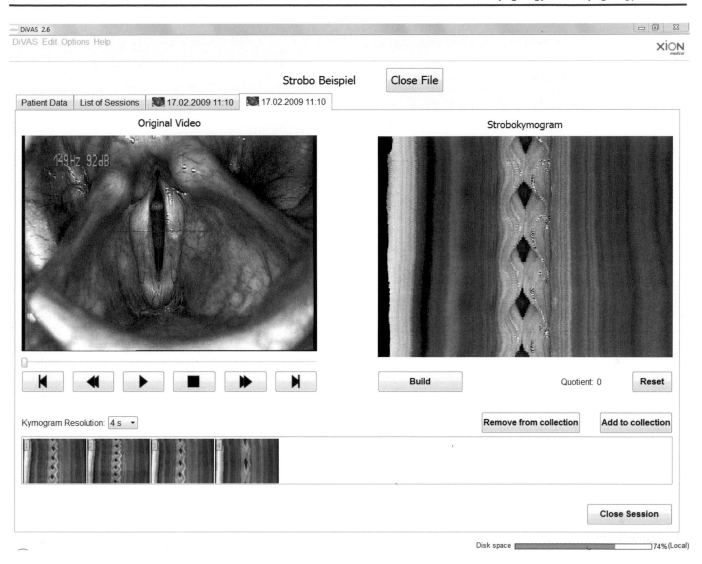

Figure 39.1   A video strobokymogram example taken from the EndoSTROB device from XION Medical. *Printed with permission* from SheffMed, United Kingdom.

regular clinical use of this tool, the characterization and discrimination power of the parameters can be explored by applying powerful data analysis techniques to see if automated discrimination between various laryngeal disorders (and stages of disorders) can be established. Data continue to build demonstrating advantages and limitations with increasing use of these laryngeal imaging methods.[8]

Adjunctive Endoscopic Optical Imaging Techniques

Other developments in endoscopic laryngeal imaging relate to emerging adjunctive optical imaging techniques attempting to exploit various properties of light, utilizing broad and narrow-band light spectra. Research has been proliferative in several related areas of this technology, with the door slowly opening to a new era of high resolution, high

accuracy (sensitivity and specificity) endoscopic imaging, which shall transform clinical diagnostics and therapeutics in laryngology, as well as a whole host of other medical disciplines and organ systems.

On the back of developments in fiberoptics, optoelectronics, applied medical optics, and photonics research, with much more powerful laser and other light sources and increasingly cheaper and miniaturized components, several potential endoscopic technologies have emerged, providing adjunctive endoscopic tools to aid the clinician in laryngeal diagnostics and therapeutics.

Optical Coherence Tomography in the Larynx

Optical coherence tomography (OCT)[10] is an emerging technology first reported for cross-sectional retinal imaging in 1991. To date, its regular use has been adopted mainly in the ophthalmology community, although with technological developments in the past 10 years, its potential for endoscopic application has been explored and adjunctive benefit slowly realized for other organ systems such as the larynx.[11] It offers a noninvasive way to visualize laryngeal tissue architecture (optical biopsy), using low-power infrared light with interferometry in an analogous way to ultrasound, with collection of back-scatter reflections at tissue layer interfaces. Up to micrometer level, resolution of morphological detail is possible, allowing a penetration depth of 2 to 3 mm into tissue. Its potential benefit as a diagnostic or therapeutic adjunct for office and theater-based clinical application in laryngology is slowly being realized as more and more preclinical and clinical studies are being reported.[12-16] Even minimal scarring from traditional glottic lesion biopsies may result in functional voice problems that do not resolve; an "optical biopsy" method would be an appropriate development for the larynx.

Wong et al[13] reports on in vivo experience using a handheld OCT probe in near or gentle contact with mucosa, for adjunctive examination of patients' larynges while under general anesthesia (normal and benign laryngeal pathology), demonstrating and confirming the findings of ex vivo laryngeal studies[12] that OCT images compare favorably with conventional histopathology. The thickness of laryngeal mucosa in various subsites is demonstrated in detail with tissue architecture clearly displaying epithelial from subepithelial layers, integrity of basement membrane, as well as microstructural features such as submucosal glands, ducts, blood vessels, and cartilage. Benign true vocal cord pathology imaged included Reinke edema, polyps, nodules, papillomatosis, mucous cysts, and granulation tissue. Others have added to this work demonstrating the ability for fiberoptic OCT to demonstrate basement membrane violation in invasive laryngeal carcinoma, as well as identify tissue transition zones at premalignant margins of cancer. These findings were limited to superficial lesions as opposed to bulky exophytic growths where tissue penetration would be inadequate to allow the basement membrane to be seen. Just et al[17] reported favorably on their unit's experience applying intraoperative OCT adjunctively to the operating microscope to define biopsy site location and resection planes precisely. Its potential for office-based application as an adjunct to flexible fiberoptic nasendoscopy for the awake patient under topical local anesthesia has recently been demonstrated utilizing a miniaturized endoscopic OCT probe passed in tandem to a flexible nasendoscope to view the larynx.[15] Rubinstein et al[16] have recently presented their experience of intraoperative OCT imaging of benign and malignant disease conditions using the first commercially available OCT imaging system for upper aerodigestive tract imaging that confirm earlier findings and provide further reliable intraoperative information to guide surgical biopsies, intraoperative decision making, and therapeutic options for various pathologies and premalignant laryngeal disease.

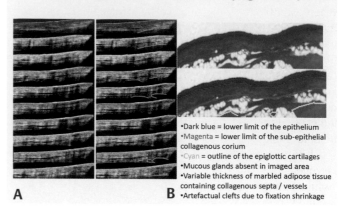

Figure 39.2 Detailed ex vivo optical coherence tomography (OCT) images versus hematoxylin and eosin (H&E) correlation: (A) A series of OCT images, which are vertical slices (B-scans) into the epiglottis at different lateral positions. (B) H&E images from the same specimen processed after OCT imaging.
Printed with permission from Tadrous P, Tatla T, Cernat R, Podoleanu A. Histopathological correlation of optical coherence tomography (OCT) images of the human larynx ex vivo. J Pathol 2012;226(S1):S.20.

Endoscopic OCT has been realized for laryngeal application, a result of imaging systems becoming cheaper and more portable, opening up potential in vivo application in the laryngologist's clinic and operation theater. Further validation work continues in this context for more accurate histological validation of ex vivo and in vivo laryngeal OCT image data, as well as development and in vivo testing of miniaturized endoscopic and handheld OCT probes with higher resolution and faster axial scan acquisition rates (**Fig. 39.2**).[18,19] Increased data acquisition rates shall generate very large OCT datasets that will require parallel improvements in digital data storage and analysis capabilities. Further improvements in instrument design and endoscopic OCT technology are on the horizon and the future holds strong promise for office-based cancer disease screening and real-time "smart surgery" be it endoscopic, microsurgical or transoral robotic application in the larynx.

Related Adjunctive Optical Imaging Modalities in the Larynx

Various adjunctive imaging modalities have been researched, adopted, and promoted in recent years by some of the major manufacturers of endoscopic imaging systems[5,20,21] in attempt to improve upon the diagnostic accuracy of high resolution, "white-light" imaging alone. Various organ systems have been studied extensively with several studies reporting individual unit's local experience in using these systems for laryngeal diagnostics.

Natural cellular fluorophores, such as flavin mononucleotide (FMN), exist as metabolic coenzymes in normal cells for aerobic glycolysis, but not in the anaerobic glycolysis pathways utilized by neoplastic cells.[22] Tissue autofluorescence is the natural capacity for tissue to fluoresce when exposed to light of a certain wavelength. Typically, filtered blue light excitation of oxidized FMN and other natural cellular fluorophores in normal cells emits a green fluorescence which can be imaged and amplified by sensitive camera systems in real time. Normal tissue appears green, whereas precancerous (dysplastic) or cancerous tissue does not autofluoresce and appear as darker fields (reddish/violet).[23] Indirect autofluorescence laryngoscopy[21,23] and flexible autofluorescence endoscopy[20] have shown increased sensitivity for diagnosis of premalignant and malignant laryngeal lesions when used as an endoscopic adjunct to "white-light" illumination, improving sensitivity levels to around 90% (a statistically significant increase of 12%).[23] Zargi et al[24] showed specificity to be lower at 71%, the findings of which were mirrored by others[23] due to some benign lesions displaying a loss of green fluorescence. Various groups have reported their findings exploring the potential additional benefits to autofluorescence in applying aminolevulinic acid (ALA) topically to the laryngeal mucosa, to preferentially induce fluorescence within neoplastic cells. Conflicting results have been noted as to whether ALA-induced fluorescence spectroscopy adds any further diagnostic accuracy to autofluorescence alone in the larynx, particularly in the context of laryngeal dysplasia and carcinoma.[25]

Narrow band imaging (NBI) is a novel, high-resolution endoscopic technique used widely to aid diagnosis of intestinal lesions, which has recently been investigated in vivo for suspected laryngeal lesions to differentiate precancerous and malignant laryngeal lesions.[5,26] The modality is based on the fact that the depth of light penetration depends on the light wavelength; the longer the wavelength, the deeper the penetration. NBI modifies the broadband white light of a xenon lamp into two narrow band beams with central wavelengths of 415 (narrow band blue) and 540 nm (narrow band green) (designed primarily to penetrate mucosa and submucosa). When used in combination they provide high surface contrast, displaying morphology of superficial capillary networks and subepithelial vessels for in vivo differentiation of nonmalignant from malignant laryngeal lesions. Ni et al[5] demonstrated that utilizing white light modes and NBI modes during office-based flexible nasendoscopy with topical local anesthesia, sensitivity of 88.9% and specificity of 93.2%, respectively, is achieved in detecting malignant lesions; significantly superior to white light illumination alone.

Raman spectroscopy provides information about molecular composition and structure and it too has been investigated ex vivo as a potential tool for noninvasive optical tissue diagnosis in the larynx.[27,28] Inelastic light scattering following excitation of target tissue using monochromatic laser light can be detected and analyzed to determine Raman spectral data, a unique molecular signature of the material. It was first described by the Nobel Prize winner Raman in 1928.[29] Good quality spectra have been obtained with ex vivo laryngeal specimens. Lau et al[28] described 5-second acquisition times, showing spectral tissue characterization and predictive sensitivities (89, 69, and 88%, respectively) and specificities (86, 94, and 94%, respectively) for normal tissue, carcinoma, and papilloma. Stone et al[27] described prediction sensitivities of 83, 76, and 92%, with specificities of 94, 91, and 90% for normal, dysplastic, and squamous cell carcinoma of the larynx, respectively. These studies support the potential for future in vivo endoscopic studies.

Rigid contact endoscopy[30,31] and confocal endoscopy[25,32] are two associated techniques that allow the surgeon to see magnified optical cellular detail in vivo of superficial tissue surfaces; studies on the normal and diseased larynx have been described in recent years but show various limitations including poor depth penetration and difficulty visualizing the basement membrane.

Other "noninvasive" in vivo optical imaging modalities are still very much in early development and presently mostly limited to research and observations on biological processes in preclinical models.[33] Of particular note, however, scanning fiber endoscopy is an emerging versatile technology for ultrathin flexible endoscope application which holds great promise.[34] It uses a single-mode optical fiber with active laser light scanning of tissue, allowing high resolution and large field of view imaging with much smaller diameter flexible endoscopes (**Fig. 39.3**). The reduced size increases furthermore the potential for developing "smart" endoscopic tools that have adjunctive optical arrangements coupling high-quality video imaging with subsurface tissue interrogation and high-resolution fluorescence imaging.

Application of Molecular Biomarkers in Laryngology

The clinical application of OCT and other endoscopic imaging modalities can be advanced further by utilizing tissue contrast and spectral data provided by disease-specific biomarkers.[11,35] Molecular imaging capabilities are poised for clinical translation in coming years, providing adjunctive disease-specific information to improve further the accuracy of any "optical biopsy" tool. Molecular imaging strategies fall into two categories: (1) endogenous molecular imaging, involving direct imaging of endogenous biomolecules, and (2) molecular contrast-imaging, involving exogenous contrast agents introduced in vivo to bind specifically to biomolecules of interest. Contrast may involve near-infrared activated fluorescently labeled antibody probes, or indeed other labeling reagents coupled to antibody probes such as submicron microspheres or nanoparticles incorporating nontoxic materials such as gold or iron oxide.[11] Presently, these are experimental only; once validated ex vivo and in preclinical animal models, they will need to undergo human trials to assess their clinical validity and safety profile.

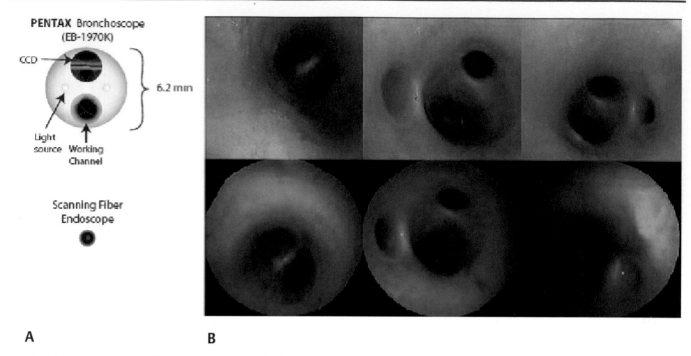

A   **B**

Figure 39.3 (A) Diagrams of a conventional Pentax bronchoscope (EB-1970K) and scanning fiber endoscope and (B) corresponding bronchoscopic images within the airways of a pig.
Printed with permission from Wiley-VCH Verlag GmbH & Co. KGaA. Lee CM, Engelbrecht CJ, Soper TD, Helmchen F, Seibel EJ. Scanning fiber endoscopy with highly flexible, 1 mm catheterscopes for wide-field, full-color imaging. Biophotonics 2010;3(5–6):400.

Multichannel endoscopes encompassing high-quality white light reflectance imaging associated with adjunctive near-infrared OCT and/or fluorescence imaging channels should soon become a reality for in vivo clinical use in the larynx, as with other organ systems.

In the context of laryngeal dysplasia and cancer imaging, the matrix metalloproteinases (MMPs) have recently emerged as potential imaging biomarkers, proteolytic "optical beacons," for both diagnosis and prognosis.[36,37] They have been studied extensively in relation to cancer of other organs in recent years but with limited studies related to the larynx.[38] They form a family of more than 20 zinc-dependent extracellular proteins, some of which are integral also to cellular membranes, acting as processing enzymes capable of degrading multiple components of the extracellular matrix (ECM) and playing seemingly essential roles in cell-proliferation, differentiation, apoptosis, and migration through degraded ECM. MMPs are well regulated and are normally expressed at very low levels, if at all. Ex vivo studies[38–40] have shown a stepwise sequential rise in MMP-2 expression (and MMP-9 to a lesser extent) with multistep carcinogenesis in the larynx, carcinomas exhibiting highest expression, atypical hyperplasia exhibiting lowest expression, and dysplasia or carcinoma in situ showing intermediate scores between these. These molecular biomarkers appear well placed for further investigation in the context of improving diagnostic sensitivity of endoscopic laryngeal cancer screening.

Advances in Lasers for Laryngeal Surgery

Following the introduction of the ruby laser by Maiman,[41] the carbon dioxide (CO_2) laser was introduced in 1972 and readily adopted by ENT surgeons following early experience of its clinical use in the larynx.[42] It has remained popular in use since then for a variety of laryngeal pathologies including vocal cord keratosis, nodules, polyps, papillomas, *carcinoma in situ* as well as early stage laryngeal cancer, due to minimum surrounding tissue damage.[43] Because water easily absorbs the 10,600-nm wavelength of the CO_2 laser,[44] it has acted as an accurate and efficient cutting/ablating laser to remove small laryngeal tumors remotely in the larynx, integrated into the mirror and lens optics of the theater operating microscope. Recent modifications include the AcuSpot scanning micromanipulator (Lumenis Ltd., Yokneam, Israel), which minimizes the focused beam diameter as well as allowing the beam to sweep the tissue surface faster; SuperPulse and UltraPulse CO_2 laser waves (Lumenis Ltd., Yokneam, Israel), which reduces surrounding tissue thermal damage by allowing tissue to cool between pulses; as well as the AcuBlade scanner software (Lumenis Ltd., Yokneam, Israel), which changes the cutting beam to a straight or curved incision line (multiple lengths and penetration depth possibilities) with improved hemostasis. These have increased the applicability and efficacy further still of the CO_2 laser.[45,46]

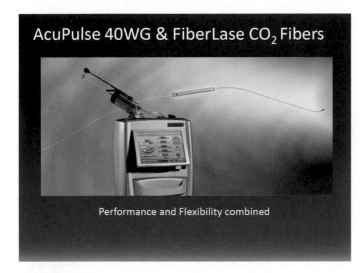

AcuPulse 40WG & FiberLase CO$_2$ Fibers

Performance and Flexibility combined

Figure 39.4 The Lumenis Surgical flexible CO$_2$ laser delivery system includes FiberLase, a high transmission flexible CO$_2$ laser fiber that purports to provide intention specific performance (cutting vs. hemostasis vs. ablation effects) where it is needed most with exceptional control and durability, combining an aiming beam with variety of hand pieces and accessories for multiple applications. *Printed with permission from* Sigmacon, United Kingdom.

The recent invention of the flexible CO$_2$ laser delivery system (**Fig. 39.4**) has expanded its use to the outpatient clinic. It offers a much more flexible system with the potential for improved ablative targeting, decreased collateral thermal damage, reduced blood loss through better tissue coagulation, and minimized smoke flume as gas flows from the distal tip through a hollow fiber core.[47,48]

Technical developments in laser technology and further recent studies have seen an expansion in the laser options available for laryngeal surgery.[49,50] Photoangiolytic lasers, such as the 532-nm wavelength pulsed potassium titanyl phosphate (KTP) laser and 585-nm wavelength pulsed dye laser, both of which target hemoglobin absorption over water, have been reported to eradicate vascular lesions very well in particular with preservation of surrounding tissue and overlying functionally important mucosa. These can be used in contact or noncontact mode. By targeting microvasculature specifically, their proponents suggest a more superior functional role in treatment of a whole host of laryngeal pathologies including papillomas, dysplasia, and early cancer.[51,52] The 532-nm KTP laser is now considered the key state-of-the-art instrument for treating phonatory mucosa lesions associated with aberrant microcirculation.[52] Both are fiber-based lasers, which deliver energy distally along thin glass fibers, and both are significantly cheaper. Innovatively the fibers can be passed through spare side-channels or incorporated into flexible endoscopes, extending the application of therapeutic options to more and more office-based surgery under local anesthesia, resulting in significant cost-savings in service delivery through avoidance of inpatient admissions.[50,52] The fiber-based thulium laser (absorption wavelength 2013 nm targeting water, with ablative characteristics similar to CO$_2$ laser) is now used and marketed as an office-based ablative laser that has various additional advantages over the CO$_2$ laser including improved coagulation, more versatile delivery system by virtue of its flexible fiber and the option of use in contact mode.[53] Its favorable endoscopic application in management of laryngeal cancer has recently been reported[54] with further larger studies in progress.

Future comparative studies (preclinical and clinical) shall build on this early experience and further define optimal operating parameters, practical advantages/disadvantages, and functional outcomes of therapeutic laser use in the larynx. The realization of fiberoptic-based and novel flexible fiber laser delivery systems, facilitating office-based applications, is happening concurrently with the development of fiberoptic imaging applications. The potential may soon be realized for the fusion and amalgamation of these technologies (based on a common technical framework involving light-based technology and lasers), to produce the "holy grail" of a single ubiquitous endoscopic tool serving accurate, precise, diagnostic, and therapeutic functions in the larynx.

Transoral Robotic Surgery—Future Laryngeal Applications

To date, no studies have been reported in relation to transoral robotic surgery (TORS) for management of benign or malignant disease of the glottis although preclinical testing in a canine model has been encouraging and hold promise for the future.[55] Present surgical practice for early stage laryngeal tumors accessible at panendoscopy is transoral laser microsurgery with good survival and functional outcomes reported,[56] although there have been no clinical trials to date directly comparing primary surgical management to radiotherapy treatment.

TORS has increased in popularity in recent years for minimally invasive management of several conditions across the surgical spectrum and increasing experience is being reported by several leading units in the context of primary management in accessible oropharyngeal, hypopharyngeal, and supraglottic malignancies.[57-59] The present generation of robotics led by the Da Vinci Surgical System (Intuitive Surgical, Inc., Sunnyvale, California, United States) (**Fig. 39.5**) provides several advantages over transoral laser microsurgery.[60] These include filtration of hand tremor, microtranslation of large hand movements increasing dexterity by the operator, as well as giving a closer, three-dimensional visualization of the surgical field which gives the surgeon true depth perception. Disadvantages of the present system include interference of the surgical arms with one another, with the camera arm, or with the retractor during the operation, lack of integrated suction, and lack of tactile feedback recognition and proprioception. This is in addition to the high initial costs of the system (presently over $ 1 million), high yearly maintenance costs, high cost

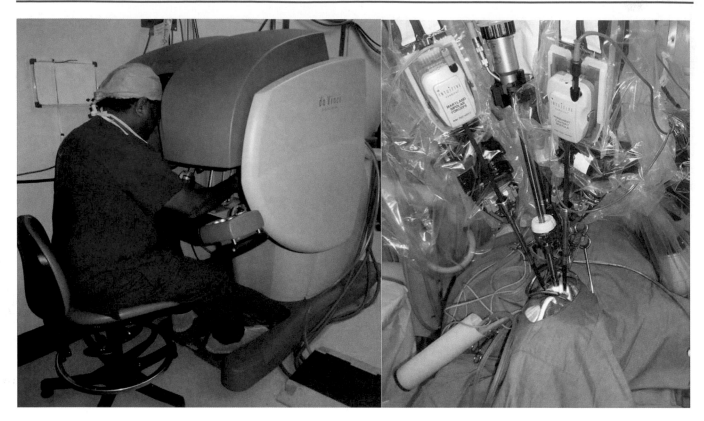

Figure 39.5 Transoral Robotic Surgery (TORS); Da Vinci Surgical System in operative set up.
Printed with permission from Dr. Suren Krishnan, Associate Professor of Surgery, Adelaide.

of individual disposable instruments, as well as required specialist training and learning curve.[61] As increasing numbers of units gain access to robotics systems and experience increases, clinical extension to precision glottic therapeutic applications under general anesthesia is likely.

Newer robotics systems such as the i-Snake (Imperial College London, London, United Kingdom) (**Fig. 39.6**), conceived and developed at Imperial College London,[62,63] shall incorporate advanced endoscopic imaging systems as well as state-of-the-art fiber-guided therapeutic lasers, providing

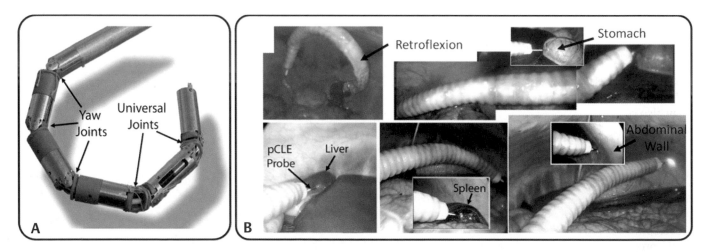

Figure 39.6 Flexible Access Platform developed using the modular joint design. (A) The 7 degrees of freedom are provided by two universal joints and three yaw joints. (B) In vivo diagnostic peritoneoscopy performed using the Flexible Access Platform via a transvaginal incision. Optical biopsy images were obtained from the liver, spleen, abdominal wall, and stomach. The entire peritoneal cavity can be accessed using the multiple degrees of freedom available, as well as the pelvis when the device is fully retroflexed.
Reprinted with permission from Noonan DP, Vitiello V, Shang J, Payne CJ, Yang G-Z. A modular mechatronic joint design for a flexible access platform for MIS. Presented at: 2011 IEEE/RSJ International Conference on Intelligent Robots and Systems; September 25–30, 2011; San Francisco, CA. © 2001 IEEE.

safe and precise management of difficult to reach endoluminal regions through a minimal access approach. The new-generation robots are likely to facilitate increased laryngeal application beyond that witnessed to date with TORS.

Nanobiotechnology

Nanotechnology is a multidisciplinary science that seeks to create and utilize novel materials, devices, and systems at the nanometer scale. It has a far reaching potential for both nonmedical and biomedical applications; in the latter for targeted drug delivery, molecular imaging, biomarkers, and biosensors.

The fundamental physical characteristics of some particles change significantly when these are reduced to an infinitesimally smaller volume, that is, nanometer. One nanometer is 1/1,000,000,000 of 1 m. For perspective, an intracellular organelle such as a ribosome is only a 20-nm particle. This significant reduction in volume of a substance changes its quantum mechanical properties. The reduction in volume of a substance exponentially increases its surface area; therefore, surface-related properties can be advantageously manipulated for diagnostic and therapeutic applications. Various nanostructures (i.e., metallic, magnetic, liposomal, and carbon based) are under investigation for innovative applications in medical and surgical practice.[64]

Plasmonic gold nanoparticle[65] appears to hold great promise among the various solid nanoparticles, nanotubes, and nanocages for its possible application in head and neck cancer therapy. Gold nanoparticles have already been applied in therapeutic trials of cancers of the head and neck in targeted therapy using tumor necrosis factor gold conjugate and photothermal therapy.[65]

Nanoparticles can be applied in diagnostic and therapeutic purposes through active and passive targeting techniques.[66] Liposomes[67] and polymeric[68] nanoparticles are different types of particles with varying functionality that hold strong promise for future therapeutic applications, while quantum dots[69] and magnetic oxide[70] nanoparticles may also contribute to a possible seismic shift in diagnostic and tumor targeting strategies.

Conclusion

Laryngological clinical practice continues to innovate in patient health care delivery through research and development, taking full advantage of the rapidly presenting and progressing technological advances of the new millennium. The next decade promises a wealth of new imaging and treatment strategies for laryngeal pathology, underpinned by huge jumps in information and data gathering that shall facilitate both improved understanding of the pathophysiology and mechanisms of laryngeal disease, as well as earlier more accurate diagnosis and targeted treatment for maximal functional and survival outcome gains. Improved patient care accompanied by large reductions in current health care expenditure, are promised.

Acknowledgment
The authors thank Dr. Suren Krishnan, Clinical Associate Professor of Surgery at the University of Adelaide, a pioneer and a world leader in the practice of TORS, for kindly providing permission to reproduce images in this chapter.

References

1. Alberti PW. The history of laryngology: a centennial celebration. Otolaryngol Head Neck Surg 1996;114(3):345–354
2. Hopkins HH, Kapany NS. A flexible fibrescope, using static scanning. Nature 1954;173(4392):39–41
3. Mafee MF, Valvassori GE, Becker M. Imaging of the Neck and Head. 2nd ed. Stuttgart, Germany: Thieme; 2005
4. Uloza V, Saferis V, Uloziene I. Perceptual and acoustic assessment of voice pathology and the efficacy of endolaryngeal phonomicrosurgery. J Voice 2005;19(1):138–145
5. Ni X-G, He S, Xu Z-G, et al. Endoscopic diagnosis of laryngeal cancer and precancerous lesions by narrow band imaging. J Laryngol Otol 2011;125(3):288–296
6. Bless DM, Hirano M, Feder RJ. Videostroboscopic evaluation of the larynx. Ear Nose Throat J 1987;66(7):289–296
7. Sung MW, Kim KH, Koh TY, et al. Videostrobokymography: a new method for the quantitative analysis of vocal fold vibration. Laryngoscope 1999;109(11):1859–1863
8. Verikas A, Uloza V, Bacauskiene M, Gelzinis A, Kelertas E. Advances in laryngeal imaging. Eur Arch Otorhinolaryngol 2009;266(10):1509–1520
9. Qiu Q, Schutte HK. A new generation videokymography for routine clinical vocal fold examination. Laryngoscope 2006;116(10):1824–1828
10. Huang D, Swanson EA, Lin CP, et al. Optical coherence tomography. Science 1991;254(5035):1178–1181
11. Zysk AM, Nguyen FT, Oldenburg AL, Marks DL, Boppart SA. Optical coherence tomography: a review of clinical development from bench to bedside. J Biomed Opt 2007;12(5):0514031–05140321
12. Bibas AG, Podoleanu AGH, Cucu RG, et al. 3-D optical coherence tomography of the laryngeal mucosa. Clin Otolaryngol Allied Sci 2004;29(6):713–720
13. Wong BJF, Jackson RP, Guo S, et al. In vivo optical coherence tomography of the human larynx: normative and benign pathology in 82 patients. Laryngoscope 2005;115(11):1904–1911
14. Armstrong WB, Ridgway JM, Vokes DE, et al. Optical coherence tomography of laryngeal cancer. Laryngoscope 2006;116(7):1107–1113
15. Sepehr A, Armstrong WB, Guo S, et al. Optical coherence tomography of the larynx in the awake patient. Otolaryngol Head Neck Surg 2008;138(4):425–429
16. Rubinstein M, Fine EL, Sepehr A, et al. Optical coherence tomography of the larynx using the Niris system. J Otolaryngol Head Neck Surg 2010;39(2):150–156
17. Just T, Lankenau E, Hüttmann G, Pau HW. Intra-operative application of optical coherence tomography with an operating microscope. J Laryngol Otol 2009;123(9):1027–1030
18. Tatla T, Tadrous P, Cernat R, et al. Development of Endoscopic Optical Coherence Tomography (OCT) for Laryngeal Cancer Screening—Ex Vivo Data Analysis. Presented at: Tri-Society Head and Neck Oncology Meeting; September 1–3, 2011; Singapore. Abstract 33

19. Tadrous P, Tatla T, Cernat R, Podoleanu A. Histopathological correlation of optical coherence tomography (OCT) images of the human larynx ex vivo. J Pathol 2012;226(S1):S.20

20. Mostafa BE, Shafik AG, Fawaz S. The role of flexible autofluorescence laryngoscopy in the diagnosis of malignant lesions of the larynx. Acta Otolaryngol 2007;127(2):175–179

21. Arens C, Reussner D, Woenkhaus J, Leunig A, Betz CS, Glanz H. Indirect fluorescence laryngoscopy in the diagnosis of precancerous and cancerous laryngeal lesions. Eur Arch Otorhinolaryngol 2007;264(6):621–626

22. Betz V, Schneckenburger H, Alleroder HP, Sybrecht GW, Meyer JU. Evaluation of changes in the NADH level between carcinogenic and normal tissue samples by use of fluorescence spectroscopy. Proc SPIE 1994;2324:284–291

23. Arens C, Dreyer T, Glanz H, Malzahn K. Indirect autofluorescence laryngoscopy in the diagnosis of laryngeal cancer and its precursor lesions. Eur Arch Otorhinolaryngol 2004;261(2):71–76

24. Zargi M, Fajdiga I, Smid L. Autofluorescence imaging in the diagnosis of laryngeal cancer. Eur Arch Otorhinolaryngol 2000;257(1):17–23

25. Hughes OR, Stone N, Kraft M, Arens C, Birchall MA. Optical and molecular techniques to identify tumor margins within the larynx. Head Neck 2010;32(11):1544–1553

26. Watanabe A, Taniguchi M, Tsujie H, Hosokawa M, Fujita M, Sasaki S. The value of narrow band imaging for early detection of laryngeal cancer. Eur Arch Otorhinolaryngol 2009;266(7):1017–1023

27. Stone N, Stavroulaki P, Kendall C, Birchall M, Barr H. Raman spectroscopy for early detection of laryngeal malignancy: preliminary results. Laryngoscope 2000;110(10, pt 1):1756–1763

28. Lau DP, Huang Z, Lui H, et al. Raman spectroscopy for optical diagnosis in the larynx: preliminary findings. Lasers Surg Med 2005;37(3):192–200

29. Raman CV, Krishnan KS. A new type of secondary radiation. *Nature* 1928;121:501–502

30. Andrea M, Dias O, Santos A. Contact endoscopy of the vocal cord: normal and pathological patterns. Acta Otolaryngol 1995;115(2):314–316

31. Cikojević D, Gluncić I, Pesutić-Pisac V. Comparison of contact endoscopy and frozen section histopathology in the intra-operative diagnosis of laryngeal pathology. J Laryngol Otol 2008;122(8):836–839

32. Just T, Stave J, Boltze C, et al. Laser scanning microscopy of the human larynx mucosa: a preliminary, ex vivo study. Laryngoscope 2006;116(7):1136–1141

33. Hickson J. In vivo optical imaging: preclinical applications and considerations. Urol Oncol 2009;27(3):295–297

34. Lee CM, Engelbrecht CJ, Soper TD, Helmchen F, Seibel EJ. Scanning fiber endoscopy with highly flexible, 1 mm catheterscopes for wide-field, full-color imaging. J Biophotonics 2010;3(5-6):385–407 (Review)

35. Weissleder R, Mahmood U. Molecular imaging. Radiology 2001;219(2):316–333

36. Funovics MA, Alencar H, Su HS, Khazaie K, Weissleder R, Mahmood U. Miniaturized multichannel near infrared endoscope for mouse imaging. Mol Imaging 2003;2(4):350–357

37. Scherer RL, McIntyre JO, Matrisian LM. Imaging matrix metalloproteinases in cancer. Cancer Metastasis Rev 2008;27(4):679–690

38. Uloza V, Liutkevičius V, Pangonytė D, Saferis V, Lesauskaitė V. Expression of matrix metalloproteinases (MMP-2 and MMP-9) in recurrent respiratory papillomas and laryngeal carcinoma: clinical and morphological parallels. Eur Arch Otorhinolaryngol 2011;268(6):871–878

39. Sarioğlu S, Ozer E, Kirimca F, Sis B, Pabuçcuoğlu U. Matrix metalloproteinase-2 expression in laryngeal preneoplastic and neoplastic lesions. Pathol Res Pract 2001;197(7):483–486

40. Peschos D, Damala C, Stefanou D, et al. Expression of matrix metalloproteinase-9 (gelatinase B) in benign, premalignant and malignant laryngeal lesions. Histol Histopathol 2006;21(6):603–608

41. Maiman TH. Stimulated optical radiation in ruby. Nature 1960;187:493–494

42. Strong MS, Jako GJ. Laser surgery in the larynx. Early clinical experience with continuous CO_2 laser. Ann Otol Rhinol Laryngol 1972;81(6):791–798

43. Yan Y, Olszewski AE, Hoffman MR, et al. Use of lasers in laryngeal surgery. J Voice 2010;24(1):102–109

44. Ossoff RH, Coleman JA, Courey MS, Duncavage JA, Werkhaven JA, Reinisch L. Clinical applications of lasers in otolaryngology—head and neck surgery. Lasers Surg Med 1994;15(3):217–248

45. Remacle M, Lawson G, Watelet JB. Carbon dioxide laser microsurgery of benign vocal fold lesions: indications, techniques, and results in 251 patients. Ann Otol Rhinol Laryngol 1999;108(2):156–164

46. Remacle M, Lawson G, Nollevaux MC, Delos M. Current state of scanning micromanipulator applications with the carbon dioxide laser. Ann Otol Rhinol Laryngol 2008;117(4):239–244

47. Wang Z, Devaiah AK, Feng L, et al. Fiber-guided CO_2 laser surgery in an animal model. Photomed Laser Surg 2006;24(5):646–650

48. Zeitels SM, Kobler JB, Heaton JT, Faquin W. Carbon dioxide laser fiber for laryngeal cancer surgery. Ann Otol Rhinol Laryngol 2006;115(7):535–541

49. Zeitels SM, Burns JA. Laser applications in laryngology: past, present, and future. Otolaryngol Clin North Am 2006;39(1):159–172

50. Zeitels SM, Burns JA. Office-based laryngeal laser surgery with local anesthesia. Curr Opin Otolaryngol Head Neck Surg 2007;15(3):141–147; Review

51. Franco RA Jr, Zeitels SM, Farinelli WA, Faquin W, Anderson RR. 585-nm pulsed dye laser treatment of glottal dysplasia. Ann Otol Rhinol Laryngol 2003;112(9 Pt 1):751–758

52. Zeitels SM, Burns JA. Office-based laryngeal laser surgery with the 532-nm pulsed-potassium-titanyl-phosphate laser. Curr Opin Otolaryngol Head Neck Surg 2007;15(6):394–400

53. Kothari P, Dhillon R. Key developments in otolaryngology. Practitioner 2006;250(1679):57–58, 60, 62 passim

54. Zeitels SM, Burns JA, Akst LM, Hillman RE, Broadhurst MS, Anderson RR. Office-based and microlaryngeal applications of a fiber-based thulium laser. Ann Otol Rhinol Laryngol 2006;115(12):891–896

55. O'Malley BW Jr, Weinstein GS, Hockstein NG. Transoral robotic surgery (TORS): glottic microsurgery in a canine model. J Voice 2006;20(2):263–268

56. Ambrosch P. The role of laser microsurgery in the treatment of laryngeal cancer. Curr Opin Otolaryngol Head Neck Surg 2007;15(2):82–88

57. Moore EJ, Olsen KD, Kasperbauer JL. Transoral robotic surgery for oropharyngeal squamous cell carcinoma: a prospective study of feasibility and functional outcomes. Laryngoscope 2009;119(11):2156–2164

58. Weinstein GS, O'Malley BW Jr, Snyder W, Hockstein NG. Transoral robotic surgery: supraglottic partial laryngectomy. Ann Otol Rhinol Laryngol 2007;116(1):19–23

59. Boudreaux BA, Rosenthal EL, Magnuson JS, et al. Robot-assisted surgery for upper aerodigestive tract neoplasms. Arch Otolaryngol Head Neck Surg 2009;135(4):397–401

60. Lawson G, Matar N, Remacle M, Jamart J, Bachy V. Transoral robotic surgery for the management of head and neck tumors: learning curve. Eur Arch Otorhinolaryngol 2011;268(12):1795–1801

61. Weinstein GS, O'Malley BW Jr, Desai SC, Quon H. Transoral robotic surgery: does the ends justify the means? Curr Opin Otolaryngol Head Neck Surg 2009;17(2):126–131

62. Kwok KW, Vitiello V, Yang G-Z. Control of articulated snake robot under dynamic active constraints. Med Image Comput Comput Assist Interv 2010;13(Pt 3):229–236

63. Noonan DP, Vitiello V, Shang J, Payne CJ, Yang G-Z. A modular mechatronic joint design for a flexible access platform for MIS. Presented at: 2011 IEEE/RSJ International Conference on Intelligent Robots and Systems; September 25–30, 2011; San Francisco, CA

64. El-Sayed IH. Nanotechnology in head and neck cancer: the race is on. Curr Oncol Rep 2010;12(2):121–128

65. Huang X, Jain PK, El-Sayed IH, El-Sayed MA. Gold nanoparticles: interesting optical properties and recent applications in cancer diagnostics and therapy. Nanomedicine (Lond) 2007;2(5):681–693

66. Wang X, Yang L, Chen ZG, Shin DM. Application of nanotechnology in cancer therapy and imaging. CA Cancer J Clin 2008;58(2):97–110

67. Sapra P, Tyagi P, Allen TM. Ligand-targeted liposomes for cancer treatment. Curr Drug Deliv 2005;2(4):369–381

68. Pridgen EM, Langer R, Farokhzad OC. Biodegradable, polymeric nanoparticle delivery systems for cancer therapy. Nanomedicine (Lond) 2007;2(5):669–680

69. Gao X, Cui Y, Levenson RM, Chung LW, Nie S. In vivo cancer targeting and imaging with semiconductor quantum dots. Nat Biotechnol 2004;22(8):969–976

70. Moore A, Weissleder R, Bogdanov A Jr. Uptake of dextran-coated monocrystalline iron oxides in tumor cells and macrophages. J Magn Reson Imaging 1997;7(6):1140–1145

Index